THE SOCIAL WORKERS' T

The Social Workers' Toolbox aims to bring order to the diversity of tools which are so characteristic of social work: assessment tools, practice tools and outcome-measurement tools. The tools described in this Toolbox can be directly put into practice and adapted to the social workers' personalized approach with their individual clients and their environments. The underlying meta-theory for Sustainable Multimethod Social Work is the 'PIE-Empowerment Theory'. This theory defines social work practice in terms of the partnership between social worker and client and is aimed at enhancing quality of life through systematically and sustainably addressing human needs and human rights. The multimethod model promotes the flexible combination of well-written evidence- and practice-based tools.

Packed full of useful checklists, the Toolbox is ideal reading for both inexperienced and more practiced social workers. The book provides a solid basis through the use of practical examples. For the more experienced social worker it offers a substantial resource and the means to legitimize a chosen course of action and social work intervention. Schools of social work will be able to use the book as an easily accessible resource for social work assessments, interventions and quality social work management.

From 1978, **Herman de Mönnink** has held a position as Senior Lecturer at the School of Social Work, Hanze University of Applied Sciences, Groningen, the Netherlands; he is in private practice as a trainer in multimethod social work (MMSW) and a trauma psychologist/ grief therapist. He believes that the strength of MMSW is that it effectively meets human needs and human rights of socially, economically and politically vulnerable people.

Herman graduated from the University of Groningen (1976) in Social Clinical Psychology (MSc), where he managed the practice research project 'Psychotherapy for the Poor'. He published several articles about evidence-based social work methods, grief support and burnout-prevention. In 1996, his first book was published, titled *Grief Support*, including Unfinished Business Syndrome (UBS) and Therapeutic Photo Confrontation (TPC). For Victim Support Netherlands he trained social workers using TPC for victims of sudden death (by accidents, homicide, suicide, natural disasters, terrorism and aircraft disaster).

In 2004, Herman published the Dutch version of this book titled *The Social Workers' Toolbox: Multimethod Social Work*. In this bestselling book he proposed a paradigm shift, working not from a one-method-fits-for-all-perspective but from a multimethod perspective. Herman trained social workers around the world about a flexible combination of 20 well-written social work methods.

Website: http://www.mmsocialwork.com
Email: monnink@home.nl

'What a thoroughly practical and extraordinarily helpful book for social workers! Herman de Mönnink has provided a treasure trove of approaches and tools for use in day-to-day practice. This is the book about "how to do social work" that social work practitioners have been waiting for many years.'

— Steven M. Shardlow, Keele University, UK

THE SOCIAL WORKERS' TOOLBOX

Sustainable Multimethod Social Work

Herman de Mönnink

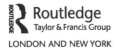
Routledge
Taylor & Francis Group

LONDON AND NEW YORK

First published 2017
by Routledge
2 Park Square, Milton Park, Abingdon, Oxon OX14 4RN

and by Routledge
711 Third Avenue, New York, NY 10017

Routledge is an imprint of the Taylor & Francis Group, an informa business

British Library Cataloguing-in-Publication Data
A catalogue record for this book is available from the British Library

Library of Congress Cataloging-in-Publication Data
A catalog record for this book has been requested

ISBN: 978-1-138-93433-7 (hbk)
ISBN: 978-1-138-93434-4 (pbk)
ISBN: 978-1-315-67807-8 (ebk)

Typeset in Bembo
by Apex CoVantage, LLC

CONTENTS

List of social work checklists   *viii*

Foreword   *ix*

Neil Thompson

Preface   *xi*

Overview of the book   *xvi*

Introduction   1

PART I

The social work approach   **7**

1 Three-step social work approach   9

2 P-I-E empowerment theory (PIE-ET)   30

3 Social workers' toolbox: overview   61

PART II

Core social work method   **81**

4 Non-directive core social work method   83

PART III
Three survival-focused methods 107

5   Bodywork method 109

6   Practical–material method 129

7   Trauma-work method 141

PART IV
Three affection-oriented methods 157

8   Cathartic method 159

9   Expression method 174

10 Ritual method 183

PART V
Three self-determination methods 195

11 Cognitive method 197

12 Narrative method 221

13 Behavioural method 247

PART VI
Six systemic methods: enhancing clients' supportive networks 265

14 Social network method 267

15 Relationship-focused method 296

16 Family work method 311

17 Groupwork method 345

18 Case management method 360

19 Mediation method 370

PART VII
Four macro methods: enhancing service delivery   377

20 Monitoring method   379

21 Prevention method   388

22 Collective advocacy method   400

23 Practical research method   420

PART VIII
Capita selecta   435

24 Human needs and human rights as an ethical guide for social work   437

25 Social work and grief support   454

26 Unfinished business syndrome (UBS): the risks of the smouldering
    peat fires   489

27 Job stress among social workers: the stress matrix   511

Appendices
1 Social casework report   *531*
2 Self-test traumatic stress   *534*
3 Trauma-reactions checklist   *536*
4 Quickscan UBS   *538*
5 Territorial inventory checklist (TICL)   *540*
6 Facing sudden death   *542*
7 Individual methods checklist: what methods match with what needs?   *544*
8 The PIE-concept in the history of social work   *546*
Literature   *548*
Index   *570*

LIST OF SOCIAL WORK CHECKLISTS

	Needs awareness checklist	14
Table 2.2	Basic resources checklist	55
Table 6.1	Problem-solving checklist: step-by-step approach to practical stress	131
	Rituals checklist: the 9w's of a proper goodbye	189
	Checklist of social support competencies	288
Table 14.4	Social support checklist: what kind of support do I need from you to optimally fulfil my needs?	295
	Relational support checklist	304
Table 16.3	Needs of children checklist	334
	Group work checklist	350
Table 20.1	Basic resources checklist	383
	Building a social work research report	430
	Checklist for therapeutic viewing of photos	485
Table 26.3	Closure tasks: finished and unfinished business	502
Table 26.4	Checklist: levels of unfinished business indicating for specific social work methods	502
	Appendix 3 Trauma-reactions checklist	536
	Appendix 5 Territorial inventory checklist (TICL)	540
	Appendix 7 Individual methods checklist: what methods match with what needs?	544

FOREWORD

I was delighted when I found out about the plan for the Dutch original of this book to be translated into English and made available to a much wider readership. From discussions with the author I knew that this book would offer an excellent resource. For far too long British social work has been moving in the direction of what I call a 'consumerist' approach,[1] with a major focus on commissioning services and rationing scarce resources. What has happened, I have kept wondering, to important ideas like 'use of self' and the recognition that the most important resource we can offer is ourselves?

When I trained as a social worker I was given a set of tools that stood me in good stead for many years. It was this grounding that prompted me in due course to develop my *People Solutions Source Book* as a set of problem-solving tools.[2] For me tools are an excellent bridge between theory and practice. They are practical in their focus, but rooted in important theoretical ideas about human psychology, society, social problems and problem-solving strategies. So, a book of social work tools was something I was very keen to see. And I have not been disappointed. Herman de Mönnink offers a fascinating set of tools to cover an extensive range of potential social work situations. His extensive experience comes shining through, as does his ability to present complex ideas clearly and accessibly.

For me what makes social work special and vitally important is its undying commitment to treating people as human beings – not cases, not statistics, not problems to be addressed, but *people*. This book, and its author, clearly share that perspective. What comes across in this volume is a wealth of experience and expertise in understanding and addressing human problems. The existential struggles, the socio-political challenges, the trials and tribulations of human relationships, these are all well represented here, admirably portrayed by an author with great skill in matching problems and unmet needs to potential solutions and strategies.

This book should be a basic primer for all social work students and a ready-to-hand reference source for experienced practitioners. This impressive tome provides an excellent grounding in a wide range of social work tools and methods, with helpful guidance on how to decide what method needs to be used in what circumstances.

Tools are not a replacement for well-informed critically reflective practice. Rather, they can be an aid to just such a positive professional approach to practice. Sadly, some social work settings seem to have settled for a narrow form of care management and rarely if ever reach out further than a fairly limited set of responses to people's problems, needs and challenges. I am aware from my discussions with a wide range of practitioners that there are very many people who would love to fulfil their potential much more fully by developing a much broader repertoire of ways of helping, but they lack the confidence and/or guidance to do so. This important book can provide much of that guidance and thereby serve as a foundation for developing that confidence and fulfilling that potential.

Dr Neil Thompson, writer and online tutor

www.neilthompson.info

Notes

1 Thompson, N. (2016). *The professional social worker* (2nd edition). London: Palgrave Macmillan.
2 Thompson, N. (2012). *The people solutions sourcebook* (2nd edition). Basingstoke: Palgrave Macmillan.

PREFACE

In 1999, when I had already spent 25 years as a lecturer at the Groningen School of Social Work (the Netherlands), I asked my carpenter: 'What are the advantages of that wonderful and well-organized toolkit of yours?'

The carpenter replied: 'I never overlook a tool, because my tools are well organized. Flexibly and efficiently, I can use the right tools at the right time for the right job to be done.'

This answer encouraged me to try to develop a well-organized Social Work Toolbox with evidence-based tools. After years of studying, testing, selecting and systematically defining the best practice methods from the rich 110-year history of social work, this resulted in the *Multimethod Social Work Toolkit* in 2004. Now, after 12 years of very favourable responses from social workers in the Netherlands who had worked with the book, I am wondering if this book might be of benefit to social workers internationally.

In writing this book I wanted to describe what a well-organized toolkit for social workers should look like. The multimethod social work (MMSW) model offers such a toolkit, which can be used to underpin the methodological approach of social work in practice. Such a toolkit is also needed for the purpose of empowering and profiling the social work profession: by describing a clear description of and by mapping out the methodological core of our practice as social workers.

In the process of conducting research for this book I discovered that the Dutch name for social worker, *maatschappelijk werker* (literally: someone who works within society), had arisen in the course of a 1903 campaign which aimed to improve the image of the profession. The then programme *Opleidingsinrigting voor Socialen Arbeid* (Educational Programme for Social Labour) in Amsterdam had come under fire for its critical stance towards society, so much so that it was thought that a change in name might be required. At that time, the term social labour (*Socialen arbeid*) was deemed to have socialist and feminist overtones. Parents from the upper (middle) classes did not allow their (predominantly female) offspring to attend such a training programme. As a result, the school, which had only been established a few years earlier, in 1899, had to close its doors for a short period of time. This existential crisis was averted by renaming it as the *School voor Maatschappelijk Werk* (School for Social Work). Social work was deemed to have more neutral overtones than 'Social Labour' and it was hoped that this name change would result in attracting a greater number of students. A century on, in 2004, the Netherlands social work training programmes and professional body were again considering a name change, but now towards *social work* (Social Work). While the 'red image' was a source for concern back in 1903, currently discussion is more around the need for an image that has 'greater appeal'. The toolkit contributes to a clear branding of 'social work' because social work methods are very distinct from those used by other professions. The toolkit will help social workers to develop a clear professional profile as distinct from that of other occupations. This is very necessary in the present day, when we find many of our colleagues in competing professions (competing colleagues) operating in the social work area. This includes specialized nurses, support workers in the social-legal arena, psychologists and 'coaches' all applying for jobs within the social work area.

I have been facilitating courses for social workers throughout the Netherlands focusing on 'dealing with loss' since 1980 and courses focusing on 'multimethod social work' from 2001 onwards. I also provide supervision to and workshops for social workers. Course participants and supervisees have shared their experiences with me: they shared how much their clients appreciated their support but also how invisible they felt. What should social workers do to rid themselves of their image of working hard behind the scenes – the so-called silent performers – and move towards a new image: that of highly visible social work professionals who not only use their heart, but also clearly described methods to maximize the quality of life of many?

Some social workers feel they are visible enough, but still struggle with a range of methodological questions: 'What methods are part of the social worker's toolkit?' 'I find it difficult to describe what I do, and this makes me insecure, but what can I do to improve my professional profile?' Questions such as these are at the core of the social work profession. This also becomes obvious when social workers become aware of the multimethod social work model through attending symposia, workshops and courses, and start to ask questions such as: 'Should we be fully conversant with all 20 methods in the multimethod model?' 'Are interpersonal communication skills part of a basic attitudinal approach or is it a separate core social work method?' 'Where does working with metaphors fit within the model?' 'Where does the solution-focused approach fit within the model?' 'Where does the empowerment approach fit within the model?' The list goes on. All these questions inspired me to write this book.

Since I am a strong advocate of social work, I have written this book to try and provide a theoretical foundation for social work practice, thus enhancing social workers' professional profile. Such an enhancement is necessary in view of cost-cutting and the advent of colleagues from other disciplines who claim to also engage in social work practice. The more clearly defined a profession, the easier it will be to convey this professional profile to others. Social work is not a clearly defined profession in all countries. I hope that the multimethod model I have developed will help contribute to a growing appreciation for the social work professional. A clearly described social work method provides clarity as to the social worker's competencies and professional practice. Such clarity will also contribute to greater appreciation of the profession. And this is long overdue if we consider all the work social workers have been doing in all corners of the globe for the past 110 years.

Social workers have tested this model from all angles over the past 15 years. Any feedback has been integrated into this new revised edition. It is incredibly satisfying for me as an author to hear how much social workers felt supported by the MMSW model in their daily practice. It seems that unnecessary professional and personal uncertainties have made way for an assured approach, inspiration and a newfound enthusiasm in their daily practice. Upon completing the course, one social worker wrote:

> When I finished my Social Work qualification it was as if I found myself in one huge methodological chaos: disordered. I tried too hard to memorise everything, but ended up not knowing how to apply any of it. This course helped me revisit these methods again and I learned about many new ones. It was fun, I learned a lot and I gained a lot of clarity. This course has allowed me to gain a better overview in my daily practice and work in a more clearly defined way. It is clear to me what methods I should use in what situations and I am aware of what to pay attention to and I am applying that knowledge more and more. So I always carry my toolkit in my workbag. I often consult the book: it provides me with the scaffolding I need.

MMSW represents the expert social worker who offers clients a range of tools that help them create order in their own lives. This is why we added the words multimethod social work to the title: social workers offer clients those tools which best fit their situation.

In Belgium the title of *maatschappelijk assistent* (literally: social assistant, the Flemish word for professional social worker) has been a legally protected title since 1946. In June of 2011, Kris Raemdonck, coordinator at one of the Centres for General Wellbeing Services (Centrum voor Algemeen Welzijnswerk) in Brussels pleaded for the empowerment of Belgian social workers, as evidenced by one of her emails to the author:

> I have just purchased your book and I can already tell you how happy I am with this book. I am a social worker. I completed my qualification in Brussels, in 1983. For years now I have been training interns at the place I work and examining final assignments/dissertations. I and others with me, have been saying for years that current social work students seem to have preciously little methodological knowledge conveyed to them. True, students are offered a great many different perspectives, but not enough guidelines.
>
> This means the social work profession (I like to refer to it as a trade) is becoming less and less clearly defined, and as a result many social work roles have started to be filled by criminologists, professionals specializing in remedial teaching, psychologists and so on. It seems to me that your book should be an essential component of social work training programmes.

There have been a lot of developments since then. A steering group was formed, chaired by Ingeborg Winters (Brussels Council for Health and Wellbeing) and its deliberations resulted in a first introductory day in June of 2012 (a year since I received that first email message) around client-focused multimethod social work. The event was titled 'Right to Social Work?! Client Emancipation . . . But What About Our Own Emancipation as Social Workers?'

It is pleasing to me as an author to see ideas from this book disseminated and contributing to social work gaining a stronger identity and image not only in the Netherlands but also in Belgium and hopefully in countries around the world now that the English edition of the book is being published as *The Social Workers' Toolbox*!

This edition will first mean connecting with the broader target audience of social work professionals. In this, I follow in the footsteps of the professional body of social workers in the

Netherlands which has called itself the Dutch Association of Social Workers (*Beroepsvereniging voor Professionals in het Social work* abbreviated as BPSW) starting from 2015.

Second, this edition contains a condensed version of the chapters on *theory*, without losing any of the content. The nine theoretical chapters in the previous edition – which preceded a discussion of the toolkit methods – have been reduced to three chapters on theory in the current edition. Again, feedback from social work students and lecturers was my guiding principle in the process of rewriting and condensing. However, I was also inspired by Kurt Lewin's famous adage: 'There is nothing so practical as a good theory!' Hence my choice for three rather than nine chapters on theory. I hope the reader will enjoy the new layout, which is geared towards improving the book's applicability in practice.

Third, the content has changed in that I have added the narrative method, which focuses on questions around identity and finding meaning in life. I have also combined the two chapters on immediate and extended family methods because there was a lot of overlap between these. Naturally, all chapters on methodology have been updated. The most striking element of this is the addition of network conferencing as part of the Social Network method. Initially there may have been some arguments against adding this technique, but social work practice has since proved that such objections have been unfounded. Years ago, it was felt that consulting a person's social network by organizing 'Own Strength Conferences' was a technique support workers should stay away from. More recently however, social workers have increasingly utilized complex social networks in particular in the form of network conferences, family conferences, community support and 'think along' conferences. This is understandable in the current environment where government-imposed cost-cutting exercises have increased calls to activate existing social networks. This is also somewhat controversial, because social workers are not responsible for implementing cost-cutting policies.

I have again elected to organize this book pragmatically: practical and methodological chapters will be followed by chapters dealing with more abstract topics. Readers are reminded that the methodological tool–based competencies so amply described in the book are not workable/cannot be understood separately from their ethical, theoretical and philosophical foundations (see the introduction).

Much has happened since 2011. As stated previously, this is the international edition of this book which will allow social workers in many different countries to use the methodological knowledge this book offers.

I would like to acknowledge the following people in relation to all four editions of the book: first, I would like to express my thanks to all my (former) colleagues in social work education all over the world: Cornelis Numan and Henk Koetsveld (Rotterdam University), Marcel Wijn (Hanze University of Applied Science), Annemiek Mellema (Windesheim University), Francis Turner (Canada), Wim Nieuwenhuijsen (European SW-Master, Netherlands), Lennart Sauer (Umea University Sweden), Michele Barber (Canada), John Fotheringhame (Scottish Borders Council, Scotland), Michael Dover (Cleveland State University, USA), Maria Rúnarsdóttir (Icelandic Association of Social Workers, Iceland), Jim Poulter (Monash University, Australia), Sherry Schachter (Calavary Hospital, USA), Tomm Attig (Canada), and Betty Davis (University of Victoria, Canada). Thank you for your valuable feedback an inspiration in a practical, theoretical and philosophical sense. I would also like to thank Pieter Hoving, Bastiaan Jurna and Joop Wolff for thinking along with me and making illustrations perfect: it has been very valuable. And all cartoonists who gave permission to 'enlighten' the texts with their cartoons, with special thanks to Fran Orford (www.francartoons.co.uk) who was a social work manager until she gave it up to become a professional cartoonist. And also special thanks to Huib van der Stelt, a Dutch painter who illustrated the Dutch and English cover (www.huibvanderstelt.nl). There are now many educational programmes, teams and institutions working from the MMSW perspective. I would like to thank them for their feedback as well, and in particular the social workers and programme leaders of two social work institutions: the foundation for social support services at Enschede-Haaksbergen (SMD E-H) and the social workers of the DOCK foundation in Rotterdam. I would also like to thank my publisher Ime van Manen, and my coordinating editor Mirjam Blom, for the great care they have provided around publishing my books. I want to thank my daughters Tessa de Mönnink and Mira de Mönnink for their assistance with PR and contracts and for never ceasing to encourage me. My team of translators also offered invaluable support with this huge project: Ineke Crezee (New Zealand) was there as a translator early on and has remained a reliable advisor on all translation matters, Ankie Mulder and Wieke and Richard Beenen, Daniel Bauer (all in the Netherlands) and Wim Stegen (Belgium). I would like to thank Neil Thompson (Wales) for checking the use of professional terminology throughout and more. And last but not least I would like to acknowledge Marlous Breukel, who always supported me by offering her thoughts and advice. Your support in this huge undertaking has been invaluable!

Herman de Mönnink
Groningen, the Netherlands
Autumn of 2016

OVERVIEW OF THE BOOK

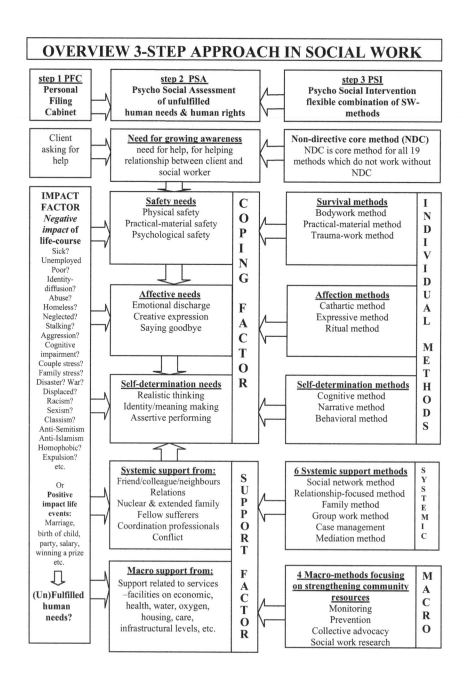

OVERVIEW 3-STEP APPROACH IN SOCIAL WORK

step 1 PFC Personal Filing Cabinet	**step 2 PSA** Psycho Social Assessment of unfulfilled human needs & human rights	**step 3 PSI** Psycho Social Intervention flexible combination of SW- methods
Client asking for help	**Need for growing awareness** need for help, for helping relationship between client and social worker	**Non-directive core method (NDC)** NDC is core method for all 19 methods which do not work without NDC

IMPACT FACTOR
Negative impact of life-course
Sick?
Unemployed
Poor?
Identity-diffusion?
Abuse?
Homeless?
Neglected?
Stalking?
Aggression?
Cognitive impairment?
Couple stress?
Family stress?
Disaster? War?
Displaced?
Racism?
Sexism?
Classism?
Anti-Semitism
Anti-Islamism
Homophobic?
Expulsion?
etc.

Or
Positive impact life events:
Marriage,
birth of child,
party, salary,
winning a prize
etc.

(Un)Fulfilled human needs?

COPING FACTOR

Safety needs
Physical safety
Practical-material safety
Psychological safety

Affective needs
Emotional discharge
Creative expression
Saying goodbye

Self-determination needs
Realistic thinking
Identity/meaning making
Assertive performing

Survival methods
Bodywork method
Practical-material method
Trauma-work method

Affection methods
Cathartic method
Expressive method
Ritual method

Self-determination methods
Cognitive method
Narrative method
Behavioral method

INDIVIDUAL METHODS

SUPPORT FACTOR

Systemic support from:
Friend/colleague/neighbours
Relations
Nuclear & extended family
Fellow sufferers
Coordination professionals
Conflict

Macro support from:
Support related to services
–facilities on economic,
health, water, oxygen,
housing, care,
infrastructural levels, etc.

6 Systemic support methods
Social network method
Relationship-focused method
Family method
Group work method
Case management
Mediation method

SYSTEMIC

4 Macro-methods focusing on strengthening community resources
Monitoring
Prevention
Collective advocacy
Social work research

MACRO

INTRODUCTION

Multiple problems require a multimethod approach.
The right tool for the right job.
If a hammer is the only tool you've got, all you will see is nails everywhere.

(Maslow, 1966)

Why do social workers need such an extensive toolkit? Why can they simply make do with an attentive base attitude and a couple of methods, rather than the 20 methods and 150 techniques introduced in this book? They cannot because social work involves issues of such a diverse nature that it requires a broad range of social work methods which can be implemented when people suffer stress due to child abuse or physical limitations, hunger, homelessness, divorce, chronic illness, domestic violence or violence out on the street, identity issues, problems with child-rearing, issues with hospital or nursing home admissions, problems at school or at work – the list goes on. This book offers the multimethod toolkit needed by social work professionals.

Structure

Part I starts by outlining a social work approach which aims to systematically and effectively utilize sources of strength (empowerment) using these to work on neutralizing sources of tension together with the client (destressing). Chapter 1 introduces three steps towards this end. These steps are summarized in this formula: Social Work = PFC + PSA + PSI. The next chapter describes the underlying social work theory, which is the PIE-Empowerment Theory. PIE stands for person-in-environment and is viewed as the core concept of social work internationally. This multimethod theory describes three factors which together determine our Quality of Life (QoL): the impact factor, coping factor and support factor. In other words, the three QoL factors can lead to problems but can also offer possibilities to overcome such problems. The interplay between the three QoL factors is symbolized by the empowerment image on the cover of the book: 'In life you have to work on fulfilling your own needs, but you don't have to do that all on your own!' This quote is an effective representation of what the three QoL factors stand for. Every human being will need to find his or her own way to adequately deal with the *impact* of the life events they experience, events which are life-changing to a greater or lesser extent and the consequences of which will follow that person. What human needs and human rights remain unfulfilled when this happens? Adequate individual '*coping*' is needed to be able to cope with such unfulfilled needs. It would not say much about the human condition if we as people had to deal with all of this all *alone* in the course of our lives. In this book, the social element is described as the '*support*' factor, the extent to which we receive support from those in our environment. Based on a careful assessment of the interplay between the three QoL factors, the social worker has to work with the client to use the positive strengths to reduce the impact of the negative factors.

Parts II to VII are the core of the toolkit, offering 20 social work methods (the non-directive core method and the 19 directive methods), which will be systematically introduced and described in Chapters 4–23. For each method, I will explain the outline, aims, historical background, indications, contraindications, techniques and so on. In this way, I will create an overview, at each level of intervention, of the objectives the social worker will be trying to achieve, working together with the client. The aim is for social workers to be able to propose appropriate combinations of methods in a flexible manner, and use these in particular situations, when specific strengths can be drawn upon, while also being able to describe the process.

The social work methods have been divided according to three different levels of intervention:

1   The individual level, with

   a   The non-directive *core* method (Chapter 4) which focuses on making contact and maintaining contact and achieving careful closure after working with clients;
   b   Nine directive individual methods which aim to engage individual strengths to reduce specific individual problems (Chapters 5–13).

2   The systemic level of intervention, with six systemic methods aimed to engage social support to reduce specific support-related issues (Chapters 14–19).
3   The macro level of intervention, with four macro methods aimed at strengthening resources in order to achieve reduction of specific structural issues (Chapters 20–23).

Part V comprises four selected topics which are discussed in a more in-depth manner: the ethical foundations of social work, which aim to help fulfil human needs and human rights (Chapter 24); social work with all kind of client groups confronted with specific losses (Chapter 25), social work involving the Unfinished Business Syndrome (UBS) in relation to clients whose symptoms are due to past hurt which they have not managed to address as yet (Chapter 26) and the social worker's own stress and self-care for social workers (Chapter 27).

The appendices provide a number of additional tools in the form of checklists with regard to traumatization, a quick-scan for UBS, information relating to people facing sudden death and PIE-concept in the history of social work. All sections contain examples from case histories to exemplify methods and techniques.

Professional expertise in terms of tools used in social work

This book describes the social worker's toolkit, and deals with the *technical* and *instrumental* side of the social work professional: how can we as social workers proceed in an effective and efficient manner? Obviously, the technical and instrumental aspects of our professional profile cannot be seen as separate from the normative and personal aspects. The professional profile of social workers in the Netherlands (NVMW, 2006) includes the following three aspects, and for good reason:

1   The *normative* aspect of our professionalism, which centres around the question of whether our actions are ethically correct (see Chapter 24).
2   The *technical-instrumental* aspect of our professionalism, which focuses on the methods and techniques available to social workers.
3   The *personal* aspect of our professionalism, which centres around the question of whether 'the social worker's methodological approach is true and genuine', in other words whether individual social workers have truly integrated and internalised 1 and 2.

Any book focusing on technical and instrumental aspects could create the impression that individual methods are of paramount importance for effective assistance, quite separate from ethics and personal competence. However it is the social worker's competence in terms of interactions and relationships – initiating and maintaining a relationship with the client – which constitutes the basis for any methodological intervention by the social worker. Methods and techniques must have become internalized, part and parcel of who the social worker is. Social workers never say: 'this is what we are going to do,' but always: 'shall we do this or that for such and such a reason', 'I suggest . . .' and 'would you agree/do you think that is a good idea?' Any social worker who uses the multimethod approach in an authentic and critical manner will interact with individual clients and a range of diverse groups of clients in a respectful way, based on the values of the social work profession, in order to 'allow people to reach their full potential'. Social workers should at all times avoid focusing disproportionately on any one of the three above aspects of the professional profile (technical-instrumental, normative and personal).

Ladder of reflection in social work

Reflection on professional practice and theory is crucial for the scientific foundation and development of social work, because as 'reflective professionals' social workers are continually acting and then reflecting on their actions. Schön referred to the ladder of reflection back in 1983 in his book on the reflective professional; the ladder of reflection in Figure I.1 is an expansion on the original one, a collaborative effort by the author and Jim Poulter of Monash University (Australia).

The ladder of reflection comprises five rungs, five levels of reflection – multilevel reflection – which serve to introduce an ever-higher level of reflection to social work (Figure I.1). The inductive or practice-based line starts at the level of social work *practice*, moving to an ever-higher level of abstraction, in an upward direction, because we can reflect on our reflections with regard to our practical actions– reflecting on reflection, and so on. And this leads to the development of an overarching social work *theory* (PIE-Empowerment Theory) on top of the *practical* theory – which is very close to the professional practice related to this case. And the overarching social work *theory* is both practice proof (usable) and theory proof (has a philosophical foundation). Theories, hypotheses and working hypotheses are tested in a downward direction: the evidence-based line. Hence reflection can occur at different levels:

1   The *practical* level: working with this client situation.
2   The *practical theory* level: what working hypothesis/es should I apply in this case?

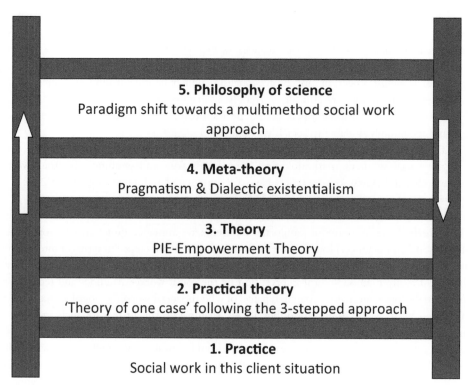

FIGURE I.1 The five-rung social work ladder of reflection

3   The *theory* level: what is our joint social work theory?
4   The *metatheoretical* level: which philosophies offer social workers both a worldview and a view of human beings?
5   The level of *scientific philosophy:* is the current theoretical social work framework restrictive or liberating?

Together these levels of reflection form the rungs of the ladder of reflection (see Figure I.1).

Within the history of social work, factors internal and external to social work kept resulting in *paradigm shifts* whenever an existing theory was overtaken by a new way of thinking or whenever social work had to meet new and different requirements.

Paradigm shift

Kuhn (1996) introduced the concept of a 'paradigm shift' within the philosophy of science, to refer to such shifts from existing to new theoretical frameworks, such changes of perspective. We need paradigm shifts because – as Albert Einstein (1946) put it – 'The significant problems we have cannot be solved at the same level of thinking with which we created them.' The paradigm shifts within social work – described below – are examples of such changes in perspective.

New theories always continued where the existing ones left off, however some of the blind spots were partly overcome by new theories. Such new theories would then be a better fit for new requirements for social work practice for a period of time, only to be in turn superseded by even newer theories, and so it would continue.

One example of such a paradigm shift was the further expansion of and more in-depth focus on *systemic* and *communicative* perspective on the client situation in the 1960s; this involved a focus on how clients communicated within their network of relationships. Rather than just focusing on individual clients, based on individual theories, attention shifted towards communication within a relationship, and within the nuclear and extended family. In other words, communication and systems theories were added on to the individual social work theory.

Another shift in thinking within the field of social work occurred in the 'rebellious 1960s' when oppressive mechanisms within society were exposed. Within this era of social criticism and rebelling against the established order, the focus shifted towards the dynamics of social oppression based on class (classism), gender (sexism), age (adultism when children are being oppressed and ageism when older adults are being oppressed) and sexual preference (oppression of gay people). Within social work the focus shifted more towards the emancipation and liberation of certain client groups. Individual and systemic social work theories were expanded on to include social *oppression* and *emancipation* theories: critical social work.

The *multimethod* paradigm in social work

> Every man is in certain respects like all other men, like some other men and like no other men.
> Kluckhohn and Schneider (1953)

Within the current field of social work, the question is how we can create more linkages and more order in the existing range of diverse theories, models, methods and techniques without throwing the baby out with the bathwater. In the course of the past few decades, 'eclectic' thinking has often been used as an overarching concept offering some sort of cohesion to this diverse range of theories and methods. However, eclectic thinking has failed to offer the field of social work the required cohesion and order, and associated theoretical and methodological transparency. The new millennium has seen the advent of a move towards *multimethod thinking* in relation to social work practical: thinking in terms of *and/and* rather than *either/or*. This multimethod paradigm achieves a synthesis of the diverse range of traditional and alternative perspectives within social work: social work has a multi-theory, multi-system, multimodal, multicultural, multi-country, multidimensional, multilevel, multifamily, multi-agency, multiracial, multi-generational, multidisciplinary, multi-method approach. Because of this *multi-perspective* there is respect for the diverse range of strengths and weaknesses in the client situation; the multimethod social work approach overcomes all manner of mono-level approaches and their associated unnecessary limitations, both in the assessment and intervention phases; this is very necessary, because 'every man is in certain respects like all other men, like some other men and like no other men'.

Every man is like all other men: respect for what is universally human

Attention is needed for what is universally human, because we are all similar in certain ways, and we share universal human needs. Life events are universal, because they occur in everyone's life. On the one hand, 'universally human' means the good times and the bad, prospering and declining, winning and losing, while on the other hand it represents the ability of the human spirit to create its own reality. People are capable to transcend their own boundaries even from the ruins of their own existence. Universal human rights are an expression of this universal aspect of human existence.

Every man is like some other men: respect for social and cultural aspects

Attention is needed for cultural resources and social networks, offering possibilities/options (or not) for channelling human needs, the space for sadness or on the contrary for denying and blocking the same grief instead. In some respects, we are similar to other people. We are similar to our parents and to people from the social and cultural group we originated. Needs are socially and culturally constructed: on the one hand they represent a reproduction of existing standards, passing on true and tested answers to life's questions, codes and conventions; on the other hand the creation of new standards, the development of new answers which may serve to overcome cultural codes which are perceived to be restrictive, and so on.

Every man is like no other men: respect for uniquely personal aspects

Attention is needed for what is uniquely personal: 'What (human) needs am I experiencing right now and which one would I like to address first? Individuals are unique in the way in which they encounter life events on their path through life and unique in how they handle such life events. What is it I need to be able to optimize my Quality of Life? Respect for individual values, strengths and the need for self-determination and autonomy is essential.

In terms of working with clients within social work the *multimethod* approach presented in this book meets the needs for transparency, justification and measurability of objectives and results, the many requirements social work needs to meet in the present time. In this sense, the multimethod paradigm in social work has a research counterpart. Just like social workers, researchers have been using mixed methods, in other words a multimethod approach, a synthesis of quantitative and qualitative methods in order to arrive at the most valid research findings.

The *multimethod* paradigm is used to build on a body of knowledge within social work. There is no longer a need for individual social workers to keep reinventing the wheel or to start from scratch. Whenever new approaches arise, we no longer have to desert the existing building but we can simply consider what contribution the 'new' can offer in terms of modifying the existing body of knowledge. This will avoid a situation where new methods are majorly attractive to individual social workers or entire social work training institutes or programme for just a short period of time. It may contribute to a situation where we critically consider whether an update or upgrade is needed from the perspective of the existing body of knowledge.

Since the appearance of the first edition of this book in 2006, we have seen the advent of new methods such as the Social Presence Theory, *solution-focused* therapy (also referred to as SFT for Solution-Focused Therapy), *mindfulness*, ACT (Acceptance Commitment Therapy), triple P, the network conferences, and the Capability Approach, to mention just a few. This is not the place for an extensive discussion of these new trends, however they do illustrate that new theories and perspectives will continue to be developed. The additional and innovative aspects of such new methods or techniques are summarized in the relevant chapters, characterized and integrated. Thanks to the multimethod paradigm we no longer have to throw the baby (existing perspectives) out with the bathwater: helpful new perspectives are the building block of the social work edifice and contribute to a solid future for the social work profession.

PART I
The social work approach

1

THREE-STEP SOCIAL WORK APPROACH

I could see no beginning and no end to it all. Using the imagery of a personal filing cabinet enabled me to see my problem areas as separate entities. It was a bit of a scare; is that me? However, my problem situation was reduced to workable proportions. Unfinished business was subsequently scrutinized and dealt with until complete closure was achieved.

(Maria, age 19)

Questions

This chapter addresses the following questions:

- What is meant by the three-step approach in social work?
- What is meant by PFC, the personal filing cabinet?
- What is meant by PSA, the psychosocial assessment?
- What is meant by PSI, the psychosocial intervention?
- What is meant by multimethod social work?
- What is meant by identifying which differential methods are indicated?

1.1 Introduction

This chapter will explain the three-step social work approach that constitutes the essential practical methods guidelines in social work for optimizing the Quality of Life (QoL). First, the three-step plan is explained, followed by a description of each of the three methodical steps. The theory is illustrated by elements from the case study of Maria.

Case study: Maria

Maria was a social work student who was not able to finish her grief support workshop, which formed part of her programme of studies as a social work student. One of her lecturers referred her to the student advisor (social worker) at her college. It appeared that her unfinished emotional business had been reactivated in the course of the workshop and as a result she found herself unable to concentrate on her studies. For a long time Maria had been struggling with her mother's unexpected death (by suicide when Maria was 5) and her brother's death (through an overdose at the age of 14) and with the fact that her father had never been there for her at the time of these life events. Maria remained rebellious and came close to having dealings with the judicial system and the police. During the college social work sessions she wondered 'Why? Why have such terrible things happened in my life? The social work sessions helped Maria sort out the troubling issues in her life. By sorting through all the problem areas she was able to deal with one specific area at a time and eventually regained her grip on life.

1.2 Sustainable multimethod social work in three steps

In order to work sustainably and in a goal-oriented way it is vital that social workers utilize a stepped plan in their thinking. By working according to a multimethod stepped plan social workers engage in stepwise and goal-oriented mapping and focusing on the pluses and minuses in the client situation.

The multimethod stepped plan in social work comprises the three following steps:

1   *PFC, the personal filing cabinet*: the social worker is mapping and visualizing the impact factor using keywords – in the client's language – to identify which minuses and pluses the client is experiencing: how do clients describe their own situation, how do clients experience the impact of life events, for example what is the impact when you suddenly lose your job (*impact* factor)? Which stressors and strengths do you experience when that happens?

2   *PSA, the psychosocial assessment*: the social worker determines a plan of action: which practical methods can empower the client situation in meeting clients' unfulfilled needs, for example how can we help clients to acknowledge the life impact (*impact* factor)? How can we help clients cope with job loss effectively (enhancing the *coping* factor)? How can we make the environment more supportive (enhancing the *support* factor)?

3   *PSI, the psychosocial intervention*: the social worker and the client work together to actually implement the plan of action to enhance personal and environmental strengths, e.g. by acknowledging the job loss, improving clients' coping style as well as support from family or friends and public resources and services. Client feedback will be measured on a regular basis to see if the actions taken are effective, if different actions are needed, and social worker and client will work through the three steps again till the Quality of Life of the client is optimal.

Case study: Maria (19)

The college social worker (student advisor) started by asking Maria to tell her own story. Maria did not really expect this to happen considering her past experiences with professionals in support services, who normally commenced by asking her to fill out various checklists and questionnaires. The social worker did not stick to any particular order when interviewing her, instead focusing on facilitating Maria to tell her story instead (non-directive core method; no filling in for the other person). Maria's first question to the college social worker was to ask how she would normally deal with a case like this. The social worker simply said she would ask: 'what support do you need to take a step forward in your life?' Answering this question was meeting Maria's unfulfilled needs (stress factors) and enhancing her strengths. In addition, they would both deal with each drawer from her 'personal filing cabinet' by easing the stress (fulfilling a need) and enhancing her strengths. Maria was encouraged to deal with one file at a time and determine her own needs (needs-centred approach). This actually appealed to Maria, who really longed for something like this after so many years of carrying such a heavy burden (sustainable approach).

This approach by social workers can be typified as client-centred and multimethod. Pluses in Maria's personal filing cabinet stand for her personal strengths and the support strength of her environment while minuses stand for stumbling blocks for optimal QoL.

Maria's social worker adopted a needs-centred approach and kept returning to Maria's needs as her point of reference. In doing so, the social worker's focus remains on the client's needs rather than on the social worker's own preferential method. By adhering to this principle, all methods and techniques can be utilized flexibly. After this overview of the three-step approach, we will now discuss each step.

1.2.1 Step 1: personal filing cabinet (PFC)

The first step for you, as a social worker, is to establish contact during the intake interview, after which you collect information about the client situation and arrange this information in the client's personal filing cabinet (PFC). In order to obtain reliable information a safe basis of interaction between you and your client is needed. Your starting point for the interview is 'where your client is'. This is where you start implementing your core method: the non-directive core method (see Chapter 3). This core social work method will be used for the duration of the whole social work interaction trajectory to maintain contact and establish a partnership (see also Chapter 4).

By making contact with your client you are also working on developing a relationship of trust. During the interview you start by mapping the client's situation. This is a preliminary inventory of the pluses and minuses, as described in the case study of Maria.

Case study: Maria

Maria's story offered the social worker a range of themes for designing a PFC, which helped her visualize Maria's story in a succinct and orderly manner, by drawing a diagram and using keywords to identify all the stress factors and empowering factors. Maria's situation became organized in a workable framework, which could be used to set an agenda and a plan of action (see Figure 1.1). Maria's PFC presented the following stress factors and empowering factors.

Client as expert

Clients like Maria draw attention to existing unfulfilled needs: a plus or a minus indicates whether the need has been fulfilled or not.

The PFC is used to summarize and reflect areas that will need to be focused on, as indicated by the client. By drawing the client's filing cabinet each area of attention is pictured as a 'drawer' from the person's filing cabinet (see Figure 1.1). The drawers contain 'troubled material', meaning the unfulfilled needs that have not yet been dealt with satisfactorily. You suggest to your client

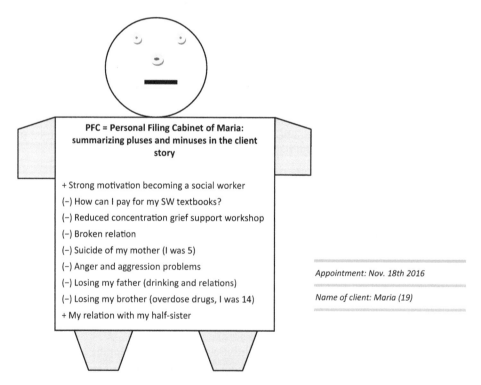

FIGURE 1.1   The personal filing cabinet (PFC) of Maria with strengths (pluses) and stress factors (minuses)

the idea of first organizing the issues in the personal filing cabinet. Your clients' strengths (pluses) will be encouraged (empowerment) to actively identify and reduce the stress factors (minuses).

The impact factor

As described earlier, three factors influence the degree of fulfilment of client needs: the impact factor, the coping factor and the support factor. The coping factor and support factor are described in Step 2. One part of the impact factor are life events. Life events cannot be influenced, because life events are part of life: 'shit happens,' and you cannot prevent tragedy and vulnerability. But life events can also be positive. You can experience successes and flow. Attention is also focused on the positive effects of these life events. There are also positive life events such as falling in love, getting married, having a child and so on. It is sufficient and essential for both the social worker and the client to first acknowledge the impact of these life events. The PFC reveals the actual and personal consequences of the client's life events, known as 'life impact'. Your clients tell their story of their life events, disclosing not only the facts of the life events but also the consequences of these life events such as their emotions and questions.

Reactions resulting from life events such as divorce, death and illness are addressed. Such reactions may be formulated as 'I feel tense,' 'I am so tired,' 'No one will help me' or 'I feel let down.' Another component of the impact factor is how the client first manages the situation or 'I don't know how to manage.' The last component of the impact factor is how the environment responds: 'I (don't) feel supported by my network.' Reflecting on these components of the impact factor in the PFC (life events, reaction-styles and support styles) will help the client identify and acknowledge these QoL issues.

The social worker acknowledges the client's issues by writing down the key words concerning the life events in the PFC. Life impact pertains to the effect that actual life events have on fulfilling human needs. To what extent have the needs for survival, affection and self-determination been fulfilled? Life impact concerns the 'dead weight', the unfulfilled needs, and the psychosocial weight that may disrupt a person's life. The death of a loved one (bereavement), illness (health domain) or job loss (work domain) may result in someone losing their footing in life. On the other hand, the impact might have been less profound if the loss had not taken such a prominent place in the client's life structure. In conclusion, life impact concerns the extent of disruption to human needs that are experienced as a consequence of one or more life events.

The impact factor: Maria

Maria was 5 when her mother committed suicide, her brother took an overdose at the age of 14 and she had recently gone through a relationship breakup. Another significant setback was the fact that she kept failing to complete the grief support seminar. For years Maria had been in a state of survival (survival needs), longing for love and attention (affection needs) and wanting to give direction to her own life (needs for self-determination). Maria was avoiding these life events and her situation deteriorated when she became confronted with her past during the grief support seminar. She was helped by her study-mentor.

1.2.2 Step 2: psychosocial assessment (PSA)

The first rough draft of the client-centred inventory in the PFC forms the foundation for Step 2, the psychosocial assessment of the client situation (PSA). Once you have mapped the pluses and minuses in the client situation, you and your client try to assess or clarify what kind of support is needed. At the same time you acknowledge and gain an appreciation of what the client discloses about positive self-care and help from informal carers in his or her own network. In doing so, the client's needs and goals can be clarified. You can use the needs awareness checklist to help the client gain more awareness about which needs and wishes can help enhance the QoL:

1   *Reality testing*: Is the client realistically observing the life-situation without being judgemental? Example: 'I was fired and I am experiencing a lot of consequences.'
2   *Feelings*: Does the client report which factors give a Yes-feeling (pluses) or a No-feeling (minuses)? Example: This job loss does not feel good.
3   *Needs*: What unfulfilled needs is the client experiencing? Example: I miss my work and therefore I miss the income, social contacts, and identity my work gave me.
4   *Wishes*: Do clients translate the unfulfilled needs in what they want from whom? Example: Can you help me to gain income, workmates and identity?

A minus suggests a No-feeling factor, a stress factor, assuming that a certain need has not been fulfilled, and thereby diminishing the Quality of Life; stress arises for instance in a situation in which a survival need has not been met (such as a safe housing situation). A plus signifies a Yes-feeling factor, an empowering factor; actual needs have obviously been fulfilled (+ having a safe place to stay). As the social worker, you are to summarize the pluses and minuses by using keywords such as ('− home feels unsafe'), labelling them as negative or positive areas to focus on. This concerns those areas on which the client wishes to focus, causing him or her distress or stress (minuses) or creating tranquillity and strength (pluses).

The impact factor was already clarified in Step 1, the PFC. The impact factor could not be influenced because life events are part of life. The next two factors − the coping factor and the support factor − can be enhanced by social work methods in a lot of situations in order to meet clients' needs.

Working hypothesis, dynamic 'diagnosis'

The PSA is needed to link 'clients' needs' to 'supportive actions', regardless of whether this is done by the clients' social network, through community resources/services or through the social worker. The PSA is the bridge between specific needs and possible intervention methods, in order to determine which practical methods best match which support needs. Once the specific support needs have been identified, the social worker can think of a specific method(s) which could be helpful.

As a social worker you have now gathered enough information and made a psychosocial assessment of the unfulfilled needs. Based on this you develop not only a way of understanding the client situation but also working hypotheses on what to do: what methods are indicated?

From client needs to social work methods

Identifying clues for employing the most suitable mix of methods is referred to as *method differentiation*. This is the formal term for distinguishing and discovering which method(s) are beneficial in a specific case. Method differentiation in social work differs somewhat from the medical term '*differential diagnosis*', used by doctors and nurses. In the case of the medical term 'differential diagnosis', the physician eliminates various possible diagnoses after careful investigation. Differential diagnosis in medicine and nursing is defined as the determination of which one of several diseases may be causing the reactions – fatigue, for instance, can be caused by all kinds of diseases; a disturbed sleep–wake rhythm, a profound emotional event, hormonal imbalance, a latent physical illness and so on. The medical professional will suggest the help which corresponds to the most probable underlying condition.

As a social worker, you are not concerned with making such a static 'definite diagnosis', but rather with formulating a 'working hypothesis' on how to go about fulfilling the client's needs. This is because problems in social work clients are multi-causal by definition, as can be seen in Maria's case. From the information obtained from the client you can differentiate all possible needs indications for selecting the appropriate method(s). In the history of social work, the working hypothesis has also been referred to as a 'dynamic diagnosis' to characterize the changeable, dynamic character of each working hypothesis.

According to the PIE-Empowerment Theory (see Chapter 2), clients in social work often present a range of needs asking for fulfilment. The following overview presents the social work methods that can be applied per specific need in social work (see Table 1.1).

This process of developing working hypotheses relating to the client's current needs may appear rather time-consuming: 'this is most likely to be the matter and these are the unfulfilled needs'. In practice, it could take seconds: sometimes a great deal of the sessions are needed to unravel the client situation.

Social workers can employ the following four types of practical methods from their toolkit:

1   *The non-directive core method*: The non-directive core method is used to provide demand-driven support and to prevent social workers from developing a patronizing attitude. This core method ensures clients' sense of wholeness and their remaining the focus of attention during the support programme. In addition, implementing the non-directive core method raises clients' awareness of their (un)fulfilled needs: what do you need to fully enjoy your life?

2   *Individual social work methods*: These coping-focused methods help clients better cope with their own needs. This is what is called 'personal empowerment': helping the client help oneself more effectively (see also Appendix 7).

3   *Systemic and macro social work methods*: How do these support-focused methods help social networks to meet clients' needs? This is what is called 'social empowerment': helping the environment help the client more effectively (see also Figure 1.1).

4   *Case management*: This overarching coordinating method helps clients by linking in with supportive specialists and coordinating the specific contribution of each specialist. The role of the social worker as case manager will be further explored later, as social workers play a specific coordinating role in relation to other professionals. The other methods are introduced in the following chapters.

5   *Case management*: This method is aimed at linking in with the right professionals involved.

Nursing staff, doctors, teachers, managers, human resource mentors and other gatekeepers also have the task to identify, counsel and screen individuals in terms of potential social problems. They may be referred to social work, offering a wide range of methods with a depth of a maximum of 5 levels (see section 1.3 on individual methods). Social work provides a social buffer when dealing with clients' uncomplicated responses to profound life events. The aim of social work is to normalize the way people and networks respond, aiming at stress reduction and helping individuals to find a new balance in life. Complications have not yet arisen, calling for more intensive and specialized help. Social workers may function as case managers if the desired progress has not been achieved, in spite of the expert use of the social work methods that have been described. For instance, in multiple problem cases, social workers may not engage in direct client contact from the start but function as case managers. In both situations, the case manager coordinates one or more specialists in the area(s) of the unresolved problems, including the financial expert, cognitive therapist, relational therapist, family therapist or physiotherapist and others (see Table 1.1).

In complex and time-consuming problem situations, social workers may refer clients to a range of specialists, who implement methods at a more profound and expert level. This concerns complications in various aspects of life, requiring intensive support programmes. Clients can also be referred to specialized social work, in which expert competencies have been developed for addressing multiple problem cases. The case management method is further elaborated on in Chapter 18.

TABLE 1.1 Overview of methods and interventions of social work and specialisms for referral

Social work (method depth 0–5)	Specialist help (method depth 5–10)
Indications for individual methods	
non-directive core method	client-centred psychotherapy
practical-material work method	debt management, discharge management
bodywork method	physiotherapy, manual therapy, etc.
trauma relief work method	trauma therapy
cathartic work method	emotionally focused therapy
expression work method	creative therapy
ritual work method	grief therapy
cognitive work method	cognitive behavioural therapy
narrative work method	narrative therapy
behaviour work method	behaviour therapy
Indications for systemic methods	
social network method	social network therapy
relationship method	couple therapy
family method	family therapy
group work method	group therapy
case management	case management
mediation method	mediation
Indications for macro methods	
monitoring	community work, labour organizations
prevention	prevention work
collective advocacy	community work, union work
practice-based research	evidence-based research

Outreach work: actively approaching clients?

Nowadays, outreach activities in social work are back again – actively approaching clients in the neighbourhood or at school or in the workplace – to see if any help can be offered. In the early days of social work, around 1900, social workers already adopted outreach strategies by directing and actively steering clients' business. They approached people directly, made home visits to those who were in need and tried to ensure that clients conformed to the prevailing rules and morals of the time. Home-visiting social workers were not only directive, but also normative and patronizing in their attitude towards clients, for example 'Is this place clean enough?' They insisted on improvements at their own discretion and employed their expertise to get things done. Social workers operated like company managers exerting power over their employees' welfare. Fortunately, this patronizing attitude was to become abandoned in the years that followed. Social casework, as advocated in Holland by Marie Kamphuis, proved an important instrument in effecting this change. Social casework, re-introduced in the 1950s, attached great importance to the developing relationship between social worker and client. Clients needed be given the opportunity to become aware of their own situation. Caseworkers interpreted clients' communications from a psychodynamic perspective (Freudian), which directed the course of interventions. The 1960s saw the introduction and rise of the non-directive method of Carl Rogers. He is a representative of human psychology, which perceives the worth of the individual as the starting point. A great number of social work training colleges included non-directive communication skills in their curriculum. At present, non-directive interviewing techniques are still an important element of interviewing skills in social work. It is considered vitally important for social workers to develop a helping relationship with their clients. All kinds of communication techniques are trained, as described in works by Rogers himself and his followers, such as Gerard Egan. Two decades later, in the 1980s, many social workers welcomed the emerging directive approach. A representative of this movement was Frederick Perls, whom many social workers considered an example of the more actively steering approach. Perls was the founder of Gestalt therapy. In addition to stressing the importance of the here and now of clients' personal experiences, he also found it essential to influence clients by confronting them. In the 1980s, Dutch social workers Roel Bouwkamp and Sjef de Vries adapted Gestalt therapy to psychosocial therapy for social work. In psychosocial therapy they emphasized the importance of direct personal response, a form of direct communication. According to Bouwkamp and De Vries (1992), the lower income groups in particular could benefit from this approach. At the time, social workers found this directive approach most appealing. Up to then they had been trained to work exclusively in a non-directive way, by for instance lending a sympathetic ear, being present and the method 'that's you'. A great many social workers found that a different approach was needed instead of the client-centred method to deal with problem situations in daily practice. They rejected the softer approach and opted for filling their toolkit with a wide range of up-to-date directive methods. By then, many social workers were already taking courses in applying directive techniques. This directive method was among others developed by Kees van der Velden. Care professionals employ the directive method by offering instructions and directives to clients. In the directive approach, assignments and instructions are essential to the relationship between care professional and client (van der Velden, 1980).

Steering or directivity has long been rejected by social work, just as setting boundaries or taking the initiative to contact a client (Jagt, 2001). Not directly seeking client contact proved to be a too one-sided approach. Not every individual has sufficient skills for self-determination and takes the initiative to ask for support. Not all clients are kind and gentle; they may sometimes be calculating or aggressive and inattentive to what harm they are causing others. Jagt argues for a work method whereby social workers take action to support involuntary service users (clients who are reluctant to contact social work or have been mandated by law to contact social work). The social worker tries to persuade the client in a directive way to participate in the support programme, for instance, by way of motivational interviewing.

At first, the client's attitude towards the social worker may be rather dismissive: 'What do you want from me?' Social workers who wish to actively offer support must first have a reason to seek contact with the client. In many cases it is society itself that calls for an intervention instead of the clients themselves. The social worker formulates the demand for care on the basis of reported incidences caused by the client or because of problems encountered by professionals (police officers, housing corporations, social psychiatrists). This demand for care is attributed to clients without their acknowledgement. Support for involuntary service users can become successful once clients acknowledge their need for intervention. The social worker takes small steps to motivate clients to participate in the support programme. This type of support, whereby the social worker takes the initiative and actively offers support, is referred to as the 'outreach approach'.

More and more voices are calling for outreach to deliver services to complex or multiple problem clients (Lohuis, 2008). It concerns people who are experiencing multiple problems and are also causing problems in their environment. A large number of them are addicts and have psychiatric complaints. The question is how to contact these groups of clients and how to maintain contact. Multimethodical social work is the most suitable approach for this target group on account of its broad and problem-oriented design. After actively approaching the client, the next step is to make contact in a non-directive way. Establishing contact with marginalized groups in society is nowadays referred to as the presence approach. Being present is considered more important than intervention (Baart, 2001). The presence approach is similar to non-directive presence, as described in the non-directive core social work method (Chapter 4).

For social workers in primary care this active support is also called 'outreach work' (van Doorn et al., 2008). Outreach work has to do with breaking the taboo to support those who do not seek help. It involves people who are at risk of social exclusion and are now given the chance to participate in society again. Examples are residents from deprived neighbourhoods, persons with psychiatric problems and alarming situations in single and family households. Examples would be, for instance, the case of the Meuse girl, whose body parts were found in the river Meuse (killed by her father), the case of Savannah (mother and stepfather killed daughter) and the Roermond case (father set fire to the house and children perished in the flames).

In their inspection reports child protection services raised the question how things could have gotten to that point and whether more active support could have been offered in these situations. They came to the conclusion that social workers should, in future cases like these, take the initiative to establish contact, instead of waiting for a demand for care. The methodical competencies involved in outreach work do not differ from those in the usual situation where clients ask for support. The only difference is that the social worker instead of the client takes the initiative to make contact. After establishing contact and formulating an acknowledged demand for care, multimethodical strategies can be implemented, as in the usual client situation. Outreach work involves all other individual methods, in addition to the non-directive core method. Furthermore, the systemic approach is regularly required, such as the family method or the social network method to strengthen the client's social supportive environment. Finally, the monitoring method and the prevention method – macro methods – are in place to identify signs of structural shortcomings, which are to be dealt with as part of the outreach programme.

1.2.3 Step 3: psychosocial intervention (PSI)

In Step 2, the pluses and minuses of PSA were identified as well as possible methods of intervention, followed by the drawing up of a plan of action. In the next step of psychosocial interventions (PSI), this plan of action can be implemented to actually reduce the minuses and strengthen the pluses. Intervention is not defined as a one-man show on the part of the social worker, but a process of informed consent in good collaboration between client and social worker. The social worker informs the client about possible ways of making the coping and support factor more effective. With the client's consent, progress can be made.

In the collaboration between social worker and clients, the question arises as to what clients define as their objectives. Also, what areas of focus and needs do they wish to address and in which order? Are there any issues they would choose to leave alone for the time being? Are there any stress factors that need not be addressed in the social work interaction? With what stress factor would your client like to start? Is it feasible to start with that particular factor in the initial session or would it be wise to address the issue in the next session? Two questions arise that are important for achieving objectives.

What is the concrete objective the client wishes to achieve? For instance, 'I have lost my way in life completely after the loss of my parents; please help me get my life back together again [Objective 1: survival] so that I will feel calm and able to enjoy life again [Objective 2: self-determination].'

What are the client's wishes as to your role as a social worker? For instance, 'I would like you to use your expertise to help me restore the balance in my life in order to move on.'

When an objective has not been formulated clearly, it is advisable to help your clients clearly express their concrete question, wish and expectation: 'What is it you wish to achieve? What do you need to take a step forwards in life in respect to this issue? What do you expect from me?' By asking questions more clearly, you aim to empathize with the client's complaints and find out what the client really wants first. Next, you need to establish the appropriate practical methods for reducing the minuses (unfulfilled needs) and enhancing the pluses (fulfilled needs) in the client situation.

This third step involves implementing specific practical methods for the identified and selected support needs for interventions on different levels (see also Table 1.2).

Scaling up and down

To summarize: you will have determined the most appropriate methods and interventions for fulfilling the client's needs, either on an individual, systemic or macro level.

- *Individual* methods are needed to enhance personal coping skills (self-care).
- *Systemic* methods are needed to enhance effective social support from informal carers.
- *Macro* methods are needed to enhance structural support from local and national resources.

If necessary, you can switch from one intervention *level* to the other. For instance, when your client tells you that he feels lonely and needs interaction with others, you can switch from the individual level to care at the systemic level, enabling you to work on strengthening the client's social network. Switching over means changing the intervention scale – as in this case, changing from the individual to the systemic intervention level. You can also switch from the individual to the structural intervention level. For instance, when the issue concerns a lack of support service for clients who have lost their parents at an early age, as in the case of your client. It is advised to switch from the individual to the macro intervention level and work on a suitable provision for a whole target group by employing macro methods that strengthen their position (e.g. support project, social meetings).

Measuring client progress

Now that your working hypothesis has yielded an indication, you can proceed to implement the plan of action. It is important that you carefully check the efficacy of the methods employed. Testing your working hypothesis is an ongoing process. Having decided which method is indicated, you may start making contact with your client in order to reduce the client's stress by fulfilling their needs.

1.3 Outcome-focused working with scaling

After establishing which methods are indicated, you, the social worker, can proceed to implement the support methods to optimize the client's quality of life. Together with your clients you work towards meeting their needs and wishes. In the process you keep an open mind to all new information that may either confirm the working hypothesis or possibly disprove it. Social work help involves regular review, and the latter constitutes an integral part of the social work process. No change of method is needed if the working hypothesis is confirmed. If disproven, certain obstacles are blocking the fulfilment of the client's needs. Together with your client you examine what is really causing the stress and then formulate a new working hypothesis. The three-step approach is both a linear support delivery process (achieving the objective) and a cyclical, reiterative process, a repeated searching process, involving shifts in methodical actions, depending on the client and the clarification or change in support demand (see cycle in Figure 1.2).

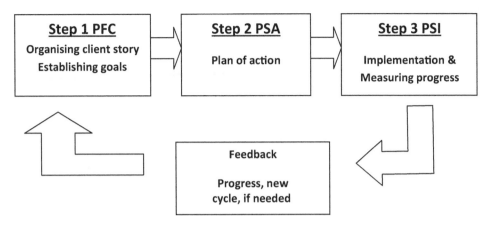

FIGURE 1.2 Repeated social work cycle: continually adapting plan of action if objectives have not been fully met

1.3.1 Preliminary and final scaling

Progress in the client situation is regularly reviewed and at the end the final review is drawn up. Have the objectives been achieved? Has the stress been reduced? Has the strength in the client situation been enhanced? Have the client's needs been fulfilled? If so, you are on the right path; if not, you need to adapt the PSA or the PSI. The stress meter, energy meter and progress meter (see Table 1.2) are useful tools for you to use:

- The stress meter (see Table 1.2) is used to establish how tense the client is feeling at different points during the session or help: has stress reduction occurred during the course of help?
- You can use the energy meter (see Table 1.2) to assess how much energy the client is experiencing at different points in the session or during the whole help trajectory: has there been an increase in energy during the course of social work help?
- The progress meter (see section 1.3.3) is used to assess the client's progress during the course of social work help.

1.3.2 Scaling techniques and measurement

Scaling techniques with so-called scale questions are utilized to measure results. The social worker keeps an open mind to new information that may either confirm the work hypothesis or reject it. Review at regular intervals is considered an integrated part of the client-centred approach. When the work hypotheses are confirmed, the same procedure can be continued. In case of rejection, something else is obviously causing the stress reactions in your client. Together, you examine what is really at the root of the stress reactions, leading to formulating new work hypotheses. You and your client regularly review the tentative results, and eventually review the final results of the client's progress. Have the targets been met? Has the

TABLE 1.2 Overview of scaling meters in social work

Aspects measured of client situation	Name meter	(see also section)
Progress in social work	Progress meter	1.3.3
Quality of life	Quality-of-life meter	2.3.1
Impact of life events	Impact meter	2.4.1
Personal strength	Strength meter	2.4.2
Adequacy of coping	Coping meter	2.4.2 + App. 7
Support level social network	Support meter	2.4.3
Level of basic resources	Basic resources meter	2.4.3
Physical condition	Condition meter	5.7.3
Stress level	Stress meter	5.7.13
Energy level	Energy meter	5.7.13

tension been reduced? Has the strength in the client situation been enhanced? If so, the social worker will find that he is on the right track. If not, either of the following actions should be undertaken:

- Adjustment to the analysis of stress and strength factors;
- Adjustment to indication and work hypothesis.

The stress level meter, the energy meter, the progress meters and other meters are useful tools in assessing and making progress measurable in the client's situation (see Table 1.2). These meters consist of scale questions, also referred to as 'working with scaling'. The stress level meter, for instance, establishes the level of tension of a client by means of the scale question, 'How do you rate your level of tension on a scale from 0 to 10, with 0 as minimal tension and 10 as maximum tension?' This question is asked at various moments of the session or social work contact, and measures differences in stress levels. The scale question is preferably posed at the end of a session and at the beginning of the next, having the client look back. In this way the social worker avoids asking all kinds of questions instead of allowing the client to tell their story. The client is invited to relate to his or her condition at two different moments. The energy meter (see Chapter 5) contains the scale question, 'How is your energy level at the moment on a scale ranging from 0 (minimal energy) to 10 (maximum energy)?' It is established by how much energy the client experiences at different moments of the session or during the whole programme: is there an increase in energy during social work? And for all mentioned scale levels in Table 1.2 the same reasoning in scaling can be used.

1.3.3 Progress meter

During the social work programme the aforementioned meters can be utilized to verify the client's progress in a certain aspect of life. The progress meter is the only meter with a scale question that explicitly assesses the client's progress during the entire psychosocial social work programme. The social worker establishes the client's progress by having the client rate their own progress on a scale from 0 to 10: 'Could you indicate on the progress scale how you perceive the progress you have made in the foregoing sessions as concerns reducing the stress factors that you have reported. Zero is the situation when we first met at the first session, when there was no progress; 10 is the moment when the sessions can be concluded'.

'What, in your opinion, is your progress at this moment?' Suppose the client rates the present progress situation as a 7. The social worker can respond to that by saying: 'We can now infer that progression has been made for 70% and that there is 30% more to go. How can we accomplish this 30% progress?' The social worker concludes the progress measurement by asking: 'What were the things that led to this progress?'

1.3.4 Functions of scaling meters

The function of the scaling meters is twofold. On the one hand, they provide the social worker with information concerning the client's actual situation at that moment, on the other, they deliver feedback as to the efficacy of social work. Should the situation arise where the client is stagnating or deteriorating, the social worker will evaluate the process so far together with the client and make adjustments where necessary. In doing so, the social worker remains close to the client's demands and needs, resulting in effective support, which is also efficient, considering that it takes minimum effort on the side of the client to attain the original or adjusted goal.

1.4 Social work interventions in practice

Table 1.3 summarizes the social work methods used in the case study of Maria, followed by an explanation of the support process, which will include all methods used by the college social worker in this case.

TABLE 1.3 Multimethod social work in the case study of Maria

Maria's needs	Social work methods used	Techniques used per method
Contact and overview	Non-directive core method	Sorting out issues with the PFC-technique and maintaining contact
Survival needs	Practical-material method	Pleading for father's contribution to therapy
	Trauma-work method	Reconstructing her life events
	Bodywork method	Assessing how to reduce her level of stress using the scaling technique
Affective needs	Cathartic method	Releasing her emotions
	Expression method	Disclosure by writing things down
	Ritual work method	Preparing and performing the ritual
Needs for self-determination	Cognitive method	Explaining and challenging her way of thinking
	Behavioural method	Learning skills
Need for social support	Relationship-focused method	Learning to appreciate each other
	Family method	Drawing family tree, family interview

The case study of Maria

The college social worker had asked Maria to choose from her personal filing cabinet the drawer she wished to discuss first. Finding the money to pay for the social work support received was a priority for her. In addition, Maria was unable to pay for her textbooks. Together they looked into the questions and options for payment, such as the possibility of a study grant. Maria also mentioned that her father could be asked to contribute financially. The social worker would inquire if Maria's college could lend financial support in urgent cases and then argue Maria's case; *practical-material work method*, in this case pleading and promoting interests. Asking her own father for help was considered with some reluctance on her side. After some exercises (how to ask such a question), and after the social worker had modelled some behaviour and had shown appreciation for her progress, Maria felt up to taking the first step towards approaching her father (*behavioural method*: social skills modelling and conditioning techniques).

Obviously, the social work methods are not always implemented as schematically as in the figure, as social workers should keep working flexibly and maintain the client's needs as the starting point. The college social worker had asked Maria which drawer from the PFC to start with first (*non-directive core method*). After sorting out the financial matters together, the social worker asked which drawer they should deal with next. Maria wanted to start by focusing on the issue of her failed relationship. She regretted the breakup but she could no longer stand being together anymore. 'What was it you could not stand?' the social worker had asked. She answered 'In fact, it was the intimacy, being so close to a person.' 'What's so difficult about that?' the social worker then asked her. 'If we had carried on, he would certainly have broken off our relationship at a certain point.' In turn, the social worker asked 'Were you afraid of losing him? Do you find it hard to become attached to someone?' to which she answered 'I do actually, I have become so disappointed in the important relationships in my life.' After these clarifying questions (*non-directive core method*) LSFQ (listening-summarizing-further questioning), Maria concluded that she was actually longing to see him again: 'What have I done, thrown something away that was really good?' The social worker asked whether Maria would prefer to talk to him alone or have her there as well. She preferred the social worker to be present during the conversation. It emerged that Maria and her ex were willing to give their relationship another go (*relationship-focused method*: assessment and focusing technique). She indicated that she wished to practice saying: 'I feel anxious' or 'Please hold me,' instead of getting upset and keeping her boyfriend at a distance. Her social worker explained that she was suffering from relational trauma on account of what had happened to her mother and brother. She explained that Maria could learn to experience safe attachment (*cognitive work method*: psychoeducation, *behavioural work method*: modelling technique). Next, Maria wished to deal with her anger, although she was having some doubts. After some further explorative talking she felt ready to deal with her anger issues (*non-directive core method*: LSFQ-technique). She came to realize that she had always been on edge in her relationship with her boyfriend. To her, the relationship had felt unsafe, although there was no reason for this. Her social worker explained that immediately responding in anger could be seen as a fight reaction, which is a survival reaction triggered in a threatening situation (*cognitive work method*: psychoeducation). Maria had known this anger all her life: the fight and flight reactions in times of crisis. Now it became clear that her anger was mainly directed at her father. 'Why did you let me down when I lost my mother? Why are you so preoccupied with yourself instead of supporting me?' Part of the anger appeared to be directed at her mother, who had committed suicide. She succeeded in writing things down (*expression method*: writing technique). She became more and more aware of what was making her angry, but also realized that talking and writing about these issues was not enough.

When the social worker invited Maria to practice expressing these feelings she found herself facing a real wall, a wall of fear. 'Am I going to lose my mind if I feel even more emotions?' Her social worker comforted her by telling her that these feelings were normal responses to a profoundly upsetting experience (of loss). As a consequence, she felt less inhibited to work on this issue (*cognitive method*: psychoeducation). During the session she expressed a great deal of anger towards first her father and then her mother, arousing profound feelings of anger but also of sadness. The social worker suggested that she freely vent her anger towards her mother and father and have her imagine them sitting on an empty chair (*cathartic method*: exposure and empty chair technique). This constructive way of releasing her anger worked very well for Maria, expressing anger towards an imaginary person rather than a real person. At first this was quite an effort for her and it made her feel very tired. At the same time she felt relieved and then more energetic. An eye-opener for her was that Maria's social worker re-labelled her anger as 'destructive right', and that she was now venting her anger towards the right persons. A child deserves to be given attention and positivity, observing a balance between giving and receiving. When there is a great deal of negativity in your life and a lack of positivity, a right to destruction arises: if the world (family members and others) treat me in such as negative way, I am given the existential right to do something back: destructive right (*family work method*: addressing technique). Then it appeared that Maria kept asking herself profoundly existential questions: 'Was I not worthwhile enough for you keep living for?' and 'Why did you leave me by killing yourself?' The social worker summed up what she had heard from Maria and paraphrased her words: 'You wonder whether you were worth living for' (*non-directive core method*: paraphrasing and mirroring technique). Maria's thought of 'Am I worth living for?' proved to be rather persistent. The social worker questioned this self-statement and did not accept it at face value (*cognitive method*: challenging technique): 'Why should you have doubts about yourself when your mother decides to end her life?' As a result, other less distressing thoughts entered her mind. 'Why should other people suffer if they behave towards me in an unfriendly manner?'

Maria was gaining more insight into her situation. The social worker suggested drawing up a family tree with the family members she had mentioned before (*family work method*: genogram technique). The loss of her mother, father and her brother as well as the disappointing responses from the extended family kept bothering Maria. On the other hand, there was also positive contact with some family members. She became aware that by being angry and aggressive she was actually taking it out on others. The real cause was the injustice inflicted upon her by her parents. 'Why did my Mum end her life when I was still so young? Why did my father abandon me when I needed love and comforting?' These questions constituted past hurt that made Maria take things out on innocent significant others who were now disappointing her, although they had nothing to do with the source of her primary anger and disappointment. Maria recognized herself in the vicious circle as described in unfinished business syndrome (UBS) (see also Figure 26.1). Like a fire smouldering beneath the surface, the existential anger burst into flames whenever ignited by another disappointment in the present. Feeling powerless to direct her anger and disappointment at the right persons, she ended up hurting others because she had to find a way of releasing the stress. She could not quite understand why she was being so unreasonable (disproportionate behaviour) but did realize now that every new disappointment (trigger) would now result in more anger. By sorting out her unaddressed feelings towards mother, father and brother, she finally succeeded in extinguishing her inner fire. A firefighter once explained to me, 'not only do you hose down the flames but also tackle the smouldering heaps to ensure the fire is fully extinguished.' Now that her anger had subsided, Maria could move on to the next drawer. She chose her mother, although she still had some doubts in her mind. She had managed to release her anger and sadness, but something kept bothering her that needed attention. The social worker asked her to explain what it was (*non-directive core method*: LSFQ technique). Maria explained that she had never really openly talked about the traumatic part of losing her mother. The social worker suggested going through the experiences she remembered as a 5-year-old child (*trauma-work method*: reconstruction technique). The story emerged in fragmented parts. Maria remembered being kept away from the scene and not being allowed to see her dead mother and feeling as if in a haze. At the time she could not talk to anyone about the events. Therefore, she was unable to recollect the whole picture, some details though, had stuck to her mind (sensory imprinting). For instance, her Dad told her that 'Mum was no longer alive' and that 'now we have to carry on without her and it's no use thinking about it.' It was a strange period of her life, instead of attending her mother's funeral, she was sent to school. She remembering sitting at her desk in the classroom and seeing the funeral procession go by. Later she put two and two together and realized that it was her mother's funeral and that she had been excluded. Sometimes she also felt shut out in the classroom situation and by her peers and by others later in life. Maria now came to realize that being excluded formed another trigger point for her feelings of anger and powerlessness. After exploring these events the social worker asked if Maria had said goodbye to her

TABLE 1.4 The ritual method in the case study of Maria

Seven of the 9 Ws	Maria's interpretations
1	What is the purpose of this ritual?	Saying farewell to mum properly after all this time
2	What things would you like to do when saying goodbye?	Go to my mother's grave, lie down on the tombstone, smoke a joint
3	What attributes do you need for this?	Joint, written letter
4	Where would you like to perform this ritual?	Cemetery where my mother is buried
5	What time of day would you prefer for this?	During twilight, on her birthday
6	Who would you like to be present, in what role?	My boyfriend, drinking a beer and listening
7	What words would you use during the ritual?	'I could not say farewell at the time, but I'm trying to do so now: Love you Mum. Farewell!'

mother in a dignified manner. It emerged from reconstructing the events that she had not said goodbye to her mother at all. The social worker proposed that Maria should as yet pay respect to her dead mother (*ritual method*: as yet technique). In preparation of the farewell ritual the social had asked detailed questions, which, Maria, retrospectively identified as 7 of the 9 Ws of the ritual method (see Table 1.4 and 'Checklist rituals' in section 10.7.1).

After Maria had performed the ritual the social worker asked her about its effect. Maria answered, 'After all those years this is the first time that I felt contact with my mother, it's alright now.'

Then she had to deal with the drawer of losing her brother. Maria reconstructed the events surrounding his traumatic death (*trauma-work method*: reconstruction technique). Maria was 14 when this took place, so that she had experienced it more consciously than her mother's death. As in the event of her mother's death, she had not said goodbye to her brother either. She also prepared a farewell ritual for him and subsequently performed it where he lay buried (*ritual method*: 10 Ws and the 'as yet' technique). With regard to her father she now felt much calmer after expressing her anger towards the empty chair and obtaining financial support from him. Still, she felt some reservations before talking about the disappointments and the contact with her half-sisters. The social worker asked about these reservations (*non-directive core method*: LSFQ technique). Maria would like to share her childhood experiences with him and voice her appreciation for financially supporting her now. This was a tough thing for her to do, considering the family culture, being one of 'every man for himself'. Her half-sisters and half-brothers were also receiving social work support, for ADHD, aggression problems and depression. The social worker suggested holding a family meeting with Maria's father and her two elder half-sisters with whom Maria was on good terms (*family method*: communication technique). After this meeting, the situation brightened up a little as they all realized that Maria had gone through difficult times and now wished to move on in life.

All things considered this social work process meant 'a huge boost to her self-confidence', as Maria put it. The social worker made Maria the starting point of the social work process (*non-directive core method*: start, follow and end where the client is) and worked together with her to reduce the stress and enhance Maria's strengths. Furthermore, she used scaling (scaling questions) to measure progress during social work sessions. For instance, she asked 'How would you rate your stress levels on a scale from 0 to 10, starting from 0 as no stress at all to 10 meaning maximum stress.' The stress scale is described in Chapter 5, the bodywork method. At the beginning of the programme she started with a 9 on the stress scale and ended with 3, energy score starting with 3 and ending with 8 at the end of the social work intervention. The main objectives had been achieved: a higher quality of living because of a reduced stress level and increased energy levels. Finally the social worker asked what had caused her to achieve such progress: 'That's simple enough, I have dealt with the troublesome drawers from my filing cabinet and my resilience, perseverance and motivation for Social Studies have been enhanced!'

1.5 Summary

The aim of this chapter has been to explain how you, as a social worker, can implement the multimethod social work approach to sustainably fulfil your clients' needs.

The current chapter described the three-step plan in social work, using the metaphor of the filing cabinet (PFC) as a structuring and empowering instrument, followed by the psychosocial assessment (PSA). The PSA was described as a step of differentiating or identifying social work practice work methods. After following the first step you, as a social worker, will have gathered sufficient information and achieved a (tentative) needs assessment of the client situation. This information forms the foundation for developing working hypotheses about underlying support needs, detecting negativity (stumbling blocks in fulfilling needs) as well as positivity (building blocks). In addition, working hypotheses are formulated about how to operate, raising the question of which practical methods can best be employed. Next, the multimethod approach in social work, psychosocial intervention (PSI) was discussed, including a wide range of individual, systemic and macro social work methods according to the client's support needs: when is which social work method most efficient in fulfilling the client's needs?

In the next chapter the PIE-Empowerment Theory will be described as the comprehensive social work theory the three-step approach is based on.

Questions

1   Apply the stepped-plan approach to one of your own cases.
2   Which social methods are you familiar with? Have you used them in practice? Which of the social methods would you like to study more closely, in theory and in practice?
3   Describe a case study and use the indication list in Table 1.1 to identify the social methods you have used and indicate which other methods could have complemented your approach.

2

P-I-E EMPOWERMENT THEORY (PIE-ET)

JONATHAN SINGER, INTERVIEWER: Why should social workers learn theory?

JOE WALSH, RESEARCHER: Well, to me a theory is simply a way to make sense out of very complex behavior, and I think that at its core, human behavior is way too complex for any of us to understand in its entirety so a theory is just a perspective or a 'lens' that we assume so that we can narrow down what we're looking at and do the best we can at understanding people and their experiences. It's sort of a way to make sense out of confusing experiences. I believe that everyone operates from a theoretical perspective whether they are aware of it or not.

(http://socialworkpodcast.blogspot.nl/2009/08/theories-for-clinical-social-work.html)

Questions

This chapter addresses the following questions:

- What types of tunnel vision may we encounter in social work?
- What two functions do useful theories involve?
- What does the PIE-Empowerment Theory entail?
- What do we mean when we talk about Quality of Life?
- What four basic needs can we distinguish in life?
- What do we mean when we talk about satisfiers and pseudo-satisfiers?
- What do the three QoL factors entail?
- What does the term 'impact factor' refer to?
- What does the term 'coping factor' refer to?
- What does the term 'support factor' refer to?
- How do we decide how to best meet the client's needs when working with different social work approaches?

2.1 Introduction

The three-step theory which was set out in Chapter 1 involves the client mapping out the positive and negative factors experienced by the client (Step 1). Next the social worker formulates a plan of approach: what positive factors (utilizing the client's own abilities) can be used to reduce the negative factors (sources of stress): this is Step 2. Step 3 involves implementing this plan and gauging the effectiveness of this approach.

So the question is, which theoretical perspectives about the dynamics in the client situation will support social workers in helping clients following this three-step approach? This chapter describes a multifactorial social work theory, the so-called Person-in-Environment Empowerment Theory (PIE-ET). The PIE-Empowerment Theory brings two central perspectives in social work history together: the Person-in-Environment perspective and the Empowerment perspective.

I will first describe the need for an overarching social work theory aimed at minimizing the risk of tunnel vision. Next I will summarize PIE-ET and in doing so I will link the Empowerment approach to two central factors: person and environment. Following this I will work out the three interrelated factors which determine QoL. Lastly, I will use a number of concepts from communicative and system approaches in social work to underpin the relationship between these interrelated factors. The theoretical concepts are illustrated by elements from the case study about Maria (19), who was a social work student and who sought help from a college social worker (this case also illustrated the three-step social work approach in the first chapter).

Case study: Maria – Multiple layers of complexity

Maria was a social work student who was not able to finish her grief support seminar, which was the final component of her social work programme of studies. One of her lecturers referred her to a social worker at the college she was training at. Maria was motivated to seek help for herself from the school social worker, in accordance with the principle of 'You cannot take others further than you have taken yourself.'

It appeared that her unfinished emotional business became reactivated during the seminar and as a result she found herself unable to concentrate on her studies. For a long time Maria had been struggling with her mother's unexpected death (by suicide when Maria was 5) and her brother's death (from an overdose at age 14) and with the fact that her father had not been there for her at the time these life events occurred.

Maria remained rebellious and came close to involvement with police and the judiciary. During the school social work sessions she wondered: 'Why? Why do such terrible things happen in my life?' The social work sessions helped Maria sort out the troubling issues in her life. By sorting through all the problem areas she was able to deal with one specific area at a time and eventually regained control over her life.

2.2 An overarching social work theory?

What overarching social work theory can be usefully implemented in social work practice? Such a theory has to be suited to the broad and often complex reality of social work. A very significant number of social work theories and subtheories have been developed to this end over the years. In this chapter I will describe PIE-ET as the overarching theory which synergistically combines the power of distinct subtheories and approaches: 1 + 1 = 3?

But before turning to PIE-ET, I will first define what constitutes a 'useful theory' and point out the danger of tunnel vision in social work, whenever theories result in a blinkered gaze and one-sided approaches. Theories are useful when they have two functions: first, useful theories offer a retrospective explanation as to how the client's issues and concerns developed; second, a useful theory helps us look ahead, to see what possible future steps the approach might entail. Therefore, social work theories are useful if they entail both the function of elucidating and offering insights, and the function of looking into the future and predicting what might happen. In an article on evidence-based social work, Bruce Thyer defined these two functions of 'theory' as 'attempts to retrospectively explain and to prospectively predict': 'The first function of theory is to explain or help us understand – to provide some insight – as to why something happened. The second function is to predict progress in the case of a particular client' (Thyer, 2001).

Theory applied to the case study of Maria

You are the school social worker working with Maria, the student who is finding it impossible to carry on with her studies. A useful theory will provide an answer to both questions: Why is this happening (*the elucidating function*) and how can she progress from here (*the predictive function*). In the course of the social work interviews it becomes clear that Maria is very much troubled by unfinished emotional business (*elucidating* the reason why she has developed problems studying). If she were to find closure for this unfinished business, she would be able to carry on with her studies (*the predictive function*).

The concept of 'useful theory' equates to the concept of 'working hypothesis' or 'working theory' which were introduced in the previous chapter. Working hypotheses also involve an elucidating function such as which life need is unmet? They also need a predictive function: if these specific client wishes are fulfilled, the client's QoL will improve. I argued that social workers always consider the need for such working hypotheses to be tested; in other words, they do not see it as simply 'the best' but are willing to replace it by a better working hypothesis if need be. This helps prevent working hypotheses or useful theories from turning into dogmas rather than hypotheses.

I will now turn to the question as to whether existing social work theories meet the elucidating and predictive requirements for useful theories. According to practitioners, a great many theories turn out to be unworkable in social work practice, while some even appear to be harmful to clients. Schön (1983) refers to this as the gap between theory and practice affecting professions such as social work. According to Schön the first problem theory posed to 'reflective professionals' is the fact that science and professional training courses teach overly abstract knowledge. Schön holds that 'Theories are the lofty highlands,' at best offering an explanation for only part of the existing problems and concerns, but not always offering practical insights as to 'what to do'. Such theories are often less useful for the professionals who have both feet in the swamp of professional practice: the 'swampy lowlands of practice' (see Figure 2.1).

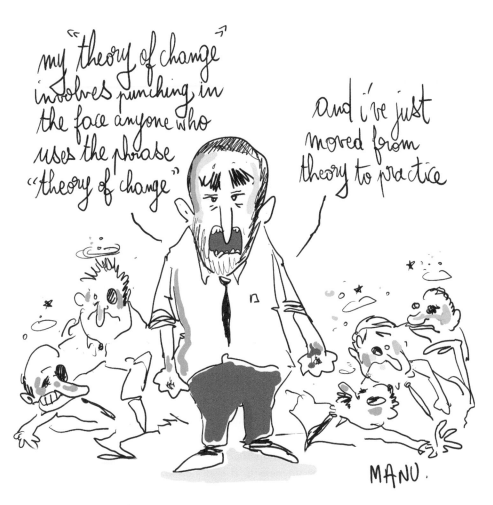

FIGURE 2.1 Theory of change

Cartoon courtesy of Manu

When applying only part of a theory, this may be harmful to the client because tunnel vision may occur. In such cases, clients can feel as if they are labelled: the focus is on only one aspect, rather than on the client's overall situation. Such a one-sided focus constitutes a major pitfall, especially when social workers keep returning to one or more preferential theories rather than focusing on all factors at play in the client's situation. That could lead to a mono-method rather than a multimethod approach: the social worker only sees what he is focusing on and addresses that. The client is subjected to a one-sided approach, because the social worker is trying to explain everything from a one-sided perspective on just a single aspect of the client's case.

Tunnel vision in Maria's case

Tunnel vision would occur if the school social worker only approaches Maria's situation from a cognitive perspective (Maria's thinking is not grounded in reality) and considers this to be the key to all aspects of her issues. In this case, the cognitive method is used to encourage Maria to think more realistically, but is not effective in issues which require a practical approach, or one aimed at addressing relationships or underlying feelings. In other words, the cognitive method is like a key which fits the cognitive keyhole, but ends up being wrongly used as the passkey to resolving all other issues.

This tunnel vision entails the risk of secondary victimization: clients feel they are not being treated with respect and this results in unintentionally adding insult to injury. A one-sided monofactorial vision underpinning a one-sided single method approach may result in the client feeling poorly understood when it comes to aspects which are not addressed, because the social worker is focusing merely on resolving only part of the issue. We may find examples of one-sided tunnel vision and unilateral approaches in many different guises in professional practice:

- Clients may feel 'blamed' when social workers apply a one-sided *person*-focused approach: 'It is all my fault.'
- Clients may be disempowered when a one-sided *environment*-focused approach is used: 'The system or social and political structures are to blame.'
- A one-sided *interactive and systemic* approach can result in downplaying the responsibilities of the partners in the interaction: 'It is all due to miscommunication; nobody is responsible.'
- A one-sided *cognitive* lens and the ensuing cognitive behavioural approach may result in placing too much value on the power of thought: 'Everything will be fine as long as the client improves his way of thinking.'
- A one-sided focus on *stress* and the associated attempt to physically de-stress may result in too much value being placed on the power of the 'physical body': 'As long as there is a reduction on physical stress, everything will improve.'
- A one-sided focus on emotions and the associated attempt to address feelings may result in too much value being placed on the power of emotions: 'Everything will be better once we get rid of these feelings.'

In short, whenever a one-sided approach is used, one gaze unduly overtakes all others – be this the social worker's own gaze, or a guideline or protocol imposed by the institution employing the social worker.

PIE-ET tries to achieve a theoretical synthesis by adopting a multifocal or multifactorial lens which underpins a multimethod approach. It combines existing models and theories from within the historical development of social work. See Appendix 8 for a brief summary of the history of the PIE-concept.

2.3 PIE-Empowerment Theory: an overview

> You should try and fulfil your own needs in life, but not all by yourself.

The social worker maximizes the client's Quality of Life (QoL) in close collaboration with the client, by engaging the power of two factors: the strength of the person and the strength of the environment (Person-in-Environment). The social worker uses scaling to regularly assess the effect of the social work approach on the client's QoL (see Chapter 1 for more information on scaling).

We first need to ask whether PIE-ET meets the requirement of a useful theory in terms of being able to explain and predict, as described in section 2.2. PIE-Empowerment Theory meets these two requirements because it not only offers a multi-factorial *explanation* for any deterioration of the QoL, but is also able to *predict* what is needed to optimize QoL. So we need to determine what is necessary, in the context of PIE-ET, to encourage the two 'actors' to positively influence QoL factors. Based on the PIE-ET framework, the social worker works with the person and the environment to utilize the positive factors to achieve a reduction of the negative factors. This shows that PIE-ET possesses the predictive function of a useful theory (see Figure 2.2).

2.3.1 Quality of life

Quality of Life (QoL) has been mentioned a few times. QoL is the final objective of social work and is therefore used as a yardstick to gauge the effectiveness of social work. So what do we mean by QoL?

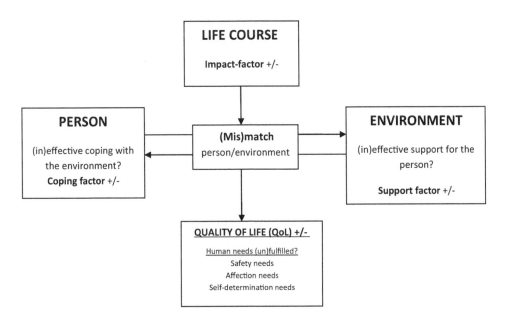

FIGURE 2.2   PIE-Empowerment Theory: empowering person–environment interaction enhancing Quality of Life

I will use the definition put forth by the Quality of Life Research Unit of the University of Toronto (2014) to define 'quality of life': 'The degree to which a person enjoys the important possibilities of his or her life: in other words: enjoying the fulfilment of natural human needs.' This definition of quality of life is based on that put forth by the World Health Organization (WHO).

It is clear from this definition of QoL that even if the client experiences all manner of limitation (of a physical, social and/or mental health nature), there can be optimal quality of life if the client enjoys the possibilities he does have, that is if he is able to live with his limitations. Such opportunities include the resources at his disposal, that is food, shelter, health, love, vitality and an outlook for the future.

How can we make 'enjoying important opportunities' more concrete when it comes to our professional practice as social workers? We can make the first definition of QoL concrete by operationalizing it as follows: In PIE-ET 'quality of life' is defined as 'enjoying the fulfilment of one's human needs'.

This definition clearly links quality of life to the extent to which the client experiences fulfilment of his or her life needs. QoL will be enhanced if the aforesaid resources such as food, love and a future perspective meet the person's needs. One can measure the Quality of Life by asking the client scale questions: how satisfied are you with your life on a scale from 0 to 10? (see also Table 1.2: Quality of Life meter) I will discuss the concept of 'life needs' in more detail later in this chapter. First, I will provide an overview of the three QoL factors which together determine QoL in every client situation:

1   Impact-factor (+/−). The *impact factor* is the first QoL factor and relates to the impact of (highly impactful) positive and negative transitions during the course of someone's life and which may be experienced as either up (+) or down (−).
2   Coping factor (+/−). Next we ask how the client is coping with the transitions which are a consequence of the aforesaid life experiences. This is the second QoL factor: the *coping factor*. Effective coping has a positive impact on QoL (+): for example saying goodbye when the need arises. Conversely, ineffective coping (−), or avoiding the unavoidable, has a negative impact on QoL.
3   The support factor (+/−). We also need to know how much support the environment offers when it comes to fulfilling human needs. This constitutes the third QoL factor, *the support factor* which can also have either a positive (+) or a negative (−) impact on QoL. Examples would be someone putting an arm around you or offering practical support, as opposed to someone being aloof or ignoring you, or not having access to essential resources.

Within PIE-ET, fluctuations in QoL are related to a combination of the aforementioned factors. Life events such as illness, being fired from a job, fleeing, a birth, success or promotion can have either a negative or a positive influence on the match or interaction between a person and his environment. Every client requires a tailored approach, which involves the social worker trying to assess with the client which factors have a positive or a negative impact on the client's needs being fulfilled. The approach involves using the client's own strengths and those provided by his environment. Once this has been done, social worker and client can see an improvement in QoL; both the individual and the environment are supported in fulfilling the person's needs. The social worker activates the client and his environment by directing his focus to the impact of the client's life (*impact factor*), how the client copes with this (*coping factor*) and any support provided by the environment (*support factor*) so as to achieve a better alignment between all factors. These are the three QoL factors which can work together to either enhance or reduce QoL.

From the early days of social work, the concepts of the 'person-in-situation', 'person-in-environment' or 'person-interaction-with-the-environment' (PIE) involved a dual focus on individual support and social reform (CSWE, 2004). The historical development of the PIE concept reflects political, social and economic concerns, as well as debates within the social work profession. PIE has been central to direct practice in particular, though there have been difficulties in applying the concept during its development within the major theoretical frameworks adopted by social workers.

I will now discuss the central concepts of PIE-ET in more detail, including the concept of 'human needs'. Which needs can be at play for clients, and is there a way in which we can rank universal human needs?

2.3.2 Taxonomy of universal human needs

The definition of QoL outlined in section 2.3.1 means that a client will enjoy life if his primary needs have been met. In other words, if there are sufficient resources (food) to meet one's needs (hunger), the client will enjoy life, and this will have a positive impact on QoL. The fact that the client presents to the social worker suggests that he may not enjoy optimal enjoyment of life. He may have unmet needs in the biopsychosocial area: he may not have adequate shelter (homelessness), he may have conflicts in his relationships or he may not see any future for himself. If we look at it from this perspective, the extent to which needs have been met constitutes an immediate gauge for QoL: if there are unmet needs, QoL will be low; if needs have been met, QoL will be optimal.

Case study of Maria and quality of life

Maria has a number of unmet needs. She feels frustrated because she is unable to complete her programme of studies (*unmet need*). She is not enjoying her opportunities. At a later stage, it will become clear that Maria has even more *unmet needs* from her past because she lost a parent when she was young and never worked through that, and this is hampering her in the present (for young parent loss, see also section 26.5). Maria was very happy about those courses she had successfully completed as part of her programme of studies (*a need that was met*). Maria is unhappy about her lack of progress in her studies (she does not have an optimal quality of life).

In other words, quality of life is the extent to which needs have been met. This is not only true for clients but also for the social workers themselves (see Figure 2.3). Quality of life is negatively impacted when one or more needs (hunger, thirst, work, an outlook for the future) are not being met. Fulfilling those needs will have a positive effect on Quality of Life.

In Chapter 24 it is explained that there is no clear evidence for a hierarchy in human needs. A hierarchy supposes that the need for survival should first be met, then the need for affection

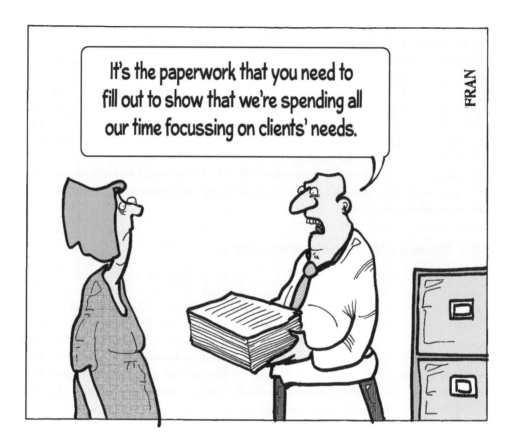

FIGURE 2.3 It's the paperwork that you need to. . . .

and finally the need for self-determination to achieve optimal quality of life. The interesting thing is that these needs can occur in sequence or simultaneously. This is reflected in the terms that initially seem to refer to the primacy of one need, but may also refer to the other three types of human needs. For instance, the word 'poverty' may initially be associated with practical-material poverty, which is the need for food and safety. However, the term 'poverty' may also refer to 'spiritual poverty' or 'emotional poverty'. Likewise, the word 'struggle' is usually associated with other struggles, such as the 'struggle for life' in survival situations. At the same time, the term can also refer to 'the struggle for meaning' (Bettelheim, 1976), the 'struggle for love' and the 'struggle for recognition' (Paradiso & Rudrauf, 2012), as well as the 'struggle for self-determination' and the 'struggle for a good life' (Kasser & Kanner, 2004). In this multiple use of the terms 'poverty' and 'struggle' we can identify four types of human needs.

So what do I mean by human needs? Human needs are defined as those biological, psychological and social needs which lead to optimal QoL when they are fulfilled by adequate satisfiers. I will start by providing an overview, explaining the four universal human needs, before discussing satisfiers and pseudo-satisfiers. The four universal human needs are:

1   Need for awareness: 'all you need is growing awareness';
2   Need for safety: 'all you need is safety';
3   Need for affection: 'all you need is love';
4   Need for self-determination: 'all you need is helping perspectives'.

This taxonomy of universal human needs is based on neuroscientific and social science research (see Chapter 24).

Case study of Maria and her human needs

Maria needs to successfully complete the current subject in order to continue with her programme of studies and she is upset at not being able to do so (unfulfilled need for self-determination). At first she does not understand why she is getting behind with her studies, however she does want to understand the reasons why (unfulfilled need for awareness). She does not feel safe in the group of students she is with. Other students forward pictures of her to a social media app as a 'joke'. She considers this to be a form of bullying. The fact that she ends up in a different group every semester is not helping either (unfulfilled need for safety). She feels she does not belong (unmet affective need).

Need for awareness

All you need is growing awareness.

There can be all sorts of circumstances resulting in clients finding it difficult to have good insight into or an overview of the situation they are in. Clients have a need to be aware of the situation they are in: the complex of problems-issues-stressors-resilience, the lack of balance between strengths (positive forces +) and weaknesses (negative forces −) at play. They feel confused when it comes to themselves. What is it I need, what are my needs, what are my rights? What steps will be in my best interests? Am I able to identify my own strengths and how can I get others to acknowledge these strengths?

Case study of Maria and her need for awareness

Maria appeals to a lecturer (career advisor) and the latter helps her gain awareness of what she needs to progress in her studies and in life, by helping her with a stocktake.

People become stressed when the need for awareness of (and insight into) their own situation is not (adequately) met. Through quality interaction the social worker helps the client develop an awareness about his or her specific needs: what is it I need to be able to take some steps in the right direction? Clients are able to develop on a personal level and grow as a person if they are aware of those needs which will result in improved QoL if they are fulfilled. The need for (self-)awareness has its theoretical underpinnings in the non-directive core social work method (see Chapter 4). Important theoretical work was done by Helen Perlman (Problem-Solving Process and self-awareness and awareness), Florence Hollis (Psycho-Social Therapy and Psychodynamic Theory), Sigmund Freud (conscious-unconscious), Erich Fromm (self-actualization), Carl Rogers (being and becoming), ACT and Mindfulness (mental state of awareness, focus and openness) and Amartya Sen and Martha Nussbaum (Capability Approach, self-flourishing, wellbeing).

Needs for safety

> All you need is safety.

Life events (losing one's job, divorce, illness) cause a disruption of physical functions; physical and situational deficits develop which are related to our physical survival (*survival*). We can distinguish three different types of needs for safety:

- *The need for physical safety (bio)*: There is a lack of oxygen, water, sleep and physical rest, warmth, food, physical activity and sex.
- *The need for psychological safety (psycho)*: There is a lack of psychological safety through anxiety-inducing, impressive experiences which have been imprinted into the senses.
- *The need for social safety (social)*: There is a lack of shelter (bed, bread and bath), work, money, practical problem solving.

When disaster strikes in the shape of floods or a fire, we can imagine these needs for survival at play immediately: the need for oxygen (we die within 5 minutes if we do not breathe), for water (we die within 10 days if we do not drink), food (we die within 2 weeks if we go without food), the need for shelter and sleep. But even small-scale incidents involve the aforementioned physical needs associated with safety and stability, and practical support in our daily lives (ensuring safe accommodation, facilities for cooking and sleeping), but also the practical aspects of saying goodbye and making arrangements for material consequences and so on.

The case study of Maria and the need for survival

Maria is behind with her studies, resulting in several practical roadblocks. From a mental health perspective, she is faced with the unprocessed traumatic loss of her mother and brother through suicide and an overdose, respectively. Physically speaking she is agitated and on red alert at all times. She does not feel safe and is not sure what to do about that.

When the need for biopsychosocial safety is not met, survival stress results. When we experience the need to survive, we almost automatically try and fulfil that need by eating, drinking and looking for material and psychological safety. Our reptile brain, also known as our stress brain, triggers the fight/flight/freeze reflex as if we were fighting for survival in the jungle. This survival pattern dates back to a previous era of human evolution.

The theoretic underpinning of safety needs is reflected in the bodywork method (Chapter 5), the practical-material method (Chapter 6) and the trauma-work method (Chapter 7). Important research in this area was conducted by Hans Selye (stress theory), Gerald Caplan (crisis theory), trauma theory (PTSD researchers), Callista Roy (adaptation theory) and others.

Needs for affection

> All you need is love.

Life events can lead to a disruption of the affective function of life, of existing social and loving and intimate relationships; this results in a lack of being acknowledged, not belonging, physical and emotional closeness, warmth, empathy and love – the building blocks of our affective social life. We can distinguish three types of affective needs:

- *The need for emotional closeness*: There is a lack of respect, feeling safe and sheltered, affection, care, love, a feeling of belonging, being taken seriously, being seen and heard, and this results in emotional pain which needs to find an outlet.
- *The need for creative expression*: There is a lack of creative expression in the shape of musical, creative, digital or dramatic expression in the presence of internal experiences which are difficult to express.
- *The need for closure and respectful goodbyes/leave-taking*: There is no opportunity for a dignified farewell in relation to experiences for which closure has not been found, due to the absence of a respectful farewell ritual.

The need for affection relates to expressing feelings (by de-stressing, creativity or rituals) with regard to our emotional hurt, our vulnerability, allowing others to share in our emotional joy and suffering, and the need to take one's leave in a dignified manner.

The case study of Maria and her affective needs

Maria has suppressed a lot of her feelings after losing her mother because as her father said: 'There is nothing we can do: life goes on.' She has never engaged in creative expression; she was hanging around the streets at an early age and her peers were people who had been through similar experiences. She has never been able to say goodbye to her mother and brother in a dignified manner.

Affective stress occurs when such social needs have not been met (as yet). When we experience the need for affection we search for emotional comfort, emotional expression and ways of saying goodbye instinctively, rather than automatically: 'Home sweet home'. Our limbic, emotional brain is regulating our emotional expression, just like military wives really benefit from expressing their feelings of having been abandoned, far away, by singing in a choir, when their spouses are away on a tour of duty. In 'Wherever You Are' they express their feelings of being physically separated from their partners.

The theoretical underpinnings of these affective needs may be found in the cathartic method (Chapter 8), the expression method (Chapter 9) and the ritual method (Chapter 10). Important contributions to the field were made by John Bowlby (attachment theory and separation distress), Harvey Jackins (re-evaluating counselling), Les Greenberg (emotionally focused therapy), Sue Johnson (emotionally focused couple therapy) and Onno van der Hart (rituals for grieving).

Need for self-determination

All you need is helping perspectives.

Life events may also cause a disruption of existing cognitive, behavioural and narrative functioning. We distinguish the following three types of self-determination needs:

- *The need for realistic information processing*: Individuals lack insight, realistic information, overview, effective problem solving, learning, personal identification.
- *The need for an existential (re)orientation*: Individuals are not able to make sense of/give meaning to, and lack a sense of identity because they cannot adequately find words for/ cannot construct an existential narrative that finds meaning in life, transforming their identity, feeling part of something bigger (spirituality).
- *The need for competency and influence*: Individuals lack assertive skills (resorting instead to sub-assertive or aggressive behaviour).

There is a need to organize things in one's mind, to see things in perspective, to brainstorm, put things into words, solve problems, make sensible choices, act assertively, find new meaning in life, engage in ongoing development, and have an outlet for spirituality.

The need for self-determination has its theoretical underpinnings in the cognitive method, the narrative method and the behavioural method. The most significant contributions in this area were made by Albert Ellis (RET), Donald Meichenbaum (cognitive behavioural therapy), Robert Neimeier (men as meaning makers), Michael White and David Epston (narrative therapy), Ivan Pavlov (Pavlov's dog and Pavlov conditioning), B. F. Skinner (the Skinner box), Albert Bandura (theory of social learning), Edward Deci and Richard Ryan (self-determination theory), Lev Semyonovich Vygotsky (social constructivism, 'co-constructed knowledge'), and Amartya Sen and Martha Nussbaum (freedom).

The case study of Maria and the need for self-determination

Maria is unable to recall a lot of what happened back then in terms of her mother and brother and she does not understand why she is so confused in the here-and-now of that time (cognitive needs). Maria wanted to start her programme of studies in order to stop being a victim by helping others (narrative need). She no longer knew how to find the words to talk about the practical consequences of her interrupted studies (need to assert herself).

Mental stress occurs when the need for self-determination is not (adequately) fulfilled. We use our logical reasoning to find helpful perspectives to turn our thoughts into helpful narratives and assertive behaviour. The logical part of our brain (the neocortex) assists us by finding helpful perspectives through (self-)reflection. As people we try to find meaning in life. If we look at our lives we can be filled with a sense of regret, but still carry on: 'Is this all there is my friend, then let's keep dancing.' (Peggy Lee)

Unmet needs and pseudo-satisfiers

What is meant by the term 'adequate satisfiers' which occurred in the definition of Quality of Life? 'Satisfiers' are resources, sources of life which adequately fulfil human needs; they can be products, activities or symbols. For example, water can be a satisfier for thirst; closeness can satisfy the need for comfort; 'helpful thoughts' can satisfy the need to find meaning in something. Social workers not only help clients become aware of their original human needs (see the Awareness checklist in section 1.2.2 of the previous chapter), but also help them identify which 'satisfier' is an effective match for the need the client experiences, because not all satisfiers will effectively fulfil these needs. So the question arises: how can clients work towards an effective fulfilment of their own needs? Social workers often notice that clients may (want to) use 'satisfiers' which do more harm than good to their quality of life. We follow Manfred Max-Neef in referring to such apparent satisfiers as 'pseudo-satisfiers' which are presented as effective satisfiers but are essentially ineffective satisfiers we are talked into trying: 'take a pill when you are feeling down'; 'bury yourself in work when you feel sad'; 'eat sweet stuff when you want to enjoy life'; 'eat junk food when you are hungry'; 'take a soft drink when you are thirsty'.

Pseudo-satisfiers in the case of Maria

Maria had regularly engaged in aggressive behaviour in the course of her life and had nearly ended up with a criminal conviction because of it. She responded like a bull in a china shop to any situation she perceived to be unfair. She started using soft drugs to try and feel a bit calmer, but realized that this only made matters worse. She perceived losing her mother (at age 5) through suicide and her brother through an overdose to be unfair, and this triggered a disproportionate response in her to anything she considered unfair in the here-and-now. Because her response was out of proportion, it did not really help her to find closure for the unfinished business in her life (for unfinished business syndrome see also Chapter 26). The use of soft drugs and aggressive behaviour acted as pseudo-satisfiers.

Once the needs have been established, the social worker's job is to work with the client to gauge which of the client's needs are as yet unmet and how the client can effectively meet these needs. The client has to carry some responsibility in all this, but so does his or her environment: in other words, this brings us back to the concept of PIE, which provides clarity about the responsibility of both actors/agents: the person and his or her environment.

2.3.3 PIE: person-in-environment

I will now discuss the PIE concept in more detail. Since the early beginnings of social work, the PIE concept has been present in the shape of 'the person in the situation', 'the person in his or her environment', and the 'person-in-interaction with his or her environment' with a dual focus on both individual support and social reform. The historical development of the PIE concept reflects political, social and economic topics and discussions within the social work field. PIE is the central concept in social work practice, but it has proved difficult for social workers to implement the concept in the course of developing important theoretical frameworks.

One of the reasons that the PIE concept has been so widely embraced in contemporary times is that it provides a format for *systemic understanding of human functioning*, crucial to the biopsychosocial perspective that is also fundamental to social work practice. Second, the PIE concept provides a basis for arguing on behalf of the social justice issues which social workers consider as providing them with an ethical mandate for their work (CSWE, 2004, NASW, 2008). Finally, PIE allows social workers to assess the existence of relationships between individuals and their environments in a way which involves a depathologized view of individual issues in social terms. The type of assessment of human functioning supported by the PIE concept supports can be used across various social work practice settings.

The person and his or her environment, abbreviated as PIE, makes mention of both the actors jointly responsible for monitoring quality of life. When a PIE mismatch occurs, a number of human needs remain unfulfilled, such as the need for shelter, to physical or emotional warmth or the need for a future. So in the case of a PIE mismatch, problems arise because person and environment are not aligned, and are unable to fulfil the existing human needs, regardless of whether this is due to the person or the environment, or due to the interaction between person and environment. This results in friction and tension in the person, the relationship and the environment. We refer to this as the psychosocial stress (−), which occurs when there is a mismatch. Due to a combination of QoL factors, the client's quality of life will go down and his or her psychosocial development may stagnate. This may occur in children, adults and the elderly.

The PIE concept and its historical development within the social work field are discussed in more detail in Appendix 8.

2.3.4 Psychosocial empowerment: its basis in personal and social resilience

Psychosocial empowerment is defined here as: 'a dynamic process that emphasizes purposefully strengthening oneself in effectively coping (personal level) and effectively strengthening social support (environmental level) both engaging needs and rights'. The person and the environment correspond with the adjective 'psychosocial.'

In the following we speak of empowerment where we mean 'psychosocial empowerment'. Gutierrez (1994) explains empowerment as the 'process of increasing personal, interpersonal, or political power so that individuals, families, and communities can take action to improve their situations'.

Minkler (Minkler, 1998, as cited in Nutbeam et al., 2010) defines empowerment as 'a social action process in which individuals, communities, and organizations gain mastery over their lives in the context of changing their social and political environment to improve equity and quality of life'.

Trained social workers are expected to have the necessary skills to empower service users to participate in assessments and decision making (coping level), and also to ensure that service users have access to advocacy services if they are unable to represent their own views (environmental level). Empowerment and advocacy are both concerned with a shift of power or emphasis towards meeting the needs and rights of people who would otherwise be marginalized or oppressed. Beyond this generalization, the concepts of empowerment and advocacy are complex and as such are almost impossible to define. Where the term 'empowerment' is used it often covers a whole range of activities from consulting with service users to involvement in service planning. Empowerment lies at the very heart of what social work is all about, as demonstrated not only by its place in the key roles for social work, but also by the term's appearance in the definition of social work, as agreed by the International Association of Schools of Social Work (IASSW) and the International Federation of Social Work (IFSW) in 2001:

> The social work profession promotes social change, problem solving in human relationships and the *empowerment* and liberation of people to enhance well-being. Utilising theories of human behaviour and social systems, social work intervenes at points where people interact with their environments.

Barbara Levy Simon (1994) argues that empowerment is only the latest term for a point of view that has been at the heart of social work since the 1890s. I will provide more historical background on the use of the term 'empowerment' within social work in Chapter 24.

2.4 More on the three QoL factors

I briefly discussed the three QoL factors in the preceding section. I will now discuss these in more detail.

2.4.1 The impact factor (+/−): does it give your life course resiliency or stress?

Life events: crisis or challenge?

In the PIE-Empowerment paradigm life events are viewed as stressors or strengths, as negative factors or positive factors for the QoL. Therefore people come in a transition process from their old life chapter to the new life chapter. Social workers often contact clients who are in the middle of a transition process from one to another life chapter. One can measure the impact of transitions by asking the client scale questions: how much impact do you experience by this transition on a scale from 0 to 10? (see also Table 1.2: impact meter).

> **Social work clients present with life transitions caused by life events such as:**
>
> Illness; unemployment; poverty; identity crisis; abuse; homelessness; neglect; stalking; aggression; cognitive impairment; relationship stress; family stress; disasters; war; removal; eviction order; racism; sexism; classism; anti-Semitism; anti-Islamism; homophobia; exclusion.

How can social workers help these clients in an effective way? Would it be helpful to look at social work helping clients with a life transition? Does this require a shift from change theory to transition theory? First, the place of change theory in social work will be described. Next, the shift from change theory to transition theory will be further elaborated.

The main strength of transition theory is that it focuses on transitions over the course of our lives, not changes. The difference between these is subtle but important. Change is something that happens to people, even if they do not agree with it. Transition, on the other hand, is internal: it is what happens in people's minds as they go through change. Change can happen very quickly, while transition usually occurs more slowly. The transition theory highlights three stages of transition that people go through when they experience change. The transition curve includes (see Figure 2.4):

1 Awareness of the transition;
2 Finishing the old life chapter;
3 Building on the new life chapter.

People will go through each stage at their own pace. It is expected that working through this transition process has more sustainable results than focusing on changes that could be more symptoms of a deeper transition process. For many years, in social work education, change theory was considered the basis of the social worker approach. This theory of 'changing' studies the conscious action-taking in a change process, the conscious changing of people. According to Donkers (1999), the word 'change' can refer to:

• Changing a situation, or helping to maintain it;
• Adding something new or maintaining something valuable;

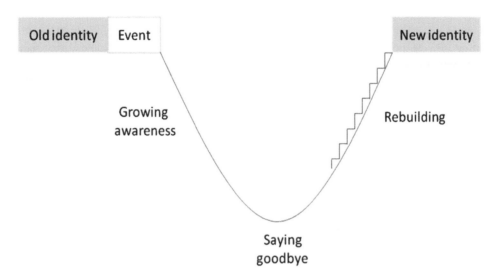

FIGURE 2.4 Transition curve – life transitions

- Learning or unlearning a certain behaviour;
- Decreasing or increasing resistance against something new.

In foreign social-work literature, the word 'change' often occurs in social work books in combination with 'planning of change'. Social-work interventions are represented as planned and desired (by the patient) changes in the client situation in certain more closely described phases. Actually, the planned-change ideas from 1960 and later, introduced by Lewin, Bennis, Benne, Chin and Lipitt, are still very topical: change is a process from unfreezing the old, moving (transition) and refreezing the new.

But can social workers really plan this change? Isn't this contribution to the changing of a client rather a matter of 'giving the process a leg-up' (van der Pas, 2008), a matter of trying to take a small step forwards so that further changes can start taking place?

In human life there is a fundamental undercurrent of stability and change which lies beneath the everyday reality. Around 500 BC, the Greek philosopher Heraclitus said that 'you never step into the same river, because the water continuously flows on'. Heraclitus was the first Western philosopher who embraced the idea that the universe is in a constant flow implying both standing still and moving. He stated:

> Everything flows and nothing stands still; everything gives space and nothing stands still . . . Cold things heat up, the heat cools down again, wet things dry up, and dry things get wet . . . It is only in change that things find peace.

How can the social worker anticipate the movement, the flow of changes? What contribution can the social worker make to this fundamental change process in the life of the client, anticipating the logics of changes taking place beneath the surface? In multimethod social work (MMSW), the social worker takes up a modest but important role in causing positive changes in the life of the client.

In his song, 'The Stone', Bram Vermeulen uses the image of stones in rivers: 'I moved a stone in a river on earth . . . its water will always find a way'. Eventually, social work is about moving 'pebbles', small rocks which cause subtle changes unnoticeable at first sight, but present nevertheless. As a social worker, you are not able to change or stop a big 'flow' or current. The 'pebbles' are the small achievable goals we set. By trying our best in this, relationships and situations which had stagnated now start to move once more. At first, these changes are small, but the acknowledgement for the efforts that were made and the attention to small changes increases the motivation in all those involved. That is exactly how a cumulative effect is started. This caused social workers to attain greater goals, which we originally did not set and did not expect, but which satisfy both the client and the social worker (see Table 5.3).

In transition theory, the change in the client's life is seen as a transition from an old to a new structure. Transition theory focuses on the term 'change' from a life cycle point of view, where change theory does not do that. How can clients' questions gain significance when seen from a life cycle perspective (see Figure 2.4)?

How do changes on the relational and organizational level acquire significance from the 'life cycle' of that relationship, family, organization or facility? Doesn't the present behaviour of the individual, relation, family and organization become more natural by looking at it from the life cycle context? De Mönnink (2008) argues for social workers to allow more space for the impact of life transitions and the existential crises they bring on an individual, relational, family and organizational level. So actually it is a plea for a shift from the *change* paradigm to the *transition* paradigm. One of the few social work models that takes into account the importance of life transitions is the one described by Germain. In the so-called life model (Germain & Gitterman, 1980), transitions in life are seen as disrupting influences causing stress. These transitions make new demands and require new answers. If human life is considered to be an interrelation of biopsychosocial components, the effects of the transitions can become visible in every one of these components.

People constantly experience transitions throughout the course of their lives, often caused by loss, trauma and chronicity, but also caused by changes in the course of life itself. This involves crises and challenges. From this point of view, clients are faced with the task of adequately managing transitions they go through: transitions from an old, existing life structure to a new one. From this point of view, social work clients find themselves in life transitions. The old footing, the old grip on life is lost when facing illness, shortcomings, debts or death. The client makes a transition from an old life situation to a new one. In the study of loss (de Mönnink, 2008), the transition from old to new includes letting go of the old and building up the new chapters of life.

Kurt Lewin (1951) described this transition process as *unfreezing-moving-freezing*: unfreezing the old, moving it from old to new, and freezing this new situation (see Figure 2.5). Mistakenly, in literature the word '*refreezing*' was more frequently used than 'freezing', while 'refreezing' may be associated with 'recovery' in the old situation.

Levinson (1978) calls this the transition of the old life structure to the new. People in the state of transition often find themselves in somewhat of a twilight zone between the old and the new. These clients often face two important transition tasks:

1   The task of *living* on: letting go of the old;
2   The task of living *on*: starting the new.

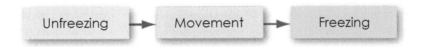

FIGURE 2.5 Transition process from unfreezing via moving to freezing

The process of letting go is called *living on*, during which someone goes through the painful experience of saying goodbye and closing the old life chapter. By arranging the mess left behind in the old and finishing unfinished business, one is actually working on building the new (see Figure 2.4).

Clients who live *on* without having had closure in the old life chapter will end up in deeper trouble. The emphasis of the Western culture on 'manipulability' and control makes the desire to live *on* understandable: moving *onward* as soon as possible. In this modern era, the increased control over all sorts of life processes – medical science and technology – only enhances the already naturally existing illusion of manipulability and invulnerability. In radical changes in life however, the illusion of control and vulnerability can no longer be sustained that easily. In an extreme attempt, the modern man can 'escape from' the transition period and hide in avoidance and denial.

A compensational grill is put over the 'void' or 'gap' that came to existence, which characterizes living *on*. Living *on* can imply 'filling up' the void by working hard, numbing oneself with the use of alcohol or drugs, and/or by disinhibited sexual behaviour. These forms of living *on* are examples of a life pattern where pain, the emotion of letting go, is avoided. In spite of this, the existing pain will not find a way to discharge itself. With the next drastic life change, a new confrontation with the old pain occurs which has a complicating effect on the new issues that present themselves.

These are the moments when social workers are called upon, to help people arrange the existing mess and to alleviate the accumulation of loss and traumas. Social workers help clients make the transition to a new balance, a new chapter in the life of the individual client, as well as in the relationship, the family and the organization. From the transition point of view, social workers help in letting go of the old on the one hand, and building the new on the other hand (see Chapter 26). Social workers help clients become more aware of the impact of life transitions.

2.4.2 Coping factor (+/–): how do you manage the impact of your life course?

> In life you have to meet your own needs *yourself*, but you don't always have to do them by yourself.

Individual coping – how someone copes with their human needs – co-determines our QoL. Adequately coping with our needs – for example adequately ensuring that we have income, relationships and an outlook for the future – will enhance our QoL, while inadequate coping will diminish it. One can measure the quality and progress of coping by asking the client scale questions: how effective do you fulfil your own needs on a scale from 0 to 10? (see also Table 1.2: coping meter and strength meter).

If we are running away we cannot stand up strong, as Brené Brown, professor in social work, says in her book, *Rising Strong* (2015). Lilian Rubin is the social work author who also shows us the importance of coping in her book entitled *The Transcendent Child* (1997). The book asks whether the past keeps us hostage forever. The subtitle of her book (*Tales of Triumph Over the Past*) suggests that it does not have to be that way. Why is it that some people manage to overcome a very damaging childhood and develop into amazing people who deserve our respect for what they have achieved at both a personal and a professional level? Why is it that these people managed to attain both success and happiness? The eight life stories recounted by the author of *The Transcendent Child* – including her own to some extent – make the reader realize that the insights proposed by psychologists, psychoanalysts and behavioural therapists are not correct, or are at the very least incomplete. Science, which almost inevitably focuses on determinism and cause-and-effect relationships, is unable to explain complex human developments, much less understand them.

The book shows how children who grew up in a pathological environment involving incest, humiliation, social exclusion and so forth have gone on to grow into adults with strong personalities, while their brothers and sisters have 'disappeared' into a life of crime, prostitution, severe depression and so forth.

These children who were able to cope effectively take control of their lives at an early stage; they take over the 'locus of control'. They want to determine what happens in their lives; they want to be in control. This is not to say that they do not feel victimized or deny or forget the past, but they do not have the time to keep pondering the past, because that stops them from living their lives. And finally, what these people have experienced comes down to this: it is not what you have experienced, but how it has affected you. What is important is the meaning you attach to it, and how you deal with it. 'When I get hit, that is nothing to do with me'. Giving meaning to what is happening, distancing yourself from it, results in these (and perhaps other) people having the insight of having a mission. This insight was usually there for these people from an early age. Continuity is accompanied by lack of continuity at that point in time. They live with a mission, be it to achieve something in science, art, sports and so forth. And for many of them there is something else as well: I don't want this to happen to other people. These people see this mission as not only transcending their origins and their environment, but also themselves. The last sentence of the book is a plea to focus more on people's coping strategies so that the past will not keep us hostage forever.

Brené Brown (2015) aims her pleas for opening ourselves up to being vulnerable, for standing up more strongly after taking a tumble, to a broad audience. She sees this as the way to re-experience Quality of Life. In her books Brown shows how vulnerability is a sign of strength, not weakness, and she underlines the courage it take to allow ourselves not to be perfect.

When we talk about the coping factor, we should not interpret the word 'coping' to mean we maintain the role of victim forever: this is the pitfall of victimism. Taking on the role of victim is very different from acknowledging your experiences as a victim, as it is important to do that. Hence we should not interpret 'coping' to mean that we should deny that we were victims, and deny our vulnerability, as that leads to the pitfall of 'controllism', the need to always remain in control.

There is a range of coping behaviour in relation to the list of human needs. We will not go into those now. In 'Individual methods checklist: what methods match with what needs?' (see Appendix 7), you will find an overview of individual methods for helping clients effectively cope with their needs.

2.4.3 The support factor (+/–): how much support do you feel you are getting?

> In life you have to do things yourself, but you don't always have to do them *by yourself*.
> In life you have to meet your own needs yourself, but *you don't have to do it by yourself*.

The *support factor* is the third QoL factor. I define effective support as follows:

> Effective support from the environment (the social network and the resources) entails support which is experienced as such by the client.

This description effectively reflects the fact that support is both a subjective and an interactive phenomenon. In the first and the final instance, it is the client himself or herself who is the best yardstick by which to gauge the quality of the support. *Support is support only if the recipient experiences it as such.* Research confirms that it is not the support received which is the most important, but *support perceived as support* (Taylor, 2011). According to Taylor social support is an important factor in terms of quality of life, for instance in terms of mental and physical health experienced.

Social support and mental health

Since the mid-1970s, researchers have explored the link between support systems and mental health and looked at what is the connection between mental illness and changes in marital status, geographic mobility and social disintegration. Researchers discovered a reduction in social support through diminishing social networks to be the common theme in each of these social changes. These studies in turn triggered an avalanche of research into the effect of social support on mental health.

Social support is associated with increased mental wellbeing in the work environment and also in terms of important life events. In times of stress, when we may be anxious or depressed, social support helps us cope. Social support appears to encourage psychological adaptation in life situations involving ongoing stress, such as chronic or progressive illnesses such as cancer, AIDS, stroke or a heart attack. People who did not receive much social support were much more likely to develop mental health issues such as symptoms of depression, post-traumatic stress disorder (PTSD), panic disorders, social phobias, mood disorders or eating disorders. People with schizophrenia experience more symptoms when they perceive themselves as receiving less social support. People receiving little social support also tend to experience more suicidal thoughts and more alcohol- and drug-related problems. Many studies into the way police officers, pregnant women, traumatized individuals and students handled stress have shown that a lack of social support negatively impacts mental health and that strong social support has a distinctly positive effect.

Social support and physical health

Social support is associated with physical health and mortality risk in many different ways. Those who do not experience a lot of social support have a much greater likelihood of dying from conditions such as cancer and cardiovascular disease (Uchino, 2009). Many other studies have shown that those who experienced better social support had an increased likelihood of survival (Holt-Lunstad et al., 2010). Individuals who lacked social support had a greater likelihood of developing cardiovascular disease, inflammatory processes and a less developed immune system (Kiecolt-Glaser et al., 2002), more complications during pregnancy (Elsenbruch et al., 2007), more functional limitations and more pain related to rheumatoid arthritis (Evers et al., 2003).

Conversely, stronger levels of social support had a positive impact in many areas of physical health, including faster recovery following cardiac surgery (Kulik & Mahler, 1993), fewer herpes infections (Cohen et al., 1988), less age-related cognitive deterioration (Seeman et al., 2001) and better control over their diabetes (Marteau et al., 1987). People who have better levels of social support have a greater likelihood of getting a cold, but will recover faster from such colds. Social isolation is almost as deadly as smoking, and exceeds the risk of premature death due to obesity or lack of physical activity. Loneliness and social isolation appear to pose a huge risk to our health.

Social isolation is detrimental to our health

NRC Handelsblad, 5 January 2016

Social isolation carries almost the same risk of dying as smoking, and carries a far greater risk of premature death than obesity or lack of physical activity. Lonely people die earlier because they are not as healthy physically, according to researchers at the University of North Carolina who published their findings in the *Proceedings of the National Academy of Sciences* this week. Their findings were based on an analysis of four longitudinal studies into health and wellbeing, which were conducted in the United States.

Up until now, any links between social isolation and increased risk of mortality had mainly been shown in snapshots, based on mean values for the population as a whole. The new study has demonstrated this link in people who were studied over a longer period of time and has shown the greater likelihood of poor health and a higher mortality risk being the result of loneliness. The team of researchers selected four indicators which gave some insight into participants' physical health: blood pressure, C-reactive protein (as a measure of inflammation), hip circumference and BMI (body mass index).

The researchers showed that social isolation had a negative effect on blood pressure and C-reactive protein (CRP), in groups ranging from young adults to the elderly. A similar link was found for hip circumference and BMI, but only in the group of adolescents.

Because the study was based on questionnaires completed by participants themselves, responses were related to the perceived 'quality' of social networks, and not so much the absolute quantity of interactions with friends, relatives and colleagues.

The research also showed that social conflicts such as arguments, or losing one's job, are bad for our health. According to the researchers, loneliness and social stress were shown to have a cumulative effect over the years, but if people managed to break through these, they were less likely to end up with chronic, life-threatening conditions.

The researchers who looked into social support and the stress buffer theory assume that receiving support from the environment (having a social safety net) impacts a person's QoL: 'My network is there for me when I need support' (see also section 14.4 about the stress buffer theory).

According to the stress buffer and social cohesiveness theories, close social networks are important for people's health. However it is precisely this social cohesiveness which does not remain the same after a loss: it diminishes over time and supportive responses follow a certain up and down pattern (Pennebaker, 1994). In the weeks following a loss, everyone talks openly about what has occurred. Social barriers disappear and people spontaneously talk to each other. Over the next 4–8 weeks they stop talking about the loss. People do think about the loss, and are willing to talk about it, but they no longer want to hear all the stories. After that, life carries on just like before.

By the mid-1980s, investigators started to notice that upheavals that were kept secret were more likely to result in health problems than those that could be spoken about more openly. For example, individuals who were victims of violence and who had kept this experience silent were significantly more likely to have adverse health effects than those who openly talked with others. In short, having any type of traumatic experience is associated with elevated illness rates; having any trauma and not talking about it further elevates the risk. These effects actually are stronger when controlling for age, sex, and social support. Apparently, keeping a trauma secret from an intact social network is unhealthier than not having a social network to begin with. (Pennebaker et al., 1988).

US researchers have also established that wound healing among rats is much slower when they are kept in isolation (Vitalo et al., 2009). Vitalo's study was the first to establish a link between life within a community and physical recovery. Rats normally live in groups, but are often kept in individual boxes in the laboratory and are visibly stressed, partly because they miss the company of other rats and partly because they like to keep busy. The study involved researchers creating a skin injury on the back of the rats.

A number of the rats received environment enrichment (EE) therapy, which consisted of offering nesting material, either when the rats were by themselves or in groups. Of the rats that were offered EE therapy, 64% healed well, while 88% of the rats who were kept in isolation still had wounds on their backs. Ninety-two percent of rats living in a group with other rats healed up (see Table 2.1). The oxytocin hormone is known to lower stress; the experiment showed that administering oxytocin was just as effective as nest building. The exact role of oxytocin in the immune system is not completely understood by researchers. One possibility is that it triggers the body's recovery process; another is that it merely lowers the level of stress hormones such as cortisol. Researchers have been speculating for a while about the influence

TABLE 2.1 Wound healing in ordinary rats under various conditions: wounds healing much more quickly in a group setting than in isolation

Intervention	Well-healed wound	Poorly healed wound
Without EE therapy	12%	88%
With EE therapy	64%	36%
Administration of oxytocin	64%	36%
EE therapy combined with living in group with other rats	92%	8%

of the mind on the body when it comes to physical recovery. Assuming that people too heal more quickly when they are in a pleasant environment and also assuming that this is due to oxytocin, social workers should help their clients to strengthen their social networks.

In principle, the client's (express) needs should be the all-important reason for offering support, but there are exceptions. Sometimes it is necessary for the environment to offer the client support they have not asked for and which the client may even consider to be a breach of privacy. However, such support may be needed in order to break through a destructive pattern (e.g. self-neglect, alcohol abuse). These are often risky situations where clients use pseudo-satisfiers which destroy more than they might like, including the things or people they love. To quote the Dutch slogan used to warn of the risks of alcohol abuse: 'It destroys more than you might like'. However, such situations also occur when desperate clients think that suicide is the only way out and are encouraged to hand over the weapon or the dangerous attributes in the course of quality/positive interactions. Another example would be people in the environment stepping in to stop clients cutting themselves or drinking themselves under the table, even though the clients initially resist.

Structural support derived from facilities

The importance of social network support has been described in the section about social support and mental and physical health as one aspect of the support factor. The support factor also concerns the support derived from facilities: how supportive are the surrounding structural facilities? Social workers contribute in enhancing these facilities as a fully integrated part of their work.

With the term 'structural support', we mean facilities such as governed by organizational policies, local policies, international laws and human rights. Whereas the delivered quality of these facilities is less directly affected by social workers, it can be vital for clients. For the fulfilment of basic needs, people need the necessary facilities and provisions in the form of shelter, but also in the form of food, clothing, money, work and social facilities.

This is about relief of universal needs for food, water, security, belonging, appreciation and self-determination. If it turns out there is a lack of a particular facility or if the quality of services does not turn out to be as desired, there is social work to do to improve these facilities. For people in vulnerable circumstances, all kinds of supportive systems were created in the history of our 'welfare states'. From maternity leave and unemployment benefits to bereavement leave if a close relative is deceased, and everything in between.

These facilities are usually the result of conflicts within the society in which workers, women, welfare recipients, the chronically ill or other pressure groups successfully stood up for their interests.

A relatively recent example of structural support for work-related problems was a man who had to go back to work after 2 days after the death of his child. Bereavement leave did not exist. He called in sick after a few days. The social worker openly discussed this with the manager but there was no such thing as bereavement leave. The social worker gave information about collective agreements (CAOs) in which this actually was arranged and because of this, bereavement leave came on the agenda in the health and safety consultation as well as the council. Ultimately bereavement leave was included in the CAO of the client's industry sector. The level of welfare and associated supportive facilities fluctuate with economic waves. There are two ways to determine the degree of support in work and private life; the degree of support from a structural angle is determined by (1) the support meter and (2) the BCL, the basic resources checklist (see Table 2.2).

TABLE 2.2 Basic resources checklist

Basic Facilities	Questions	Availability (V = sufficient, O = insufficient)
1	Work and income	
2	Housing	
3	Food	
4	Clothing	
5	Health	
6	Education	
7	Childcare	
8	Family and parenting	
9	Personal care and relaxation	
10	Transport: in what form: bus, train, taxi or car?	
11	Other signals about facilities	

The checklist may be completed based on a case or in the SW-team as a result of multiple cases. Was every facility available in the last year (V = sufficiently available; O = insufficiently available)? Discuss this with each facility.

A second way to determine the quality of the facilities is the support meter. The social worker asks the client how he or she evaluates the support at an operational level as well as from laws and procedures on a scale from 0 to 10, where 0 is no experienced support and 10 is the maximum experienced support. If there are any possible gaps in the level of facilities for a group of clients, the macro methods are appropriate methods to improve this.

The following facilities enhance what is needed for an improvement of 'the quality of health care, regulations and policies for the benefit of vulnerable citizens who need support from society.' Facility upgrades could include:

- Methods for signalling the structural needs in society (relationships with colleagues or neighbours and so forth);
- Preventive services for vulnerable groups whose situation would worsen without these facilities;
- Facilities for collective representation of interest for frustrated and angry client groups who wouldn't find an adequate place for their grievances without such facilities;
- Research facilities to identify what needs and requirements exist within client groups and to assess the effects of existing facilities.

Facilities: improvement programs

> My parents were getting support – they received benefits for living expenses.

By 'facilities' we mean the support that is derived from a health care institution, a rule of policy or law. If the support does not function optimally for a group of clients, an improvement is needed – as in the following example of parents of a stillborn child.

The parents experienced unnecessary pain when they wanted to register the birth of their stillborn child. The official told them this was not possible, because the law does not provide for lifeless children to be registered. Political pressure with contributions from social work – a form of collective representation – has ensured that the registration of stillborn children is possible through the new Burial and Cremation Act declaration (public support base). Another form of political pressure in which the collective position of social work was important was in an example of American social work. The House of Representatives initiated a hearing on 'the state of social work in the United States'. This hearing has contributed to the achievement of social work becoming less invisible to the public.

Within the existing institutions that are providing these services, there is always a need for feedback about the effectiveness of the facility so that services can be made more fitting. But in reality, bureaucracy may get in the way of things so that the institutions become 'deaf' to the signals or react sluggishly. In a bureaucracy (Sheafor & Horejsi, 2003), there exists an implemented division of labour in which operations are clearly defined and assigned to specialized workers; a hierarchy of strata managers, sub-managers and executive employees. A formalized set of rules and regulations are applied rigidly and work is performed in an impersonal atmosphere which is not adjusted to the uniqueness of the individual. Bureaucracies are characterized by justice and equality, but they also suffer from a lack of flexibility and an inability to individualize. They are stable and consistent, but slow in their ability to change.

At the other end of the continuum of organizational structures are the 'adhocracies'. These are institutions with an internal structure that makes them able to respond to each question individually – more ad hoc. The employees have a lot of autonomy and do their job with few rules and regulations. They are flat organizations in which there is as little hierarchy as possible. Ad hoc settings are weak both in structure and stability, but they are able to respond to new demands quickly. They are particularly effective when the nature of the work is dynamic or fluid.

In some cases improvement programmes are needed to have the existing facilities respond better to questions from groups of clients. A movement of bureaucracies to adhocracies can be beneficial in this improvement. For this purpose, the social worker deploys four methods: detection, prevention, public advocacy and applied research.

The provisioning level in society depends on the structure and the executive authorities such as laws, facilities and whether or not these things meet the vital needs of clients.

Since the client and its surroundings are always subject to change – such as economic and political developments – adjustments are always needed in the policies and facilities. The social worker has to be alert to make sure there is no deterioration in laws, social policy and social organizations. It may be desirable to work on the strengthening of good quality housing, employment, anti-discrimination procedures and legislation, the infrastructure of neighborhoods and communities and the functioning of organizations. The social worker can promote improvements in the social and health sectors that clients use: hospitals, nursing homes, rehabilitation centres, shelters, psychiatric institutions, social work in neighborhoods, social services within companies and other labour organizations.

2.5 The intertwining of QoL factors explained

The aforementioned three QoL factors – impact, coping and support – determine in conjunction the fluctuations in QoL. In each client's situation it is the coincidental mix of present factors that determines how the client experiences his own life. The last question is, how can the interaction of the described QoL factors be understood? What does systemic, causal and circular biopsychosocial thinking say about this nexus of factors that is so characteristic of social work clients? The multifactorial theory of PIE-ET is based on multi-causal system thinking and distances itself from mono-causal, individual thinking.

2.5.1 Systems or systemic thinking

The client constantly interacts with the people around him, regardless of whether those people belong to his social network or represent collective resources. PIE-ET assumes that there are interactive connections between these actors: they form a communicative system. This is known as systems thinking (which is often confused with *systematic* thinking).

The question is whether this 'systems or multicausal thinking' is fully integrated into social work practice. There could be a difference between theory and practice. In theory, systems thinking is the core concept of social work, as shown in the international definition of the social work profession (IFSW, 2014, http://ifsw.org/get-involved/global-definition-of-social-work/):

> Social work is a practice-based profession and an academic discipline that promotes social change and development, social cohesion and the empowerment and liberation of people. Principles of social justice, human rights, collective responsibility and respect for diversities are central to social work. Underpinned by theories of social work, social sciences, humanities and indigenous knowledge, social work engages people and structures to address life challenges and enhance wellbeing.

This definition may be amplified at national and/or regional levels.

The commentary on this definition is that

> The social change mandate is based on the premise that social work intervention takes place when the current situation, be this at the level of the person, family, small group, community or society, is deemed to be in need of change and development.
>
> It is based on holistic biopsychosocial, spiritual assessments and interventions that transcend the micro-macro divide, incorporating multiple system levels and inter-sectorial and inter-professional collaboration, aimed at sustainable development. The PIE concept in this social work definition is clearly reflected. For the social worker it is still difficult in practice to stay flexible between working from personal, systemic and macro perspectives.

Several notions have been derived from the circular or systemic view. Terms such as 'system' and 'subsystem' are used to indicate the existence of a larger entity of people that can be subdivided in subsystems or component systems. For example, the nuclear family is a system, where the parents make up one subsystem and the children make up another. The Person-in-Environment Theory (PIE-ET) assumes that every client situation is a system where there is a constant interaction between the subsystems: the personal system and the environmental systems. Every one of these systems influences the others, but also consists of subsystems which, in their turn, continuously influence one another. Every subsystem can be a pretext for change. Especially when there are several stressors within the client situation, there are several possible pretexts for change as well.

A client situation can be considered as a system with multiple levels and spheres of influence. Within a personal system as well, several subsystems are active which mutually influence one another and eventually determine the behaviour of the person: the emotional system, the cognitive system, the behavioural system, the physical system, the creative-expression system and so on. The personal system also interacts with the social systems in the direct or broader environment (see Figure 2.6). Subsystems in proximity are the relational system, the nuclear family system, the family system, the social network (school system included), the companion-in-adversity system and the case management system of professionals who are involved in the client situation. These are all social subsystems that, once again, mutually influence one another. On the macro level too, there are subsystems acting as a facility for the client situation, such as district facilities, labour organizations, social services, hospitals, nursing homes and rehabilitation centres, but also the political and legal systems. The macro subsystems too are constantly interacting with one another.

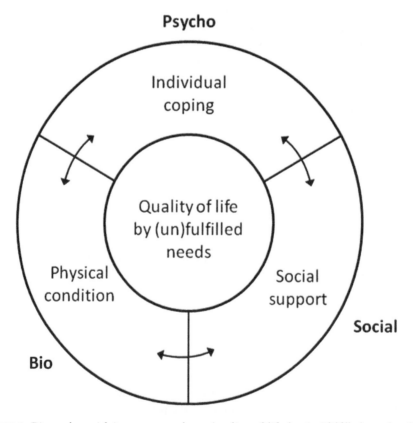

FIGURE 2.6 Biopsychosocial interconnectedness (quality of life by (un)fulfilled needs, physical condition, individual coping, social support)

2.5.2 Biopsychosocial thinking

Another well-known principle in social work is biopsychosocial thinking. The term biopsychosocial (BPS) means that our physical condition is associated with our mental state, but also with the social situation in which we live, and that these three forms are a dynamic unit.

BPS thinking underpins the framework of the ICF – the International Classification of Human Functioning – which aims to describe the situation in which a person functions. Instead of pinpointing one cause for one issue (causal thinking), ICF assumes there is an underlying interconnectedness between all BPS factors at play (circular causality). The specialist perspectives which viewed these as factors separately from one another are now largely a thing of the past, because at some point they tend to result in a type of tunnel vision. Hence the building blocks of our lives are of a biopsychosocial nature, and they are all interconnected. The issues people experience in life when they suffer a loss affecting one of these factors – that is in one of the building blocks which form the structural underpinning of our lives – will have repercussions on other building blocks connected to the one that was affected (see Figure 2.6).

Seen from this systemic definition, the quality of the client's BPS life will suffer when his needs remain unmet. Conversely, when human needs are fulfilled, this improves their quality of life (they will enjoy life again).

2.5.3 Circular causal thinking

The point of departure in the biopsychosocial interrelation is that the forces in the client situation on all levels – client factors – are constantly influencing one another; this is called the multi-causal or systemic view. The client factors in the client situation are interconnected. A life event, such as the death of a loved one, causes the client to have trouble sleeping and concentrating. This in turn causes him to make errors at work, resulting in missing out on a promotion. He is constantly on edge and tensions rise in social relationships, and this leads him to contact the social worker. This client is confronted with a tangle of stressors and sources of tension. Causes and effects are not clear-cut. The things that initially are a normal response to illness (sleep disturbance, loss of concentration), can become sources of tension at work and in social relationships.

The example with the death of a loved one clearly shows that it is unrealistic to analyze the client situation, starting only from the so-called cause-and-effect thinking: assuming that there is one problem with one because that has to be solved. It is not realistic to assume one core problem (or better, one stressor) as the cause, because the chronology of events teaches us that there is often a whole accumulation of stressors. Circular or multi-causal thinking (originating from system theory) is in order: every link in the chain of events can be a consequence of a previous event (cause), as well as the cause of a successive event. This is also called *circular causality* or multi-causality. There is a continuous interaction between different elements in a social situation. In biology, there is the notion of the natural cycle, a large chain in which nature and man are linked. In general system theory, the holistic starting point is seen in the interdependency (mutual dependency) of the parts in a system: a change in one part of the system affects all other parts – the ripple effect.

The social worker focuses on inventorizing and disentangling the intertwined and ever-increasing problems together with the client. The circular view on reality originates from general system theory (von Bertelanffy, 1968). During the 1960s, this theory led to an explosion of so-called systemic approaches which have been integrated into the social workers' toolbox under the heading of 'systemic methods'.

So the question is how all the different methods in the social workers' toolkit, including the non-directive basic method, the individual, systemic and macro methods, can contribute to the fulfilment of the client's natural needs by influencing the two PIE factors. I will try to answer this question in the next chapter, in which I will discuss the 20 social work methods in more detail. I will discuss how each of these 20 methods promotes optimal QoL by addressing the QoL factors (impact/coping and support) discussed previously.

2.6 Summary

This chapter described the PIE-Empowerment Theory as a practical theory for social work: the match of the Person-in-Environment. It began by describing what is meant by 'a useful theory' before moving on to the potentially harmful effect of non-overarching theories. Then the PIE-ET was introduced with an explanation of three QoL factors. Then the three QoL-factors in the client situation were explained, along with two empowerment actors which can fulfil our needs. The theoretical concepts are illustrated by fragments from the case study of Maria, who was a social worker student herself, and asked for help from a college social worker. In the next chapter we will introduce the 20 practice methods social workers can use in close collaboration with their clients to enhance QoL.

Questions

Look at a case study or focus on your own situation as an example.

1   Can you identify the three QoL factors in your case study?
2   Which life needs were most under pressure in the case study (or in your own situation)?
3   Can you identify satisfiers and pseudo-satisfiers?
4   Can you identify possibilities for influencing the three QoL factors so as to achieve optimal QoL for the client?

3

SOCIAL WORKERS' TOOLBOX

Overview

Questions

This chapter addresses the following questions:

- In what respect does the philosophy of pragmatism support social work practice?
- In what respect does the philosophy of dialectical existentialism support social work practice?
- What can outcome research tell us about the effects of psychotherapy?
- What can outcome research tell us about the effects of social work?
- What 20 methods are included in the toolbox?
- How will the descriptions of these 20 methods allow for comparison between them?

3.1 Introduction

Chapter 1 introduced the three-step approach, while Chapter 2 described the theoretical underpinnings of this approach: the PIE-Empowerment Theory. So the question is: what does a handy social work toolkit look like? One that can help social workers optimize the client's QoL? Which methodical model offers an easily accessible toolkit in relation to the complex issues social work clients present with? How can pragmatism, dialectical existentialism and outcome research underpin the multimethod approach?

This chapter will present a social work toolkit consisting of an overview of 20 practical methods. What method should social workers use for what issues? And what does each individual tool (method) look like and what taxonomy should we use if we want to compare the various methods?

I will start by describing pragmatism and dialectical existentialism as a philosophical perspective which supports the social worker's practical, flexible approach and engagement. Next

I will provide a summary of outcome research for psychotherapy and social work: what do we know about the effectiveness of the various social work methods? Do social work methods contribute to outcomes to such an extent that they justify the development of a multimethod toolkit? Next I will present an overview of the 20 different methods, and I will conclude by presenting a summary of the chapter.

3.2 Pragmatism and dialectical existentialism

Social workers often describe themselves as pragmatic people who are engaged with the tragedies that happen to other human beings. What are the philosophical trends underpinning the social worker's pragmatic and engaged approach?

Philosophy has the ability to bypass existing theories, functioning as a sort of meta-theory — a theory about theories. As such, philosophies can integrate a number of client- or method-related theories in such a way that these form a synergistic whole rather than simply the sum of separate theories. Together, the pragmatic and dialectical-existentialist philosophies offer one philosophical scaffolding for social work.

First I describe pragmatism as something social workers can identify with, reflecting their practical-pragmatic attitudes and their flexible attitude around making use of a range of methods and techniques. Next I will describe dialectical existentialism as a philosophy which provides theoretical support to engaged and critical social workers who assist clients and their networks in their 'struggle for life' — their existential struggle.

3.2.1 Pragmatism

> Social workers start, follow and end where the needs of the client are.

Social workers have a pragmatic attitude: how can my interventions contribute to improving my client's life situation? Social workers are doers. This pragmatic attitude is also reflected in the philosophical movement of pragmatism. In William James's pragmatism, the question was not does something make sense logically speaking (is it true), but what practical application could this philosophy have in terms of our life and our best interests? The philosophy of pragmatism makes statements about the struggle for survival and the struggle with nature. Pragmatism comprises four principles: usefulness, dynamism, pluralism and scepticism (see Table 3.1).

TABLE 3.1 Pragmatism as the philosophical basis for multimethod social work

Features of pragmatism	Reflected in these social work principles
1 utilitarism (usefulness)	Contributing to improving the client situation: what will help the client most?
2 dynamism (study of forces)	Dynamics of the mutual influence between individual clients, in client systems/networks and the outside world
3 pluralism (multi-)	Multitheory, addressing diversity, multiculturalism, the multidimensional
4 scepticism (open-mindedness)	Continually responding to any new client situation with an open mind, delivering tailored services, heuristic social work, the critically reflective professional

In *What Pragmatism Means* (1907b), James sets out the actions of a pragmatist:

> A pragmatist . . . turns away from abstraction and insufficiency, from verbal solutions, from bad a priori reasons, from fixed principles, closed systems, and pretended absolutes and origins . . . turns towards concreteness and adequacy, towards facts, towards action and towards power.

In short, pragmatism follows the evolutionary view about knowledge: research is done to allow people to get a grip on their environment. In this sense pragmatism is realistic: it acknowledges the existence of an external world which we will have to interact with.

Principles of pragmatism

1 *Usefulness:* the view that knowledge should contribute to a better life. The principle of usefulness helps the social worker to contribute to improving their clients' lives: what will help the client most? Obviously the *caricature* interpretation of William James's usefulness principle does not apply to social workers, because they cannot identify with the slogan that 'Truth is where you make dollars from.'

2 *Dynamism:* the world is considered incomplete, a continual work in progress. Our thought processes too are like a stream, a system of relationships. The dynamic principle helps the social worker to understand the ongoing dynamics with regard to individual clients, in client systems and in the outside world, which influence each other. Within PIE-ET theory this refers to the dynamic force field which occurs in every client situation and which determines the client's quality of life.

3 *Pluralism:* the world cannot be explained based on just one principle, as reality comprises many different independent areas. The world is not a *uni*-verse, but rather a *multi*-verse. Within this world, which is the arena/platform for many opposite forces, humans have the opportunity to introduce their own volition and their own strengths into this force field. The pluralistic principle provides social workers the *multi*theory underpinning the *multi*, a multitheory which requires social workers to be flexible and creative when addressing diversity, multiculturalism, multidimensional forces, rather than the illusion of one monotheory to cover everything. The pluralistic principle again emphasizes that reality comprises more than one truth, and underlines the need for alignment with the client's reality. To this purpose social workers have a range of methods at their disposal to tackle a diverse range of problems – just like the carpenter does not equate every single problem with a 'nail' so as to be able to use the hammer as his only tool.

4 *Sceptical open-mindedness:* we do not hold that our own views, or our human way of knowing in general, are the only ones possible and valid. The principle of scepticism helps social workers to work based on their personal professionalism, continually addressing every new client situation with an open mind, using a tailored approach, providing heuristic social work, in other words continually creating a customized theory for a particular case, 'a theory for one case', rather than embracing standard solutions, following protocols and following an automatic approach. The scepticism principle requires every social worker to have a critical-reflective attitude, to go on learning from each and every case. Thus, in a sense pragmatism underpins ongoing multimethod social work in a number of ways.

3.2.2 Dialectical existentialism

> In life, you have to fulfil your own needs and rights, but you don't have to do so all by yourself.

Dialectical existentialism is a philosophy with regard to human existence, one which is not only critical as to the extent to which the social context is in control, but also of the extent to which individuals are in control. This explains why social workers can identify with this philosophical movement. Dialectical existentialism considers the crises which occur in our human lives, the big questions about being and the meaning of life, questions which arise in response to significant losses, traumas, significant changes in life, which leave us feeling vulnerable or confused. Thompson (2004) formulated this vulnerability as follows:

> Feelings of loneliness, emptiness, meaninglessness are typical features of periods of crisis, in other words, these are in fact an existential experience where a sense of safety and equilibrium are replaced by doubt and existential insecurity.

Dialectical existentialism introduces the concept of 'bad faith' and its opposite, 'authenticity'. Authenticity means the client takes responsibility rather than becoming dependent on the social worker (or his own social network), and rather than accepting the problems as permanent and unchangeable. Clients who turn their backs on freedom and responsibility, taking refuge in stories and excuses, are told that they have the freedom and the opportunities to choose alternative options.

Jean-Paul Sartre was one of the existentialist philosophers. In his *Critique of Dialectical Reason* (1960), he tried to achieve a synthesis of his critical-existentialist analysis and a sociological analysis. In this book he tried to connect the concepts of human freedom and responsibility to an analysis of specific structures of oppression in a in a social, economic and political sense.

Sartre operated from the central principle that man exists in the universe in which he lives. Man exists together with the world. Man influences the world and the world influences man. Within a social framework, dialecticism involves humans both forming social, political and economic forces and in turn being influenced by these. Human freedom is an important component of dialectical existentialism, also as a counterpoint for determinism and fatalism which hold the view that human beings are determined by their environment or external developments. As such, Sartre opposed repression of the individual by social structures. To Sartre dialectical existentialism is social humanism which involves engagement.

However, dialectical existentialism as a philosophy also reflects the dialecticism of changes. There is a tension between history and human beings, which could be seen as a vicious cycle, but which is more like a spiral enabling human beings to act first. Human beings create the world and are created by it at the same time. This provides human beings with the freedom of movement which is so characteristic of people in the modern age: human beings design, and in the freedom this gives them, they are both ahead of themselves and of the actual situation. Modern man can identify with this dynamic game of freedom and determination. In the philosophy of existentialism, the emphasis is not so much on the structure of science but on the actual being of humans in the world. When human beings are confronted with borderline situations, struggles, suffering or death, they will start to wonder about the meaning of life. This happens in communication, because human beings are essentially dependent on other people. It is only when human beings communicate with others that they are able to get down to the deepest level with their own questions. In *Phénoménologie de la perception* (1945), Merleau-Ponty tries to think of the consequences of the situation human beings find themselves in, in the world. He explicitly assumes that there is a unity of body and spirit. There must be this unity, and it has to be reflected in all our actions. Observation comprises both perceiving something with the senses and also being aware.

Dialectic existentialism comprises six principles: (1) personal choice and responsibility, (2) ontology (the study of being), (3) connection between the personal/individual and the social/collective, (4) critical attitude, (5) uncertainty and (6) dialectical reasoning (Table 3.2).

Principles of dialectical existentialism

1   *Personal freedom of choice and responsibility.* The principle of social workers helping enhance client self-reliance on the one hand (not accepting victim behaviour), while on the other hand pointing out that everyone is responsible for their own actions (not accepting *blaming the victim*). In this sense, the principle of responsibility encourages independence and discourages dependence.

2   *Ontology.* The study of being, which help social workers to cope with the crises and situations of loss so frequently encountered in their work. The questions about being, existential questions which demand a personal focus, rather than technical, 'plastic' answers.

3   *Connection* between the personal/individual and the social/collective. This principle of connectedness underpins the social work focus on the interaction between person and environment. It helps social workers place freedom of choice and responsibility within the broad social context of class, race, ethnicity, gender or age. Individual factors (freedom, values, behaviour and so on) and social factors (oppression on the basis of gender or race), which mutually influence each other are in a dialectical relationship to each other and continually impact each other.

TABLE 3.2 Principles of dialectical existentialism as the philosophical underpinning of social work

Features of dialectical existentialism	Recognizable principles from social work
1 Personal freedom of choice and responsibility	Enhancing people's self-reliance/autonomy and getting them to take responsibility for their lives
2 Ontology (study of being)	Existential crises and loss leading to questions of a truly existential nature
3 Connection between the personal/individual and the social/collective	Placing the individual within the broad social context of class, race, ethnicity, gender or age and getting social agencies to take responsibility for facilitating individual happiness
4 Critical attitude to all that is taken for granted: understanding and challenging oppression as a lived experience (*le vécu*)	Eliminating/reducing discrimination and oppression, which violate and dehumanize reality
5 Uncertainty	Uncertainties in the work of social workers in the everyday swampy lowlands in contrast with the theoretical and abstract highlands
6 Dialectical reasoning	Change and conflict, as recurrent theses and antitheses which transcend each other in syntheses

4   *Critical attitude* in relation to whatever is taken for granted; a critical understanding of and a critical challenging of oppression as a lived experience. This critical principle helps social workers to gain insight into the complex processes of discrimination and oppression, which violate and dehumanize human reality. Critical social work comprises ongoing reflection and self-reflection about the client and the environment, both as part of the issue and as part of the solution.

5   *Uncertainty.* This principle helps the social worker deal with the uncertainties of working in the swampy lowlands, rather than hiding behind the abstractions, the beautiful theoretical highlands. Here the critically reflective attitude demonstrated by social workers (learning from each case) bridges the gap between theory and practice in social work.

6   *Dialectical reasoning.* This dialectical principle helps the social worker deal with change and conflict and the many other dilemmas social workers are faced with; according to dialecticism, the tension or contrast between thesis and antithesis transcends both, resulting in synthesis. Dialecticism is a philosophical vision of the developmental nature, that is the dynamic nature of reality, according to Schaaf (2007):

> A permanent development, an ongoing development can never be captured in its entirety. It is the thesis in conflict with the antithesis, resulting in a new unit, the synthesis. This is at the heart of dialecticism. Connections are very much intertwined through interaction, the action of opposite 'poles' impacting on each other. When using the word poles, this sounds as if there are only two, but in fact an infinite number of actors and factors can be at play, exerting their influence all at the same time. Nothing is, everything exists in relation to. This is at the heart of (material/materialist) (materialistische) dialecticism. Relating to, therefore evolving. Something or someone exists in relation to another or to something else, although also possessing its own individual features, such as a certain connection to the other (things).

As far as social work is concerned, dialecticism underpins the many conflicting and tense situations, involving opposing theses and antitheses, where the goal is to work on achieving a synthesis. This not only applies to working with clients, but also to the many methods and theories/models in social work which may appear to be in conflict with each other, but where an overarching theory may achieve a synthesis.

3.3 The strength of outcome focused methods

> All have won, all must have prizes.

Outcome research into 'common factors' considers the contribution of methods to the overall results when supporting clients to be relatively low. However, in practice this is different for social work, when compared to psychotherapy.

3.3.1 Outcome research in psychotherapy

Based on outcome research into the strength of various psychotherapy methods in relation to anxiety disorders and depression (what effects do the various psychotherapy methods have?),

TABLE 3.3 Common factors and their contribution to the outcome of psychotherapeutic interventions

Common factors	Definition	Contribution to result in %
1 Client factor	the client's strength, social support, life events in the course of the therapy process	40%
2 Relationship factor	empathy, warmth, encouragement	30%
3 Therapist factor and method factor	specific methods/techniques	15%
4 Placebo factor	expectations and the placebo effect	15%

the researchers concluded: 'All have won, all must have prizes' (Lambert 1992). This is the metaphorical pronouncement made by the dodo in *Alice in Wonderland* when the wet animals have dried themselves by running around the pond. After exerting themselves by doing those laps around the pond, they ask the dodo who the winner is. The dodo replies with the famous pronouncement, oft cited by researchers: 'All have won, all must have prizes'. Psychotherapy researchers used this statement to indicate that all psychotherapy methods showed an equally strong effect for a number of mental health disorders. They also found that there were a number of common factors, aside from the methods used, which may have had a stronger effect in psychotherapy than suspected thus far. Four factors were found to have an effect in psychotherapy (Lambert, 1992) (Table 3.3). Both the client factor and the relationship factor turned out to have a very significant effect (70%) on the outcome of psychotherapy.

It will be clear from Table 3.3 that shared factors make the most significant contributions to positive outcomes of psychotherapeutic interventions – the *client factor* and the *relationship factor*, the so-called *non-specific factors* – and this applies to all types of psychotherapy, when compared to factors related to specific methods/techniques.

Within the field of psychotherapy this has prompted the conclusion that all specific methods are equally useful, as long as the relationship factor and the client factor are adequately safeguarded. If 70% of the result of therapeutic interventions is due to the client and to the relationship between therapist and client, it makes sense for special emphasis to be placed on the client's strengths and on facilitating a safe and effective therapist–client relationship. If specific psychotherapeutic methods and techniques only make up 15% of the effect of a therapeutic intervention, it would appear that methods are needed, but contribute less to the overall outcome than previously thought. This finding came as a shock to psychotherapists. Specific approaches such as cognitive-behavioural therapy, communication skills, relationship therapy and so forth all turned out to be less important than previously assumed! It appeared that the competition between specific 'psychotherapeutic movements' had been decided in favour of non-specific factors. These findings resulted in a more liberal way of thinking: everyone was able to follow their own approach, as long as client and relationship factors were adequately safeguarded.

3.3.2 Outcome research and social work

So what do these research findings mean for social work? What are the effective factors within social work? Unfortunately no comparable outcome research has been done in the field of social work. One of the underpinnings for writing this toolkit for social workers was the Dutch proverb: 'Good tools are half the work'. Can we conclude that social work methods contribute to 50% of the outcome of our support? In reality, no one knows what percentage to attribute to the contribution of social work methods and techniques in relation to the final outcome. It is very likely that *attention for the client and the relationship factor* are of great importance in social work, just as they are in the field of psychotherapy. It is for good reason that the non-directive core method in social work – which focuses on such client and relationship-related factors just as it does in psychotherapy – has constituted the *core method* in social work from the very beginning. What remains is the question of whether the non-committal conclusion contained in the dodo's verdict – it does not matter which method you choose, because all are equally effective – also applies to social work.

Because the fields of psychotherapy and social work are very different, for now I do not think the same conclusion applies. The psychotherapist addresses specific mental health disorders such as anxiety and depression, and this is a much more narrow domain than the broad psychosocial domain of the social worker. A toolkit comprising a wide range of tools and methods may be much more applicable to social work practice with its diverse range of issues and problems, relating to divorce, poverty, marginalization, abuse and so forth.

Numerous objections can be raised against indiscriminately extrapolating the dodo's verdict from psychotherapy-related outcome research to the field of social work. The first objection relates to the aforementioned argument that psychotherapy practice and social work practice are too dissimilar; the common factor study was aimed at outcomes (effects) within the area of psychotherapy which aimed to address mood disorders and symptoms of anxiety.

This argument was confirmed by Reid (1997), the only one to examine the question of whether all methods/interventions in social work are equally effective. Reid (1997) concluded that there was not enough evidence to warrant generalizing the 'dodo bird effect' from the narrow field of psychotherapy towards the broad domain of social work which involves a very diverse range of problems and interventions. We follow Reid's argument: there is a persistent and widely held belief – referred to as the 'tie-score effect' or the 'dodo's verdict' – that different types of intervention have equivalent outcomes. However, the research supporting this belief has been limited largely to comparing methods drawn from different schools of psychotherapy with emphasis on treatment of the emotional problems of adults. A review of relevant meta-analyses published in the past decade ($n = 31$) was undertaken to determine whether this verdict applied to the broader range of problems and interventions typically found in clinical social work. The majority of these meta-analyses reported differential effects associated with different types of interventions. There proved to be little basis for extending the dodo's verdict to the range of problems and interventions of concern to social workers. Moreover, several patterns of differential effectiveness occurred that could help guide the practitioner's choice of interventions. The meta-analyses examined in this article give little support to the dodo's verdict when that verdict is applied to the broad range of problems and interventions of concern to social workers. The meta-analyses suggest what kind of interventions may be effective for a range of problems with indications of what kind may be more effective than others. A second pattern of differential effects can be seen in the advantage enjoyed by multicomponent interventions over their rivals. This pattern occurs in eight meta-analyses across seven problem areas (bulimia, obesity, child internalizing disorders, drink-drive offenders, drug abuse, juvenile delinquency and panic disorder/agoraphobia).

Multicomponent intervention

Even if true, the finding could be given a 'so what?' dismissal because many interventions should accomplish more than one intervention. In my view, the result is by no means self-explanatory. A multicomponent intervention provides more tools to help the client, but breadth and variety may sacrifice depth. There is no obvious reason to assume that practitioners are more successful in using an assortment of methods than in concentrating their efforts on one. Nevertheless, given that multicomponent interventions appear to do better, one might speculate why. One reason may be lack of knowledge as to which intervention is the 'correct' one for a given client or problem configuration. If such knowledge is lacking, a multicomponent intervention might do better because it would increase the chance that clients with differing needs would at least get the social work help best suited for them. Another reason may lie in the multifaceted nature of most problems brought to human services practitioners – juvenile delinquency is a prime example. Different facets of a problem may require different components.

Therefore, the conclusions of common factor research cannot be extrapolated from the field of psychotherapy to that of social work one by one. The narrow mental health domain of mood disorders cannot be compared to the broad psychosocial domain of social work problems. According to Reid (1997), research into social work might show that methods and techniques play a much more important role in social work, precisely because social workers have to address both material and immaterial questions, individual as well as systemic issues, and have to engage in prevention as well as client work. Social workers' focus on this broad range of psychosocial stress-related issues in cases of illness, loss, trauma, practical and material matters, divorce, identity crises, relationship problems as well as those related to nuclear and extended family, burglary, theft and violence could well dictate the need for a broad range of methods. The sheer biopsychosocial breadth of problems requires a toolkit which offers a broad range of methods. One method is not enough, because how can one method be useful for this entire range?

Another objection to the statement that social work methods/techniques do not make much of a contribution to the outcome of the intervention lies in the fact that common factor research emphatically underlines the importance of specific methods. Common factor research has shown that specific methods play a small but essential role, constituting a common factor which therapists have to have at their disposal. If therapists do not implement a specific method, other common factors will lose their effectiveness as well. For therapists working in a client-focused manner, which means that they invest a lot in their relationship with the client, this means that they must have specific methods and techniques at hand. For therapists working with a specific method/technique, this means that they should also include the common factors in their toolkits. It is not a matter of 'either/or' but of 'and/also': it is essential that the therapist has a good relationship with the client, otherwise the specific method used will not get through to the client. However, when therapists are not using a clearly defined method, there is no added value, because the other three common factors will not be effective unless a specific method is used. In other words, methods and techniques are also part of the common factors in psychotherapy. According to common factor research, it makes no difference which method the psychotherapist utilizes, as long as he has a preferred method he or she believes in. When baking yeast bread, the amount of yeast to be added is tiny compared to the amounts of flour, fats and water, but even so, the yeast is an essential ingredient!

We can therefore conclude that specific methods/techniques are an absolute must for social workers, on the proviso that they not think these methods will be of any use without the non-directive core method which will guarantee that they are utilizing the client's strengths.

3.4 Twenty social work methods: an overview

The social worker's toolkit comprises one non-directive core method (NDC method) and 19 directive methods (see also the overview following the Preface). The underlying principle is that the directive methods are only effective when combined with the NDC method. The question as to whether social work is a profession based on non-directive listening or one which directively coaches the client has met with different answers over the lifetime of the profession. There were alternating periods in which either directiveness or non-directiveness dominated. It was as if the wheel needed to be reinvented over and over again, without ever arriving at a synthesis. At a certain point in time, a new generation of social workers criticized the highly 'accommodating and non-directive' attitudes of some of their social work colleagues. This was the start of a directive era in which 'giving directives' became the norm. More and more social workers attended directive therapy courses, learning all manner of directive techniques. The innovators stated: 'You are the expert, so you do not need to shy away from suggestions, advice and giving clients tasks to complete.' However, eventually directive social workers realized that giving one-sided directives simply was not effective.

The multimethod social work (MMSW) model constitutes a synthesis of the non-directive and the directive client approach: an 'and/also' rather than an 'either/or' approach, as both have their good points (see Figure 3.1). The MMSW model involves non-directive communication skills as a core method, in addition utilizing 19 directive methods, each of which can be used when specific issues are involved. One-sided listening and directiveness are no longer appropriate in the modern social work era: their time has passed. Social workers need to be able to flexibly use multiple methods, combining non-directive and directive social work.

3.4.1 Non-directive core method: acknowledging the impact factor

> Start, follow and end where the needs of the client are.

The non-directive core method enables us to provide support as requested by the client – non-paternalistic. The client is at the heart of non-directive core social work method. In fact, it seems odd that we speak of client-focused support, when in fact every form of support should be client-focused by definition. In practice, however, the focus is (often) on either the method or the protocol. Social workers helping clients take on an attitude of 'professional innocence', asking questions such as 'what do you mean by that?' or 'what does that mean for you?' By asking these questions, social workers take nothing for granted. Everything the client says or does requires attention and requires the client to explain.

The non-directive core method is the core method in social work, the basic tool used by the social worker at all times. The NDC method refers to a method which allows for the development, maintenance and completing of a positive working relationship between social worker and client. The underlying principle always entails the client's story and stresses

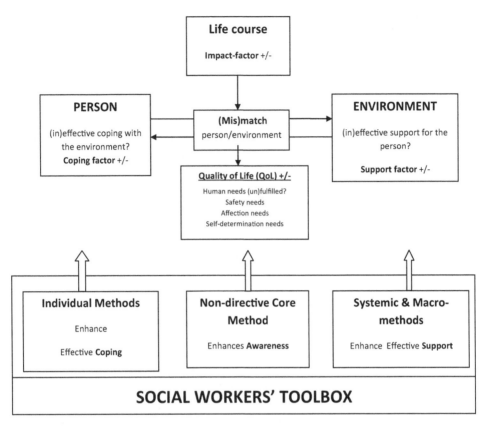

FIGURE 3.1 Social workers' toolbox optimizing PIE: social work methods help the person and the environment to interact optimally with each other

'Starting Where the Client Is', as Goldstein (1983) named his seminal article. I expanded on this motto: we should not just start where the client is, but also follow and finish with the results experienced by the client. Specifically adding the client's human needs as a starting point − 'Start where the needs of the client are' − is the result of the growing realization that the client's QoL will improve when his human needs are met. In other words, client-focused work is further specified: it should focus on the client's needs.

The social worker starts the process of helping the client become aware of (as yet un)fulfilled needs by using the non-directive core method: 'What is it you need for you to be able to achieve an optimal enjoyment of life?,' because what strikes us about the definition of human needs is that the concept of unfulfilled needs implies an *experienced* wish, which presupposes an awareness on the part of the client in terms of his or her unfulfilled need(s) and wishes. To this end, the three-step approach (Chapter 1) included a checklist to assess the awareness process, because we cannot take it for granted that the client will be aware of his or her needs at the start of the social work interaction. Clients do not always present to the social worker with a well-defined request for help; they are often in trouble and do not know how to get out of trouble. It is part of the social worker's jobs to use the NDC method to help the client to formulate a conscious request for help or to help the client become aware of an underlying human need.

3.4.2 Nine individual social work methods: improving the coping factor

> Every human being has *to fulfil his own* human needs, but not all by himself.

It will have become evident from the client story what the client's specific individual human needs are: but how adequately do they cope? In other words: how adequately is the client dealing with his or her need for survival, affection and self-determination? The checklist for indications for *individual* social work methods (see Appendix 7) allows you to assess the status of all 'needs' items: what needs are present and how adequately is the client himself or herself coping with the fulfilment of these needs? The social worker uses pluses and minuses (+/−) to indicate to what extent an area of need creates strength or tension – in other words, whether or not the need is fulfilled.

The client's story will help provide clarity as to the client's resilience (the coping factor): is the client able to provide their own needs using their own strengths? How about self-care and self-management? How effectively can the client surf the waves which will inevitably keep rolling in?

The mere fact of the social worker mapping out both self-care issues and client strengths is enough to kick-start a constructive process. The client's strengths are reinforced by expressing appreciation for his resilience up until that point and the results which have been achieved since the start of the interaction. Careful communication skills during every stage of the social work interaction will result in the client feeling respected. This in itself encourages the level of self-respect and self-care on the part of the client: 'I feel acknowledged and I am being taken seriously and I am better able to cope'.

Now that is has become clear what individual methods can be used to improve coping, the question remains which methods are available to improve support from within the person's environment.

3.4.3 Six systemic and four macro methods: improving the support factor

> Every human being has to fulfil his own human needs, *but not all by himself.*

In the course of interacting with the client, social workers gain an insight in the extent to which the former receive support from people in their environment when it comes to fulfilling the client's needs. The same question applies to every client: what is the quality of support from the client's social network as regards his private life, work situation and public resources or services (structural support received by the client by way of resources or services, legal provisions, social policy)? How much support do caregivers provide with regard to helping the client fulfil needs.

When drawing up a psychosocial assessment (PSA), support from the client's social network can be mapped out using the overview in the Overview of the book. This overview can be used to quickly map out support factors in the client story, making it clear which methods would provide the best alignment.

3.5 Taxonomic principles per method

A multimethod approach involves the social worker aligning himself with the client story on the one hand, while on the other hand influencing the client in a focused manner. It is as if the client is put on a psychosocial intravenous drip (the core social work method) so as to allow the administration of the right medication (implementing directive). This cannot be done the other way around: directive approaches are only effective in the presence of a good collaborative relationship and positive interaction.

Multimethod social workers are skilled in the use of the 20 tools, using the right tool at the right time and to the right extent. The social worker feels competent to act because he is working from an unambiguous methodological model, which provides an easy overview.

Being competent to act means that the social worker is implementing a multimethod rationale and possesses the relevant technical skills to do so. Social workers who are competent to act are self-aware, secure in what they are doing, and know what to do in what situation. From this they draw strength, both on a professional and on a personal level. And this is exactly what social workers who have become familiar with the multimethod approach say.

> I have become familiar with our toolkit. I know what to do and I am not afraid to take a more directive approach, because I know what I am doing. I am also clearer about describing the boundaries between social work and specialist support.

3.5.1 The methodological profile as the standard

Part II will describe 20 social work methods according to a fixed structure: starting with the definition and historical background, then moving on to the goals, indications, contraindications, techniques, results, evidence and pitfalls. This serves to create a methodological profile, or methodological standard, for each method. Since no two situations are the same and because there are always different factors involved, the standard can only ever be a 'guideline to guide our thinking'. Therefore the methodological standard does not contain any mandatory provisions. Standards leave us more room for autonomous professional decisions than do protocols (which prescribe uniform actions). To put it broadly, establishing a standard still allows us to work from the special features of each individual case. In practice, social workers use these methodological profiles to describe and assess their interventions.

This book will use the systematic approach and a fixed structure, like that used in nursing protocols (Cuperus et al., 1995). A protocol prescribes the way one needs to work when carrying out a certain action, in accordance with what is considered best practice at that point in time. An example would be the nursing protocol of what to do when patients are put on an intravenous drip: a prescribed way of doing things.

I prefer the term 'methodological profile' over the term 'methodological protocol' for two reasons. First, the social work profession involves a lot of talking: many of the social worker's actions are of a more verbal nature. Verbal actions do lend themselves to descriptions of what these should ideally look like, but they do not lend themselves to a fixed, prescriptive form of practical implementation.

The second reason why we talk about 'profiles' instead of 'protocols' is that the implementation of the method very much depends on the client's situation. It is easy to describe the core social work method in clear terms for social workers – as a general standard – but how a session is implemented in practice depends on the client's psychological status and the situation he or she is in, and cannot therefore be turned into a protocol as easily. Social workers align themselves with the client and adapt the method to this unique situation. Hence the choice for this way of structuring the description of the methodological profiles: to create a standard for the possible implementation of the method in question. Thanks to these methodological profiles, methods can be recognized/identified and defined.

I will start by explaining the nature and structure of the methodological profiles by means of the following:

1 Methodological profiles
2 Methodological profiles social work
3 Objectives
4 Structure
5 Principles
6 Rationale.

Methodological profiles

A 'methodological profile' is the description of the method's individual characteristics, all in accordance with current insights into that method at that point in time:

1 Definition of concept and elucidation
2 Historical background
3 Goals
4 Indications
5 Contraindications
6 Techniques
7 Outcome of intervention (results)
8 Evidence
9 Pitfalls
10 References.

Methodological profiles social work

Whenever the concept of *methodological profile* is extrapolated towards the social work profession, the definition of a social work profile will be as follows:

> A methodological profile in social work involves the description of the features of a specific social work method including the historical background, definition, indications, contraindications, techniques, outcome of intervention, evidence, pitfalls and references, in accordance with current insights concerning that particular social work method.

This definition helps us define what is meant by a *social work method*:

> A social work method is a set of specific techniques used by the social worker to reduce or eliminate a client's stress. Social work methods stem from targeted actions aimed at

reducing stress and to enhance the client's strength in specific areas: on the individual, systemic and macro level.

This last definition includes each and every methodological intervention – from giving the client one-off information and advice, up to and including long-term support.

At the current time the profession of social worker has not yet been included under the BIG legislation in the Netherlands: this Act regulates professionals providing individual health care. The BIG register is an actual register for pharmacists, doctors, physiotherapists, health care psychologists, psychotherapists, dentists, midwives and registered nurses, and records any limitations in their scope of practice. Only those professionals registered in the BIG register are allowed to use the legally protected title and are entitled to exercise the powers associated with that title.

Since this book offers a very clear description of social work practice, this may bring us a little closer to the social work profession being included in the BIG register.

Goals

The aim of describing a particular action in a profile is primarily to provide clarity around when to carry out a specific action, based on state-of-the-art knowledge and experience. The prior objectives consist in: standardizing actions and testing/assessing those actions.

The foundation for providing a declaration of competence for carrying out a particular action in social work is a description of that action in the profile. It may be necessary to describe certain actions in other situations as well. Therefore, profiles may serve the following goals:

- Assessing, monitoring and promoting the quality of the support;
- Adequately inducting new colleagues;
- Learning new approaches (education/professional development);
- Defining tasks and responsibilities.

Structure

Each profile contains a number of items. Relevant information for each of these is provided in a particular order, making it easy to find what one is looking for. All methodological profiles include the following components:

- Name of method
- Definition of concept and elucidation
- Historical background
- Goals
- Indications
- Contraindications
- Techniques (overview and elucidation)
- Social work result
- Evidence
- Pitfalls.

I will now provide some specific information relevant to the description of each item. Information is always described in very general terms, and examples provided.

Name of method

The name of the method must cover the subject: the name should provide a clear indication as to what set of actions must be carried out to achieve a specific purpose described in the profile. So we should have 'Profile of the core social work method' rather than the more abstract 'Profile of the methodological approach'.

Definition of concept and elucidation

This includes a description of the method and an elucidation of the term(s) used.

Historical background

The historical background includes a brief overview of the historical context for a given method, the most important initiators/proponents, references on application of the method within social work and key concepts.

Goals

These tell us what the method is trying to achieve: what is the outcome we are aiming for? Goals can be formulated at various levels of abstraction. As an example, the goal of the cathartic method is to achieve a release of any hurt that may be present. This is an abstract, indirect goal. A more concrete and direct goal would be to allow the client to cry. The latter can be a sub-goal to achieve the abstract goal.

Indications

The indication is the reason for or the situation in which a method can or should be followed or carried out. These include the most frequently occurring situations. One example of an indication for a particular core social work method is, 'Client tells a story involving a complex range of intertwined issues. Core social work is indicated to achieve a stocktake, unravelling and localization of these accumulated issues.'

Contraindications

Contraindication includes the reason why or the situations in which a method cannot or should not be implemented. These include the most common situations. One example of a contraindication for a particular core social work method is, 'Client is under the influence and inaccessible/incapable of self-reflection.'

Techniques

The techniques of methodological profiles involve the entire set of actions needed to achieve the objectives. A number of techniques will be described for each method. I will start by providing an overview. Next I will elucidate each technique separately and provide an example of this technique in practice. In describing a technique I am assuming that social workers will adhere to and implement the usual guidelines in terms of privacy, safety and comfort (informing clients when a technique is implemented). One example of a behavioural method technique is the social skills technique, which allows clients to practice new behaviours in terms of social skills.

Social work result

The outcome of an intervention refers to the effects of a particular method: what is the outcome of the intervention? One example of an outcome of an intervention as part of the cognitive method is, 'Client has more realistic thoughts about himself.'

Evidence

Evidence refers to the extent to which we have scientific proof as to the effectiveness of the method described: has research shown this method to be effective? One example of evidence in relation to the bodywork method is, 'In terms of the outcome of the activation technique, when encouraging people to be more physically active, we know that people feel better when they are more physically active.'

Pitfalls

Pitfalls refers to errors social workers can potentially make when applying a particular method. One example of such a pitfall in terms of the ritual method would involve social workers imposing their own preferred rituals on the client, instead of allowing the latter to develop their own rituals.

Principles

The methodological profiles are structured as follows. I have outlined the general and specific features of the way I have structured each methodological profile.

- I have written a separate profile for each method, even when two methods are often implemented at the same time in practice – such as the core social work method in combination with the cognitive method.
- When formulating each profile, I have worked from the assumption that the reader has never implemented a certain action or approach: the information provided is unambiguous and complete.
- I have given a practical example after formulating the techniques.
- I have worded everything in a brief and succinct manner.
- All headings show the same terminology and order: title, definition of concept and elucidation, historical background, goals, indication, contraindication, techniques, outcome of results, evidence, pitfalls.

Rationale

In developing the methodological profiles, I used the principle that all profiles should be written by someone who has extensive theoretical and practical experience with the method in question. Every one of the theoretical profiles has been tested in practice by experts in the specific field of a given method and by social work teams. Each profile has been underpinned by the available literature and based on expertise in the workplace. The definition of what a methodological profile entails contains the statement 'in accordance with current insights concerning that particular social work method'. This part of the definition of the methodological profile implies that actions or approaches may change due to fresh insights. This will require an ongoing testing of existing profiles to see whether they are still in accordance with current insights. I therefore strongly recommend that the practical approaches described be continually tested to see if they are still appropriate.

3.6 Summary and questions

This chapter has described the social worker's toolbox by providing an overview of 20 useful methods, and elucidated the multimethod approach in social work.

First, pragmatism and dialectical existentialism were described as useful philosophical principles for social workers. Next the findings of outcome research were summarized based on factors which are effective in the interaction with clients. It was apparent that there is no clarity around the contribution of certain methods in achieving the result of social work support. Next I briefly introduced each of the 20 methods. Finally, I described the taxonomic principles which have been used to describe each method or tool in the remainder of the book, to make it easy to compare them.

Questions

1   Do you recognize elements of pragmatism and dialectical existentialism when you think about what motivated you to become a social worker?
2   Examine a case study or take yourself as an example. Now try and describe the relationship between the core method and the other methods.

Parts II to V: ten individual methods: enhancing individual coping

Parts II–V deal with describing 10 methods that strengthen the coping of clients. Reinforcing clients' coping contributes towards optimally meeting clients' universal needs for safety, affection and self-determination. Coping can be defined as 'effectively managing one's own human needs', realized in social work attention for the impact and coping factor. Ten coping methods are described, distributed in four parts.

* Part II: The *non-directive core social work* method for developing a relationship with the client and enhance acknowledgement of the impact of life transitions (Chapter 4).
* Part III: Three *survival-focused* methods for helping the client effectively meet their safety needs: the bodywork method, the practical-material method and the trauma-work method (Chapters 5–7).

- Part IV: Three *affection-focused* methods for helping the client effectively meet their affective needs: the cathartic method, the expression method and the ritual method (Chapters 8–10).
- Part V: Three *self-determination* methods for helping the client effectively meet their self-determination needs: the cognitive method, the narrative method and the behavioural method (Chapters 11–13).

PART II

Core social work method

4

NON-DIRECTIVE CORE SOCIAL WORK METHOD

Support can only be defined as support if the person in need feels supported.

Questions

This chapter addresses the following questions:

- What is meant by the non-directive method?
- What is meant by a client-oriented approach?
- What is the meaning of the concepts of congruence, empathy and unconditional positive regard?
- What is the function of the PFC technique?
- What are the effective components of social work?

4.1 Introduction

This chapter describes the non-directive method as the core method of social work. First, the term 'non-directive method' is defined. Then, the non-directive method as the core method in social work is elaborated. The three components of the client-centred approach are elucidated, those being congruence, empathy and unconditional positive regard. In addition, non-directive interviewing techniques are described. The chapter concludes by presenting a summary.

4.2 Conceptual definition and elucidation

4.2.1 Conceptual definition

The non-directive method is the core method in social work, the basic tools for the social worker to work with at all times. The non-directive method (ND method) in social work aims at developing, maintaining and finalizing a positive work relationship between social worker and client. By describing the non-directive method as the core method, it is emphasized that the relationship between client and social worker forms the basis of all social work interventions.

For a relationship-based practice, then, 'relationship' can be the primary means of intervention, that is the end in itself or, as it is more commonly utilized, as 'a means to an end' (Network for Psychosocial Policy and Practice, 2002). For this reason the ND method encompasses elements from a range of successful methods in social work history (elaborated later on). Contact with the client is essential to the non-directive approach. The client's verbal account is always the starting point. The ND method underpins the starting point in social work: 'Start where the client is,' reflecting the title of Goldstein's historic article (1983). We will extend this to 'Start, follow and end where the client is,' in order to emphasize that the safe work relationship between social worker and client is to be maintained during the entire process.

The non-directive approach facilitates individually tailored care without patronizing the client. One of the key trends in social work has been the rise of bureaucratically driven models in social work practice and managerialism. Managerialist perspectives on social work emphasize meeting administrative requirements at the expense of time spent looking at casework (Hafford-Letchfield, 2009). The danger of proceduralized practice is that it runs the risk of being insensitive to and inappropriate for individuals' circumstances and becomes 'a substitute for human contact and exploration, denying the necessity for professional judgement in assessing high risk situations' (Hughes & Pengelly, 1997).

The client is central to the non-directive method. It seems somewhat odd to use the term 'client-centred', considering that each form of care should be directed at the client. Practice shows that the professional's own preferential method or protocol often holds centre stage instead of the client. A social worker who is helping the client in a non-directive way will assume an attitude of professional 'ignorance' (see Figure 4.1). Nothing is obvious for the social worker, and by asking questions such as 'What do you mean by that?' and 'What does that mean to you?,' the client is given the social worker's undivided attention.

4.2.2 Elucidation

The ND method is a method of 'self-exploration'. It encourages the client to focus on the following issues:

- Self-searching
- Making an inventory of areas of attention
- Identifying problems and obstacles
- Acquiring more self-knowledge
- More self-respect
- Analyzing strengths
- Controlling one's own life
- Gaining insight into one's demand for care and wishes.

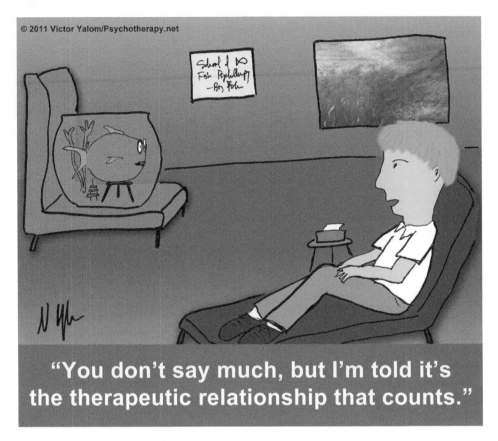

FIGURE 4.1 The relationship that counts...

Image courtesy of Psychotherapy.net

By approaching the client in a non-directive way, new information will emerge that will contribute to analyzing the client situation. The following components of the ND method are described in the social work literature: sensitivity, warmth, understanding, acknowledgement, trust and acceptance. The core attitude of the ND method encompasses empathy, unconditional positive regard and congruence. The ND method as the core method in social work facilitates a caring relationship. The client is the key focus of attention during all phases of the psychosocial help. The ND method is utilized by the following action points:

- Gathering information
- Interpreting observations
- Drawing up work hypotheses
- Monitoring client's work on the areas of focus that were inventoried.

In doing so, the social worker is helping the client to help himself. In order to make an inventory of the areas of focus the ND method employs 10 different techniques: the safeguarding technique, sandwich technique, the archive cabinet technique and the SLVP techniques. The inventory and identification techniques are used to analyze the problem issues, for which directive methods have been indicated.

Two methods from social work history have yielded the structural elements of the non-directive core method, which will be elaborated in section 4.3 together with social casework:

1   Rogerian counselling
2   Narrative or constructivist method
3   Social casework.

Rogerian counselling

Rogerian counselling – named after Carl Rogers, the founder of the so-called reflective listening technique – is the method in which the work relationship between care worker and client is the key principle. According to psychologist Carl Rogers, adequate care can only be offered by assuming a client-centred and non-directive attitude. He explains that non-directive means that a social worker does not approach the client from his own perspective but from the client's perspective. He does not act according to his own agenda, diagnoses or help options. On account of the profound influence of client-centred counselling and extensive research on Rogerian counselling, the Rogerian body of ideas will be examined more closely in this chapter. Periods in Rogers's thinking can be typified as follows: the non-directive period (1940–1950), the reflective period (1950–1957) and the experiential period (1957–1970). In this section, I will describe how Rogers made the change from a psychoanalytical to a non-directive orientation.

Active listening

Rogers first worked as a child psychologist. At the institute where he worked he was asked to counsel a woman with complaints about her son's behaviour. Both mother and son were receiving help and Roger treated the mother. During therapy he tried to convince the mother that she was treating her son badly by rejecting him. The team of experts had arrived at this diagnosis. On multiple occasions he tried to show her the pattern of rejection. Nothing seemed to be working, and after 12 sessions Rogers suggested stopping the sessions. The mother left the room and returned asking: 'Do you offer counselling to adults?' First he did not know how to deal with the question, but then answered that there were indeed some known cases. The woman returned to her seat and poured out her heart about the serious problems between her and her husband. Rogers just listened to her and after a few sessions her marriage relationship improved and gradually, also her son's problem behaviour. Rogers concluded his story by saying, 'This was an essential learning moment for me. I had followed *her* path instead of mine. I had just listened instead of moulding her into a diagnostic concept that had already been there before we met.' (Rogers 1951)

In the ND method the client determines the direction of the social work sessions; the social worker determines the final direction. The interviewing techniques – extensively described in section 4.7.1 – are aimed at understanding the client from his own frame of reference. This is called the core empathic attitude.

Training schools

The training schools teach social workers the basics of the client-centred approach by instructing them in interviewing techniques. Books are used such as Gerard Egan's *The Skilled Helper* and Alfred Kadushin's *The Social Work Interview From 1976*. Social workers are trained in a list of core skills (Trevithick, 2012) including non-verbal communication skills, observation skills, listening skills and interviewing skills. These skills can also be summarized as 'people skills' (Thompson, 2016) or interpersonal skills (Koprowska, 2010). In order to emphasize the client-centred orientation in social work, the term 'non-directive core attitude' is preferred to 'training the aforementioned skills'. These skills deserve to be given a framework within the important non-directive method.

Gendlin and Ivey

Former students of Rogers, Gendlin and Ivey followed in his footsteps. Gene Gendlin made a name for himself by introducing the notion of 'focusing', encouraging the client to concentrate on the physical sensations representing the world as they perceive it (see section 5.7.8). Allen Ivey became known for his so-called microcounselling, a number of core counselling skills for a wide range of person-centred professionals.

Narrative or constructivist method

The most recent method in which the work relationship between social worker and client occupies centre stage is the narrative or constructivist method. (The narrative method will be dealt with separately in Chapter 12.)

The narrative method starts from the principle that a person's history, the story about oneself or someone else, does not represent a random collection of events. Individual stories reflect our culture (a pattern), not only our folklore (random frills). Personal stories help us become conscious of our history. The adage 'start where the client is' becomes more concrete when the social worker has the client tell their own story.

4.3 History of the non-directive core social work method

The history of social work variously has yielded a number of methods that highlight the importance of the relationship between professional and client, as in Rogerian counselling and the narrative or constructivist method, both of which are still widely applied in practice. The application of the ND method in social work is, however, still in its early stages.

4.3.1 Social casework

Social casework is considered the oldest method of social work. In the early days of social work the focus of attention was placed on the relationship between the social worker and the client. At a later stage more attention shifted to the systematic and structural aspects. Social casework tried to break with the patronizing and judgemental assistance provided by charities and churches, by starting from the principle of an equal relation between social worker and client. In 'What is social work? Marie Kamphuis (1972) states the following 'What used to be "no charity, but a friend", now converted to the notion of a partnership, is a practical ethical principle, influenced by psychology, and is now perceived as fundamentally significant in helping other *people*.'

In social casework clients are stimulated to enhance their self-reliance. Social casework has been strongly influenced by Freud's psychoanalytic body of ideas on psychodynamics. Therefore it has also been typified as psychological social work. Freud was the first to introduce the concept of the working alliance, the helping relationship (Hubble et al., 2002). According to Freud, this work relation gave rise to transference, counter-transference and positive associations. Transference occurs when a client recollects problematic memories from a previous relationship, for instance with mother and father, and projects these memories on the care worker and then processes these memories. This process was said to produce healing effects. By counter-transference it is understood that the care worker himself projects someone of his own relationships (parents, partner, children) on the client. Positive association (positive transference) means that the practitioner evokes positive associations in the client by using the client's positive experiences from the past.

4.3.2 The client is centre stage

The ND method as the core method in social work facilitates the realization and maintenance of a helping relationship. The client remains the starting point during all phases of psychological help. The basic assumption in social work is that 'the customer is always right'. The client-centred principle assumes that a person is free and that their behaviour results from deliberate choices from alternatives. Social worker and client are equal. As a social worker you can help clarify the demand and help think about the way to proceed. Eventually, clients will make their own choices, having you or someone else to guide them. So, the pillars of the client-centred approach are individual freedom and responsibility, on the side of both the client and social worker. A client-centred approach in social work is characterized by congruence, empathy and unconditional positive regard (Geldard, 1993). It was Carl Rogers (1951) who first described these three characteristics (see Table 4.1).

A first characteristic of the client-centred approach is congruence, or authenticity. For a professional to be congruent, you have to be honest with yourself and allow yourself to feel and think freely about your client, including the negative aspects. Being genuine does not imply spontaneous communication of these thoughts and feelings: 'You are a difficult person' or 'This is horrific'. The important thing is that you acknowledge these feelings and find out how they influence the contact. This supposes an awareness of the roles you play as a parent,

TABLE 4.1 Client-centred core attitude

Characteristics of client-centred approach	*Description*
Congruence = authenticity	You, as a social worker, are aware of what you really feel and you accept those feelings
Empathy = ability to feel what your client feels	You understand the client from his frame of reference
Unconditional positive regard	You approach the client in a non-judgemental way

friend, brother, patient, client or professional and the differences in the way you behave in each of these roles in different situations. As a social worker you remain congruent by listening sensitively and precisely without being overwhelmed by your client's outpouring of feelings. In case you do feel moved, you are to isolate these feelings to avoid anxiety or pity. You can only help a person by being who you are, without feeling sorry for this person.

Empathy

A second characteristic of the client-centred approach is empathy, or the ability to acknowledge and understand someone else's feelings. Imagine that your client is walking along a path. Sometimes he abandons the path, walks into the woods, climbs over rocks, walks through valleys and crosses streams, and explores his surroundings. At times, the client will walk around in circles and return to the same starting point. As his social worker, you are supposed to follow him rather than guide him. Most of the time you will walk beside your client. You accompany him to where he wishes to go, where you can sort things while being warm, open, friendly, caring, nurturing, genuine and realistic. In doing so, a basis between you and your client will develop and you will be able to see the world through the eyes of your client. This is what is meant by empathy. As a social worker you are capable of perceiving the client's world as your own events and experiences, without losing sight of the 'as if' (Lang & Molen, 1991). Your client will notice that you are able to feel with him and understand what's going on in his mind.

Unconditional positive regard

The third characteristic of the client-centred approach is unconditional positive regard. That means that you accept your clients as they are, in a non-judgemental way. You accept them with all their weaknesses and vulnerabilities and all their strengths and positive qualities. Approaching your client with unconditional positive regard does not mean that you have to agree with your client all the time. In this way you help you help your clients accept themselves. Giving someone your unconditional positive regard is not easily done. As an accepting social worker this will prove quite challenging if your own inner conflicts have not yet been resolved. As an accepting social worker you acknowledge the feelings of the other person, you understand that feelings may be bewildering and that anxious persons are capable of acting irrationally.

4.3.3 Non-directive method: mapping the situation together with your client

Assessing the factors of the life event situation lays the foundation for planning, designing and implementing the supply of social work. In many cases the client will not come forwards with a formulated demand for social work. Instead, you, as a social worker, are expected to identify your client's suffering due to one or more life events and their need for support. There is often no well-considered and motivated demand for care. Instead of expecting the clients to ask for the care they need, it is more realistic to assess the condition they are in and together formulate what is needed now and later, considering the circumstances.

In Chapter 1 the stepwise approach was covered in great detail. In this chapter the focus of attention is on describing the strength of the personal filing cabinet as a client-centred social work technique.

Structuring the client's story

The ND method provides the tools for the client-centred approach, non-directivity, by presenting a number of interviewing techniques. There are two main indications for utilizing these techniques:

- When the client is need of order and structure ('I see no beginning and no end to it all');
- When the client is facing existential questions ('Why me?').

Basic interviewing techniques (SBVP) and the personal filing cabinet are important instruments for both indications. SBVP stands for listening and mirroring techniques, and with the use of the PFC the client is able to sort out obstacles and problem issues per area of attention (see sections 4.7.1 and 4.7.2). The social worker utilizes a range of interviewing techniques. The narrative method (see Chapter 12) is employed to help the client deal with existential questions. These questions pertain to the way persons perceive their own place in life.

'Who am I?', 'What do I want with my life?' 'What is the meaning of my life'? The problem is that these questions about the meaning of life – 'Why me?' – often arising from life events, cannot be answered. It concerns questions about how to cope with these life events and the emptiness that has been created. Applying interviewing techniques such as mirroring and summarizing, you, as a social worker, are primarily concerned with arranging all the issues and drawing up an inventory. How much was the client attached to what has been lost (past), how is the client's situation now (present) and how does the client wish to move forwards (future)? This inventory will help the client mentally adapt to the new situation following the life events. It is essential to identify and acknowledge the client's existential issues and the psychological earthquake they are experiencing. Through communication skills the disruptive impact of these life events can be shared and given a place. The pointlessness of it all is given a place.

4.4 Goals

General goals

- The client identifies the factors causing anxiety and tension.
- The client experiences less negative tension.

Specific goals

- The client is given more clarity on the situation.
- The client identifies areas of attention.
- The client gains more insight into their coping skills.
- The client feels respected and experiences that someone is taking an interest in their story.
- The client identifies the stress factors causing tension, to be dealt with by more specific methods.
- The client learns to acknowledge their own positive qualities.
- The client gets a better grip on the coping process.
- The client is moving forwards, in the right direction.

- The client formulates their own demand for care and goals (articulation).
- The client explores the world as they perceive it (exploration).
- The client becomes introspectively more skilled.
- The client dwells on existential questions.

4.5 Indications

- The ND method has been indicated for every session.
- The client is seeking help on account of psychological turmoil, has no clear understanding of the cause.
- The client has insufficient insight into areas of attention.
- The client has no clearly formulated demand for care.
- The client's condition needs addressing, for instance, when feeling restless, tense or hurt.
- The client is facing existential questions such as: 'Why me?', 'I'm stuck' and 'I don't know what to think'.
- The client is showing signs of resisting the social work process: shuns intervention and exploration of problem issues.
- The client is unable to express themselves (insufficient introspective ability).

4.6 Contraindications

- Insufficient cognitive ability (by dementia, mental disability, brain injury).
- Being severely confused.
- The client is under the influence.
- Concrete informative question.
- Attributed demand for care.
- Continuity insufficiently guaranteed.
- Individual problem issues/obstacles needing a directive approach.
- Systemic indications (not just individual social work, for instance, when there are problems in the relationship with the partner).
- Macro indications (more is needed than only individual or systemic interventions, for instance, when more clients are having problems with services).

4.7 Techniques

1 Basic interviewing techniques: SBVP (silence, body language, verbalization, practical assistance)
2 Personal filing cabinet (PFC) as a structuring tool
3 Safeguarding confidentiality technique
4 Sandwich technique
5 Inventory technique
6 Identification technique
7 Scanning technique
8 Main theme technique
9 Empowerment technique
10 Motivational interview technique.

4.7.1 Basic interviewing techniques: SBVP

The client-centred, non-directive approach involves a number of techniques that facilitate the actual implementation of the core social work method. In practice, this non-directive basic attitude can be also referred to as 'Listening, Summarizing and Further Questioning (LSFQ)', 'Not Filling in for the Other Person (NFOP)' and 'Matryoshka'. A Matryoshka is a Russian doll containing a number of wooden dolls of decreasing size placed one inside the other. The Matryoshka stands for the client, who, in a safe environment, opens up and, layer by layer, unravels the meaning of their life events.

Assuming the client-centred core attitude alone is not enough, the basic techniques are the tools you need to be equipped with in order to employ the client-centred method in social work practice. The four basic skills are summarized in the abbreviation SBVP: silence, body language, verbalization and practical assistance (see Table 4.2).

TABLE 4.2 SBVP-interviewing techniques

Technique		Description
S = silence	1 Silence technique	A good social worker is a good listener
B = body language	2 Physical presence	Physical presence showing involvement and proximity
	3 Physical distance	Sitting at an appropriate physical distance
	4 Eye contact	Giving confirmation by eye contact
	5 Physical listening attitude	Body posture conveying engagement
	6 Minimal encouragements	Saying 'yes, yes', humming as short confirmation that you understand and follow
	7 Touch	Holding client's hand or any other body part that is appropriate
V = verbalization	8 Starting technique	Trustworthy start. Proceed with an open agenda; 'I have noticed or heard that ... and then I thought it would be an idea to sit down with you.'
	9 Inviting questions	'Is there more you could tell me? What does that mean to you? What exactly do you mean by that?'
	10 Paraphrasing the content	Mirroring the issues one by one as presented by the client
	11 Summarizing	This is done over a longer period of time; mirroring all the formulations together
	12 Reflecting feelings	'I can see that this affects you a bit/a lot'
	13 Normalizing	Your depressed mood is a normal reaction to life events
	14 Giving information	'You keep saying: "I have to stop crying," but crying is considered a good way of releasing tension'
	15 Confronting	'You say you are doing fine, but you sound despondent when you say it'
	16 Re-labelling	'It keeps you awake and is always on your mind, but it is indeed a heavy burden to bear'

Technique		Description
	17 Meta-communication	'What I sense is that your expectations do not correspond with mine' (evaluating what's been said)
	18 Appreciation	'I appreciate that you are willing to discuss this with me . . . that you are dealing with this respectfully'
	19 Humour	'We have been rather dramatic, haven't we?'
	20 Functional self-disclosure	'What's been troubling you has also been troubling me for some time now'
	21 Rounding off technique	'We are now going to conclude; what you have been telling me . . . how does this conversation end for you?'
P = practical assistance	22 Practical techniques	Making a cup of tea/coffee to make client feel more at ease, 'Would you rather have me make that phone call?,' etc.

Source: de Mönnink (2015)

Silence

When you keep quiet by not speaking a situation is created in which the client can grieve. This is called helping by listening or therapeutic silence. As Mark Twain (1835–1910) put it: 'If we were supposed to talk more than listen, we would have two mouths and one ear.' As a social worker you are helping your client by listening because you are attentive to what they are saying. Human attention is the most powerful kind of encouragement. During the interview there are moments of silence, pauses, during which the client can relax, cope with their feelings or find encouragement to move forwards. As a consequence, your silence may produce a therapeutic effect. Being silent is much harder than it seems because the right timing of the pauses is essential to the process. A subtle sense of judgement is required as well as the ability to suppress your own tendency to break the silence in the conversation. Assuming a listening attitude as a professional does not warrant unconditional regard, attention that is devoid of your own biased thoughts.

As Suzuki (1980) shows,

> When you are listening to someone you are to abandon your biased thoughts and your subjective opinions, the only thing you do is listen to your client, only perceiving what he is conveying. . . . Most of the time when you are listening, the words you hear echo your own thoughts. You are, in fact, listening to your own ideas. If both views correspond you will accept the other person's view, if not, his opinion gets rejected or you stop listening altogether. A mind full of preconceived ideas, subjective intentions or habits cannot be open to how things are.

Listening is an art. By observing silence the client is allowed to dwell on their own situation. Your listening attitude encourages your client to sort out their own affairs and feelings. Accept that not everything can be adequately put into words. Therefore we realize what cannot be spoken of remains best unspoken. Still, a deadly silence is to be avoided at all times.

Body language

Body language as a social work skill refers to conveying physical messages of compassion and engagement, accompanied by touching or not touching. Your body language shows that you are engaged in your client. You communicate the extent of intimacy and involvement with your client through your physical distance, your eye contact, your physical listening attitude, minimal encouragement, your touch (see Table 4.3). Your body language is constantly conveying messages, rendering what you say less important than your body posture and tone of voice. Of all human communication, 55% is determined by non-verbal language, 38% by the tone of our voice and only 7% by our spoken words (Hargie, 1986). Body language never lies.

As a social worker you choose a form of physical contact appropriate to the client–social worker relationship and stage of the social work process. Touching can be admissible within the limits of well-defined codes, for instance, shaking hands, walking hand in hand, a tap on the shoulder, putting an arm round the shoulder. However, some people will experience touching as emotionally charged. By touching you are showing your involvement in a physical way. Touching can also be associated with 'comfort'. An arm round the shoulder, a hand on the shoulder, a hand on the knee. In doing so, you, the social worker, are showing respect for both your own and your client's boundaries. At your training college you have learned to explore your own boundaries by self-searching in order to become free from your own experiences of the past. Therapeutic touch – touching without physically touching – is a method that reduces pain and tension (Busch, 1993). By sensing the patient's energy field with the hands – 5 to 15 cm away from body surface – changes in temperature, pressure and tranquillity can be established. Numerous American nursing training colleges teach the workings of the therapeutic touch.

TABLE 4.3 Basic technique body language

Body language	Adequate	Inadequate
Physical distance	At an appropriate distance, not too close, not too far away	Too distant or too close
Eye contact	Looking at the other person, at regular intervals	Staring
	Occasional blinking	Looking away
	Occasional glancing over the person	Losing eye contact at critical moments
		Gazing alongside the client
Physical listening attitude	Slightly leaning forwards	A rigid posture
	Relaxed face and attitude	Arms crossed before chest
		Posture lacking energy
	Close to the client	Tense facial muscles
	Smooth, quiet movements	Wobbling and fidgeting
	Occasional nodding	Constantly nodding
Minimal encouragements	Hmhm.	Artificial use of hmhm, yes, etc.
	Yes.	
	And?	
	And then?	
Touch	Touching in an appropriate and desired way: functional touching	Inappropriate physical contact, overstepping professional boundaries
Therapeutic touch	Deliberate exchange of energy through your hands	Exchange of energy with a hidden agenda and subsequent manipulation

Verbalization

Apart from the use of body language, support can be given by talking to your client. Reassuring words, such as 'nothing can be done about it,' 'it's the way things are' and 'time is a great healer' can produce different effects in a variety of situations. What may be reassuring in a certain situation may be a cliché or worn-out phrase in another. What also applies here is that consolation is only given when experienced as consolation by the receiver. Applying the technique of verbalization encompasses inviting your client to talk, paraphrasing what's been said, reflecting feelings, summarizing, normalizing, giving information, meta-communication, confronting, positive labelling and functional self-disclosure. Table 4.4 presents a summary of these components.

TABLE 4.4 Basic technique 'verbalization'

Verbalization	Adequate	Inadequate
Invitation to talk	Clarifying open questions, brief, unequivocal, asking way of repeating the client's words. 'What would you like to talk about?' 'Could you tell me more about it?' 'What do you mean by tired?' 'How are you feeling now?' At suitable moments closed questions may invite the client to respond to difficult questions or encourage silent clients to talk: 'Who was involved?' 'Where is this leading to?'	Closed question at an inappropriate moment with an inhibiting effect, long-winded obscure conclusions containing questions, rendering the feeling of being cross-examined and only to be answered by a yes or no
Paraphrasing	Organizing and complementing factual information; mirroring factual information provided by the client. Ensure that you are listening closely and stimulating the client to be specific.	Incorrect paraphrasing will make the client feel misunderstood.
Reflecting feelings	Mirroring the client's feelings by putting them into words helps the client identify underlying feelings: 'You say that you are tired and you look somewhat despondent.'	Incorrect way of mirroring by reserved use of language, interspersed with interpretations and prejudices that are long-winded, abstract and boring: 'That fact you feel powerless shows that something else is bothering you, isn't it?'
Summarizing	Various elements from the conversation are brought together into a meaningful whole; the key issues are clear; the client feels understood and invited.	Incorrect summary of a longer part of the interview or of what was said before (see paraphrasing)
Normalizing	Telling your client that their reaction is the normal way of reacting to a life events	Making everything seem normal, even in case of disturbances

(Continued)

TABLE 4.4 (Continued)

Verbalization	Adequate	Inadequate
Giving information	Individually tailored approach to giving information to actual questions, enabling the client to feel more at ease: 'Should I report this to the police now?' Social worker: 'That won't be necessary at this moment.'	Reacting to coping questions by providing factual information. Client: 'Why is this happening to me?' 'Because you have a festering tumour.'
Confronting	Pointing to the remarkable, odd or contradicting aspects in their feelings, thinking and acting: 'You seem rather upset by this.'	Questions concerning remarkable, odd or contradicting aspects are asked in a rude and inappropriate way: 'Why are you feeling so tense?'
Re-labelling	Putting a gloomy view into a different perspective, at all stages of the contact. Client: 'My life has become a tragedy.' Social worker: 'The life event has had a profound impact on you.'	Contradicting the client and trying to reverse the situation from the beginning, turning all that is negative into something positive
Meta-communication	Evaluating what's been said in order to tune mutual expectations	Evaluating the conversation without a clear purpose in mind
Functional self-disclosure	Social worker is sharing their own reactions, for instance, by talking about their own experiences, as confirmation or eye-opener	Moralizing and bringing up one's own experiences in order to reject or coerce
Rounding off technique	Announcing that the social work session is to end soon, calmly breaking off contact	Concluding the session by stating: 'Time is up, we have to stop,' allowing no time to round off session

Practical assistance

The practical techniques are well-developed in most social workers (see Table 4.5). Clients derive a great deal of support from the correct and well-considered way in which you as a professional operate in their interest. If this were not the case, the result would be the effect of the revolving door, where clients keep returning due to the lack of adequate support. Moreover, clients will greatly benefit from your technical knowledge. In fact, there are many ways to lend a helping hand, both practically and materially, varying from delivering bad news correctly to providing immediate assistance, intervening in a crisis situation, signposting to other services, providing care and aftercare.

Learning process

A great deal of support can be derived from adequate implementation of these daily routine tasks, as shown in the following chapter. As a social worker, you can work in a client-centred

TABLE 4.5 Basic techniques for practical assistance

Practical guides	Adequate	Inadequate
Assistance in arranging and managing financial, legal, domestic, parenting and relational issues and other matters	Appropriate and timely support, as by writing letters, filing requests for debt relief, promoting client's interest at services	Inappropriate and untimely support: social worker determines tempo and activities by client, particularly the extent of self-determination

TABLE 4.6 Learning process of basic techniques in social work

Stages		Description
TP	technique-person	technique first, client as a person in the background
TP	technique-person	varying prominence of technique and person
PT	person-technique	client first, technique still recognizable
P	person	client first, technology integrated

Source: Adapted from Hogan (1964)

way if you utilize the skills of the SBVP technique. Learning to counsel clients with life events goes through a number of phases (see Table 4.6). In the first phase of the learning process the focus of attention is on the technique. During the last phase the technique has been fully incorporated and doesn't need to be focused on any longer. As a result, you, as a social worker, can then be fully attentive to your client.

4.7.2 The personal filing cabinet (PFC) as a structuring tool

The PFC-technique is an inventory technique aimed at sorting out and reflecting the areas of focus (see Figure 1.1). Together with the client you discuss whether this inventory has been made correctly. Next, you both decide on which drawers to deal with, in which order and for how long. The modelling of the PFC encourages the client to actively tackle unfinished issues from the recent or distant past. The technique helps clients visualize the areas of focus by means of an archive cabinet with drawers, each drawer representing a single area of attention. By arranging these areas by way of a 'drawing of the archive cabinet' the social worker stimulates the client to face his or her own situation and be in control over 'what to deal with at what moment'. The metaphor of the archive cabinet enables the client to consciously deal with his or her own situation: in doing so, the internal chaos becomes organized 'externally'. The PFC technique is a model for client-centred and emancipatory social work. A client-centred approach involves starting from where your client is and staying near your client during the process, at an appropriate distance. By emancipatory social work we understand social work based on an equal partnership, whereby the social worker creates the right circumstances for the client to start working on the grieving process. The PFC technique does not model the social work relationship as being 'know-it-all' versus 'ignorant'. Social worker and client are in an equal relationship.

How can the PFC-technique be utilized as a structuring tool in social work? During the first session, the cabinet in Figure 1.1 helps you, the social worker, explain the imagery and workings of the archive cabinet. You explain that each area of attention is to be stored in each of the imaginary drawers. After your first contact with your client, you take the first step in mapping the painful stories of life events and trauma. Next, you categorize these stories into different drawers. These drawers are then organized and summarized for the client, who corrects, complements and adds further details. This organizing is a necessity, for these carelessly suppressed profound events concerning life events and loss have generated a mental, physical and relational turmoil. As one client put it: 'The archive cabinet sorts out the chaos in my mind, the whole mess floating around in the imaginary cabinet.' The client is no longer able to cope with their mental, physical and relational situation by themselves. Social work helps the client focus on the problem areas and create mental ordering and tranquillity.

Active and conscious process

Tranquillity can be accomplished by applying a wide range of social work methods. These methods are to be appropriately implemented, encouraging the client to actively, consciously deal with unfinished business, at their own PFCe, in a safe environment. When the client indicates that they have come terms with the life events, the moment has come to conclude the social work process: 'I have more peace of mind now'. Clients tend to appreciate the structure offered by the PFC technique, which stimulates the client to actively keep on working. There is a lot of work to be done; the cabinet needs clearing up and every drawer has be cleaned. A client reports, 'It makes me feel calm to deal with one drawer at a time. As a client you help decide which drawer to tackle. You are working in a structured way.' This method of continued working on the material from the drawers facilitates effective review. To what extent has the turmoil been reduced in the drawer, both in your opinion and your client's opinion? How much progress in what area has been made per session? A client reports: 'It is an efficient way of sorting out the chaos and offers clear understanding of the work method and the steps forward: working directions are straightforward. By clearing up the drawers one by one, you are the one who's doing the job.'

According to the metaphor of the personal filing cabinet the client engages in archiving, cleaning and tidying activities. The collection of all the unfinished and painful business has been stored in imaginary drawers of someone's archive cabinet (memory) and needs processing. This metaphor enables the patient to go through the grieving process in an active and self-conscious way. Metaphors generally help persons structure their experience, understand and define their reality (Lakoff & Johnson, 1980). Coping with life events can now be seen as working through the life events. It concerns an active and conscious process which clients can go through successfully at their own PFCe and with your help. Thus, the metaphor of the personal filing cabinet offers clarity and structure in social work.

Emancipating

Your attitude of facilitating the core conditions produces an emancipating effect on the client, who is now actively working on the bereavement issue and is therefore gradually getting his feet back on the ground. At the same time, you are to be creative in selecting the most appropriate method of social work and also observe your own boundaries, by way of self-care. (de Mönnink, 1998b). This core attitude stresses the responsibility that you and your client have. Balancing this role is illuminated by an example of Perls's (1969) famous 'Gestalt Prayer', where he was describing one's (existential) responsibility and the tension between autonomy and interference in phrases like: 'I am I and you are you. ... I do my thing and you do your thing.'

4.7.3 Safeguarding confidentiality technique

Social work introduces the basic rules of confidentiality and voluntariness; basic rules that enhance the client's sense of safety. The first rule of confidentiality observed in social work is that no personal information is to be disclosed to a third party without the client's explicit consent. The second rule of voluntariness that applies to social work contact is that there is no coercion involved on a personal level, the client should not feel coerced to do anything during contact with the social worker. The third rule is transparency in working methods and assignments during contact with the social worker. An inventory of the areas of focus is drawn up by the client and social worker, after which the client proceeds to deal with the issues by utilizing the suitable combination of methods.

4.7.4 Sandwich technique

The social worker divides the session into three parts: the initial phase, the middle phase and the final phase. This format of each session warrants the experiential, close-by approach, as expressed by the phrase: 'Start, follow and end where the client is.' The initial phase is devoted to introducing the rules of the sessions, conveying all the information that you, the professional, have received so far. You make an open start by asking: 'What brings you here?' In later sessions you welcome the client at the start and offer him or her something to drink and then ask 'How are you doing?' The principle remains 'Start where the client is.'

In the middle phase – the in-depth phase – a suitable combination of non-directive core method and directive techniques are to be applied. Each session starts by applying the inventory, identification and indication technique. What also applies here is 'follow where the client is'.

The final phase consists of introducing the rounding off of the sessions – it's a good thing to round off – and then gradually work towards concluding the session and towards the transition to the daily life situation. The session also ends by asking 'How does this session end for you?' and if desired, 'In what way was your contribution positive today?' 'What are your plans for today?' *End where the client is.*

4.7.5 Inventory technique

The social worker observes the client carefully during the session and takes notes (keywords), if desirable, of the areas of attention as presented by the client. In doing so, the social worker can draw up an inventory of the areas from the client's story, and also name the issues that are experienced as stressful by the client.

Inventory technique

In this interview you have as a client so far mentioned three areas of attention: (1) the attitude of the doctors, (2) the life events of your child and (3) the past.

4.7.6 Identification technique

Together, the client and social worker identify the problem areas and obstacles in each area of attention.

> ## Identification technique
>
> In area of attention 1 you report being frustrated and angry with doctors. In area of attention 2 you state that you feel sorrowful and that you miss your wife. In area of attention 3 you say that you have experienced a childhood trauma.

4.7.7 Scanning technique

The next step for the social worker is to scan each identified problem area to find out what obstacles need to be removed in order to reach the desired goal. (What do you wish to accomplish?) This approach leads to unravelling the initial area of attention.

> ## Scanning technique
>
> In area of attention 1, 'attitude of doctors' the social worker asks the client: 'what doctors are we talking about?' What went wrong in the contact with doctor 1? What went wrong with doctor 2? The client has become rather frustrated and angry because of doctors' indifferent attitude during his wife's hospital admission. Scanning further revealed that the client was even planning on reporting the matter to the disciplinary tribunal. This information points to potential indications for further social work (identifying the real stress factors), release and expression and mediation. In the current case, the social worker proposed writing a letter in which the client could exactly formulate all his grievances.

Social work is here combined with the expression-oriented method. The underlying stress factors have now been clearly revealed, facilitating further differentiation of the most suitable combination of methods.

4.7.8 Main theme technique

Social work operates in a goal-oriented way by starting from the zero line, an inventory of the areas of attention (see section 4.4) and then, by working with tentative results and eventually working towards a satisfactory final result for the client (see Figure 1.1). The results from the previous contact are always the starting point for each following session. Between times new areas of attention are often presented and written down. In the following session the social worker and client return to this issue. The final results are recorded during the final contact, in a verbal or written report. In doing so, the client's stress levels can be reduced by working in a goal-oriented way (see Figure 4.2).

At the end of each session and the start of the follow-up sessions the practitioner should always stay focused on the key issues. At the beginning of the session: 'What can contribute to stress reduction?' Or at the end of the session: 'In what way has this session contributed towards stress reduction?' At the end of the social work the results are compared with the starting situation.

4.7.9 Empowerment technique

The social worker asks the client: 'What do you wish to accomplish with the issue we have talked about? What do you need to achieve this goal?' These questions will stimulate clients

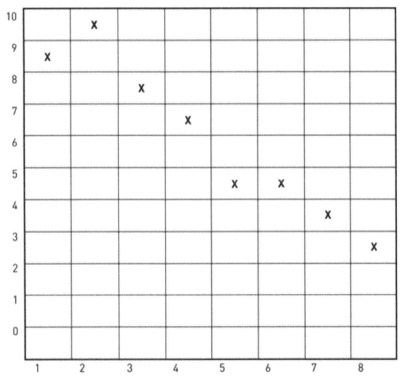

10 = Maximum stress

0 = No stress

FIGURE 4.2   Stress scaling in SW-sessions: Extent of tension etc. Extent of tension experienced during the social work programme, measured per session by stress meter (maximum stress – no stress)

to determine the direction of the social work process themselves. In doing so, clients' actions can be monitored during and between sessions to establish whether the desired targets have been met.

Empowerment technique

The client wants to express his frustration to the doctors. Due to a succession of medical errors he feels that his wife has unnecessarily suffered. The question is now: 'What do you need to achieve this goal?' The practitioner proposes writing a letter first so that client can ventilate his grievances, and focus on the doctors without having to actually send the letter. The client will now feel stronger because of having addressed his frustration by writing the letter.

4.7.10 Motivational interview technique

Motivational interviewing is a technique that works on facilitating and engaging intrinsic motivation within the client in order to change behaviour. Motivational interviewing is a goal-oriented, client-centred communication skills style for eliciting behaviour change by helping clients to explore and resolve ambivalence. The practitioner realizes that the client is facing a dilemma that they are at the crossroads of choosing the right direction. The practitioner restates what both choices are and evaluates the pro and cons as perceived by the client. These pros and cons are to be written on a large sheet of paper, so that the client is given a clear view of the options. If desired, the client can be asked to attribute values to these pros and cons (scores from 0 to 10). The final score turns out to correspond closely with the client's own deliberation and they will now feel more confident about the way they have handled the dilemma. Next, the question arises whether more information will be needed to support the right choice. Finally, the client is asked to express his or her feelings after the choice. In addition, practitioner and client discuss the necessary practical steps involved (see also section 6.6.3 Advising technique).

4.8 Social work results

General goals

* The client reports identifying factors of negative tension.
* The client reports experiencing less stress.

Specific goals

* The client gains more insight into his or her own situation.
* The client reports having control over social work process.
* The client reports having clear view of the areas of attention.
* The client has reviewed the process so far.

- The client formulates a clear demand for support.
- The client acknowledges the demand for care (not attributed by someone else).
- The client reports feeling psychologically calmer.
- The client says that he feels good about the contact.
- The client feels less resistance to interventions (less process resistance).
- The client can express him or herself more easily (is more introspective).
- The client is able to give more direction to his or her life.

4.9 Evidence

Scientific research on social work methods is still in development. The effectiveness of the non-directive method in psychotherapy has been extensively studied and has yielded compelling evidence. From meta-research (study on existing research), encompassing 40 years of psychotherapy it has emerged that (Hubble, 1999)

- 40% of the success of psychotherapy can be attributed to client factors (events in life outside the sessions of social work, such as accidental encounters, positive experiences with friends, stroke of luck at work, reading a good book and so forth);
- 30% of the success of psychotherapy can be attributed to relational factors (relation between social worker and client);
- 30% of the success of psychotherapy can be attributed to specific methods, 50% of which is placebo effect (an encouraging demeanour increases the success rate by another 15%).

When considering this last-mentioned percentage it should be borne in mind that this concerned a group study and therefore it cannot be established which method proved successful in which session. However, a specific method from the group study that was accountable for this 15% could prove vitally important to this particular client during this session. The success of psychotherapy can for 30% be accounted by 'relational factors', also called *common factors* or non-specific therapy factors (Miller et al., 1997). This is exactly what social workers do in practice: start from where the client is and respond to their demand. Because of its relationship-oriented approach, the non-directive method underpins the core attitude in all social work. When the results of psychotherapy are generated to social work, and there no reasons not to do so, two conclusions can be reached:

- You, as a social worker should be competent at implementing the non-directive method.
- You should be adequately trained in multimethodical skills.

You will be able to support clients with problem issues that call for a more directive approach. The non-directive core method of social work as indicated can be combined with one or more of the 19 directive methods. Sheldon and Macdonald (2009) report that service users want social workers to demonstrate:

- Non-possessive warmth
- Genuineness
- Accurate empathy.

Healy (2012) also pointed to the importance of the perception that social workers are non-judgemental, willing and able to help the service user. Several studies have found that service users appreciate social workers being willing to go the extra mile, that is, being sufficiently flexible to offer help in a way that is appreciated by service users.

Motivational interviewing is a well-known, scientifically tested method of helping clients developed by Miller and Rollnick and viewed as a useful intervention strategy in the help of lifestyle problems and disease. Motivational interviewing in a scientific setting outperforms traditional advice giving in the help of a broad range of behavioural problems and diseases. Large-scale studies are now needed to prove that motivational interviewing can be implemented into daily clinical work in primary and secondary health care.

Meta-analysis (Rubak et al., 2005) showed a significant effect (95% confidence interval) for motivational interviewing for combined effect estimates for body mass index, total blood cholesterol, systolic blood pressure, blood alcohol concentration and standard ethanol content, while combined effect estimates for cigarettes per day and for HbA(1c) were not significant. Motivational interviewing had a significant and clinically relevant effect in approximately 3 out of 4 studies, with an equal effect on physiological (72%) and psychological (75%) diseases. Psychologists and doctors obtained an effect in approximately 80% of the studies, while other health care providers obtained an effect in 46% of the studies. When using motivational interviewing in brief encounters of 15 minutes, 64% of the studies showed an effect. More than one encounter with the patient ensures the effectiveness of motivational interviewing.

4.10 Pitfalls

There are two pitfalls in the ND method:

- Missing directive indications: more active directive social work interventions are needed; the social worker, however, fails to recognize the indications;
- Continuation of the non-directive method without making progress.

Compliance may result in a situation where the social worker is drawn into the client's story and expressions. A client-centred approach does not mean going along with the client, but also involves confronting the client when resisting personal deepening.

4.11 Summary and questions

This chapter has discussed the non-directive method as the core method in social work. The characteristics of the client-centred core approach were described, notably congruence, empathy and unconditional positive regard, which are no longer self-evident in helping clients. By being emphatic, being and remaining who you are, and accepting your client, you are working in a client-centred way, and can be guaranteed that supply and demand for care are adequately tuned. The non-directive techniques were described that form the basic tools for the client-centred approach. Important are the elements of the SBVP (silence, body language, verbalization and practical assistance) and the structuring and emancipating function of the personal filing cabinet (PFC technique). Then, attention was focused on safeguarding, the sandwich technique, inventory, identification, scanning, main theme technique, scaling, empowerment and cost–benefit technique. In conclusion, we have further examined the efficacy and pitfalls of the non-directive method.

Questions

1   Select a case study. Determine how client-centred your approach was. Which of the three client-centred core components can you identify?
2   Design a personal filing cabinet of the areas of attention as put forth by your client.
3   Which of the SBVP skills did you utilize at what moment? What is your most proficient skill and least proficient skill?

PART III

Three survival-focused methods

'All you need is safety'

Part III describes the role of the social worker when a client has a survival reflex: How do you survive a situation when your physical, material or psychological survival is being threatened? How can a social worker help leverage the client's personal power for optimal security?

The following three survival methods are discussed in order to help to optimally fulfil the biopsychosocial security needs of the client:

* The bodywork method helps fulfil the need for physical security (bio) in Chapter 5.
* The practical-material method helps to fulfil the need for practical-material security (social) in Chapter 6.
* The trauma-work method helps to fulfil the need for psychological security (psycho) in Chapter 7.

Chapter 5 describes the role of social worker when a client struggles with physical survival. It describes how a stress reflex is generated from the brain in case of physical survival threat. How can a different form of 'threat to life' cause physical stress? And what can the body method offer to alleviate the resulting physical (and therefore mental) stress?

Chapter 6 deals with the role of the social worker in practical-material survival. It describes how life events can cause practical-physical stress and what the practical-physical method can do to reduce this stress.

Chapter 7 describes the role of the social worker with trauma survival. A traumatic experience causes trauma stress. The trauma-work method can help to invoke the existing personal resilience in order to reduce the traumatic stress.

In this and subsequent paragraphs the role of the social worker is illustrated with reference to the case of Mr. Stack. His name was chosen to indicate that tension sources accumulate during life events. Any similarity to actual persons, to madness or psychiatry is a coincidence.

The case of Mr. Stack: stress and resilience

Mr. Stack is 52 years old. He has been walking around for decades with the unexpected stillbirth of his son, as well as the disability of his second son caused by an accident at the age of 4. He never even shared his grief with his wife. Every now and then he vented through some misplaced black humour. His attitude turned bitter and he was overly critical towards social workers, as a survival mechanism and to fill the void. Because of this he never came to a proper grieving process and its relationship with the involved social workers turned problematic. Because of the core social work method Mr. Stack finally made a neat stack of his 'messes' and room was created to closely look at the futility and the elusiveness of his losses. The psychological film was moving again and he stopped dwelling on the 'why' question. Mr. Stack gained more control over his life.

5

BODYWORK METHOD

Questions

This chapter addresses the following questions:

- What is the role of the survival brain in life events such as loss and trauma?
- How does physical stress arise in clients?
- How can the bodywork method contribute to reducing physical stress and restoring one's strength?

5.1 Introduction

This chapter describes the physical survival response to life events such as loss and trauma when they are perceived as (life-)threatening. The bodywork method, which the social worker can use to ease physical stress, is also described. The chapter also looks deeper into several questions. What is meant by physical stress and what are the consequences of persistent stress?

The case of Mr. Stack

Mr. Stack is looking for support amid the chaos he finds himself in. Without any help, he will not get out of that chaos. First he talks about the setback at work. After years of working on a higher professional education level – without a corresponding degree, however – the promotion he was promised had been called off. He was very angry because of this and had called in sick. There were also tensions in the relationship with his partner, tensions so profound that he feared it would result in a divorce. Mr. Stack also reports that he was never able to process the stillbirth of his first son; nor was he able to process his second son becoming disabled (at age 4) due to a shovelling accident in front of their home. On top of that he was also angry with his doctor at that time, who prescribed sedatives a bit too fondly, causing Mr. Stack to wreck his newly bought car. Mr. Stack has a friend and a colleague to support him.

By using the personal filing cabinet (PFC) technique you reformulate the starting situation as follows: 'Mr. Stack, I hear a collection of complaints and problems, which can be divided and put into the seven drawers of your imaginary personal filing cabinet in the order in which you have just named them':

(−)　the severe disappointment in your employer (cancelled promotion);
(−)　tensions in the relationship with your partner (fear of divorce);
(−)　the stillbirth of your first son;
(−)　your second son becoming disabled;
(−)　anger towards your general practitioner (because of the incorrect dosage of sleeping pills and lack of support);
(+)　support coming from a friend;
(+)　support coming from a colleague.

From this inventory, you leave the choice up to Mr. Stack as to which of the seven drawers he would like to focus on first, and which drawers he would like to elaborate on later and in which order. This social work plan is then executed during eight 1-hour sessions over a period of 4 months. Social work interventions allows Mr. Stack to create order into the 'mess' and gives him space to further investigate the meaninglessness and impalpability of his losses. The psychological film is no longer paused at the 'why' question: he gains a better grip on his life.

5.2 How survival brain regulates the survival reflex

5.2.1 Safety first

Given a 'loss'-signal (regardless of whether this loss is caused by death, job loss, illness or divorce) the survival brain is activated (see Figure 24.2), because losing a loved one causes fear: 'Something is amiss, there is danger!'

Some threatening situations require a lightning fast reaction from our brain because it is a matter of life and death, for example a loss of oxygen. The amygdala will produce a fast, conditioned fear response following signals of extreme threat. Additionally, the amygdala (see Figure 5.1) plays an important part in managing other emotional reactions through the autonomous nervous system, partly via the hypothalamus that is situated below the thalamus. There is an amygdala situated on either side of the brain right in front of the hippocampus, which has a memory function. The amygdala is considered to be important in learning and remembering emotional information.

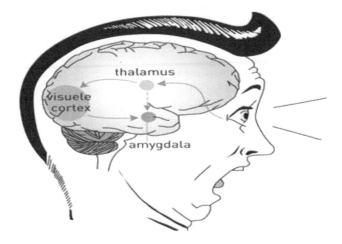

FIGURE 5.1 LeDoux and the fast and slow route direct or indirect to the amygdala

LeDoux (1996) discovered that processing fear signals occurs via two routes, a fast route and a slow one. The fast route runs from the thalamus in the cognitive brain directly to the amygdala in the survival brain. The slow route runs from the thalamus via the visual cortex of the cognitive brain to the amygdala in the affective brain. Because the emotional information goes via the cognitive brain, there is more time for complex analysis.

Presented with a physical threat – though also given a social or psychological threat, as we shall see in the following chapters – our need for survival causes our survival brain to immediately engage the *fight–flight–freeze* mode in our stress-systems (see Figure 5.1). This stress mode exists in animals and humans to protect themselves from danger. The survival brain maintains our continued physical existence, and from an evolutionary standpoint is the oldest area of the brain. It is a reflexive and instinctive brain that responds impulsively to physically, psychologically and socially threatening situations, so not only to physical shortcomings, but also to emotional and social pain. In traumatic experiences, it is activated by the traumatic occurrence (violence, accident), especially if there is actual physical danger. And the survival brain does not only respond to actual pain, but also to imagined pain. This means that when we are emotionally 'wounded', this brain 'overreacts', so to speak, as if your life were in danger.

5.2.2 Physical stress in life events such as loss and trauma

The question here is how to define physical stress and how to reduce it. Physical stress arises when we need to let tensions which have been evoked flow away (desired condition), but when we actually bottle them up (actual condition). This causes us to enjoy life less.

The 'physical aspect' requires specific attention in social work contacts because the pain coming from life events such as loss and trauma also affects our body directly or indirectly. Before we elaborate on clients' physical stress signals, we first define what is meant by physical condition:

- The physical state of health (illness, amputation, aging);
- The degree of pain (chronic pain);

- The energy level (fatigue, strain, exhaustion, chronic fatigue syndrome, fibromyalgia);
- The degree of physical stress signals;
- The degree of physical addiction (to work, alcohol, drugs, internet, pornography, shopping).

During every social-work session the client is constantly emitting physical signals which say something about his or her physical condition. The most common physical perceptions after life events such as loss and trauma are (Worden, 1992):

- Feeling of an empty stomach;
- Tightness of the chest;
- Having trouble swallowing;
- Oversensitivity to sound;
- Feeling of depersonalization: 'I roam the streets and nothing seems real, including myself';
- Feeling short of breath;
- Feeling weak;
- Lack of energy;
- Dry mouth;
- Headaches.

Psychosomatic reactions to life events such as loss and trauma have been determined by a number of researchers (Lindeman, 1944, Parkes, 1972, Rudestam, 1977, Winn, 1981, Guy, 1982). Research on the evolution in the long run shows a steady decrease in depression and motor symptoms. Around the third year of grief, most symptoms disappear (Epstein et al., 1975).

Normal depression

The signs of a normal dejection after life events such as loss and trauma are reduced energy, reduced interests to complete apathy, limited concentration, limited emotional depth, sleep interruptions, feelings of emptiness and irritability (Rando, 1993). Dejected people are often treated for 'depression' without paying attention to their life events such as loss and trauma.

Attention for body signals

In every demand for help concerning life events such as loss and trauma, the body plays a direct or indirect role:

- The stressed employee, who is in the middle of a reorganization, complains about over-tiredness and headaches.
- The abused client (life events such as loss and trauma of the physical integrity) complains about sore body parts.
- The client who experiences tightness or even pain in the chest when discharging the pain (crying).
- The client who was raped (life events such as loss and trauma of sexual integrity) reacts in a jittery manner to physical approach.
- The client with parting anxiety who has relationship problems and talks about missing sexuality.

- The client with traumatic life events such as loss and trauma who cuts himself or herself (self-mutilation).
- The client who had a leg amputated after a car accident and now experiences phantom pains (pain in the missing body part).
- The client recovering from a heart attack (life events such as loss and trauma of trust in your own body).
- The client who has cancer and is very tired, and feels as if his own body has let him down.
- The traumatized client with sleeping problems.
- The client who uses psychopharmaceutic drugs (sleeping pills, sedatives and anti-depressants) and experiences some kind of buzz during the session.
- The client struggling with back problems as a sign of overstrain of the back, but also as a sign of psychological overstrain.
- The client who has a negative body image because he or she was born with a deformation or was maimed in an accident (burns, amputation, etc.).

In short, every client requires alertness and attention for the body if desired, even if it were only for a quick screening. As far as medical knowledge is needed, consulting a doctor is the right thing to do. Since social workers often deal with people who are ill or impaired on a daily basis, basic medical knowledge is indispensable for them as well. Social workers also play a role in the early diagnosis of illnesses. The book *Medische kennis voor hulpverleners* (*Medical Knowledge for Social Workers*; van Endt-Meijling, 2008) provides such information.

Muscle tension

The social worker paying attention to the body signals coming from the client is useful because clients very often suffer from physical tension complaints. That is why the social worker has insight in the tension levels of muscle tissue. The point of departure is that human tissue is a lot more elastic and plastic than is generally assumed. When a muscle is used normally, it contracts and then relaxes again, while the muscle gains force in doing so. A normal muscle can contract and relax whenever humans want it to. When tissue has sustained a certain injury, elasticity decreases in due course. This is the case for distortion due to an accident, because of abnormal emotional tension or because of the permanent state of tenseness which the client needs in order to compensate for a certain disruption in the body's balance. A muscle becomes stiff and rigid in order not to feel this anymore. This is a physical equivalent for the psychological defence mechanism. When such things happen frequently or in case of a very severe event, the muscle gets into a state of chronic tension. Life events such as loss and trauma affect the muscle's ability to react appropriately. Strain put on this muscle then becomes painful, because the muscle cannot appropriately process the strain, namely by yielding. Not taking into consideration the cases where tissue has been permanently altered due to an operation, there are four possible states for tissue (Schutz, 1975).

1   *Healthy and normal muscle tissue* can process high levels of strain without pain. The client is able to relax and contract his muscles at his own willing. This kind of tissue does not suffer from injury or blockings. So to speak, this tissue says: 'I relax whenever I'm asked to do so'.

2   *Lightly tense muscle tissue* experiences some strain, but when physical stress is applied from the outside and the client's awareness is focused on the pressure point, the client is able

to relax this muscle by will and process the strain without pain. This type of tissue has sustained light injury and has stiffened up to avoid repetition of that same injury. However, tension is so low that support, help and trust from an outsider suffice in enabling the client to relief the tension at his own will. So to speak, this tissue says: 'I will relax when you comfort me and help me'.

3 *Highly tense muscle tissue* is disabled due to an experience so frightening that it simply cannot be neutralized by supporting the muscle from the outside alone. The psychological and physical level interact. In this case, a combination of psychological support and physical pressure from outside may succeed in relieving the tension. Tension is a means of protection against fear, anger or sadness, and when treated physically, emotions will surface since they are no longer blocked. The wall behind which the client was hiding is broken down and the client's anxious attitude becomes visible. Good therapy may help him in processing his anxieties so that he no longer needs that barrier where he keeps his muscles so tense. So to speak, this tissue says: 'I will relax when you give me enough support and force me to relax at the same time'.

4 *Chronically tense muscle tissue* is so tense that it cannot be relaxed, not even with the strongest help from outside. This tissue still reacts so heavily to the trauma that it takes more than help and pressure from outside alone for the client to give up this state of permanent tension. A state of chronic tension has arisen in a muscle or entire muscle group, in order to block out a feeling from the client's consciousness. Whatever the client is trying to protect with this tension, psychotherapy or other help will most probably be needed in order to render the client's situation so safe and secure that he can let himself go and show his vulnerability. So to speak, this tissue only says: 'I refuse to relax'.

In tension levels 2 and 3 the social worker is advised to pay attention to the body to reduce stress, whereas referral is required in case of tension level 4 (depending on the competence level of the social worker) (see Figure 5.2).

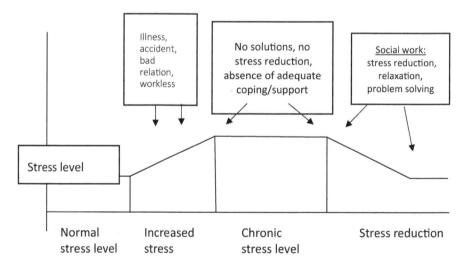

FIGURE 5.2 The intervention of a social worker results in stress reduction

5.2.3 Segment-reflex and psychosomatics

According to the holistic, biopsychosocial take on psychosocial assistance, body and mind are interconnected and form a unity. Changes in one segment cause a ripple effect in other segments. It is really a reaction to a stimulus from one tissue to another tissue, for example the coercion attitude in case of a renal colic. The complaint is: 'When I push here, it hurts there'. In medicine, this ripple effect is called 'segment-reflex'.

Two types of complaints are important for the bodywork method (Meijer, 2001): psychosomatic complaints and conversion complaints. A psychosomatic complaint indicates a psychosocial problem, while a conversion complaint is a sign of intrapsychic trauma.

Psychosomatic complaints

We speak of psychosomatic complaints when the client somatizes (experiences psychosocial unease which is displayed through physical complaints), while the doctor cannot diagnose any illness. A doctor draws the conclusion of a psychosomatic complaint:

- When there are somatic or functional complaints;
- When adequate research does not find any physical anomalies explaining the complaints;
- When he trusts that there are no such deviations (tension headaches are an example of a psychosomatic complaint).

Conversion complaints

Conversion complaints take their name from their nature: a subconscious, repressed psychological injury which is turned into the disruption of a physical functionality. Conversion complaints are pain complaints, blindness, deafness, paralysis, nausea, vomiting, dizziness or fainting. The complaints are the consequence of a traumatic event. Loss of functionality is very real and not an act. There are no simulants (who consciously have a goal for their so-called complaints) or hypochondriac clients (who claim to suffer from complaints they do not have, but also do not consciously pretend).

5.2.4 The chronically stressed body: psychoneuroimmunology

Physical stress may – as described earlier – trigger an unhealthy physical downward spiral. Persistent stress which remains unprocessed may eventually have unhealthy consequences. Longer-lasting psychosocial pressure points like unprocessed life events such as loss and trauma may lead to health issues or may aggravate already existent health issues. Stress then becomes unhealthy stress. Unhealthy stress is the result of a persistent imbalance between strain and bearing capacity. People with unhealthy stress will describe their stress situation more as a situation with negative consequences, which is not or inadequately suggestible, where all results are blocked, energy fades away, skills and competencies do not grow and mutual relations deteriorate.

Chronicity as a stress factor

The life events mentioned, such as loss and trauma-events and traumatic events, may become chronic due to all sorts of causes. An illness, for example, may be incurable. Life events such as loss and trauma may also be inadequately processed, causing the corresponding complaints to become chronic. All of these cases imply chronicity, which involves chronic tension. Below, chronicity is defined as customary in the context in which it occurs: biopsychosocial chronicity. Medical, psychological and social chronicity are defined as an illness:

- With a long course;
- With little prospect of full recovery;
- Often for the rest of one's life;
- With a high chance of progression: intensification of care;
- With a phased course: often variable, sometimes stable.

Weakened immune system due to persistent stress and problems

Psychoneuroimmunology has made decent progress over the last few years in terms of knowledge about the connection between the psychological, neurological and immune system. In the long run, chronic stress seems to weaken one's immune system (Davis et al., 2003). Persistent stress causes fewer defensive cells (leukocytes) to be released. All physiological processes are focused on action, a fight or flight reaction. The mechanisms which have a caring function are then put on the backburner.

When the body remains in the alarm phase for a longer time and thus produces fewer defensive cells, it causes health issues to arise. Examples of stress-related illnesses are cardiovascular diseases, disruptions in the digestive system or in the skeleton. Other possible consequences of chronic stress are tense muscles, fatigue, high blood pressure, migraine, a stomach ulcer or chronic diarrhoea. Chronic stress can damage nearly all body parts and bodily functions.

The steady drop erodes the hardest stone

How is the weakening of the immune system established? Stress research has discovered mechanisms explaining how long-lasting stress can lead to health issues. When stress persists for a long time, in other words when it becomes chronic, possible health issues must be taken into account (see Figure 5.3).

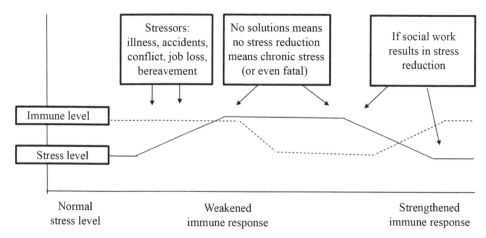

FIGURE 5.3 Chronic tension weakens the immune system; stress reduction by social work intervention empowers the immune system

As long as someone is able to fully recover before living life to the fullest again, there are no negative consequences for his or her functioning and health, no matter how hard a certain strain has been – work pressure, conflicts, fatigue (Krahn, 1993). Research shows, without exceptions, that effective support – meaning support which is also experienced as support by the involved person – has a positive effect on, for example the processing of life events such as loss and trauma (Silver and Wortman, 1980). A longitudinal study of employees' reactions to being fired after their companies were shut down showed that social support from partners, family members and friends relieved the pain coinciding with life events such as loss and trauma (Cobb and Kasl, 1977).

Higher risk of illnesses is the consequence of persistent stress: when someone experiences long-lasting and unhealthy stress, a downward unhealthy stress spiral is created. The client walks into a trap which cannot easily be escaped. The psychobiologic balance is disturbed more and more, causing psychological and psychosomatic complaints and pathophysiologic (pathogenic) processes to arise. On the psychological level, problems arise in terms of:

- Concentration: easily being distracted, not having any energy;
- Personal behaviour: overcontrol through pacing, fidgeting, being irritable, smoking and/ or drinking more, eating disorders;
- Personal thoughts: overcontrol through worrying, overthinking, puzzling;
- One's own body: overcontrol causing headaches, dizziness, stomach complaints, hyper-ventilation, nervous twitches, stuttering, shaking hands, sleeping problems.

Long-term processes of unhealthy stress are easily illustrated with the example of the thermo-stat and its role in the central heating system (Gaillard, 2003). The thermostat is a sensor which sends a signal to the central heating boiler: temperature in the living room is lower than the pre-set minimum. The boiler starts heating until the desired temperature in the living room is reached. This closed circuit is broken when someone leaves the window open. The heating boiler 'desperately' keeps working until the desired temperature is reached. A disruption in the regulation of all subconscious physical processes such as blood pressure and heart rate takes place in a similar way. When the sensor reads a value which is too high, the regulating centre will try everything to even out the pressure peak. This *will* happen automatically, unless our emotions or thought processes *overrule* these actions time after time. Chronic stress leads to a decreased sensitivity of pressure receptors (baroreceptors) in the carotid artery. This causes the regulating system to continuously calibrate using varying values, also causing the control values (e.g. while asleep and at the beginning of a workday) to be higher. Eventually it leads to chronically elevated blood pressure (hypertension). Elevated blood pressure which came about in such a way is very difficult to treat with medication because the problem does not lie in elevation, but in regulation. Administering medication may be interpreted as opening a window to lower the living room temperature. As long as the central processes interfere in the regulation (e.g. because someone feels threatened), help will not work. The help must focus on removing negative feelings and emotions, in combination with relaxation, but also on learning new coping strategies in order to deal with problems.

Previously we illustrated the harmful effect of persistent stress. The opposite effect is known as well: relaxation induced by a social worker may induce strengthening of one's immune sys-tem. When one's stress level is reduced, his or her physical immune system becomes stronger (see Figure 5.3). People seem to develop a stronger defence against illnesses and ailments when they relax. To put it briefly: people who find themselves in the wrong social situation are more susceptible to illnesses, but may also physically regenerate when their psychosocial problems are alleviated, for example by an effective social-work intervention.

Social workers working on alleviating problems and relaxation also indirectly help in recovering the immune system and thus the prevention of neglect and a higher quality of life.

5.3 History of the bodywork method

> Every man is a house with four rooms: a physical, a mental, a social and a spiritual room. Most of us are prone to spend most of their time in only one room, but as long as we do not go to another room once every day, even if it were just to air the place, we are incomplete.
>
> (Indian proverb)

In social work, the bodywork method focuses on tension signals coming from the client. Physical tension signals are experienced by the client himself or herself, such as tightness in the chest or stomach pains (direct signals). The social worker may also notice physical signals or changes during the session, for example a sweaty handshake, forehead beaded with sweat, red spots, a deflective body posture, frowning eyebrows and so forth (indirect signals). Indirect signals may be the physical expression of emotion or tension. The latter may have miscellaneous causes: life events such as loss and trauma, a conflict, a reprimand or a chronic disease. There is a good reason for the expression: 'What the mind represses, the body expresses'.

The social worker's primary aim in this is 'de-stressing'. One of several direct de-stressing methods is the bodywork method. A contraindication for the bodywork method is 'inadequate exclusion of medical causes'. It is very important for the social worker not to start 'doctoring' without having medical causes ruled out first.

The origin of the bodywork method is hard to trace. For centuries, oriental philosophies such as Zen, yoga and Sufi have been emphasizing the importance of care for one's body, the consequences for one's consciousness and the connection with stress. In the twentieth century it was the work of Wilhelm Reich, originally a student under Sigmund Freud, which stimulated Western mental health care's interest in the interaction between body and emotion. Two modern therapies which regard the relation between body and emotional stress are Fritz Perls's gestalt therapy (1996) and Alexander Lowen's bio-energetics therapy (1998). Both forms focus on increasing awareness about one's own body. In gestalt therapists' books, hundreds of exercises can be found to increase awareness about the body. In bio-energetics books, the separation between body and mind is removed through physical exercises which may bring up powerful emotions. In the latter sense, bio-energetic exercises are not suitable for social work practice. The aforementioned body-related approaches are collectively denominated as emotional bodywork (EB). The point of departure in EB is that emotions which cannot be expressed or experienced freely will attach to the body in the form of muscle tension. This may be observed in the contorted posture and exhaustion of energy. By doing body exercises, the client learns to become more conscious of his own body and things going on inside. This enables the client to free the body from tensions. Life energy can start flowing again. Paying attention to the client's body is emphasized too little in social work, which is mainly a 'talking profession'. Physical complaints and body signals were only given specific attention by social workers who had enjoyed additional training out of personal interest. For example, they had taken a course in the gestalt approach, bio-energetics or EB. In social work, the client's body is not regarded as a social worker's area of competence, but rather as the expertise of physiotherapists and doctors. Not surprisingly, only little attention is paid to the body in social work literature. In the 1960s, attention for working with the body grew during the second feminist wave. While working in the *Feministische Oefengroepen Radikale Therapie* (*Feminist Exercise Groups Radical Therapy*) or FORT-groups, apart from mental and emotional consciousness, the emphasis was also on physical consciousness by means of body exercises. Body posture and nutrition were broadly discussed, and all sorts of (then still regarded as alternative) exercises were performed in yoga and massage. A small number of social workers integrated these exercises into their work, however still off the record. Nowadays we see a more systematic integration of the physical aspect in social work, among other things the growing attention for *mindfulness*.

The blind spot

Since 1980, more and more social workers are being trained who, through their thesis, plead for more attention for the body in social work contact. Almost all of the social work students conclude that attention for the body is a blind spot in social work, and that a clearer vision (if any) must be developed on it in training programmes. They criticize the training which unilaterally pauses at the verbal aspect while thinking in dualistic terms (e.g. separation of mind and body). According to the students, methodology books should include more information about non-verbal communication and the importance of the physical condition in the anamnesis.

5.4 Goals

General goal

- Reducing or removing negative tensions in the body.

Specific goals

- Making the client more aware of his own body signals;
- Reducing the client's tension level;
- Letting the client take his body signals seriously;
- Helping the client to no longer physically contort;
- Encouraging the client to start exercising again (e.g. by going for a walk more frequently or by practicing sports).

5.5 Indications

- The client states suffering from physical stress complaints such as unpleasant, increased physical tension, headaches, stomach aches, fatigue and so on.
- The client exhibits noticeable body language (through changes in voice pitch, mimic or physical expression by turning away, shaking and/or red spots appearing in the neck or face).

- The client states noticing these physical changes himself or herself as well (e.g. strain, stiff muscles, nausea, more headaches, more stomach aches, queasiness and so on).
- The client asks attention for physical signals or complaints (e.g. psychosomatic complaints: 'my upper legs are so tense').

5.6 Contraindications

- Medical causes have inadequately been ruled out;
- The use of certain medication;
- The client does not wish to perform bodywork exercises during sessions.

5.7 Techniques

1 Self-touching technique
2 Relaxation technique
3 Breathing technique with visualization
4 Activation technique
5 Physical awareness technique
6 Body image technique
7 Biofeedback technique
8 Focus technique
9 Diary technique
10 Touching technique
11 Decontamination technique
12 SNARE technique
13 Scaling techniques (stress meter, energy meter)
14 Use of medication.

5.7.1 Self-touching technique

When the client indicates suffering from something in a certain part of the body, the social worker may ask the client to put his or her hand on that body part. With this intervention, the client learns how to pay attention to physical sensations, for example right before or after a pain discharge. An example: a client experienced terrible pains in the sternum after a car accident. However, there was no medical explanation. By means of the self-touching technique the client's bottled-up anxiety and grief come to the surface.

5.7.2 Relaxation technique

A second physical social work technique is working with relaxation exercises. Every individual has specific areas in the body where physical and emotional tension are tangible. Everyone has weak spots where sensations and complaints arise first in case of tension and emotion. Even physical illnesses may be activated by the stress of life events such as loss or trauma. Asthma attacks, migraines and numerous other diseases may also occur and aggravate under the influence of stress. As a social worker you can observe body signals through body language without the client actively talking about this. For one client, this tension may primarily be observed in the head, for another client in the stomach, and yet another client will suffer from emotional pain in the back or the sides. Related to the emotional pain of life events such as loss or trauma, this may be a physical parallel to emotional pain. Provided that body and mind are one, these signals are to be taken seriously by a social worker such as yourself. Without having to play doctor, specific attention for specific areas in the body may be a straight blessing. It is recommended, however, to verify with the client whether the physical complaints have already been medically examined.

The case of Mr. Stack

Mr. Stack was immediately admitted to hospital because of heart problems. Medically speaking, there didn't seem to be any problems. However, his heart had reportedly been 'broken' by the accumulation of losses and disappointments. The accumulated physical tension is reduced by means of relaxation exercises.

5.7.3 Breathing technique with visualization

The instruction goes as follows:
Sit down comfortably (sometimes lying down is preferred) with both feet on the ground and lay your arms down in a comfortable position. For example, rest your arms on your legs or on the chair's armrest. Close your eyes. Concentrate on your breathing. You can see your breathing as if it were the sea washing up the shore, pause, recession, pause, washing up again: inhale, pause, exhale, pause. Everyone has a different breathing rhythm, it happens automatically. Try following this rhythm without forcing it. Next, we will relax all parts in your body, working from the bottom up. Let's start with your feet. Tension flows away from your feet while exhaling . . . your left foot . . . your right foot . . . your left ankle . . . [and so on].

From the ankles you work your way to the top: lower legs, hip and pelvis area, bottom, lower back, belly, trunk, middle and upper back, chest, shoulders, upper arms, elbows, fore-arms, wrists, hands, fingers, neck, mouth, cheeks, nose, eyes, forehead, temples, ears, crown, hair and cranium. The client relaxes more and more parts of the body. When the client reaches the fingers, for example, the social worker indicates that tension is ebbing from his legs, arms and upper body (up to the neck). At given times, the social worker asks the client to breathe more deeply from the stomach. Upon exhalation, tension disappears from the legs, belly, trunk, arms and head. He concludes the relaxation exercise by telling the client to open his eyes again whenever he is ready.

Relaxation exercises can be found in *The Relaxation and Stress Reduction Workbook* (Davis et al., 2003). In order to record how the client feels before and after relaxation exercises, the social worker can use the tension gauge (see section 5.7.13).

5.7.4 Activation technique

The social worker informs the client – upon saying they exercise too little – on the importance of exercising and determines which sports and other types of exercising best suit the client. Together they look at the reasons for stopping or cutting down on exercising. The client is activated to gradually pick up sports and other types of exercising again. A form of biofeedback may be linked to this activation in order to measure and visualize progress in stamina (see section 5.7.7 and Table 1.2 Condition meter).

5.7.5 Physical awareness technique

The social worker lets the client perform exercises which increase one's physical awareness of the body (Davis et al., 2003). Two examples are internal and external awareness and body scan.

Internal and external awareness

The instruction goes as follows:

> First, focus your attention on the outside world. Start every sentence with: 'I am aware of ...' (e.g. 'I am aware of the sun shining at this moment and ...'). Now shift your focus to your body and physical perceptions and to your inner world (e.g. 'I am aware that my back hurts, that I am hungry'). Continue by switching between internal and external awareness.

When the client performs this exercise several times per day, at different moments whenever he finds the time, he will become more aware of the real distinction between his inner world and the outside world.

Body scan

The instruction goes as follows:

> Close your eyes. Think about every single part of your body. Start with your toes and ask yourself whether you are tense. As soon as you encounter a tense area, flex it a bit more so that you are more aware of it. Feel which muscles are tense. Then say to yourself: 'I am flexing my neck muscles. I am hurting myself. I am creating tension in my body'. Let it get through to you that all muscle tension is caused by yourself. In your thoughts, try to figure out which situation in your life causes tension and what you can do about it.

5.7.6 Body image technique

When the social worker notices that the client is sending signals of dissatisfaction with his body, he asks:

- What do you mean by that signal? (e.g. 'You say that your burns have deformed you – what do you mean by that?').
- What bothers you the most about that physical aspect?
- What do others see when looking at your body?
- To what degree does this physical aspect play a role in your life?
- What do you worry about specifically?
- Bring along some photographs from before the physical change.
- Look at your own body in the mirror while squinting and let the corresponding emotions or thoughts out.

By means of the cognitive method (see Chapter 11), the social worker tries to improve the client's way of thinking about his own body.

5.7.7 Biofeedback technique

If desired, the social worker can provide the client with feedback on bodily functions by measuring the client's heart rate. This may be done to activate the awareness of the client's physical condition or physical reactions to stress. Generally, biofeedback is used in impact studies or medical check-ups. Say, for example: 'Place your finger on your wrist and count your heartbeats for 15 seconds. By multiplying this number (e.g. 25) by 4, you get a heart rate reading (in this example 100 beats per minute [bpm]). While in rest, a normal heart rate would be 80 bpm'. In case of several measurements, you can draw up a heart rate curve showing its fluctuations. In case of abnormalities or worries about this, you refer the client to a doctor.

5.7.8 Focusing technique

The social worker sees to it that the client becomes more aware of physical perceptions: what is happening inside his body and what is this sensation connected to? Focusing was introduced by Eugene Gendlin (1999), a student under Carl Rogers. Gendlin understood that the social worker could teach people to listen to their body more, and could change their lives by doing so. The focus technique consists of six steps.

1 Making room for physical sensations. Example: 'Become aware of the signals in your body'.
2 Focusing on physical sensations which arise when encountering a problem. Example: 'What do you feel in your body when you think about the pressure point you just mentioned? Where in your body do you feel it?'
3 Finding a word, sentence or image describing the sensation.
4 Letting the client follow the sensation with his attention.
5 Ask questions such as: 'What is the worst about this feeling? What need does this sensation represent?'
6 Let the client understand a message which he recognizes. Example: 'I have to do something about this conflict, my body is protesting'.

Suitable forms of focusing, and playing games in the case of children, may be deployed to pay direct attention to the body or physical resistance. Many surveys point out that paying attention to the person behind the illness has a great influence on the progress of the illness itself, as do visualization techniques in cancer treatment and yoga techniques as part of one's rehabilitation after a heart attack.

5.7.9 Diary technique

The social worker gives the client homework: in a diary (see Figure 5.4), the client must write down the time when a stressful event occurs and the time when he notices a physical or emotional signal which could be related to the event. This provides insight into frequency, circumstances and effects. This is also called 'monitoring' or 'self-registration', which is why this technique is also called the 'monitoring technique'.

Stress diary: _____

Day: _____

Day of the week: _____

Time_____Stressful life event_____ Physical reactions_____

_____

_____

_____

_____

_____

_____

_____

_____

_____

_____

_____

_____

_____

FIGURE 5.4 Stress diary

The social worker asks the client to keep the diary for a few weeks. From the diary we deduce how certain stress situations may lead to unpredictable physical reactions. Confrontations with others may cause tensions in the stomach. Hastiness may result in narrowing blood vessels, causing irritability and headaches (Davis et al., 2003).

By means of this journal, the client gradually learns where muscle tension arises in the body. When he becomes aware of it, he can look for ways to relieve this tension, resulting in more energy and a better mood.

5.7.10 Touching technique

A touch may mean positive proximity to a client. Upon greeting and saying goodbye, people usually shake hands. Physical proximity may also be a form of therapeutic touch – touching without touching.

As a social worker, you yourself may also physically touch the client as a way of comforting him and on condition that it 'feels right' for both of you. Whether a touch feels right isn't always predictable. From your perspective, it requires you to be yourself and to be aware of your own physical signals as much as of the client's. In some social work situations, for example with young persons, physical contact may also occur while playing around and taking a child on your lap in order to comfort him. Physical contact in social work offers the ability to confirm and ratify one's personal and physical boundaries. For clients with a past of physical and sexual abuse or an abusive past, physical contact may be confronting and cause a lot of emotion. As a social worker, you are sensitive to signals of rejection and show all due respect for the client's boundaries. If the client agrees, this may also become subject of a conversation.

5.7.11 Decontamination technique

The social worker focuses attention on the part of the body which became physically or psychologically burdened ('psychologically contaminated') by an accident or a violent or abusive experience. He wonders what type of 'contamination' may have taken place and what the consequences are for the client.

The case of the washing compulsion

A woman had experienced her mother to have 'taken' her body away from her because of a physical disability. The mother always said: 'Don't you worry, *I* will take care of your body'. The social worker made the woman dig into the meaning of her washing compulsion (she compulsively washed her hands). The client found out that she 'wanted to be clean again' from the 'overcare' which was her mother's continuous meddling. Becoming aware of this psychological contamination and saying out loud 'I want to be free from you' had a cleansing effect. It had also caused her need to wash her hands to go away: her hands were freed from her mother's meddling.

5.7.12 SNARE technique

There is danger that people start living more unhealthily in times of crisis. As a guideline for a healthy lifestyle, you can sum up the SNARE factors:

S   no Smoking;
N   healthy Nutrition;
A   moderate with Alcohol;
R   Relaxation and Recovery;
E   sufficient Exercising (at least half an hour a day, moderately to intensively).

With this lifestyle programme, the client improves his or her own health. Not only do they deal with fixed habits, they also actively work towards changing their lifestyle. The result of it all is that they become healthier and more active. The SNARE factors have an influence on people's vitality and health. For each topic, the client is given concrete attention – in combination with aforementioned body techniques – in a positive and inviting way.

- Quitting smoking: what is the best way for the client to quickly cut down on smoking and eventually quit?
- Healthy nutrition: how can the client determine what healthy nutrition is and how it can be incorporated by making small changes? The healthy nutrition guideline advises consuming products from the five main categories on a daily basis: (1) bread, cereal products (rice, pasta, couscous), potatoes and legumes; (2) fruit and vegetable; (3) dairy, meat, fish, eggs and meat substitutes; (4) fats and oils; and (5) water.

- Less alcohol: how does the client become aware of his habit and how can he break free from his drinking pattern? The healthy nutrition guideline advises limiting consumption of alcoholic beverages to maximum one glass (adult women) or two glasses (adult men) per day.
- More relaxation: how can clients learn how to relax in a way that suits them best? People who experience stress often show compensational behaviour such as unhealthy nutrition, smoking or excessive alcohol consumption. Stress from work and stress from private life occur when there is an imbalance between situational demands and the individual's capacities and needs. It is important that clients are able to recover from their work and private life efforts. This can be achieved by relaxing by means of movies, books, poetry and other types of leisure activities.
- Keep on exercising: how can the client have fun while exercising again? Frequent physical activity has a positive influence on one's physical and mental condition. The advised 30 minutes of daily exercising need not be done in one go, but may also be divided into shorter periods, such as three periods of 10 minutes each.

5.7.13 Scaling techniques

Tension meter

When using the tension meter ('stress-o-meter'), the social worker asks the client to indicate the tension level he experiences at that very moment on a scale from 0 to 10 (see also section 1.3.2), with zero being no tension at all and 10 being maximum tension. For example, the social worker may ask: 'What was your tension level at the beginning of the session?' When noticing progress or decline, he asks the client to point out what is making the difference.

The tension meter contributes to the client becoming aware of his own tension fluctuations and is also a part of the impact study because the social worker can verify whether his interventions induce a reduction in the client's tension level. It is also an assessment instrument to determine whether existing pressure points are actively being dealt with or whether they are being avoided.

When using the tension gauge it is important to know that it may read a higher level at first, and indicate a lower tension level later on in the session (or in the week), when the client has already done a lot of hard work.

Energy meter

When using the energy meter, the social worker starts from the experienced energy level. He asks the client to score his energy level at that moment on a scale from 0 to 10, with 0 being no energy at all and 10 being the maximum energy level. For example, the social worker may ask: 'What was your energy level at the beginning of the session?' Next he observes whether there is progression or decline after which he asks the client to point out what is making the difference.

The energy meter contributes to the client becoming aware of his own energy fluctuations. It is also a part of impact research, because the social worker is able to verify whether his interventions induce an increase in the client's energy level. When using the energy gauge, it may be interesting to inform your client that the energy level may have low readings at first, and higher readings by the end of the session (or week) after the client has done a lot of hard work.

5.7.14 Use of medication

Lastly, it is important to inform with your client whether he is taking any medication. Medication may have such psychological side effects that it hampers an effective social work intervention.

The case of Mr. Stack

For a year, Mr. Stack used a powerful sleeping medicine which had the side effect of 'numbing one's feelings'. Upon agreement with his general practitioner, his prescription was cut back and Mr. Stack was instructed to no longer resist his sleeping problems, but to use that time to write down what went through his head and to find some distraction. This in combination with relaxation exercises seemed to reduce the sleeping problems very quickly.

5.8 Social work results

- The client is more aware of body signals.
- The client can more easily indicate the immediate cause for certain physical reactions.
- The client listens more closely to his body signals.
- The client is more relaxed.
- The client is satisfied with the bodywork method ('I feel lively and fit').

5.9 Evidence

No known research has been conducted to investigate the bodywork method in social work. It is a known fact, however, that running and jogging act as antidepressants (Bosscher, 1996). A psychoneuroimmunology research also shows that relaxation exercises have a strengthening effect on our immune systems (Ader et al., 2001).

5.10 Pitfalls

- Insufficiently ruling out medical causes;
- Lingering on body signals for too long and neglecting timely consultation of a physiotherapist or haptonomist;
- Initiating physical fixation (somatization) as if the stress situation were only of a physical origin;
- Forcing your own interpretations of body signals upon the client;
- Forcing your own style of physical contact (with examples from your own family experience) upon the client, as if it were the only right way;
- Being infatuated with the client and sexualizing physical contact;
- Engaging in unacceptable physical contact;
- Making misplaced remarks about the client's body (e.g. trying to cheer up the client by making positive remarks about the body, which the social worker finds repulsive himself).

5.11 Summary and questions

In this chapter we described the physical survival response when life events such as loss and trauma have a life-threatening effect on the client. This may have physical (violence), psychological (trauma) or social (resignation) causes. The following question was answered: what can the bodywork method do to relieve physical stress?

First we described how physical stress arises and what may be the consequences of unprocessed life events such as loss and trauma. In conclusion we described how the bodywork method contributes to increased physical (and mental and social) peace.

In the next chapter we proceed to a description of the situation of clients who struggle with practical-material consequences: how do I practically and materially survive life events such as loss and trauma?

Questions

1 Do you recognize situations of physical survival where your own life was at stake, for example life events such as loss and trauma?
2 How does *your* body react to stressful situations?
3 What seems to help you in these situations, and what doesn't?
4 What makes people start doing exactly the things that are unhealthy for them when they find themselves in an unhealthy stressful situation?
5 What causes people to avoid giving their bodies the attention it needs?
6 What do you have to offer in paying attention to body signals coming from the client?

6

PRACTICAL-MATERIAL METHOD

I lurched from one crisis to the next. On top of which I had a lot of money issues. Got hooked on alcohol. I filled the emptiness with a void. This made me so restless that I could only give half my attention to the tasks at hand.

Helping clients with money problems, housing and employment is very supportive.

Questions

This chapter addresses the following questions:

- How does practical-material stress take place?
- What is meant by the 'problem-solving cycle'?
- What practical-material method can contribute to the deployment of the client's own power to reduce physical stress?

6.1 Introduction

This chapter describes the practical-material survival response looking at the following: When can the client's situation be called threatening in the practical-material sense? When do practical-material bottlenecks deliver stress because the practical needs are not met or not enough?

This question is answered: what can be offered by the body method to provide more calmness in the practical-material stress component?

First there is an indication of what we mean by the term 'practical-material stress', followed by a description on how to deal with this practical-tangible threat: practical-material coping. After this a description is made on how the practical-material method contributes to more mental and physical rest.

The practical-material method focuses on disentangling practical and procedural knots in the areas of housing, money and provisions, in order to reduce its burdens. This involves thinking along with the client, providing a helping hand or bringing the client in contact with a content expert in a particular field. The practical method contributes to positive practical-material coping.

The case of Mr. Stack

Mr. Stack has numerous practical problems: the company that was responsible for the shovelling accident of the second son, is not willing to compensate the damage. Years of legal battle demanded strong juridical and practical support. The remuneration of Mr. Stack's therapy costs raised concerns, but a conversation with the employer brought answers.

6.1.1 Practical-material stress

What is practical-physical stress and how can it be reduced? Practical-material stress happens when there is a need to solve problems (desired situation) but in reality it has not been solved yet (actual situation). As result, we don't enjoy life so much anymore.

There are many issues that need to be settled because of the actual impact of a life event. In case of a loved one's death, getting professional help might be considered such as for organizing the funeral, the death announcement, inheritance issues, and so on. Also other life events might cause a lot of paperwork and organization too, such as with divorce and dismissal. Labour of grief also means 'doing work' in the literal sense of the word. It can happen that people are solely focused on organizational tasks and controlling practicalities during loss situations. But it also happens that the plethora of unfinished organizational stuff in addition to the already existing stress of the life event causes a lot of physical stress.

In the growing complexity of society it can happen that a client is completely unable to solve practical and material problems, for example, money, housing or food and drink. Especially if there are insufficient coping skills present ('how do I cope with this?'). This creates a downward spiral. Practical representation of interests gives the client a better livelihood.

6.1.2 Conceptual definition and elucidation

The practical-material method focuses on reducing tensions due to clients' problems in managing their practical business. The method entails making an inventory of all the practical problems and possible solutions as well as a stepwise reduction of the material problem areas. Material problems involve questions and problems concerning rights, provisions and legal obligations. The practical-material method helps persons solve their practical-material problems and fulfil their needs, which contributes to reducing clients' stress levels.

Elucidation

Clients feel greatly supported by practical assistance. One of my former students reported that she had become homeless in her second year as a general social worker, as the service where she worked had suffered bankruptcy. She said:

> Now I really feel what it's like to lose your job and what kind of practical issues my clients were talking about.

Persons with financial problems often encounter problems in other areas as well, such as housing, employment and leisure activities. In addition, they may also struggle with identity problems, loneliness, and relationship and family problems. Social workers first establish priority issues for the help programme, known as *integral debt support*. They can employ services that specialize in specific sub-areas of housing, employment or finance. Situations differ across countries. In industrialized countries, we often see a patchwork of specialized agencies. Every social worker has a social map (overview of community services in a certain region) of the many local services that provide material support. Apart from social services, there are municipal credit banks, building societies and organizations for employment and labour market integration. Some services employ social workers; others use professionals who are specialized in debt support.

The social worker helps the client with solutions in multiple problem areas. For this the 7 steps of the problem-solving cycle are useful. Table 6.1 summarizes the steps of the problem-solving cycle and the present necessities and the role of the social worker for each step. It is clear that several problem areas call for a combination of methods: for example, the cognitive method (how realistic does the client think?), social network method (how much support is given to the client from the local network?), the narrative method (how much space does the client experience for meaning making?) and the case management method (how can different professionals work together with the client situation?).

TABLE 6.1 Problem-solving checklist: step-by-step approach to practical stress

Problem solving in 7 steps	Need of stress reduction step by step	Role of the social worker in problem solving
1. *Trigger*: is reliable, false or incomplete information available on the cause of the problem?	Need realistic information from the environment	Helping, honest and complete coverage in information
2. *Problem definition*: is the interpretation of the external and internal informational signals realistic?	Need realistic interpretation of the external information and inner reactions	Helping realistic interpretation of the informational message and called on all physical and emotional reactions (personal failure, guilt, shame, hallucination/dream and concentration problems)

(Continued)

TABLE 6.1 (Continued)

Problem solving in 7 steps	Need of stress reduction step by step	Role of the social worker in problem solving
3. *Goal setting*: can the client move from a victim perspective to a director's perspective?	Need for helping perspectives, for meaning and recording life event in life event, help give language to the shift from identity 1.0 to identity 2.0	What is your future your perspective? From 'Why me?' to 'Why not me?'
4. *Brainstorming* about possible scenarios: how to convert needs into wishes?	Need to brainstorm how to fulfil 'What can I do?' What options are there for the impact of life events to be in control?	
5. *Decision making*: are you able to choose an alternative?	Need for a decision	Helping realistic decisions: what makes you doubt? What do you need to get out of a dilemma?
6. *Action*: are you able to convert your decision into action?	Need for action, assertive behaviour	Helping behavioural actions: take practical steps, practice skills
7. *Review*: what is the result? Attained goals?	Need for review whether the goals have been achieved (in full); decrease/increase in quality of life (QoL)	Helping self-reflection: successful action; adjusting goals; increase the QoL

6.1.3 Debts

The social worker will identify which problems have priority in social work contact. This is called integrated debt management – assuming a dominant money problem.

The following kind of debts can be distinguished (de Greef, 1992):

- Survival debts are the result of a structurally low income.
- Compensation debts occur when a household compensates a deficit by purchasing luxury articles, expensive holidays and so forth.
- Adaptation debts occur when households do not (or are unable to) adapt to a changed financial situation due to dismissal, illness, divorce or death of a partner.
- Overextensions of credit are the result of households spending too much money beyond their means.

Broadly speaking, there are three forms of debt support (von den Hoff, 2004):

1   *Debt management* involves a strategy of considering the debtor's financial options and making a proposal for an instalment plan to (partially) pay off the debt. The debtor has to pay back a certain percentage of the outstanding payment. If creditors agree to this proposal, the parties have reached an amicable settlement.

2   *Debt restructuring* is quite similar to debt management. The only difference is that financiers make the money directly available, for which clients need to save money for a period of 3 years to pay off the total amount of debt.

3   *Budget help* involves learning new spending behaviours. Clients receive social work in how to plan their expenses and how to save money (see section 6.6.5).

6.2   History of the practical-material method

Dating to 1899, the practical-material method was established in the early days of social work in poor urban areas. In those days, social work consisted of a combination of practical philanthropy and community work. The first generation of social workers assisted the poor by providing improved housing, employment and money management. Material and immaterial support were linked together in ways that were later considered unacceptable. From this point on, we will further elaborate on the history of Dutch relief for the poor. A general description on relief for the poor would not do justice to the differences across countries. Before World War II, relief for the poor was perceived as a phenomenon consisting of both 'physical' and 'spiritual' elements, now referred to as material and immaterial problems (Engbersen & Jansen, 1991). According to Adriani (1932), poor relief workers were to thoroughly investigate clients' individual conditions to determine the cause of poverty:

> Scrutinising the needy person's personal situation would certainly always involve a certain extent of blaming. Persons in financial need were fundamentally distrusted. '*Poverty*' was always inextricably linked to '*guilt*'.

Whenever possible, financial need would be related to non-financial issues. Financial support was always given in concert with spiritually or morally uplifting aid. When needy persons received church aid, it meant that their poverty could be associated with sinfulness. The only remedy was conversion. Those helping the needy were fundamentally distrustful of those in need. In practice, the poor were consequently subjected to intense scrutiny to blame them for their own predicament. After World War II, it became more and more difficult to link financial support to moral 'uplifting' or 'elevation'. One of the main reasons was the increasingly important role of government authorities in delivering financial support.

According to van Loo (1981), in 1955 church and private institutions only made up 3% of the total care for the poor. It took about 20 years after the war to officially separate religious and financial care. As late as 1965, the separation became institutionalized by the introduction of the Dutch Assistance Act, (*ABW, Algemene Bijstandswet*). This Act came into effect on January 1, 1965, and was considered a welcome change to the Poor Relief Act from 1912. A totally new terminology was created, including 'social security', 'social security entitlement', 'clients', 'minimum income', 'social services' and 'authorities'. Old terms were consequently abandoned, such as 'the poor', 'cases', 'poor relief' and 'committees for the poor', 'charitas' and 'deaconate'. The ABW was designed to disconnect material support from poor relief and charity.

Former Dutch Secretary for Social Affairs Marga Klompé reported:

> Mr. Chairman, my aim was to create a law that would allow every citizen to appeal for support, while holding their heads up high and feeling assured of their sense of freedom, preserving their sense of dignity and humanity. Those were my principles.

The Act marks the transition in social thinking in terms of 'charity' to 'social feeling'. In the old way of thinking, financial support was perceived as a favour, arbitrariness, humiliation and charity. It was a time when relief for the poor went together with stigmatization. The new way of thinking was marked by social feelings.

In the explanatory memorandum to the ABW, the change in social thinking was stated explicitly by the politician proposing the law:

> Individual expressions of charity have been replaced by expressions of social justice by the government.

In other words, the Dutch Assistance Act signified the end to the stigmatization of financial help (Engbersen & Jansen, 1991). Financial help and spiritual guidance were now officially disconnected. The care delivery services – government authorities – no longer perceived clients with fundamental distrust but rather with fundamental trust. Nevertheless, the old sense of charity still lives on, considering that the ABW does not objectify the minimum sustenance (Engbersen & Jansen, 1991). The social assistance officer assesses 'the necessary cost of living' of each applicant. This is what the ABW calls the individualization principle. Determining the amount of benefit is an activity whose success depends on those conducting the assessment. One person (the officer) has to assist the other (person entitled to benefit) to the best of his ability. The good thing about the introduction of the ABW is that it has separated financial help from social work. The government is responsible for financial assistance, while non-government bodies and church organizations provide social work.

Debt support has been part of our society since the 1970s. Debts emanate from important social-cultural and macro-economic developments (von den Hoff, 2004). In the post-war years, the average Dutch person was distinguished as being thrifty, diligent and modest. In the decades that followed the level of prosperity rose, and more and more citizens were seeking ways to benefit from this development as much as possible. Market participants readily responded to the changing situation. A good example of these developments is the creation of consumptive credit, which was a rare phenomenon in the 1950s. In the 1980s, the normal thing to do was to borrow money to buy a new car. At the same time, people were feeling less and less morally obligated to pay back the amount borrowed. The 1980s also saw mounting pressure on the much-praised Dutch system of social security. In times of high unemployment, people had to live on a low income and at the same time, they wished to share in the prosperity. It is not hard to imagine that debts became the logical result of this situation.

Work procedures have become gradually professionalized under the auspices of the Dutch Credit Bank Association (von den Hoff, 2004). This association compiled the Code of Conduct for Debt Management, which is widely used and perceived as reliable by a large number of creditors. According to this code of conduct, debtors are to live on 94% of the minimum sustenance level for a period of 3 years and devote the rest of their income to paying off their debts. Creditors are offered a repayment settlement, based on a percentage of the total repayment sum. Preferential creditors – receiving preferential help as stipulated by law – are given a double percentage of the total sum due. If all creditors agree to this proposal, they will have reached an 'amicable settlement'. In the late 1980s, the Mijnssen Committee ruled that a legal settlement was needed to offer debtors a way out, in case an amicable settlement would prove unachievable.

Politicians supported the proposal, convinced that the increase in debt problems were causing too much damage to society. Nearly 12 years later, on December 1, 1998, the Debt

Restructuring Act for Natural Persons (*WSNP, Wet Schuldsanering Natuurlijke Personen*) came into force. The WSNP served as a forceful measure for reaching amicable settlements. The idea behind this legislation was that debtors would eventually go for their money, and, though reluctantly, agree to an amicable settlement. It should be noted that there was an important difference between the WSNP and an amicable settlement. Implementation of a WSNP measure involved payment priority to the cost of debt restructuring, including legal expenses and the cost of appointing an administrator. If all goes by WSNP rules, debtors are given a clean slate after a period of 3 years.

6.3 Goals

General goal

- Reducing or eliminating negative tension caused by practical-material problems, such as financial, housing and work problems.

Specific goals

- Alleviating or solving clients' practical problems and removing practical obstacles;
- Alleviating or solving clients' material problems and removing material obstacles.

6.4 Indications

- Signs of negative tension because of clients' practical and material problems;
- A practical-material problem or obstacle, such as lack of shelter, housing problems, unemployment, money problems and parenting problems;
- Requesting information.

6.5 Contraindications

- Clients' refusal of practical or material assistance;
- Clients' demands are too specialized.

6.6 Techniques

1. Inventory technique
2. Information technique
3. Advising technique
4. Advocacy technique
5. Budgeting technique
6. Job search support technique
7. Referral technique.

6.6.1 Inventory technique

Social workers directly address clients' practical-material problems. There is no need to focus on underlying causes at all times. After drawing up an inventory of the problems at hand, it is examined whether there are any further interconnected issues that need addressing. For instance, a demand for money support may be linked to a demand for care concerning tensions in the home situation (a demand for care that is more difficult to formulate). A demand for care concerning parenting may be related to disagreement between spouses. Dealing with housing problems may also involve health-related issues that need addressing.

6.6.2 Information technique

Social workers encourage clients' information-seeking behaviour. Clients are assisted in obtaining all relevant information on their practical problems, concerning money, housing, employment and parenting. These information sources include local councils, libraries, local services and the internet. Social workers may also make information available from their own media centre, such as brochures, folders, books and audio-visual materials. An informative handout explaining rules and regulations can also be quite helpful.

6.6.3 Advising technique

Social workers are confronted with questions such as 'What am I supposed to do?' and 'What is your advice for me?' Questions for advice are directed at solutions and decisions (Witte, 1997). A potential pitfall is to advise clients based on limited client information. Working along the lines of the problem-solving cycle helps social workers avoid these pitfalls:

1 Cause, signs (for instance, from medical social work: My wife died due to medical malpractice);
2 Problem definition (for instance, you can only find peace when the doctor admits his mistake);
3 Defining targets (for instance, it is your wish that the doctor apologizes);
4 Brainstorming about solutions (for instance, you can go see (a) the doctor, (b) the complaints officer, (c) the complaints committee or (d) the medical disciplinary board).
5 Deciding on the solution (for instance, interview with the doctor);
6 Implementing the decision (for instance, the social worker calls the doctor on behalf of the client);
7 Evaluating the outcome (for instance, unsatisfactory interview; client wishes to see the complaints officer).

A new cycle is utilized to deal with the remaining problems (see also section 11.3.1). The social worker assesses the place of the request for advice in the problem-solving cycle. Advice given to clients too soon may adversely affect their interests. In addition, some clients would be better advised to acquire problem-solving skills, rather than receiving concrete advice. For instance, 'Could you help me find a house, because I can no longer stay with my parents?' The social worker points out that he can only offer his advice after the client has explained his reasons for moving out. In addition, it should become clear what kind of situation has led to the client's request for assistance.

6.6.4 Advocacy technique

Social workers serve individual clients' interests by cooperating with a range of service organizations and relevant persons. Individual client advocacy may consist of a telephone call or a supportive letter directed to services, such as housing agencies, social services or the Dutch

Centre for Employment and Income (*Centrale Organisatie Werk en Inkomen, CWI*). In consultation with their clients, social workers organize support for clients' daily routine activities (ADL) and daily household activities (HDL). Buddy support can be given to the chronically or terminally ill. For instance, buddies may assist clients who are unable to dress or wash themselves or go shopping on their own. Volunteer agencies organize daily support for clients at fixed times. Home care for the terminally ill can be provided by a wide range of buddy services that are attuned to clients' wishes. Social workers start by making an inventory of clients' housing needs and wishes. Their role is to act on behalf of their clients in order to fulfil their needs. It concerns clients of diverse ages who need (new) housing, due to leaving the parental home, death of a loved one, domestic violence or following a hospital admission. Clients are referred to other expert services if it concerns complex housing problems (see section 6.6.7).

6.6.5 Budgeting technique

The social worker proposes to get a clear picture of the financial situation. An inventory is made of the client's expenses, income and debts. If clients are facing relatively simple money problems, a debt-structuring plan can be devised to help clear the amount of debt. Social workers and clients work together on making a careful analysis of the debts (see Table 6.2). An inventory is drawn up of the cost items, expected bills, financial capacity per item and amount of debt per month. The social worker advises clients to pay off large bills and debts. They need help on how to cut down expenditure or increase income, or both. The purchase of goods by credit card or on credit must be stopped immediately. In addition, goods should only be purchased that are essentially needed. Outstanding bills that cannot be paid should not be ignored. Never advise clients to neglect an outstanding balance and advise them to explain the situation to the creditor. Once creditors understand the client's situation and feel convinced that that the debt will be settled, they are mostly willing to adjust the terms of payment. Some creditors are prepared to spread the payment over a longer period and agree to a lower interest rate. Clients should not avoid contact with debt collection agencies. An open discussion should be stimulated, since these agencies do all they can to facilitate payment by the debtors. Creditors will appreciate debtors' genuine intention to pay off their debt, even if it involves paying off by small monthly payments. Should repayment not be effected, collection agencies will proceed to legally confiscate clients' possessions. Clients can be advised to sell unnecessary possessions and make the proceeds available to pay off their debts. Budgeting support may also involve advising clients to put their money in envelopes. All envelopes are

TABLE 6.2 Budget plan

Cost items	Expected bills	Realistic monthly instalment	Debt per month
Loans			
Credit card payments			
Rent			
Energy, phone bill, etc.			
Car expenses			
Insurance cost			
Other cost items			

Total debt per month

to be kept in a box, including an envelope for high expenditure items. Clients facing complex debt problems are signposted to specialized services for debt support, such as city banks, credit unions or other debt support organizations (see section 6.6.7).

6.6.6 Job search support technique

When dealing with unemployment or practical work-related issues, an inventory is first drawn up of what actions clients themselves have undertaken so far. A cost–benefit analysis of these actions is also made. It concerns clients who seek employment after leaving school, removal from active duty, discharge or because of reintegration needs. A strength–weakness analysis of the clients' qualities is drawn up to help clients become aware of their own work-related wishes. Clients are also stimulated to explore the job market systematically. Clients with complex reintegration problems are referred to specialized agencies for recruitment and job reintegration (see section 6.6.7).

6.6.7 Referral technique

Social workers always try to direct clients' questions to the right service provider. A referral is an intervention aimed at matching clients with the service providers they need. Referral is indicated when social workers find themselves unable to offer the support required. In the light of their expert knowledge of the social map, social workers emphasize the need for clients to seek contact with the new care provider. Clients may feel ambivalent about the referral. Even though the referral to the new care provider may seem logical, clients may feel anxious and hesitant about taking this new step. Social workers help clients communicate their ambivalence and correct any misunderstandings concerning the new service provider. For some clients a referral causes hardly any stress at all, whereas others experience a great deal of stress. Careful social work towards accepting the new care delivery service is essential for those who hesitate. Social workers offer clients maximum assistance to ensure successful contact between clients and care providers. Clients receive the name, address and phone number of the new care delivery service and, if needed, detailed instructions of how to get there. In addition, clients are informed of the contact person of the organization. In a letter addressed to the new organization, the social worker formulates clients' needs for support and request for employing the agency's expert service. Clients are always present when the social worker establishes contact by phone. After speaking with the contact person and explaining the need for referral, the phone is handed over so that clients themselves can make arrangements with the agency for a first interview. Clients are instructed to ask the right questions and be assertive during these first contacts with the new organization.

6.7 Social work results

- Practical problems have been alleviated or solved and obstacles removed.
- Material problems have been alleviated or solved and obstacles removed.

6.8 Evidence

Limited research has been conducted on the relation between debts and health problems. A range of studies do point out that problematic debts may result in prolonged stress.

A combination of the following stress factors may explain the occurrence of prolonged stress (von den Hoff, 2004).

- Any phone call may be from a pushy creditor;
- Any parcel post may contain legal warrants and notices;
- Every time the doorbell rings, it may be the debt collector;
- The electricity supply or telephone can be cut off at any given time;
- Expenses for three meals a day, clothes for the children, pocket money, school money, school trips, birthday presents and contributions to medical expenses and legal support;
- The tendency to pay off one debt and create another, be overly cautious in money matters and pay the creditor who is most forceful;
- Worrying about the day to come;
- Struggling hard not to show what is going on;
- Cutbacks in health care by the government, resulting in persons (certainly those in debt) neglecting their health problems.

Part of evaluating the Debt Restructuring Act for Natural Persons (WSNP) included a study on indebted households. Those participating in amicable settlements showed the following characteristics (Jungmann, 2006).

- A mean age of 37; 60% of the debtors varied between the ages of 27 and 45.
- More than half the debtors (53%) were men.
- Nearly half were single person households: 22% were single parent families, 10% were two-person households without children and 19% of two-parent households with children.
- Of the debtors under study, 61% received benefit support, 37% had employment income.
- Regarding household income, 70% lived on an income lower than €900 a month and 33% lived on an income lower than €680 a month.
- The average amount of debt was just below €10,000, distributed over seven creditors.
- The majority of the creditors were financial institutions (16%), tax authorities (9%), building societies (7%), energy companies and health insurance companies (both 6%). The amount of debt owed to financial institutions, 39%, by far exceeded the amount of debt owed to other creditors.

Creditors have appeared to find WSNP arrangements more appealing than amicable settlements. As a result, the success rate of amicable settlements has been decreasing since the introduction of the WSNP, instead of increasing. A striking development is that employers are employing corporate services to offer workers debt support. So far, there have been no scientific data supporting the effectiveness of the practical-material method.

Homeless

Van Laere et al. (2009) found that the recently homeless in Amsterdam fit the overall profile of the homeless population in Amsterdam: single (Dutch) men, around 40 years, with a mix of financial debts, addiction, mental and/or physical health problems. Contacts with services were fragmented and did not prevent homelessness. For homelessness prevention, systematic and outreach social medical care before and during homelessness should be provided. To improve homelessness prevention practice, we met with recently homeless adults to explore their pathways into homelessness, problems and service use, before and after becoming homeless.

There is little evidence on good practice in caring for homeless people in the medical literature. It has been reported that for homeless people life expectancy averages around 45 years, and that lack of access to health care services has too often proved a barrier to recovery, and, as a result, contributes to a downward spiral of deteriorating health and premature death. Therefore, public services strategies should include homelessness prevention. To prevent and reduce homelessness, strategies that address the general population and/or a targeted population could include housing benefits, welfare benefits, supplementary security income, supportive services for impaired or disabled individuals, programmes to ameliorate domestic conflicts, programmes to prevent evictions, discharge planning for people being released from institutions and (outreach) care programmes for homeless populations.

Household financial debt in the United States has risen dramatically in recent years. While there is evidence that debt is associated with adverse psychological health, its relationship with other health outcomes is relatively unknown. Sweet et al. (2013) investigated the associations of multiple indices of financial debt with psychological and general health outcomes among 8,400 young adult respondents from the National Longitudinal Study of Adolescent Health (Add Health). The findings show that reporting high financial debt relative to available assets is associated with higher perceived stress and depression, worse self-reported general health, and higher diastolic blood pressure. These associations remain significant when controlling for prior socioeconomic status, psychological and physical health, and other demographic factors. The results suggest that debt is an important socioeconomic determinant of health that should be explored further in social epidemiology research.

6.9 Pitfall

- Being overzealous in controlling clients' business in order to save them.

6.10 Summary and questions

In this chapter, the practical-physical survival response was described: when are the practical-material events life-threatening? And the question was answered: what can the practical-material method do to provide calmness in the practical-material stress component?

It was explained what the term 'practical-material survival' means, then described how to deal with this practical-material threat: practical-material coping. Then it was described how the practical-material method contributes to a more practical-material calmness or peace.

Questions

1 Do you recognize situations in which there was a lack of bed-bread-bath?
2 Which survival reactions do you recognize in the situation of flight, poverty, war?
3 What kind of support should a social network and connected services give in such circumstances?
4 What do you have to offer in the practical-material support of people who feel grief?

7

TRAUMA-WORK METHOD

Questions

This chapter addresses the following questions:

- How does traumatic stress arise in clients?
- What is meant by survival in case of trauma?
- How can the trauma-work method contribute to reducing traumatic stress and restoring one's strength?

7.1 Introduction

From previous chapters we have learned that clients can experience physical and practical-material stress. We also described the outlines of how to methodically help clients to 'survive' in both physical and social ways.

In this chapter we describe how we can help clients in traumatic life events. As it happens there are situations, apart from missing the person one has lost, that can be experienced as being threatening because of the circumstances in which they took place, as is the case for accidents and suicide.

First we define what is meant by the notion 'trauma survival'. Then we describe how to deal with this traumatic threat: trauma coping. Subsequently we illustrate how the trauma-work method contributes to mental (and physical and social) peace. In conclusion we summarize the chapter. In section 27.3.1 we further explore Post Traumatic Stress Disorder (PTSD) where we cover in this chapter Post Traumatic Stress Reactions (PTSR).

Trauma relief focuses on taking first care of clients who have experienced an exceptional and striking event. This form of care may take place directly after an acute extreme situation, but also several years later when at the time of the traumatic event, poor or even no care was provided. Trauma work method is not the same as trauma therapy.

The case of Mr. Stack

We saw that Mr. Stack was looking for support amid the chaos he finds himself in. He states that he was never capable of processing his first son's stillbirth. The same thing goes for his second son becoming disabled at age 4 because of a shovelling accident in front of the house. Of all seven drawers of Mr. Stack's personal filing cabinet (PFC; see Chapter 5), there are two drawers which may be an indication for an extreme experience:

(–) his first son's stillbirth;
(–) his second son becoming disabled.

By using to the safety-net technique, the company doctor and loss social worker actively spread a 'psychological' safety net by reaching out to Mr. Stack. A controlled reconstruction is performed: practically and perceptively, he is given the opportunity to gather the facts about the traumatic circumstances in losing his first son (stillbirth) and his second son becoming disabled (shovelling accident). Keeping a view over your own situation is an important cognitive support. Putting sensory details into words and telling the story make that the client is given some breathing space, both literally and figuratively speaking. Eventually, factual storytelling contributes to the implementation of these 'trauma chapters' into one's mental life story. Using the check-up technique, the involved person is checked up on during contact moments. A pitfall for relief workers may be that 'checking up' is confused with 'pulling up' the involved person. No one profits from obtrusive contacts with a relief worker who decides that 'It's good for you to talk now'. Such a patronizing attitude in trauma relief is counterproductive. Trauma relief contributes to positive trauma coping.

7.2 Traumatic stress

> Losing her was something I could deal with, but the murderous way in which she died. . . . *That* I cannot process.
>
> (sister-in-law of a raped and murdered woman)

In traumatic loss we speak of an unexpected and violent way in which the loss occurred, as is the case for accidents, homicide, suicide and sexual violence. Violent loss experiences are 'burnt into one's senses', so to speak. Because of their alarming nature they induce reactions such as: 'How will I survive this?,' 'This is too violent' or 'No words can explain this'. In these cases, recognizing traumatic reactions is of great importance: avoidance, frequent reliving and increased vigilance are normal reactions to an abnormal situation (see section 7.2.3). When the need for relief after a traumatic experience is not fulfilled, we speak of traumatic stress.

7.2.1 Traumatic loss situations

It is important for professionals and fellow citizens to be familiar with the tangle of processing actions a traumatic loss experience entails. Traumatic losses entail grief processing *and* shock processing. In grief processing we distinguish three components: the RSB-components of Realization, Saying goodbye and Building memories and a new life. In trauma processing, three additional components can be distinguished: the FAI-components of Frequent reliving, Avoidance and Increased vigilance. All three processing components are part of a post-traumatic stress reaction (PTSR) (see Table 7.1).

For many shocking loss experiences, it is unclear how many of the persons involved develop complications in the form of post-traumatic stress disorder (PTSD). A PTSR turns into PTSD in due course. It has been calculated that for severe traffic accidents, 1 in 5 victims develops a disorder. On a yearly basis, about 10,000 to 20,000 people are struggling with PTSD as a direct consequence of a traffic accident. Research shows that, by frequently being confronted with shocking events alone, 7% of police officers suffer from complete PTSD and 32% suffer from partial PTSD (Carlier et al., 1994).

Inventorying research states that 60.7% of men and 51.2% of women experience at least one potentially traumatic event in their lives (Javidi & Yadollahie, 2012). The occurrence of post-traumatic stress experiences varies from 0.3% in China up to 6.1% in New Zealand. The average PTSD percentage for the general population is 4%, and this rate is significantly higher in women than in men; the rate after rape is 80%; the rate for victims of violent crimes is 19%–75%; direct victims of disasters show a 30%–40% rate; for rescue workers the percentage is 10%–20%; for police officers, firefighters and other emergency services the rate varies from 6% to 32%. Rescue workers and aid providers show a rate varying from 5% to 32%. We find the highest PTSD rates in search and emergency workers (25%), firefighters (21%) and workers without any training on how to deal with disasters. War is one of the most intense stressors. In the army, the rates for PTSD, depression, addiction and anxiety-related disorders are relatively high. Even more frequently than in adults, PTSD occurs in children who were abused or who have survived natural disasters.

Apart from general knowledge about shock processing, it is important for social workers to have insight in differences between several types of shocking loss events. It is unfeasible to describe all traumatic life events. In the following sections we further discuss traumas caused by traffic accidents, homicide, suicide, disasters, wars and other physically, psychologically and sexually violent experiences.

TABLE 7.1 The processing actions in traumatic losses

Processing type	Topic	Process components	
1 Grief processing	Missing a loved one	R	Realization
		S	Saying goodbye
		B	Building
2 Trauma processing	Unsettling circumstances	F	Frequent reliving
		A	Avoidance
		I	Increased vigilance
3 Processing of traumatic losses	Missing and circumstances	Combination of grief processing (missing) and traumatic processing (circumstances)	

Traffic accidents

In traffic accidents we focus on physical injury and material damage. Though, traffic accidents have several other consequences as well. For example, psychological complaints may arise due to brain injury (post-concussion syndrome). Post-concussion syndrome involves complaints such as headaches, dizziness, fatigue, touchiness, emotional instability, anxiety, memory disturbances, concentration problems and slowness.

Homicide

The range of consequences following the murder of a loved one is underestimated too often. For the people involved it is an act of violence combining suffering and sorrow with a feeling of injustice, distrust and helplessness. In the Netherlands, there is an association for mutual support from the relatives of violence victims: *Niet Dood als een Dodo* (*Not Dead like a Dodo*). In the United States, a therapy programme was developed by Redmond (1989).

Suicide

In suicide cases, relatives characteristically experience the 'present absence' of the dead person. Although a person has committed suicide, their presence is still strongly felt. The unexpectedness, hastiness and often gruesome circumstances of suicide may thoroughly complicate the processing of it all. Remaining relatives can often only guess at motives and experience strong feelings of rejection caused by the suicidal person. Emotions of fear for 'heredity' may arise. Relatives may experience a strong sense of guilt, or feel great anger and shame because they were left alone. There may also be less social support when suicide is considered an unmentionable loss, a taboo. For mutual support among relatives, there are regional support groups which are sometimes guided by prevention departments of mental health care institutions.

Disasters

Disasters such as plane crashes, train accidents and large-scale industrial calamities trigger a contingency plan in which care initiation and coordination must be implemented. Disasters may lead to strong and permanent disagreements among friends and families about who is to blame and what should have happened. When compared to other areas, more social conflicts and distrust is recorded in areas where disasters have occurred. Feelings of vulnerability, survival guilt and anger often lead to finding a scapegoat: when the community does not unify against an enemy from outside, or when they do not support a common goal, victims will turn on each other.

War

Very often war situations cause transgenerational traumatization, that is long-term damage for second, third and further generations to come after those who have witnessed the terrors of war. The symptoms of PTSD fall short to describe the consequences of war. Some survivors suffer from concentration camp syndrome: anxiety, fading of emotions, depression, dysphoria, somatic complaints, psychosomatic complaints, cognitive disorders, memory disorders and sleeping disorders are the most frequent complaints.

Strikingly, the children who take great care of their traumatized parents are rarely satisfied with their own efforts. Extreme idolization or extreme rejection of the traumatized parent often occurs as well. Psychotherapists consider both types of behaviour to be two sides of the same coin: insufficient psychological autonomy in relation to the parents. Furthermore, addiction and relation problems occur relatively frequently in later generations.

Other loss situations

We have already discussed several traumatic loss situations. However, there are also clients who are weighed down with (profession-related) traumatic experiences without losing a loved one, for example when having witnessed a severe traffic accident, a violent attack and so forth. When we mention traumatic experiences in the next section, both categories of clients are implied: those who have witnessed a traumatic event and those who have experienced traumatic loss.

7.2.2 Characteristics of a traumatic experience

Many people deal with shocking or traumatic experiences in their lives. A traumatic experience may lead to complications when there is no timely care, or even no care at all. The client is deeply affected, unsettled, and needs primary care. In this context, 'trauma' is defined as a psychological injury. Even though the term 'trauma' is often used in this sense, a more correct term would be 'psychological trauma', because in many cases physical trauma is not the only type of trauma. Of course it is possible for someone to sustain both physical and psychological trauma, for example after a traffic accident.

Traumatic experiences often involve:

- An extreme, exceptional event: an event which unexpectedly takes place and strongly differs from everyday events;
- An event related to the line between life and death (or when there was a threat);
- An event evoking extreme powerlessness;
- An event leaving sensory traces in the form of images, sounds, touch, smell and taste (sensory perception);
- An event which personally affects the involved individual: physically, psychologically or both;
- An event having an unsettling effect on one's professional and private life: the client is completely upset, confused, disconcerted, put out;
- An event after which the involved individual shows one or more of the 17 post-traumatic stress reactions (see Table 7.2);
- A certain degree of dissociation: no emotions, someone behaves like a zombie, or a certain period is erased from one's memory;
- A triggering effect causing specific stimuli to re-evoke (parts of) the shocking experience (e.g. touching brings up the sexual assault in one's mind).

Although it doesn't have to be a characteristic of every trauma incident, many trauma clients get insensitive reactions from their surroundings, causing secondary victimization due to *undercare* (insufficient or wrong care) or *overcare* (wrong and misplaced care) (see Chapter 1).

TABLE 7.2 Post-traumatic stress reactions (PTSR): The FAI components

Three types of reactions	Stress reactions	
Frequent reliving	1	Recurrent and intrusive memories
	2	Repeatedly having bad dreams
	3	Acting or feeling as if the trauma happens again (e.g. looking for cover)
	4	Intense grief when reminiscing
Avoidance	5	Avoiding relevant thoughts or emotions
	6	Avoiding relevant activities or situations
	7	Memory loss (partial or complete) about trauma
	8	Decreased interest
	9	More solitary, withdrawn behaviour
	10	Not expressing emotions, being more indifferent
	11	Being more depressed (in this case the feeling of having a limited future)
Increased vigilance	12	Having trouble sleeping
	13	Irritation, anger outbursts
	14	Concentration problems
	15	Being on edge
	16	Excessive shock reactions
	17	Functional physical complaints (perspiring when remembering disaster)

Sensational media attention and delayed legal or insurance cases are examples of unnecessarily mistaken help by one's surroundings, causing secondary victimization.

7.2.3 Post-traumatic stress reactions (PTSR)

In case of traumatic (loss) experiences, our natural protective armour appears not to be resistant against the extremeness of the event. Every individual has a psychological armour – also called the 'illusion of invulnerability' – which mean that, every day, we do not worry about the tragic and cruel aspects of our existence. This armour is broken after a shocking event. The person involved feels vulnerable and anxious, and is thrown off guard. The life of this person is (temporarily) thrown upside down. The loss social worker recognizes a traumatized client by the way they leave a sensitive impression, and is obviously worrying about the trauma. There are two types of traumatization: type 1 and type 2. In type 1 traumatization there is a once-only traumatization (e.g. a traffic accident). In type 2 traumatization we speak of multiple traumatization (e.g. sexual abuse or war), and dissociation disorders often occur. For both types, trauma relief is recommended. For type 2 traumatization, it is necessary to subsequently refer the client to a trauma psychologist. The trauma-work method is the social work method assisting people during the first crisis after a type 1 traumatic experience.

Many requests for help are related to similar situations the clients have been confronted with. Normal reaction to abnormal events – such as homicide, suicide, violence, sexual abuse – are summarized by the acronym FAI: frequent reliving, avoidance and increased vigilance. Being shocked by abnormal events is a normal reaction. After a shocking event, we call this a post-traumatic stress reaction. The psychiatric classification system DSM-5 distinguishes 17

PTSR symptoms. These reactions to abnormal events are regarded as being normal during the first period of time. In due course – some say after 3 months, others after 6 months or more – PTSD is diagnosed when six complaints from the FAI components persist. People experiencing these persistent complaints qualify for more intensive forms of help. We speak of full PTSD when in the long run, complaints keep occurring in a certain combination of the FAI components:

- Frequent reliving: at least one complaint;
- Avoidance: at least three complaints;
- Increased vigilance: at least two complaints.

When complaints do occur, but not in this combination, we speak of partial PTSD. When there was a drastic incident involving extreme powerlessness and acute disruption where complaints persist over a longer period in time, we speak of complicated processing which can be treated very well.

7.2.4 Survival reactions and traumatization

The following *fight–flight–freeze* reactions are distinguished in traumatization.

Flight (avoidance)

Losing a person, animal, object or symbol can be traumatizing when circumstances are especially frightening. Defence keeps fear out of your consciousness at first instance. This normal reaction acts as an automatic emergency brake stopping the full intensity of physical and emotional pains from getting directly through to you. This defence mechanism is not part of your conscious perception, as it occurs completely involuntary.

The best metaphor to describe how defence mechanisms work is that of wound healing: an unarguable and unimpressionable autonomic biological process. Defence mechanisms are reaction patterns of emotions, thoughts and behaviour to the perception of an intra-psychological threat. In a positive processing process, one's defence decreases and consciousness increases. Eventually you fully acknowledge the actual impact of traumatization. This is part of the task of raising awareness in case of loss (see Chapter 2).

Many loss-related defence mechanisms are described in literature, such as numbness, denial, searching, bargaining and dissociation. We look further into two defence mechanisms: numbness and dissociation.

Numbness

Numbness may vary in terms of intensity. The intensity is dependent upon the possible acuteness of loss and the possibility to prepare oneself for loss (Freud, 1925; Shontz and Fink, 1961; Shontz, 1965; Hertz, 1981; Rando, 1984). Numbness is the defence mechanism which lasts the shortest, though it is very intense and is remembered for a long time afterwards.

Reactions of individuals who were confronted with loss show that numbness is inevitable, that it is a natural way of adapting to loss. It is imperative to mobilize emotional resilience in this new and grave situation. On a behavioural level, this reaction becomes visible by shutting out the world.

Dissociation

Dissociation is the most direct and practically automatic defence mechanism against the extremely threatening and overwhelming nature of a shocking loss experience. The individual can dissociate the shock in roughly two ways. The first way is completely: someone mentally escapes the shocking event by imagining being somewhere else. This causes another part of one's personality to experience the event, and afterwards the personal consciousness suffers from complete loss of memory about the shocking experience. The second way is called 'partial dissociation'. Partial dissociation is when the individual witnesses the things happening to him, but from a distance. Emotions and physical perception are dissociated during this experience, not the visual and auditory images. Afterwards there is only memory loss in terms of emotions and sensations (van der Hart, 1991).

Dissociation hinders the integration of loss events into one's life and is often diagnosed in people who have witnessed terrible tragedies such as train or airplane disasters, earthquakes and especially wars. It also occurs in different types of trauma, such as sexual and other types of child abuse, ill-help and neglect.

One's defence system is armed to take on the first grief task: becoming aware of the facts about loss and acknowledging the impact of loss. When the defence mechanism is active, the individual temporarily functions on autopilot, so to speak, causing him to distort the reality of loss and deny the facts. Still, temporary defence is a form of survival which prevents you from decompensating, which is why it is considered unwise trying to break through this defence. It is better to allow someone the time to let loss get through to him at his own pace.

In case of persistent defence we speak of negative coping with loss. When someone keeps avoiding things related to the traumatic loss, or even starts mummifying them (by leaving a room or certain things intact and building the entire life around it), the first task to raise awareness is blocked. We see the same blockade in people taking refuge in substance abuse as a means of artificial numbness or deflection of the loss reality.

The following forms of avoidance can be distinguished (see also Table 7.2):

- Avoiding relevant thoughts or emotions: doing your best or forcing yourself not to think about the event;
- Avoiding relevant activities or situations: avoiding people or things which remind you of the event (e.g. shops, restaurants, movie theatres, airports, parties);
- Memory loss (full or partial) about trauma: not being able to remember the event; you feel as if the event never really happened;
- Reduced interest: taking less joy or interest in things you used to like (e.g. hobbies, leisure activities): since the event you go out less with other people;
- Withdrawn behaviour, expressing less emotion: you feel less involved in other people's lives; you have lost your sense of emotion, so to speak;
- Being more indifferent and depressed (feeling as if your future is limited): you think more pessimistically about the future (e.g. 'I don't expect all too much from life, my work or relationships with people');
- Taking refuge in substance abuse (alcohol, drugs, medication), gambling, work (workaholic), drifting.

Fight (increased vigilance)

A 'fight reaction' after a traumatic situation is caused by the state of increased vigilance people find themselves in. Some fight reactions:

- Excessive shock reactions and being on edge: you have become more nervous and are scared more easily (e.g. by an unexpected sound); you feel less at ease or even unsafe;
- Sleeping problems: you experience difficulties sleeping (e.g. having a hard time falling asleep, or waking up in the middle of the night and not being able to get back to sleep);
- Irritation, anger outbursts: you tend to lose your temper more often and more easily become angry;
- Concentration problems: you find it difficult to concentrate on something (book or paper, work);
- Memory problems: you have become more forgetful;
- Functional physical complaints: when thinking of the events, you feel yourself physically deteriorating (chest pains, tremors, perspiration, nausea, headaches).

Freeze and unfreeze

Usually the survival reaction is characterized by the *fight–flight* response, though it would be more complete to also discuss the *freeze* reaction in traumatization. A freeze reaction occurs before or after the fight or flight reaction. Freeze behaviour is a reaction which is usually seen in prey animals. When a prey is caught and finds itself under complete domination of the predator, it can try to escape by playing dead so that the predator will cease the attack. Freeze reactions are characterized by changes in blood pressure, crouching, increased heart rate, perspiring, or asphyxiation symptoms.

The victims of Robert M.

In the sexual abuse scandal in Amsterdam where 27-year-old Robert M. sexually abused 83 children aged 0 to 4, many children were diagnosed to have had freeze reactions. The offender carefully selected his victims based on their age: they were too young to autonomously tell their story, but they did show freeze reactions: the stony face, the psychosomatic reactions. Fighting or fleeing was not possible for these young children. On April 26, 2003, Robert M. was sentenced to 19 years in prison and civil commitment with compulsory admission.

Experience shows that the freeze can be breached in unguarded moments and that unfreezing and corresponding reliving reactions are possible. All sorts of reliving reactions are observable in unfreeze moments:

- Recurrent and intrusive memories: you often think back to the event, even if you do not want to, and sometimes images from the event come back to you;

- Repeatedly having bad dreams: you repeatedly dream about the event, and sometimes wake up screaming or bathed in sweat;
- Acting or feeling as if the trauma happens again (e.g. looking for cover): you feel as if you are reliving the event or certain moments;
- Intense grief when remembering: you feel bad (sad, angry, afraid) or are upset when the radio, television, newspaper, people or situations remind you of the event.

7.3 History of the trauma-work method

A client who has experienced one or more extreme events may not be able to deal with it adequately, or may not be able to deal with it at all. Avoidance occurs very often in these cases. Even though avoidance initially is a normal reaction to an abnormal event, it may have a counterproductive effect when it persists. Frequent reliving is normal at first, but continuous frequent reliving is no longer normal in the long run. The same goes for increased vigilance: it is normal at first, but persistent increased vigilance is not.

The first step towards adequate trauma coping is the grief social worker orientating the client. The next step is letting the client experience the trauma at his own pace, and in a monitored environment. Referral to one of the many types of trauma therapy may be a final step and a good alternative for adequately learning to deal with the trauma.

The trauma-work method aims at providing relief for clients experiencing a crisis after a traumatic experience. The method stimulates recovery of the client's stability and sense of safety. In that way the trauma-work method encourages the client's adequate trauma coping. In this method we assume that a client receiving timely trauma relief support is less at risk for complications such as PTSD.

For civilians who experience accidents and crimes, for several years now there have been victim support centres where voluntary workers and case managers provide primary practical and mental support (http://www.victimsupport.org.uk). The Dutch victim support organization (SHN) is deployed more and more frequently in large-scale disasters as well, for example after the Bijlmer disaster in 1992 when an airplane crashed into two apartment buildings, the 2000 firework disaster in Enschede and the 2001 pub fire during New Year's Eve in Volendam. Together with social work organizations, the SHN provides first support on a practical, material and personal level. The lesson learned from the Bijlmer disaster was that there was a hiatus within the victim services for information and advice. That is why an information and advice centre was established in Enschede where social workers from the entire region took turns in providing support. Also, more and more general social work institutions are assigned as disaster institutions by the government, meaning that they can be deployed in case of small- or large-scale disasters. 'Crisis aid' is most in line of the trauma-work definition: intervening in the client's urgent crisis situation. Providing aid after a disaster requires a specific skill set (Berendsen, 2003).

The origin of the trauma-work method dates back to World War II. Not surprisingly, the realization that people need trauma relief came during wartime. Wars make people more at risk of witnessing or experiencing multiple shocking events. When not experiencing them, they are often witnesses. In many countries social work institutions were providing support to World War II victims. Afterwards social work was also used for all kinds of traumatizing situations on both large and small scales, such as war and disaster situations, airplane crashes, tsunami, nuclear disasters, flooding and volcanic eruptions, but also domestic violence, traffic accidents and sexual violence.

Of course, apart from practical support, victims need trauma relief as well. In some cases victims never received such support until many years later, after which the social worker provided this support. Quite evidently, the social worker would refer clients to a trauma psychologist when they needed trauma therapy. Generally, World War II veterans never received any type of support and would struggle with all kinds of trauma complications for years to come.

Meanwhile, aftercare for military men returning from a mission has improved. Nowadays, by default, soldiers get a so-called psychosocial debriefing when returning from a mission abroad. The debriefing is a personal review to determine whether or not aftercare is needed. Additionally, when bad news must be brought to a soldier's family, the Ministry of Defence's corporate social workers are deployed to fulfil the task. Defence's corporate social worker is also responsible for aftercare. The need for trauma-relief work is also acknowledged in other trauma-prone sectors such as police forces, fire departments, emergency medical technicians and nurses and in medicine. Trauma-work teams help their colleagues in processing the first shock. Corporate social workers are very often added to the relief-work team or are the first instance trauma-work teams may refer to. Social workers also play an important role in the picture line-up, particularly after airplane disasters. The picture technique is further explained in Chapter 11.

7.4 Goals

General goal

- Reducing and removing negative tension linked to the traumatization.

Specific goals

- Giving the client better mental and physical stability;
- Letting the client find (cognitive) control over his own life again;
- Reducing the FAI components: frequent reliving, avoidance, increased vigilance.

7.5 Indications

- The client experiences an actual, recent traumatic event.
- The client is struggling with a traumatic event from the past.

7.6 Contraindications

- Physical or psychological impotence of the client;
- The client displays inadequately stable or uninhibited behaviour;
- There is a type 2 traumatization (multi-traumatization);
- The client is suffering from PTSD (trauma complications);
- The client does not want support.

7.7 Techniques

1 Trauma intake technique
2 Stabilization technique
3 Director technique

4 Reconstruction technique (factual level, perceptive level)
5 Follow-up technique
6 Indicated techniques from other methods.

7.7.1 Trauma intake technique

After the firework disaster in Enschede on May 13, 2000, a condensed intake form was developed by the Social Welfare Centre Enschede-Haaksbergen. This shortened version of the intake form can be used in the acute phase after a disaster (see Figure 7.1).

7.7.2 Stabilization technique

The loss social worker proposes to look for a quiet and undisturbed room where the client feels safe. When the client is very upset and/or confused, the loss social worker actively takes charge in taking the client to this room. It is determined what the traumatized client needs most. For example, after an explosion all of the witnesses are invited to gather at a local pub. They do this to investigate whether anybody else must be informed about the event. Witnesses are also taken care of with a cup of coffee, tea and something to eat. By means of securing the relief location, the rules of trauma relief are stated (confidentiality, informality, equal participation). Going over these rules provides structure and control.

7.7.3 Director technique

The loss social worker starts with the client's needs and desires. He asks the client what he needs after a certain incident ('don't drag, but check'). It is very important to tell the client that the event may be accompanied by loss of control, and that he decides for himself what will happen during trauma relief: he has control over what happens. That way the client becomes the director in his own situation and is given control over how to deal with the event. The entire story is worked through again in a way the client determines. The client is the director during the trauma-work sessions and the loss social worker is in charge of the 'final editing'.

Name: _____

Address: _____

Phone number: _____

Birth date: _____

Name of social worker: _____

Date and location of social work appointment (SWA): _____

Length of time for SWA: _____

Exposure to the disaster: _____

Physical wounds/health impact: _____

Lost loved ones/animals/goods: _____

Referred by (name, person, institute): _____

Stressors: _____

Advice/actions: _____

Appointments/referrals: _____

FIGURE 7.1 Intake form for the acute phase after a disaster

7.7.4 Reconstruction technique

At first, all of the facts are structured, after which the perceptions are arranged, unless the client needs something else.

Factual level

The social worker lets the client draw up a factual reconstruction of what happened. This detailed reconstruction regards all facts which are relevant for the involved person: from before the incident to directly or even longer after. It is taken into account that the client may be missing some fragments, which will probably come back to him later. Overview of the facts provides cognitive control: in his mind, the client reorganizes what happened, creating order from chaos. Questions about the facts may arise and may even be presented to other involved colleagues and/or instances in a later stage.

Perceptive level

The social worker lets the client reconstruct how he experienced the incident. This detailed reconstruction regards all perceptions which are relevant for the involved person: from before the incident to directly or even longer after. It is taken into account that the client may be missing some fragments, which will probably come back to him later. Reconstructing perceptions provides the client with a sense of order and awareness. Overtones on the event may also arise in the form of sadness, anger or fear. Eventually the client may come to peace, even when many perceptions alternate in short periods of time.

7.7.5 Follow-up technique

At the end of help, the social worker proposes to make a new appointment to check up on the client after a while. This is a way for the social worker to spread a fitting net around the client. If the client denies this appointment, it is enough for the social worker to propose a check-up by telephone anytime later. Actively offering support and follow-up support acknowledges the client's status as a victim.

7.7.6 Indicated techniques from other methods

Of course a loss social worker will deploy other techniques when indications point in that direction. He opts for social work techniques when 'why me' questions arise or when there are many problems to be dealt with. He uses the cathartic method in case of emotional discharge, the cognitive method when the client needs information, the bodywork method in case of physical tensions, the ritual work method when there is the need for a ritual providing closure (see Chapter 10) and so on.

7.8 Social work results

- The client is mentally or physically more at ease.
- The client is in a decreased state of vigilance.

- The client experiences fewer uncontrolled relivings.
- The client shows less avoidance behaviour.

7.9 Evidence

There are no scientific data from research on the trauma-work method in social work. Debriefing exhausted police officers after the Bijlmer disaster seemed to do more harm than good in the long run (Carlier et al., 1995). Officers appeared to be suffering from trauma complications even more than their colleagues who did not get any support. Researchers say that this effect is due to lacking willingness of police officers to take aftercare *after* trauma support, while it was needed all the while. Researchers also point out that the technique which was used, the Critical Incident Stress Debriefing (CISD) technique, focused too strongly on emotional ventilation rather than focusing more on cognitive control. CISD was developed as a fast and effective form of group trauma support (van der Velden, 1997).

A trauma-support programme for children showed that post-traumatic complaints had decreased significantly in children from the trauma project during the last meeting (Eland et al., 2000). However, the children's complaints also appeared to decrease without any intervention. Because there was no control group, researchers could not determine whether complaints disappeared more quickly because of the programme. Children seemed to have picked up the thread in life again, did not feel tense or afraid anymore, were able to sleep again and could talk about the event without too many problems. Shocking events which the children in the trauma-support programme had witnessed include violence by parents or others, being the victim of violence, being the victim of abuse with physical injury, one-off or repeated sexual abuse, sudden loss of a parent, arrest of the mother, a sister being burned and a car accident.

Initial research on loss and potentially traumatic events has been dominated by either a psychopathological approach emphasizing individual dysfunction or an event approach emphasizing average differences between exposed and nonexposed groups (Bonanno, 2011). Researchers consider the limitations of these approaches and review more recent research that has focused on the heterogeneity of outcomes following aversive events. The review of research showed that resilience is not the result of a few dominant factors, but rather that there are multiple independent predictors of resilient outcomes.

7.10 Pitfalls

- The social worker is pushy and 'drags things out of the client' instead of 'checking up on the client'.
- The social worker quits when the client gets angry or in case of other emotions.

7.11 Summary and questions

This chapter described how a traumatic experience brings about a survival response. Sometimes there are life events which have a traumatizing effect and are thus experienced as being threatening, as is the case for accidents and suicide. The trauma-work method may provide mental (and physical) relief by normalizing and reconstructing as a social worker 'the normal reactions to traumatic incidents'.

First we defined the terms 'trauma' and 'survival after a traumatic experience'. Subsequently we described how to deal with different types of traumatizing, threatening situations. We also pointed out some situations which may have a traumatizing effect. Special attention was paid to violent situations, after which we described how the trauma-work method may contribute to increased mental (and physical and social) relief.

In section 27.3.1 we address complicated reactions (PTSD) to traumatic incidents.

Questions

1   Do you recognize examples of traumatization?
2   How do you recognize traumatic stress (FAI components)?
3   Which examples of trauma support do you know, and how do they work?

PART IV

Three affection-oriented methods

'All you need is love'.

Part IV will describe what the role of the social worker is when the client instinctively is looking for affection in a natural way: such as seeking for attention, belonging or love. How can a social worker help mobilize the clients own power for the purpose of developing an affective balance?

The following three affection-directed methods are discussed to optimally help to fulfil the need for emotional cleansing of the client:

- The cathartic method helps to fulfil the need for emotional release (Chapter 8).
- The expression method helps to fulfil the need for creative expression (Chapter 9).
- The ritual method helps to fulfil the need for finishing things in a ritual way (Chapter 10).

Emotional expression contributes to making the most of life (optimal Quality of Life). How can a social worker help deploy the affective power of the client to address internal barriers to emotional ties?

Chapter 8 describes the role of the social worker with emotional discharge. What emotions are evoked with the loss of a loved one(s) or with other situations of loss and how can the emotional cathartic method offer closeness to reduce emotional stress?

After this, the role of the social worker in creative expression is being described in Chapter 9.

What can the expression method offer to reduce creative-expressive stress? Finally, Chapter 10 talks about the role of the social worker in saying farewell in a dignified way. The ritual method can help reduce stress connected to saying goodbye by mobilizing the emotional power of the client.

8

CATHARTIC METHOD

Talking about pain is not the same as the release of that pain.
Sometimes 'talking *about*' pain can even mean avoiding true catharsis.

(de Mönnink, 2015)

Questions

This chapter addresses the following questions:

- What is the role of the affection brain in life events?
- What causes emotional stress in clients?
- How can the cathartic method help reduce emotional stress and restore strength?

8.1 Introduction

In this chapter the role of the social worker is described when emotions are released. What emotions are evoked during the loss of loved ones?

First, the function of emotional release in a loss situation is described. After this, it is made clear how the affection brain operates during the regulation of emotions (see Figure 24.2). Then it is outlined how the cathartic method can contribute to reducing emotional stress. Finally, a summary is made.

The case of Mr. Stack

Twenty years later, Mr. Stack is still walking around with a prescription in his wallet. The general practitioner had asked to be paid 'cash in hand' for the prescribed medication. This caused Mr. Stack lot of pain. Although Mr. Stack felt a lot of anger, he could not release it. His plan to visit the doctor with whom he was angry was strongly discouraged by his environment. His close friends were afraid of Mr. Stack because he was harbouring a lot of disinhibited aggression.

Through the cathartic method, Mr. Stack was invited to work on his anger with the 'empty chair technique'. The supervised way of 'addressing the internal aggression' in the social work room in a non-damaging way was a relief for him. After detailed preparation Mr. Stack took the step and contacted the former general practitioner. All possible scenarios were taken in account to prepare for every possible reaction in a confrontation with the doctor and how the client was going to deal with the situation. The case was dismissed with an apology from the doctor after it was talked over in a mutually satisfying way.

8.2 The affection brain regulates attachment

> There are so many different kinds of grief; I am not going to begin to mention them all. I am only going to mention one, separation and divorce. It's not the cutting that hurts so much, but to be cut off.
>
> (Vasalis, 1954)

During life events such as loss, emotional pain is being brought to the surface. It hurts to be left, to lose love, care and protection. When we are faced with life events our affection brain is triggered. The affection brain regulates our emotional ties, our mutual affection, the attachment and detachment from loved ones, but also our creative power, our creativity. Our affection brain (see Figure 24.2) is also referred to as our 'limbic brain', 'mammalian brain' or 'emotional brain'. Brain scientists often speak of the 'emotional brain' because this is the part of the brain that regulates our emotions. The regions that are involved in the affection brain are the hypothalamus, the amygdala, the hippocampus, the olfactory bulb and the cingulate cortex.

8.2.1 Terminology

The term 'affection brain' is preferable to the 'emotional brain' for two reasons. Emotions are not isolated ('I feel happy or I feel sad') but they have a relational context ('I feel something for you' or 'I felt so much for you'). The term 'emotional brain' suggests that there is a brain that regulates all emotion, while it's actually multiple 'brains' that are cooperating in the regulation of emotions; fear, for example is well regulated in the affection brain as well as in the survival brain.

8.2.2 Oxytocin

From an evolutionary perspective the affection brain is younger than the survival brain, but just like the survival brain it is instinctive of nature. Every person has instinctive need for affection, belonging, love relationships. In short, everyone has emotional needs. Our affection brain takes care of finding and maintaining interpersonal contact. That is an innate, primary motivating principle that works for life. From birth on, our emotional bonds, connections with important others, are vital. Infants give signals by crying: 'come closer, help me in my need for food, warmth and love'. If that closeness is given, physical and mental peace is created. If not, anxiety and disorganized attachment is created. So we build our lives on safe and secure attachment relationships. The bonding hormone oxytocin plays a positive role in the development of these emotional ties. Oxytocin is created by people who have a positive mutual contact, such as eye contact, touching, cuddling and making love. A high level of oxytocin is associated with a sense of confidence and belonging. The underlying mechanism is most likely that oxytocin is a stress reducer (Neumann et al., 2000). Oxytocin inhibits the activity in the right part of the amygdala, a portion of the brain that is involved in emotional responses. In a confrontation with fearful and angry faces oxytocin takes care of weakening the amygdala response, thus facilitating positive social interaction (Domes et al., 2007). The higher the oxytocin levels are, the more resistance to stress and addiction a person will have, and the body also recharges faster. Anxiety is more easily suppressed, or felt less. At the same time oxytocin also causes people to behave more aggressively towards people from a competitive group.

8.2.3 Attachment

Connection is deeply embedded in our brain. It is possible to influence the affection brain system so that positive emotional relationships get a chance with people who are unhappy in their relationship. Developing more intimacy, security, and trust is based on learning to deal with separation, pain and life events. This creates a safe harbour for a lasting love relationship. Sue Johnson, relationship therapist and relationship researcher, shows based on brain research how to feel love (love sense) and how people can develop the ability to build long-term relationships (Johnson et al., 2013). Love turns out to be a wise prescription for survival. The need for affection is in its important instinctive need. Mature love is an example of attachment such as also exists between a parent and a child. Emotional interaction with a partner provides a buffer against stress and makes us stronger in confronting the challenges in life. Touch and intimacy stimulates mirror neurons, which help us to 'read' the signals from the partner and respond to them. A good relationship is the best recipe for happiness and good health, and those without secure attachment relationship usually live shorter lives.

8.2.4 Seven affective systems

Our emotions not only play an important role in making connections, but also in detachment processes. Upon being left because of, for example, a divorce, death or dismissal, the same kind of emotions are evoked. These emotions can be explained, because it 'hurts' to lose a beloved other or someone else. It evokes a scale of emotions such as sadness, fear or anger. But these emotions in life events can also be understood as an attempt to get back close again.

There are seven distinct affective systems (Panksepp, 2010):

- The search system regulates search behaviour for necessary survival sources.
- The anger system is turned when freedom is limited by others, escalated by having angry outbursts.
- The fear system is intended to protect against pain and devastation.
- The pleasure system regulates sexual behaviour.
- The care system regulates maternal nurturance.
- The sadness separation pain system regulates the demand for care and nurturing through intense crying, giving attention to posterity, acute separation anxiety.
- The game system evokes positive feelings.

Life events can influence the affection brain by inhibiting the negative systems and stimulating positive systems. The care and the game system could be encouraged to generate positive feelings. This principle is used in the expression method (see Chapter 9).

John Bowlby (1988) was first one to notice that depressed moods were related to loss situations. His insights about the essential role of separation pain – acute protest or panic in response to losses, especially in young animals – and neuroscientific findings seem to support each other.

8.2.5 Emotional stress in life events

Stress occurs when there is a need to let emotions of loss flow away (desired state) but you actually keep these emotions inside (actual state). This makes you enjoy life less. The loss of a person, animal, object or symbol brings emotional pain. Through defences you unconsciously keep this pain out of sight at first. This normal reaction acts as a kind of automatic emergency brake that ensures you to not directly feel and be hit by the physical and emotional pain. This defence mechanism is beyond your conscious perception, which is involuntary. Defence mechanisms are response patterns of feelings, thoughts and behaviour on the perception of an inner psychic or external threat. In a positive process the resistance is decreased and acceptance is increased. Eventually you fully recognize the actual impact of the loss. With this the awareness task is completed (see Chapter 2).

8.3 Conceptual definition and elucidation

The cathartic method is used when the client is indicating he wants to get rid of his emotional pain, is experiencing pain or is about to release pain. Different techniques can be used when the client is about to release pain. The cathartic method is focused on a constructive release of pain that may take the form of laughing, crying, being angry or even trembling with fear. This method enables the client to discharge the pain that is present: as a result, the client will no longer keep his emotions hidden, but instead will be 'an open book' and vulnerable at the same time. By releasing this pain, related personal stress or emotional stress will also be reduced. In this respect, emotional catharsis will result in reduced stress and emotional strength.

If not expressed, emotional, physical and social pain remain and can create stress in the individual's personal and social systems. Therefore constructively 'venting' emotions should decrease tension and subsequently the negative psychological experience and symptoms. The greater the constructive expression of negative emotions, the greater the relief should be (APA, 2007). This so-called hydraulic model of emotions uses the analogy of fluid flowing through a system. If the flow of fluid is hampered/impeded, destructive tensions can build up. Thus the cathartic work method facilitates the venting of pain, reducing stress. Viewed from the multimethod social work model perspective, the cathartic work method allows the social worker to work together with the client in reducing the destructive misfit and enhancing the constructive fit between person and the environment by influencing the personal part of the PIE dynamic (the person-in-environment): assisting the client with constructive emotional coping. The client being facilitated in adequately emotionally coping feels happier and develops more fit with their own environment.

8.3.1 Elucidation

Pain can be described as becoming conscious of vulnerability of a physical and/or psychological and/or social nature. Physical pain occurs when your body tells you that someone is treading on your toes or pricking you with a sharp object. Psychological and social pain occur when hurtful comments are made or when hurtful behaviour occurs, but also when receiving bad news or experiencing a loss or trauma. Oppression because of race, gender, sexual orientation or religion may be experienced as pain. Experiences of social rejection or loss have been described as some of the most 'painful' experiences that we may face as humans, and perhaps for good reason. Because of our prolonged period of immaturity, the social attachment system may have co-opted the pain system, borrowing the pain signal to prevent the detrimental consequences of social separation. Research (Eisenberger, 2012) has shown that experiences of physical and social pain rely on shared neural substrates.

Sexual and physical abuse is a combination of physical, psychological and social pain, however illness or amputation can also cause psychological hurt, quite aside from the physical pain. Finally psychological pain can also be physically experienced as pain, for example when a bereavement causes so much physical pain that it results in headaches or stomach aches.

Pain does not simply cease without release, but may be internalized and made invisible. At a later stage the pain that was swallowed will come out and may demand our attention in whatever way, in order to be released.

Talking about pain is not the same releasing it. Sometimes 'talking about' pain can be seen as avoiding release. Some authors cast doubt as to the release effect. The argument for this doubt is specifically that 'venting anger' creates more problems relating aggression with clients. There is as yet no research to support this.

8.4 History of the cathartic method

In psychosocial care, what happens is that one may practice in a 'cathartic' way, but under a different name. Ramsay (1979) and de Mönnink (2001), in their description of grief therapy, refer to techniques such as 'flooding' and 'imaginary exposure', whereby the client is exposed to 'stimuli', in other words 'linking objects' (photos, letters, music) all connected to the specific painful life events related to separation or loss. According to the authors, extinction or 'neutralizing' the grief linked to bereavement, in other words 'catharsis', is worked towards by therapists and clients together, which boils down to the release of built-up or rejected pain.

Re-evaluation counselling particularly focuses on allowing through allowing them to break out into an anxious sweat, allowing them to cry, shake and cry out in anger. Fear, anger, sadness and happiness are basic emotions in all people (Leijssen, 2001). Avoiding, suppressing and denying emotions is a form of self-deception that always has a way of creeping back, seeking revenge, because the elementary energy in some or other distorted way tries to find a way out. Most of the time this leads to (self-)destructive behavioural patterns. The only healthy option is to enable the emotion to come to the surface again, recognizing the fact that the emotion has resurfaced and letting it out. Obviously negative emotions such as fear, anger and sadness in particular are often blocked or distorted, yet they are forces that serve an important function for human beings. Fear keeps us protected by keeping us on the alert, anger can be used for self-defense and strength while grief can provide release and cleansing. But even emotions we experience as positive may be suppressed; for example, when love with its essential function of connecting people has no chance. When basic emotions cannot find an outlet, they lead to inadequate responses and these can be particularly poisonous or explosive. The cathartic method is used whenever the client indicates that they want to get rid of pain, is currently experiencing pain or is at the point of release. More than one technique can be used when the client is looking for catharsis.

I should, however, sound a caution with regard to using the cathartic method. The social worker cannot take the client beyond the point at which the social worker finds himself or herself at that moment in his or her life. Social workers who do not recognize their own sadness, fear or anger are advised against using the cathartic method with their client. As a matter of course, a learning process around the social worker's own release issues is required in these instances.

Historically, the cathartic method is difficult to place. In theory, numerous existing methods appear to pretend to work with release of feelings such as may be the case in psychoanalysis (where the word 'catharsis' is sometimes used for 'appear to pretend to work towards insight') and Rogerian counselling ('exploration of experiences'). In practice this is good because space is created for someone's imagination, which in itself is better than denying such imagination. Although, attention for the imagination *can* result in becoming stuck at 'talking about' or 'exploration of feelings' and not aimed at living through or release of the corresponding pain.

The word catharsis is derived from the Greek word κάθαρσις, which is translated as 'cleansing' or 'purification' (Powell, 2013). Most of the definitions emphasize two essential components of catharsis: the emotional aspect (strong emotional expression and processing) and the cognitive aspect of catharsis (insight, new realization and the unconscious rising to the level of conscious awareness) and as a result, positive change. Aristotle defined catharsis as 'purging of the spirit of morbid and base ideas or emotions by witnessing the playing out of such emotions or ideas on stage'. Breuer and Freud described catharsis as an involuntary, instinctive body process, such as crying. Schultz and Schultz (2004) followed the psychodynamic tradition and defined catharsis as 'the process of reducing or eliminating a complex by recalling it to conscious awareness and allowing it to be expressed'. The American Psychological Association (2007) also associates catharsis with the psychodynamic theory and defines it as 'the discharge of affects connected to traumatic events that had previously been repressed by bringing these events back into consciousness and reexperiencing them'. Scheff (2001) emphasized both essential components of catharsis: emotional-somatic discharge and cognitive awareness which he called 'distancing', when the person experiencing catharsis is maintaining the 'observer' role rather than that of participant, which involves a sense of control and full alertness in the person's immediate environment. Scheff indicated that the detailed, vivid recalling of forgotten events and insights most often occur towards the end of somatic-emotional discharge. There is a certain amount of confusion and misunderstanding about the definition and interpretation of catharsis: some of the researchers perceive catharsis as an emotional discharge, equating it with the behaviour of expressing strong emotions, while others emphasize the cognitive aspect and the new awareness that emerges after reliving traumatic events from the past.

Harvey Jackins (1965) is the founder of re-review counselling. The term 're-review' refers to the client's need to rethink their distressing past experiences after the emotional hurt in those experiences has been discharged, thereby regaining ('re-emerging' with) their natural intellectual and emotional capacities. In 1969 in Seattle, Jackins started a way of working so that in a focused way sustained emotional pain could be released. This way of working is called re-evaluation counselling, which is also known as co-counselling (Heron, 1998).

The original theory of co-counselling centres around the concept of distress patterns. These are patterns of behaviour, that is, behaviour that tends to be repeated in a particular type of circumstance, that are irrational, unhelpful or compulsive. The theory is that these patterns are driven by the accumulated consequences in the mind of (not currently) conscious memories of past events in which the person was unable to express or discharge the emotion associated with the event in an appropriate manner. Co-counselling enables release from the patterns by allowing 'emotional discharge' of the hurtful past experiences. Such cathartic discharge includes crying, feeling hot and perspiring, trembling, yawning, laughing and relaxed, non-repetitive talking. In day-to-day life, these 'discharging' actions may be limited by social norms, such as taboos around crying, which are widespread in many cultures.

Greenberg (2002) concluded that emotional arousal and processing within a supportive therapeutic relationship is the core element for positive change. He argued that a combination of awareness, healthy emotional expression and cognitive integration of emotions tends to produce positive change. It appears that emotion-focused therapy appropriately addressed the cognitive component of catharsis and safety issues. Emotion-focused therapy developed techniques to help clients recognize and validate their strong feelings, and enabled clients to express hurtful emotions safely, as well as to find meaning for their experiences through coaching and support.

At the graduate Amsterdam School of Social Work IVABO, emotional release techniques were used for years in the 2-year 'Women and Wellbeing' course through practicing co-counselling. It was thought that that people who are *not* given opportunities to work through tensions and painful experiences hold on to this pain in their feeling and thinking processes, for example when psychopharmaceuticals are used. This pain influences their perception negatively and keeps them from responding in an adequate and effective manner (see Figure 8.1).

The cathartic method assumes that people by nature are able to take out their tensions and frustrations. The release comes with laughing, crying, shaking, sweating, yawning, stretching and the urge to visit the toilet. Everyone is born with this 'skill', but our culture teaches us not to use it by feeding back the wrong information during the parenting process (boys do not cry, girls do not get angry), punishment/discipline and by ignoring such unwanted behaviour ('I'll come back when you have stopped crying'). The cathartic method assumes that all individuals can fully regain their freedom to act if there is sufficient space and attention to still let go of the painful emotions and tensions.

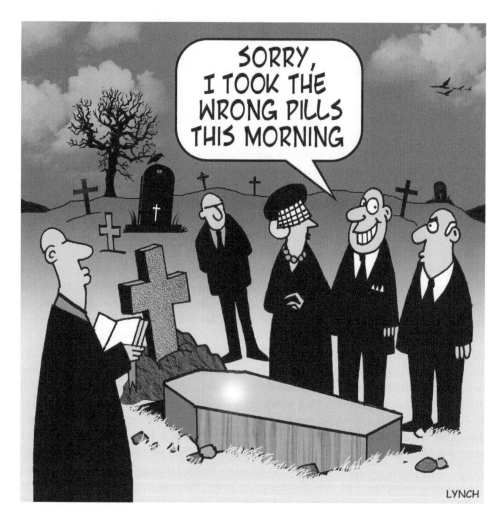

FIGURE 8.1 Effects and side-effects of psychopharmaceuticals

Cartoon courtesy of Mark Lynch

Viscott, a US psychiatrist (1996), has spent three decades engineering therapeutic break-throughs for his patients; in nearly all of these cases, it was the acceptance of some previously concealed truth that opened the way for healing to begin. Hurt and loss constituted the first topic covered in his work *The Language of Feelings* (1977). Viscott recognized that hurt can occur every day and is more intense the higher the value of whatever is lost. Hurt is natural and can help clarify what is important to a person. Although good can come out of hurt, it is not always that way. Hurt becomes a negative result when a person does not manage that hurt correctly. Some people do not allow emotions to run their natural course. By not expressing one's hurt in a feasible and rational manner, it may accumulate and destroy a person emotion-ally. Hurt is the fertilizer that helps all other negative feelings to grow. Viscott recommends that a person should 'be entirely honest' when hurt and 'identify the original source of hurt and to suffer and grieve for the original loss that caused it.' By allowing time and expression to heal the hurt, a person will be able to move past the hurt. However, many people do not and regress to deeper negative feelings.

In *Emotional Resilience: Simple Truths for Dealing With the Unfinished Business of Your Past*, Viscott describes his cardinal rule: resolve any pain at the moment it arises and resolve what's getting in the way of your sense of freedom and happiness now. Telling the truth and making positive choices can become a way of life.

When the past invades the present and your future experiences, emotional debt is 'an unexpressed or unnamed feeling that is held onto, distorted, and becomes a symbol for any similar loss or painful event' (Viscott, 1996, p. 130ff).

> You know you are storing a feeling in Emotional Debt when you find yourself making excuses, explaining away your guilt, justifying your anger, blaming others and making them the cause of your problems or behaviour, or pretending not to care. Your suffering is not because you have been hurt – you suffer because the way you chose to deal with the hurt has kept it from resolving naturally. When hurt or pain is not expressed at the time it occurs, the feeling of hurt/pain is stored. The purpose of current anxiety is to help you determine how real the danger is and what you need to do to avoid it. When the danger has passed, you determine how close the danger was, learn from it and let go of your fear. The key to managing your Emotional Debt is to decide not to let unimportant things upset you and to accept what you cannot change without taking it personally.
>
> *(Viscott, 1996, p. 279)*

'Toxic nostalgia' is when emotional debt is full and you are emotionally overdrawn (Viscott, 1996). The stored unexpressed, unnamed, unfinished emotions get triggered in similar situations and this is when you overreact: toxic nostalgia. We repeat this pattern and can't figure out why things are always the same. Toxic nostalgia

> is a subtle mixture of feelings, attitudes, perspectives and needs from different ages all showing themselves at once as the unresolved past attempts to define the present. Your capacity for Toxic Nostalgia limits your freedom to be who you are, to act in your own best interest, or to be open in expressing yourself.
>
> *(Viscott, 1996, p. 279)*

Toxic nostalgia happens when some trigger awakens the old hurt and you are presented with another opportunity to feel your loss, examine your hurt, accept the intense feeling, and come to acceptance and peace.

> How you see your past is how you feel about yourself. Because toxic nostalgic intrusions overstate the negative legacy of the past, they tend to undermine your confidence. They do this because you see the return of old feelings as confirming your worst beliefs about yourself. These returning emotions are another opportunity on the way to acceptance and letting go of the loss and hurt by changing the old beliefs about yourself. Accepting what happened to you reflects your willingness to accept others and yourself. You accept that you have weaknesses. You know you can fail but realize that no single failure can define your worth as a person.
>
> *(Viscott, 1996, p. 279ff)*

For many social workers the cathartic method is an important addition to the concept of encouraging/allowing the client to 'talk'. In social work, it was thought for a long time that 'talking about feelings' equals the release of pain.

Historical anecdote

When Jackins took in a friend, he was amazed that his friend improved after a long good cry (Roggema, 1979). The intensity of the crying shocked him, but he considered this as a symptom that would pass. When the crying kept coming back, Jackins became really worried. But then he noticed his friend was getting better, becoming more active, taking the initiative. Jackins realized that the crying was not so bad after all. He became interested in the release function and he set up a group that considered release as something perfectly normal: the human capacity to release pain.

8.5 Goals

8.5.1 General goal

- Reducing or taking away negative tension and enhancing emotional strength by allowing to release pain.

8.5.2 Specific goal

- Allowing the client to release his or her emotional and physical pain by means of crying, trembling (with fear) or shouting out in anger.

8.6 Indications

- Signals of negative tensions through pent-up grief, fear and anger.
- The client wants to let go of the pain.
- The client is about to release his or her pain.

8.7 Contraindications

- The client uses sedative medication.
- The clients' physical stability or psychological capacity is insufficient for him or her to be able to manage the release of the pain.
- The client is unstable or exhibits uncontrolled behaviour (arguing with everyone).
- The clients is asking for or exhibits a range of attention-seeking behaviours.
- The client dramatizes (the client abuses emotions in order to seek attention).
- When talking to the social worker, the client does not want to concern him or herself with pain and does not want to be confronted by pain and release (I do not want to cry now, because I have to pick up my daughter in a moment).

- The social worker is unable to provide sufficient continuity.
- During the course, the social worker has gained no insight and experience in respect of their own release issues and does not adequately recognize and acknowledge fear, sadness and anger.

8.8 Techniques

1 Reflective technique
2 Normalizing technique
3 Permission technique
4 Exposure technique
5 Attention balance technique
6 Scanning technique
7 Contrast technique
8 Contradiction technique
9 'This hurts' technique
10 Repetition technique
11 Empty chair technique
12 Replacement technique
13 Role model technique.

8.8.1 Reflective technique

The social worker mirrors the emotional load he thinks he can observe. For example he will say: 'Is it having a profound effect on you, is it not?' or 'I can see you are touched by this.'

8.8.2 Normalizing technique

The social worker says that the release or the embarrassment that occurs is normal, so that the client feels stimulated to let go, or to release. For example he may say: 'What happened to you/what you experienced must be quite painful' and 'You say you are embarrassed, but it is normal to feel like that.'

8.8.3 Permission technique

The social worker gives permission for the client to let go of his or her pain if they sense that the client is at the point of release. The social worker may say: 'Let the pain come out, that's better' and 'Please take your time, you don't have to talk yet.'

8.8.4 Exposure technique

The social worker uses exposure to painful triggers, which he is aware that the client will experience as painful. Repetition of triggers brings out feelings of grief/sadness, anger or fear. He says, for example: 'You say you really miss your wife?' 'Would you take a look at that picture for me?' 'Would you mind listening to the music?' or 'Could you please read out that poem from book X?'

8.8.5 Attention balance technique

The social worker ensures there is a balance between the 'intraverted attention' and the 'extra-verted attention' so that the level or 'dosage' of pain release/relief remains appropriate for the client.

8.8.6 Scanning technique

Bit by bit, layer by layer, step by step, the social worker will let the client explore a certain theme by asking what the clients' associations are with tears, laughter or feelings of fear and anger. It becomes apparent through this 'scanning' what kind of experiences the client has with crying and which constraining or stimulating experiences there have been. As a result the client may become aware of the extent to which he feels constrained from crying. That will allow him to actively get rid of blockages/constraints and any burden he may feel he is carrying. Release/relief is or was often ignored or not allowed during childhood, at school, or even in our current environment, and this may result in the client deciding to not release his pain any further. At a later stage, it could be said/argued that these impediments, which may initially be externalized and later on internalized to be released are unhealthy, because the pain, anger or fear are demanding to be released.

8.8.7 Contrast technique

The social worker can bring out the joyous and loving side of a relationship or life period the emotion is linked to. Through this the client experiences the contrast with loss or trauma in a much stronger way and is able to let go and move on. When dealing with a divorce, the social worker asks: 'How did you two meet/get to know each other?'

8.8.8 Contradiction technique

The social worker will keep the contact light-hearted, for example by letting the client name the opposite emotion or by referring to a heavy subject as 'light'. He may for instance ask someone who has a negative view about themselves: 'What did you think were your strong points?' Thereby the pain caused by someone undervaluing themselves is allowed to surface. The social worker proposes a 'direction' which may be opposite to what the client is experiencing.

The social worker may also say to a man who refers to himself as emotionless: 'I am a sensitive man.' The release can be put in motion because of the contrast with what the client is experiencing. Or he can challenge the client who feels burdened by something, by calling that burden loud and in a light manner, contrasting the heavy burden. The use of humour could bring about the release of laughter in the client, because it is in contradiction with the serious character of a topic which is rather heavy going.

8.8.9 'This hurts' technique

The social worker instructs the client not to talk about the pain they have experienced and suggests instead that the client says: 'This really hurts' whenever the pain is coming to the surface. He may also instruct the client to say: 'You can simply say, "Ouch, this hurts!" when you are in pain.'

8.8.10 Repetition technique

The social worker asks the client to repeat what he has just said. For example, he may tell a client whose mother has died: 'Repeat the phrase, "I miss her so much," once.' Once the phrase is repeated by the client, the release can occur.

8.8.11 Empty chair technique

The social worker directs the client to talk to another person with whom he experiences a lot of pain. This person is imagined to be sitting in an empty chair beside or across from the client. This helps the client to experience and understand the feeling more fully. Thus, it stimulates the client's thought processes, highlighting his or her emotions and attitudes. For example, the social worker may say, 'Imagine your father in this chair, see him vividly, and, now, talk to him about how you felt when he was. . . .'

8.8.12 Replacement technique

The social worker suggests he plays the role of a person the client may associate with pain (mother, partner, child, colleague or boss). This is called an 'address or 'projection screen'. Because the social worker more or less conducts himself as the real person, the release is stimulated. During the session, the social worker will ask the client which behaviours or which remarks the client finds so painful.

8.8.13 Role model technique

The social worker demonstrates a form of release by taking the place of the client. For example, he says: 'I believe that I would get angry on the spot if I was hearing what you went through.' The client will notice that expressing anger is a normal reaction in his situation.

8.9 Social work results

- The client feels a sense of inner tidiness.
- The client has more energy.
- The client is clearer about their own situation.

8.10 Evidence

In the social work domain there is no particular research demonstrating the effectiveness of the cathartic method. It is more a matter of clinical evidence relating to social work clients who have released their pain and who feel relieved and have more space to take the necessary steps to move forwards. Steinfort (1999) undertook exploratory research examining the added value the cathartic method offers social work by means of a questionnaire that cannot be classified as representative, which was distributed among teachers and social workers. She concluded that according to all respondents, the cathartic method does have an added value, because the method focuses particularly on the release of sustained pain and that the method fully deserves a place next to social work methods aimed at improving client insight and methods aimed at a change in client behaviour.

Emotionally focused therapy (EFT), very comparable with the cathartic method in social work, has proven effectiveness for individuals suffering from moderate depression, the effects of childhood deprivation or abuse, and a variety of general 'problems of living', including interpersonal problems (Paivio & Greenberg, 1995, Greenberg & Watson, 1998). In addition, psychotherapy process research has shown that the 'depth of emotional processing' (which EFT emphasizes) is strongly correlated with lasting therapeutic outcome.

EFTs have been shown to be effective in forms of therapy aimed at both individuals and couples in a number of randomized clinical trials (Johnson, 1999, Elliott et al., 2004). A manualized form of EFT of depression in which specific emotion activation techniques were used within the context of an empathic relationship was shown to be highly effective in treating depression in three separate studies (Greenberg and Watson, 1998, Watson et al., 2003, Goldman et al., 2006). EFT was found to be more effective in reducing interpersonal problems than either Client-Centered (CC) or Cognitive-Behavioural Therapy (CBT), in promoting more change in symptoms than the CC treatment, and highly effective in preventing relapse (77% nonrelapse; Ellison et al., 2009). EFT also has been found to be effective in treating abuse (Paivio & Nieuwenhuis, 2001), resolving interpersonal problems and promoting forgiveness (Paivio and Greenberg, 1995, Greenberg et al., 2008). Emotion-focused couple therapy is recognized as one of the most effective approaches in resolving relationship distress (Johnson, 1999, Baucom, 1998). EFT also has generated more research than any other treatment approach on the process of change, having demonstrated a relationship between outcome and empathy, the alliance, depth of experiencing, emotional arousal, making sense of aroused emotion, productive processing of emotion, and particular emotions sequences (Damasio, 1999, Elliott et al., 2004, Pascual & Greenberg, 2007).

From around the year 2000, researchers have started to entertain doubts as to whether the 'working through and venting' of anger is adequate, and more specifically the question of whether a client's situation might not go from bad to worse if the client were encouraged to express his or her anger. Unfortunately, there are no examples that this possible outcome would be a contraindication and a reason to pursue a certain line of treatment.

8.11 Pitfalls

- The social worker projects their own style of release onto the client.
- The social worker 'waltzes over' and transgresses the threshold of the client instead of using communication skills to explore the resistance behaviour.
- The social worker approaches the release of the client in a 'technical' way without having the essential therapeutic tools or having learned those and self-reflection into their own ways of release.

8.12 Summary and questions

In this chapter the role of the social worker was described when emotions are released. What emotions are evoked during the loss of loved ones?

First, the function of emotional release in a loss situation was described. After this, it was made clear how the affection brain operates during the regulation of emotions. Then it was outlined how the cathartic method can contribute to reducing emotional stress. In Chapter 9 the role of social worker will be described using the expression method.

Questions

1 In which respect is the affection brain working differently from the mind (cognitive brain) and the survival brain? Is it very different from the mind or the survival brain?
2 Do you know examples from the animal world in which mammals like horses, elephants, cats and dogs show mourning behaviour?
3 Do you recognize examples of yourself or others of emotional release?
4 Which discharge form is your 'favourite' (crying, shaking, anger) and what do you find the most difficult form?
5 Why was 'talking about' emotions not the same as 'unloading' emotions?
6 What is happening within yourself when some else is emotional (crying, anxious, angry)?
7 What do you need for being really open to the emotional release of others?

9

EXPRESSION METHOD

Questions

This chapter addresses the following questions:

- What role does creative expression play in stress reduction?
- How does stress arise in clients?
- How can the expression method contribute to the reduction of expressive stress and the recovery of someone's emotional wellbeing?

9.1 Introduction

> I came to peace and found solace in being creatively active during the darker days in my life, especially in times of grief.
>
> (Jennie, on http://www.recover-from-grief.com)

Creative social work methods aim at using the power of art and spirituality through symbolism, metaphors and stories. The goal lies in alleviating the psychological and spiritual pain of not only clients and stressed out family members but also that of the professionals who play a stimulating role in this process. Being able to express one's creative potential is as relevant as any other social work method. According to Bertman (1999) there is a strong tradition associated with using fiction, poems, photography and audiovisual art to address emotional obstacles and moments of loss. Creative social work techniques are based on the use of pictures, videotapes, assorted symbols, writing, drawing, sculpting, acting and music. Creative activities can help people process many of the emotions associated with grief. The expression method contributes to the constructive expression of emotional strain.

The case of Mr. Stack

As a means of reflecting closure to his social work contact, Mr. Stack has made a picture of a hand holding a candlestick. This image illustrates his renewed grip on his own life. This piece of art speaks to one's imagination, as did Escher's picture of two hands holding a globe.

9.2 Creative expression

9.2.1 Sources

Clients who have a difficult time verbalizing their problems and emotions can use alternative forms of expression. This can often be done by stimulating and using the client's hobbies or creative skills (be it writing, composing poetry, photography or painting). Stress linked with a life event can be channelled in this way.

There are many ways of expressing stress. Talking is just one of them. There is no right or wrong way of processing stress associated with life events. There are, however, many possible ways of lightening the burden and working towards closure of a difficult chapter in one's life. This life event can be dealt with by drawing and painting, by modelling clay, by making music or simply by writing. Using your hands, an action which does not require difficult thinking processes can lead to the release of pain and to catharsis, thereby allowing such creative expression to provide a 'cleansing' function. Drawing, painting and clay modelling are ways of coping with grief that can put the client in touch with their emotions. Essentially, the expression method is meant to help clients to move on in one's blocked expression in the coping process. A social worker uses the client's creative skill set as much as possible. It then comes down to stimulating this expression through hobbies, such as writing or drawing, so that the client can relieve a larger part of their stress through non-verbal forms of expression.

A source for creative expression in grief can be found at http://www.recover-from-grief .com, a website which describes a wide range of creative techniques: writing, visual arts, music, poems, creating memorials and books. The main advice when applying creative expression techniques is to find the expressive form that is right for the person experiencing the grief.

9.2.2 Types

Plastic expression

Free plastic expression entails making images or sculpting objects in clay, wood or other materials (Wertheim-Cahen, 1994a). It offers the following options:

* Communicating bereavement and traumatic experiences in a non-verbal manner;
* Unconsciously bringing up memories of traumatic events in cases of amnesia;
* Providing tangible elements which can be used in rituals for processing grief and loss.

Music

Musical expression of grief reactions is based on what is emotionally spoken strongly present. When someone is depressed or anxious, these feelings are connected negatively, and this negativity is attempted to be changed in a playful manner. Not only can the piano be used for this, but other instruments as well. An instrument can be used to identify what clients find beautiful or ugly, good or bad. Musical expression can be a means for people to connect with their emotions or even discover something entirely new. Similarly singing – be it alone or in a choir – and listening to music can also have a stimulating effect on the grieving process. As Ramses Shaffy used to sing: 'Sing, fight, cry, pray, laugh, work and admire.'

Bibliotherapy

Bibliotherapy is described as using a selection of texts as a guide in solving personal problems to complement other therapeutic means. In literature, several reasons are identified as an explanation for the therapeutic effect of bibliotherapy. The most important one is the identification process: the reader identifies himself with a person or situation in the story and learns that he is not alone and that others are dealing with the same problem. Identification can have a curative effect and can release hidden emotions.

Other possible explanations for the therapeutic effect of literature include:

- Insight in one's own situation arises through being immersed in someone else's situation.
- The story provides solutions different from the ones that have already been tried.
- The story teaches the reader that everything we go through still has a certain value.
- Seeing how others respond gives someone the courage to tackle their own situation.

9.3 Phases

A letter or a gesture can sometimes speak more than a thousand words. The expression method is meant for clients who feel the need to express their sorrows and emotional stress but who cannot do so verbally. It is also helpful for those people experiencing grief whose verbal skills are completely blocked or diminished, offering a way for them to release emotional stress. These people can include those with a limited vocabulary, but also traumatized or apathic clients who can no longer verbally express themselves for psychological or physical reasons. The expression method reduces negative tension because it allows clients other channels of expression, apart from the verbal one, which they can use to relieve tension themselves. The expression method assists people in reducing tension in a non-verbal way. The expression method (Wertheim-Cahen, 1994b) entails four phases:

- *Doing and experiencing*: all forms of expression (writing, drawing, acting) can render 'experiences' visible where verbal expression exercises do not achieve this.
- *Result*: a letter, diary, drawing or poem makes the client's situation visible.
- *Interpretation of the result*: the client's inside world is brought to the surface and allows there to be some detachment from the result and which enables it to be looked at more calmly. Expressing the meaning of this piece of work in words can also increase the client's awareness.

- *The relation between client, piece of work and social worker:* the social worker follows the meaning which the client attributes to the creative product and asks questions such as 'How did it feel drawing this?' or 'How does it feel seeing it, now that it's finished?' The moment where this triggers something in the client, the social worker can, verbally, continue their core social work or cathartic work.

9.4 History of the expression method

However many social workers already use simple expression techniques in their work, education and training could pay more attention to these expressive techniques. Many social workers are hesitant to use the expression method's non-verbal techniques. This is understandable as the social workers themselves may not enjoy drawing or may not have used any other forms of expression since primary school. Social workers often draw diagrams and genograms during training, but they do not use these creative types of drawing to allow clients to express themselves. When language causes difficulties – which can be the case when clients are children, adolescents, immigrants or when something is difficult to discuss, for example grief – the expression method can facilitate communication (Scheller-Dikkers, 1998). The basic principle is that images are a natural way of expressing thoughts and emotion, just like words. Expression and visualization of experiences through a variety of alternative mediums enhances the recovery process. Offering clients ways of expression, other than verbal, means a unique opportunity for dealing with problems in both alternative ways and in another language. The list of expression forms is inexhaustible: playing with animals, dolls or toys; acting; talking to a picture; making animals talk to one another; performing vocal exercises; singing.

The origin of the expression method in psychosocial support dates back to the 1950s. The curriculum then encouraged all sorts of playful activities as a means of preparing social workers for youth welfare work. In 1956, aside from the general theoretical formation, the social work education programme in the Netherlands also featured handicraft, folk dancing, playing the recorder and so forth (Buys, 1956). By utilizing handicraft, possible client resistance towards the social worker would be easier to overcome. Nowadays it is mainly the creative-expressive disciplines that are interested in these alternative expressive techniques.

9.5 Goals

General goal

- Reducing or removing negative tension by encouraging creative expression.

Specific goals

- The client explores their own fields of experience.
- The client exposes their own inner processes (e.g. describes experiences).
- The client makes their pressure points or blockages visible, audible and tangible.

9.6 Indications

- The client experiences difficulties expressing himself verbally (due to traumatic events, limited vocabulary, inadequate introspective skills, aphasia, removal of vocal cords, etc.).

- The client prefers expressing himself in a non-verbal manner (complementary to or as a replacement of other methods).
- The social worker observes that the client is talking 'around' something in an evasive manner.
- The client no longer speaks/does not speak.

9.7 Contraindications

- The client does not wish to work expressively.
- The client hesitates to work expressively.
- The social worker himself feels a resistance towards the expression method.

9.8 Techniques

1 Writing technique
2 Plastic techniques
3 Biographical technique
4 Play techniques
5 Diverse techniques.

9.8.1 Writing technique

The social worker proposes to the client that the stressful event or experience be addressed during the course of the sessions by writing. This may be in the form of a report, but also as a letter, a poem or a combination of these. Upon agreement the client can send the text by post or email before the next session. The social worker can also encourage the client to write an abusive letter or to keep a reflective diary.

Letter

A man saw his wife drown to death before his own eyes and cannot find the words for this experience. He and the social worker have agreed that he will write a letter in which he describes the effects of the session and which emotions it triggers inside him. For him, this is a small step towards the next session where he can describe bit more of what happened, more than explicitly talking about what he has seen.

9.8.2 Plastic techniques

In plastic techniques, psychological and relational tension is expressed by making a drawing, collage, painting or clay model. The social worker proposes to the client that they make a drawing, of the event or problem, for example.

Globe

A client was asked to paint something (painting was his hobby) as a way of bringing closure to a very intensive course of therapy in which he had dealt with many losses. He painted a dark frame with a floating globe, with a hand that found a new grip.

Rebirth

A woman processing her incest experience was asked to make a drawing that fitted her current feeling as to what point she had reached in therapy. She drew a child being born again.

9.8.3 Biographical technique

The social worker suggests the client make a 'life book' or biography which contains a chronological lifeline and all relevant events (Kuin & Bieman, 2002). In a biography, four lifelines are used:

- Health and sickness
- Family, friends and relationships
- Work/education
- Ideology and spirituality.

Every event is identified with a different symbol and graded according to its emotional value. Special events include, for example, festivities or travels. Milestones in one's life might be graduation, a promotion or a wedding day. Moving away, the passing of a relative or acquaintance or a divorce are also major life events. Decisions and choices in life are crossroads. The client uses symbols to draw the events on his age continuum (a horizontal line with age indications) with an emotional value up to 2 inches above (positive emotional value) or up to 2 inches below (negative emotional value). The client also uses key words to indicate or describe the event.

Boxing

A man was referred to a social worker by a sparring partner who thought he was losing his normal self; according to this friend, the man had some emotional processing to do. The man had been taken away from his family as a young boy and had been moved from foster family to foster family, ending up in the Netherlands again after having lived as a drifter. The man was asked to visualize his life story. He was also asked to write linking text between events. During the next session, this visualized life story was the main subject.

9.8.4 Play techniques

For particular audiences the social worker can use various play techniques, like acting or games. For children the game called 'All the Stars Above' (http://www.allthestarsabove.com) can be used to gently set them thinking about a death. For adults the social worker can use play to non-verbally portray their struggle with a particular problem. These play techniques are primarily used in group sessions.

9.8.5 Diverse techniques

The social worker can also use other expression-stimulating techniques that fit with the client's hobby or profession. Examples can include photography, video, drama or music.

9.9 Social work results

- The client releases negative tension.
- The client gains clarity of their inner thoughts.
- The client comprehends the pressure points which he experienced.
- The client experiences progress.

9.10 Evidence

Not much research has been done on the use of the expression method with different target audiences. Such research is hampered by methodological limitations, such as small sample, non-experimental settings, unconfirmed diagnoses, homemade instruments with limited psychometric validity, inadequately reported interventions and results that cannot be linked to the intervention. We provide a few instances where the effect of the expression method has been substantiated.

9.10.1 Expressive writing

Pennebaker (2014) researched expressive writing. His project 'Words That Heal' provides research results, in layman's terms, which demonstrate how and when expressive writing can improve health. It explains why writing can often be more helpful than talking when dealing with trauma, and it prepares the reader for their writing experience. The book looks at the most serious issues and helps the reader process them. From the instructions: 'Write about what keeps you awake at night. The emotional upheaval bothering you the most and keeping you awake at night is a good place to start writing.'

In *Expressive Writing: Words That Heal*, Pennebaker and Evans offer a basic writing assignment like this:

> Over the next four days, write about your deepest emotions and thoughts about the emotional upheaval that has been influencing your life the most. In your writing, really let go and explore the event and how it has affected you. You might tie this experience to your childhood, your relationship to your parents, people you have loved or love now, or even your career. Write continuously for 20 minutes.

Mother of a deceased child

A mother's personal grief experience when losing her child shortly after labour, or even later, is profound. Coping with sadness and the incomprehensibility of loss heightens her risk of feeling vulnerable and isolated. When a woman expresses her sadness and grief, she is better able to cope with the loss of her child. This grief stops the mother from taking practical steps in overcoming the loss of her child. Harr and Thistlethwaite (1990) introduce some creative, but non-traditional, approaches which can be used to help these mothers accept such a loss and feel complete again.

Life-threatening diseases

Creative therapy and other humanistic intervention strategies have become increasingly popular when working with clients and their relatives who are suffering from life-threatening diseases, particularly when children are involved (Perach, 1989). Creative therapy stimulates conscious and unconscious expression of the grieving process in both adults and children. Children are more prone to risk not only because their grief is less visible but also because it can resurface months or years later. Group therapy is used to standardize the expression of grief and to encourage the normal grieving process.

Nursing home care

The therapeutic use of expressive and creative methods is becoming increasingly popular in nursing homes and care of the elderly (Phillips et al., 2010). Artistic and other creative expression related activities, such as the *TimeSlips Storytelling* programme, improve communication, attention and fun, as well as neuropsychiatric symptoms. Several randomized controlled trials have proved that physiotherapy and musical therapy can result in significant improvements in levels of agitation, general neuropsychiatric symptoms and speech.

Multimethodical loss guidance

Over a period of 3 months, multimethodical grief therapy was offered in a Dutch health centre in the form of a behavioural and artistic therapy programme (Schut et al., 1996). Researchers found a systematic positive progress in terms of participants, symptoms measured on the general health questionnaire.

Grief groups

The literature on bereavement and grief focuses primarily on the grieving process and the emotions after loss (Ferszt et al., 1998). Little has been written about the 'transformation power' in cases of loss. Creative therapy used within a 'grief group' for adults appeared to help participants to express their emotions and gave them the opportunity to reflect on their own perceptions about death and their lives in general.

Social work

Involving people in creative forms of expression has the potential to create change at a personal level as well as facilitate social development (Gray et al., 2010).

Health information

Technology and storytelling can be combined to help improve health (Wyatt & Hauenstein, 2008). Stories, in all of their forms – books, plays, movies, poems, songs – are appealing to all ages but especially children. Children become easily engrossed in stories, however the current generation expects interactive and multimedia environments. Storytelling, reading and playing as a means of learning and teaching are frequently used in the classroom, but they are not always used as a method of coping with grief or encouraging health and wellbeing.

9.11 Pitfalls

• The social worker offers only their favourite type of expressive work.
• The social worker pushes their own interpretation of what the expressive work could possibly mean.

9.12 Summary and questions

This chapter described the role of the social worker in creative expression. First we looked at the contribution of creative expression in helping to address emotional stress. Then we described how expression methods may contribute to the reduction of emotional stress.

Questions

1 Do you recognize some of the examples of creative expression in yourself or in others?
2 Which expression category is your favourite (writing, drawing, digital, music) and which category do you find difficult? Why?
3 How can creative expression allow you to grasp a situation in a way that cannot be put into words?
4 What happens to you when others express themselves creatively instead of using words?
5 In the event that you do not, either fully or in part, believe in creative expression, what can you do to accept other people's creative expression?

10

RITUAL METHOD

Questions

This chapter addresses the following questions:

- What is the function of saying goodbye in case of loss?
- How does farewell stress arise in grieving individuals?
- How can the ritual method contribute to the reduction of farewell stress and enhance one's Quality of Life?

10.1 Introduction

In this chapter the social worker's role is described in relation to a proper goodbye; what does a 'proper goodbye' contribute to the reduction of emotional stress? First we look at the need and purpose of saying goodbye to lost loved ones in a worthy way and the effect this has on the bereavement process. Then we will explore how the ritual method can help reduce emotional stress and aid emotional wellbeing. Because as Sonia Ricotti (2015) said: 'surrender to what is, let go of what was, have faith in what will be.'

The case of Mr. Stack

Mr. Stack wishes to say goodbye to his stillborn son, something he hasn't done yet. What are the actions he wishes to undertake? Where? With whom? When? He decides to visit the place where his son lies buried and read aloud a poem he has written himself and to sing a song he used to sing to his other son. Those were the 'good' days, Mr. Stack said.

10.2 Proper goodbye and changes in emotional bonds

Farewell stress arises when the grieving client did not get a chance to say goodbye or when the farewell was not favourable, for example the last words were an argument being said in anger. Stress is caused by the natural need to say goodbye and the lack or inability to do so. When this situation is perceived to be less than desirable, for example a sudden death, the fulfilling of this need can have a tremendous influence.

10.2.1 Turning to a 'next page'

Almost anywhere in the world, important life events such as births, coming of age, marriage and death are marked by ceremonies, festivities and rituals. Even 'negative' events (e.g. divorce, resignation or illness) emphasize the importance of some form of ritual. Rituals are meant to make the transition to a new situation visible, perceptible and possible, for example to close one life chapter and start the next. Rituals also serve to wish the individuals or groups a 'safe journey' (van der Hart, 1987). How many people left behind by loved ones feel inconsolable or experience years of unexplainable complaints because they did not have a chance to properly say goodbye? Family, friends and work colleagues are left behind to struggle with the emptiness after such a drastic change. Increasingly more attention is being given to the need for people to express themselves at such times, even in organizations and companies that undergo downsizing or reorganization.

Births are also events that can cause feelings of loss, and birth rituals can be useful. The birth of one's first child fundamentally affects the lives of those involved. No one is thinking about the aspects of loss when a new life comes into existence, but with the coming of a newborn baby the lives of those involved are changed entirely: interactions change, the family system has grown and is expanded. Both parents' parents suddenly become grandparents; brothers and sisters become uncles and aunts. They are all placed in a new position and their relationships are given a new dimension.

10.2.2 Definition

A ritual is an action or series of actions that mark the transition from an old phase to a new phase in life and involve 'verbal formulas', words that express the closure. Whether someone performs a ritual is a matter of personal preference. More and more individuals have their own custom-made rituals; one of the advantages of this freedom of expression is that people are able to give their own meaning, form and content to their ritual.

Farewell rituals are not only meant for funerals but also for a finished relationship, loss of one's employment, loss of one's expectation of a healthy child and loss of one's proper health. After all, loss isn't only – as described in this book – about passing away. We just don't have any rituals or traditions for losses unrelated to death.

Custom-made rituals can help clients in the transition from the previous situation to the new. 'Burying' a lost relationship, health or expectations is an important element in this. One's focus on the past can then be changed into a focus on the present and on the future.

10.2.3 From traditional rites to custom-made rituals

Traditional rituals have an ordering and channelling function, partly because of the references to the past. Actions taking place as part of a ritual are generally of a symbolic nature. They find meaning not in themselves, but refer to the larger picture which is ideology or faith. They also induce collectiveness and confirm relationships within a group or community.

In an individualistic culture, such as the Western European, the number of customs and habits 'prescribed' by culture is decreasing. Whether someone performs a ritual when saying farewell has become rather a matter of personal preference. More and more individuals have custom made rituals where they can give their own meaning, form and content to the ritual. While this is an advantage in that people are free to give their own meaning to the farewell or reunification ritual, it also means that the support, originating in the collective ritual, is gradually eroded away.

Lately the interest in therapeutic rituals in the social work of uncomplicated and complicated grief has grown.

Processing grief requires time, but also active coping and farewell, in brief: loss demands grief work. The fact that the client is not themself when dealing with grief is a huge issue in itself. Clients who deny or trivialize their loss or who take too little time to process their grief hampers their healing process. Acknowledging loss is of great importance when dealing with grief. Holding on to the past is ineffective, as is forcedly looking to the future when the past is unresolved. The question is therefore about the meaning behind performing ritual actions in farewell or seeking closure.

Grief processing is seen as a gradual transition process, the transition from a previous life chapter to a new one. The factual relationship had with the lost loved one does not all of a sudden disappear: the grieving process is not as simple as a push of a button or the flipping of a switch. In grief there is rather a gradual transition process of *fading away*, the old relationship's gradual shift to the background by means of a metaphorical *dimmer* working step by step towards the transformation to a new meaning in the relationship with the person or thing lost.

10.2.4 Grief instinct

In loss, instinctive farewell behaviour is induced, as can be seen in many mammals (Brown, 2010). This farewell behaviour is a sign of attachment and is necessary in the realization that someone – in case of the deceased – is no longer alive. Instinctive farewell behaviour is seen in elephants, chimpanzees, dogs, cats and dolphins as they carefully approach the mortal remains and take in the situation with all of their senses. This instinctive pattern could be similar to the affective *reality testing* our brain needs: emotionally, is this really true? This happens in order to make the reality of the situation more tangible and to come to grips with it. How many times has this need been blocked because people are steered away from the reality of loss? The empirical fact for many therapists is that many people come to therapy with years of vague biopsychosocial complaints as an indirect consequence of unprocessed grief and insufficient reality testing. Performing a ritual can reduce the amount of emotional stress in those cases.

10.2.5 Three-phase structure of life transitions

How do people make the transition to this new stage in life? How can such a transition be accomplished? The basic pattern of change is described by Lewin (1951):

- Unfreezing
- Moving
- Refreezing.

The triphase structure and corresponding rituals are schematically depicted in Figure 10.1. The old structure is 'unfrozen' and after a period of time a new structure is found and 'refrozen'. This remains so until this structure is once again tested by a new life event where by the same cycle is completed again.

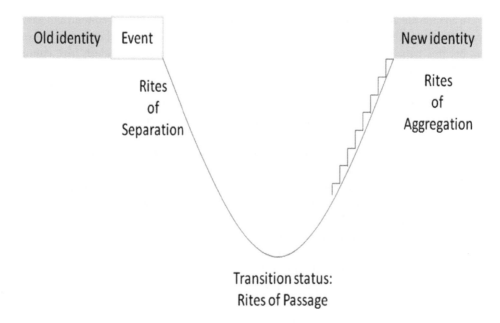

FIGURE 10.1 Three-phase structure in transitions with rites

    The farewell ritual is mainly about symbolic actions, indicating that the person is freeing them self from the original status quo, in the same way that in a wedding ceremony the bride can be taken away from her family's home, thus marking her breaking away from her family.

    This transition ritual is meant to provide guidance through the area between the old and the new. The old is no more, the new is yet to come. According to van Gennep (1909) one finds himself in a 'threshold situation'.

    In the reunification ritual the main focus is on the beginning of a new life. The reunification ritual is tied up with starting over after loss, by means of reunification with the remaining people, animals and things. Reunification means taking part in 'normal' life from a new position, status or situation.

10.3 History of the ritual method

By ritually saying goodbye to people or situations, one can leave the past behind and make a fresh start. The ritual method aims at identifying and completing activities or 'tasks' which provide a sense of closure, the completion of which symbolically indicates the transition to a new stage in life, but also goes hand in hand with verbal social work techniques. Ritual-oriented social work techniques consist of encouraging the client to think of an appropriate closure ritual. Depending on the stage the client is at, the ritual can be of a farewell, transitional or reunification nature. Despite receiving specific grief support (by a means other than the ritual method) and engaging in lots of soul-searching, a client can still experience unresolved feelings. Therapeutic rituals can then have a powerful effect by channelling both the emotional and behavioural sides of loss. The ritual method contributes to a constructive transition towards a new chapter in one's life through an individualized and custom-made ritual.

The social worker assesses the client's unresolved or *unfinished business* (also Chapter 26) and the actions they have taken in order to bring about a sense of closure. This is done by constructing a detailed description of the tension factors related to the farewell. Afterwards a ritual work technique is used to bring about a transition (see also Figure 2.4).

Using rituals only comes into play when other solutions do not provide the desired peace of mind, as was the case for the woman whose husband sustained brain damage, as a result of a cold sore virus, in the movie *Mind Machine*. In this case – and when thinking of using a ritual work technique in general – the following method indicators need to be considered. The social worker must first identify whether there are indicators for other methods and only then can he use the ritual method. The client:

- Has a headache: indicator for bodywork or cathartic method (Chapters 5 and 8);
- Would like to 'paint it out': indicator for expression method (Chapter 9);
- Wonders how to tell his friends: indicator for behavioural method (Chapter 13);
- Cannot adequately express pain and sorrow: indicator for cathartic method (Chapter 8);
- Cannot let go of the event: indicator for ritual method.

The ritual method assumes that an individualized custom-made ritual brings peace because it meets that person's need for a 'proper goodbye'.

Onno van der Hart (1987, 1992) has written a lot about the use of rituals in mental health settings. In present-day Western society there are fewer and fewer rituals when compared to the past and more traditional societies. We still know the primary rituals, such as weddings, customs around childbirth and funerals. Van der Hart believes that therapeutic farewell rituals constitute a modern substitute for what were once traditional transition rituals. Nowhere do we see this as clearly as in the social work of adolescents struggling to free themselves from their parents. The resemblance between modern psychotherapy and traditional transition and healing rituals is even clearer when the therapist 'prescribes' a ritual for his clients. These rituals are not invented by the therapist, but are constructed in collaboration with the client.

A therapeutic farewell ritual is a specific action or series of actions with a symbolic meaning marking the transition to a new phase in life, accompanied by verbal and non-verbal techniques, and performed during grief counselling or grief therapy.

For a person in grief, a therapeutic ritual can be structured to enable a client to come to grips with the loss, to remember the thing or person lost, to examine, clarify, integrate and express his feelings and thoughts; it can enable the client to say goodbye and move on.

10.4 Goals

General goal

- Reducing and removing negative tension related to unresolved/unfinished business (loss events or traumatic events).

Specific goals

- Allowing the client to separate themselves from the old situation with the person or thing lost and letting them focus on the new situation without the person or thing lost;
- Providing the client with closure over an intensive period;
- Letting the client find closure for a shocking (life-disruptive) event.

10.5 Indications

- The client indicates not being able to let go of the old situation, not being able to move forwards despite the effort put into the other methods (incidental loss).
- The client finds himself in a drastic life transition and indicates not being able to move on (transition loss).
- The client has unresolved/unfinished business (from the past).
- The client cannot let go of a traumatic event after trauma work.
- The client is at a point of closure in intensive social work. Here too, it is necessary to take the time to say goodbye.

10.6 Contraindications

- The client denies or fights against the loss.
- The client freezes during rituals because of previous experiences with them.
- The client performs the ritual as dictated by others.
- The client has insufficient (physical or emotional) strength.

10.7 Techniques

1 Farewell technique
2 Yet-still technique
3 Suspension technique
4 Trauma-closure technique.

10.7.1 Farewell technique

The farewell technique is used in cases of actual loss. The social worker proposes to make the actual transition from the old situation to the newly arisen situation by performing a farewell ritual. The client knows exactly what happened, thanks to social work sessions, and has changed their unrealistic thoughts (by means of the cognitive method), has discharged himself by crying (discharge method) and has released bottled-up tension (body-oriented method). Despite all of this, they cannot let go of the person or thing they have lost. That is why the social worker proposes performing a ritual.

When the client agrees to this proposal, they are asked whether they can think of a ritual, whether they have performed any other rituals, and if so to name examples of what worked and what did not work in these rituals. The three phases of the farewell technique are:

1 Preparation of the ritual
2 Execution of the ritual
3 Assessment of the ritual.

Phase 1 entails some brainstorming around rituals and which ones might be appropriate. Often clients cannot think of a suitable ritual straightaway. Repeating the question and letting the client brainstorm can help. For instance, the social worker asks: 'What does the person or thing you have lost remind you of?,' 'What was valuable?,' 'How was the attachment realized?' and 'What would be an appropriate way to say goodbye?' The following questions are answered: 'In what way can you say a proper goodbye to the person or thing that was lost?,' 'Which attributes of symbolic value (pictures, booklets, jewellery, etc.) belong to it?,' 'When and where will the ritual be performed?,' 'Who will be present, who will say what, at which time does it start and when does it end?' and 'When is our next appointment?'

When this is finalized with all the necessary attention given to all of the details (the social worker checks everything very precisely), phase 2 can be initiated: the execution, where the ritual is actually performed. The social worker points out to the client that performing a farewell ritual can be emotional and that it is perfectly normal.

Then comes phase 3, the farewell ritual is discussed and assessed during the next session. How does the client feel? What was it like performing the ritual? Are there any loose ends? A letter to the social worker about the execution of the ritual and its effects can be a useful way to look back and to verify whether all goals were attained. If not, the remaining aspects are determined and further action is undertaken. It may also be useful to ask which 'skeletons' are still left in the 'closet' after the execution of the ritual. This can be done before or after the ritual has been performed. Often an internal critic negates the performed ritual's effect afterwards. A question about what the client expects to think or encounter in the period after the ritual and disproving or confirming any fantasies about the future can eventually ratify the outcome of the ritual. A checklist such as the one that follows may be useful in the detailed preparation of a ritual.

Rituals checklist: the 9 W's of a proper goodbye

1	What is the purpose of the ritual? Which specific goals does the ritual serve?
2	Which actions (symbolic) can help in providing closure for this old and unresolved/unfinished chapter in the person's life?
3	Which attributes are required for these symbolic actions?
4	Which verbal formulas does the client want to utilize (for example supported by words [letter] [expressive work method]). Which message is symbolically expressed by the ritual?
5	Who does the client want next to him during the ritual and what is that person's role?
6	Where does the client wish to perform the ritual? What is the most appropriate location and ambience?
7	When does the client wish to perform the ritual? Is the execution of the ritual being worked towards?
8	Was the ritual effective? What was the ritual's influence before, during and after the execution?
9	Which unfinished affairs remain? Are there any remaining aspects requiring attention?

The letter Mr. Pieterse wrote to his father is an example of a farewell ritual.

The case of Mr. Pieterse

Mr. Pieterse was feeling very oppressed in his relationship with his father. He had also lost the sense that his father was protecting him and lost his own self-worth. In order for him to win back his self-esteem and respect for his father (who was still alive), some unresolved/unfinished business with his father was still to be finished.

Mr. Pieterse was fully aware that he made an active contribution in going along with his father's expectations and continuing to play along as if 'everything was OK'. Medical complaints had brought him down, and after a few therapy sessions it was clear that there were still some painful feelings originating from the past that needed to be addressed. The therapist and Mr. Pieterse agreed upon him writing a letter to his father as a starting point. He read it aloud during the next session. They arranged when, how and with what expectations he would read the letter to his father. During the next session he would think about an appropriate way of dealing with the reactions from his father. The session after reading the letter to his father the client came in clearly relieved, as if an enormous burden which he carried with him for years had been lifted from his shoulders. After reading the letter to his father, his father said he had never intended to be so dominant. At that point, Mr. Pieterse and his father agreed that from now on they would use the word 'father' to refer to the severe and oppressive person his father had been, and the word 'Dad' to refer to the positive, new parent.

10.7.2 Yet-still technique

The yet-still technique is applied in cases where there is old, unprocessed grief. The social worker walks the client through the same phases as in the farewell technique. The client, however, is not dealing with an actual loss but with a loss from the past in which there was no farewell or an improper farewell. By calling the ritual a 'yet-still ritual', it becomes clear that it concerns a retrospective event. The client goes through the same three phases as in the farewell technique.

10.7.3 Suspension technique

Sometimes it is impossible to say goodbye because the physical evidence associated with the loss is missing, for example in cases of missing persons. The social worker suggests that the client prepares and performs a ritual for their own peace of mind. This ritual symbolizes the emotion associated with the loss, that is the person who has gone missing and who will never return. The missing thing or person is placed in limbo, so to speak. There is no final farewell because it is not possible in these types of situations where lack of evidence continues to raise uncertainty.

10.7.4 Trauma-closure technique

The social worker proposes to start a closure ritual after a client has had to deal with an extremely traumatic situation or extreme event. A commemorative ritual can be performed to pay respect, at the same location where the extreme event took place (e.g. where people died or were badly injured). Here too, the three phases of the farewell technique are followed.

Fatal accident

A client had run over a man at night; he felt himself suddenly driving over a 'bump' on the road. Even though he was not to blame, he still felt sorry for the deceased victim. After trauma-work he found more peace, but he could not let go of the event entirely. He felt as though there was something 'unfinished' between him and the victim. Grief support had taught him that it may be helpful to perform a closing ritual in order to bring closure to the unfinished business. The client was receptive to this idea. The question was, how can you give shape to this? The answer came rather quickly: by visiting the location with his girlfriend, standing there and laying down some flowers while saying the words: 'Sorry, I didn't mean to take your life'.

10.8 Social work results

- The client has symbolically put an 'end' on the past.
- The client experiences a sense of closure for the extreme event.
- The client experiences more peace of mind.
- The client is at peace with the (loss) situation.
- The client experiences the beginning of a new period.
- The client says he is able to move on.

10.9 Evidence

There has been little research done as to how the ritual method is applied in grief counselling. The only evidence-based ritual research conducted to date was done by Norton and Gino (2014). First we will summarize the research, after which we will have a closer look at the experimental design and the results as they were published in the science supplement to the Dutch *NRC Handelsblad* newspaper (De Bruin, 2014).

In a number of studies the effect of mourning rituals on grief reduction have been examined, including after instances of losing a loved one or losing the lottery. The subjects who were instructed to reflect upon the performed rituals, or those instructed to write a story after experiencing loss, reported being less sad. According to researchers the stronger feelings of control experienced by subjects after the rituals take place could be a result of using such rituals. The advantages of performing rituals did not only apply to those who believed in the meaning of rituals, but also to those who did not believe in them. Furthermore, while specific rituals vary between cultures, religions and studies, this research suggests that there is a common mechanism at play: the renewed feeling of control.

This survey on the effects of farewell rituals is so unique that we incorporate an abstract in the form of the newspaper article, as follows.

Rituals provide sense of control over loss

Tearing up pictures, burning letters: Makeshift rituals help in processing grief, even for people who do not believe in rituals, as long as you call it a ritual.

'I gathered all the pictures from our time together and shredded them to pieces. Even the pictures I loved so much. Afterwards I burned those pieces in the park, where we shared our first kiss.'

The above was written by one of the participants in an American survey on mourning rituals, recently published in *Journal of Experimental Psychology: General* (February 2014). When people lose a loved one, for example when a relationship comes to an end or when someone has passed away, many people come up with their own personal ritual for processing their grief.

The rituals are seldom of a religious nature: 76 people were asked how they processed their grief after losing someone, and only 5% of the rituals appeared to be related to religion. Most rituals (95%) were performed alone, and 90% without anyone else even seeing it. People really do it for themselves: according to researchers at the Harvard Business School, rituals help people to regain a sense of control. And they feel less sad because of this.

The rituals described by participants were very diverse – and touching. One participant has been lighting a candle every year for 21 years on the day his loved one passed away. Another one went to the hairdresser's on the first Saturday of every month, 'like we used to do together'.

Even the mere thought of the rituals they had performed after losing a loved one, retrospectively gives people a stronger sense of control. This was shown by researchers in an experiment where half of the participants were asked to only describe their grief, while the other half were asked to describe their grief plus the ritual they had performed to process it. There were no significant differences, but the less control people reported to feel at the time, the emptier their lives appeared to be without the person in question. So the less control they felt, the more grief they felt.

In another experiment, researchers showed that an artificial ritual can help as well, even for people who do not believe in rituals. Participants, young people, came to the lab in small groups and were told that one of them was about to win $200 and would be excused straightaway. And so it was, leaving the participants to cope with a certain loss. Obviously not as bad as losing a loved one, but of course this type of tragedy cannot be induced in an experimental setting.

Half of the participants were told to draw their feelings on a piece of paper, but this was not referred to as a ritual. The other half were instructed to perform a ritual: also drawing their feelings, then pour some salt over it, tear the paper into pieces and silently count to 10 five times. Subjects who performed the ritual, felt more in control over the situation and were less sad, regardless of whether they believed in rituals, performed them often or thought that the researchers expected them to feel better after the ritual.

The essence, according to researchers, is in performing an action which you refer to as a ritual. What you do exactly does not really matter. Not surprisingly, Hindus shave their hair when mourning, while Jewish men let their (beard) hair grow.

(Summary from de Bruin, 2014)

10.10 Pitfalls

- Prescribing ready-made 'McDonalds rituals' (instead of letting the client brainstorm).
- Exceeding the client's thresholds.

10.11 Summary and questions

This chapter described the role of the social worker in facilitating a proper goodbye; it also described how a proper goodbye contributes to reducing emotional stress as well as the different types of techniques that can be used based on the loss experienced. The conclusion was that the ritual method can help reduce emotional stress and boost someone's personal strength.

Questions

1   Do you recognize examples of farewell rituals carried out by yourself or with others?
2   What do you see as the difference between traditional and therapeutic farewell rituals?
3   Which ritual actions mean a lot to you, and which rituals are difficult to relate to?
4   What makes self-constructed, personalized rituals stronger than prescribed ones?
5   What is your opinion on the following statement: 'There is no such thing as saying goodbye, because in loss you don't have to let go. It's a matter of "holding on differently"'?
6   If you do not believe in farewell rituals, what can you do to open your mind to them?

PART V

Three self-determination methods

Part V describes three methods which social workers can use to work with the client in order to find helpful perspectives to deal with problem situations. The aim of these perspectives is to help fulfil our universal need for self-determination, our need for autonomy.

The concept of perspectives is here used to refer to 'thoughts, reflections, attempts to find meaning in and help with actions' which originate in our neocortex, the rational part of our brain. The social worker uses three specific methods to assist the client in developing helpful perspectives:

- The cognitive method, used to develop *helpful thoughts* (Chapter 11);
- The narrative method, used to develop *helpful narratives* (Chapter 12);
- The behavioural method, used to develop *helpful skills* (Chapter 13).

Helpful perspectives contribute to our optimal enjoyment of life at the mental level (optimal Quality of Life). All three cognitive-behavioural interventions employed by the social worker are aimed at influencing the client's thought processes (cognition) in a constructive manner. So how can social workers utilize the client's mental strength to help convert factors which impede his self-determination into helpful perspectives?

Chapter 11 looks at the role the social worker plays in effectively addressing the 7 steps towards mental problem solving. When our need for helpful thoughts is not (sufficiently) met, cognitive stress results. We will see how social workers can utilize the cognitive method to enlist the client's own cognitive ability to reduce this cognitive stress.

Chapter 12 looks at the social worker's role in helping to develop a helpful narrative, starting from a story which had real impact. Stress around trying to make sense of our lives results when our need to find a positive meaning in our life is not sufficiently met. We will see how the narrative method can be employed to enlist the client's cognitive ability to reduce this type of stress.

Finally, Chapter 13 will describe how social workers can help clients to assert their own needs, because behavioural stress is what results when the client's wishes are not adequately met due to his or her lack of behavioural skills. This chapter will focus on how the behavioural method can help to use skills training to enlist (the client's) social strengths to reduce such behavioural stress.

11

COGNITIVE METHOD

Questions

This chapter addresses the following questions:

- What role does the rational brain play in life events?
- What needs do clients have at the cognitive-behavioural level?
- What does helpful and non-helpful problem solving entail?
- How can the cognitive method contribute to enlisting the client's cognitive strengths in order to reduce cognitive stress?

11.1 Introduction

This chapter will describe the social worker's role in helping meet the client's need for *helpful thoughts* in and about life. How can social workers teach clients to deal with life experiences in a constructive manner?

I will first turn to the role of the rational brain, which is of importance to the three cognitive-behavioural methods, which will be described in the next three chapters. This chapter will then look at the development of cognitive stress and its role in potentially impeding the problem-solving cycle. Next I will describe the cognitive method which helps contribute to the development of helpful thoughts. Cognitive stress can be reduced with the aid of the client's own cognitive strength. I will then provide a summary of the chapter.

11.2 Role and function of the rational brain (neocortex)

The way in which people learn from their life experiences is very much influenced by their ability to reflect, self-reflect and self-control/self-direct, by the way they think, in other words, through cognitive processes. Clients can 'self-obstruct' when their cognitive processes (i.e.

thought processes) are disturbed/disordered. This can lead to unhelpful perspectives (negative, unrealistic or dysfunctional thoughts), which in turn can result in cognitive stress. Cognitive stress entails the lack of balance/the disequilibrium between helpful thoughts around certain life events ('I want to have a job') and the actual situation ('I lost my job'), resulting in the need to restore that balance. Where life events are irreversible (e.g. someone has died), the only thing that remains is the opportunity to think of a way to say goodbye in a dignified manner, and create memories. In that case, cognitive stress will be reduced as helpful thoughts will occur, rather than stressful thoughts. Cognition involves all mental processes, including thoughts, attention and focus, memory and the ability to observe and assess. To quote a popular saying: it involves whatever happens in the top two inches. The term 'cognition' itself, originates from the Latin word *cognitio*, referring to 'knowledge which can be acquired either through the senses or through thought processes'. Cognitive science views people as information-processing systems, with reference to processes which play a role in acquiring, storing and reproducing information. The three most commonly studied cognitive processes are attention, interpretation and memory (source).

Life events such as a loss regulate the rational brain (see Figure 24.2) to go through the transitional curve by means of cognitive processes. In brief, the rational brain plays the role of information processor. Ideally, the rational brain controls the adequate processing of information (see Figure 11.1). And like any other information processing system, the rational brain involves a cycle of *input–throughput–output*.

What information do clients receive about a particular topic (input), how do they interpret that information (throughput), what do they communicate and how does this eventually translate into client behaviour (output)?

In brief, the client responds to external (*input* = e.g. bad news) or internal information-type stimuli (e.g. a rumbling stomach) which are observed, interpreted and made sense of

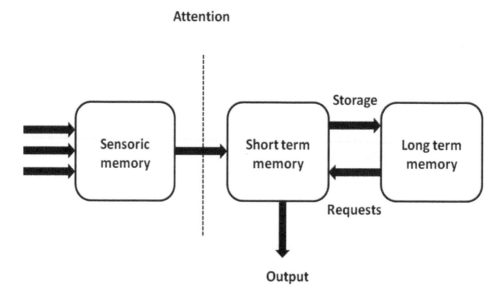

FIGURE 11.1   The information-processing model: input–throughput–output

using both the short- and long-term memory, and which result in certain behaviours (*through-put*). The client processes this information and makes certain choices which are translated into grief-related behaviour (*output*).

In the course of this cognitive process, the client adds new information to the existing database of knowledge in the brain, making use of three types of memory: the sensory memory ('What were the exact words used by the person who gave me the bad news?'), short-term memory ('How did I respond when I lost my job?') and long-term memory ('Have I been through a job loss and emotional responses in my life previously, and how did I cope at the time? Can I live without a job when work was such an important part of my identity?'). To this end clients will code and rationalize information, a process that is invisible to the world around them. We often refer to the *black box* in relation to such *throughput* thought processes, precisely because they remain invisible. The client systematically observes and interprets events based on previous experiences.

Our rational brain is located in the neocortex, which is the most recently developed part of our brain in an evolutionary sense (see Figure 24.2). Whenever we receive a signal to warn us of a threat (such as a loss), all three parts of our brains (survival, affective and rational) are activated. Eventually it is our rational thought which shapes the collaboration between these three parts of the brain. Does our rational brain always pay close attention to our internal responses? Or does it not always do so when we are faced with certain threats? At times, our survival and affective brains will be activated more quickly than our rational brain. This happens because certain dangerous situations which are a matter of life and death (e.g. when we experience a lack of oxygen) require a superfast response from our brain (see Chapter 5). In extremely threatening situations, the amygdala will show a rapid, conditioned, fearful response (survival brain). As stated previously, LeDoux (1996) discovered that fear-inducing signals can be processed along two routes: one fast, one slow. The fast route runs through the thalamus in our rational brain, directly to the amygdala and the survival brain. The slow route runs from the thalamus via the visual cortex in the cognitive brain through to the amygdala and the affective brain. When emotional information is processed through the rational brain, there is more time for a complex analysis.

Our rational brain uses logical reasoning to regulate questions in accordance with the problem-solving cycle: signals are responded to as information which requires processing, the brain processes this information, reflects on it all (which includes self-reflection), finds the language, starts to plan, makes decisions and ensures these are acted upon (behavioural actions).

Life events require both external (the environment) and internal adaptations (within the person), leaving the client with a lot to deal with: 'I feel overwhelmed,' 'Everything has changed,' 'All these things that need to be done, I feel like I have a mountain to climb,' 'So many feelings going through my head, how can I carry on?'

In such instances, everyone needs helpful perspectives on the world around us, on life events, changes in identity, and on actions. These are our cognitive, existential and behavioural needs. The rational brain ensures that we cope in a rational manner by interpreting information from our two more intuitive brains – our survival and affective brains – and using that information to plan and execute certain behaviours. Physical and affective threats are regulated by the other parts of our brain, but are 'read' by our rational brain. This part of our brain is able to put our instinctive impulses into words: 'How unsafe is my current situation?' (survival brain), 'What are my feelings right now?' (affective brain), 'What is the best action to take (or should I not take any action)?' (rational brain).

Table 11.1 shows the seven steps of the problem-solving cycle (see also Chapter 6):

TABLE 11.1 Helpful cognitive-behavioural methods in the problem-solving cycle

Information processing cycle	Problem-solving cycle	Helpful methods
1 Input	1 Trigger, signals/flags (*example from social work in the medical setting: My wife died as a result of a medical error*)	*Cognitive method* (realistic thoughts: was this due to medical error, how could this have happened?)
2 Throughput	2 Defining the problem (e.g. *You won't rest until the doctor admits he was wrong*)	
	3 Formulating goals (e.g. *You want the doctor to say he is sorry*)	*Cognitive method* (solution-focused: what do I want, how can I move forwards?)
	4 Brainstorming about solutions (e.g. *You can go see (a) the doctor, (b) the patient advocate, (c) the complaints committee, (d) the Medical Council disciplinary committee*)	and *Narrative method* (I want to carry on with my life, I don't want to be a moaner.)
	5 Decision on solution (e.g. *talking to the doctor*)	
3 Output	6 Acting on the decision (e.g. *social worker helps client make an appointment: meeting takes place*)	*Behavioural method* (assertive behaviour: how do I say what is on my mind?)
	7 Assessing the outcome (e.g.: *meeting was unsatisfactory; client wants to see the patient advocate*)	*Cognitive method* (reflecting on whether the goals have been achieved or not)

11.3 Cognitive stress: unhelpful problem solving

It is clear that our rational brain can assist us in developing helpful perspective, so the question remains: how do cognitive stress and unhelpful thoughts develop and how can we develop more helpful ways of thinking? We will take the various steps in the problem-solving process outlined in Table 11.1 and will use them as a guideline for identifying and reducing unmet cognitive needs.

11.3.1 The problem-solving cycle and our cognitive needs

How can an awareness of the problem-solving cycle help reduce cognitive stress? What parts do information and information processing play in problem solving?

Information processing can either contribute to or deduct from your quality of life:

> Adequate information processing in relation to life events entails interpreting bad news and the associated consequences in a realistic manner, so that eventually, you learn to enjoy the opportunities life offers you again.
>
> *(Eisma et al., 2013)*

Cognitive stress results when the client's need for adequate information processing remains unmet to a greater or lesser extent. Stress occurs when the client is not given any or incorrect information, interprets information in an unrealistic manner, makes the wrong decisions, takes the wrong actions or is unable to readjust his identity following the life event. Unrealistic information processing – in the form of unrealistic thoughts or avoidance behaviour – has been shown to significantly hamper the problem-solving process.

Before I go on to look at the needs in the problem-solving cycle step by step and how these can be met, I would like to briefly comment on solution-focused support. I will describe the *solution-focused* technique as one of the cognitive techniques discussed elsewhere in this chapter; it is an example of working to achieve a solution, rather than ruminating on problems. The solution-focused approach holds that it is wrong for support workers to merely focus on issues, spending too much time on exploring those. By contrast, the solution-focused technique stresses that good support involves working on the future: what is it you need to carry on? In Chapter 2, which dealt with theory, we saw that a good theory does not only look at how to move towards the future (prospective predicting), but also entail gaining insight and understanding into how the current situation arose (retrospective understanding). If we argue that the strength of the client in his environment should always be considered the engine that helps us progress, this can only occur on condition that we look both back into the past and forwards into the future. Therefore, all the steps of the problem-solving cycle are conditional for growth if applied in a flexible manner, without patronizing the client, and the focus should be on resolving the problem, that is, solution-oriented.

Step 1 Cause of the problem: the need for realistic information

The aim of informative messages is to provide adequate information:

- Make sure that a given situation is conveyed to the recipient in a realistic manner, thus ensuring that the news remains manageable;
- Provide information that the recipient needs to be able to make decisions.

As an example, when you give someone bad news, you should do this based on the assumption that the recipient is entitled to the bad news being conveyed in a direct manner: so a succinct informative message, given in an empathetic manner/tone of voice, followed by a brief additional explanation.

Where things go awry is when bad news is being conveyed using clichés:

- Postponing the real message (leaving the recipient to guess);
- Leaving things hanging ('So there is something wrong');
- Downplaying the severity ('But things could have been worse');
- Justifying the bad news ('It is better this way');
- The person giving the bad news starts to talk about himself ('I am finding this difficult as well').

When bad news is given the wrong way, information processing is also off to a bad start. In instances where information has been kept back, clients can feel as if the bad news has come completely out of left field. Take the employee who carried on working hard for his employer right through to the weekend, and who was told that the company was doing well ('Not to worry') only to receive a letter in the mail the next morning (on Saturday) to say he had lost his job. This can be very disturbing: the client/former employee can remain stuck in those initial feelings of shock or go on being angry about the way in which he was notified of his dismissal.

Step 2 Defining the problem: the need for realistic interpretations

The next step in the information processing process is the interpretation of (bad) news. To what extent is the client able to interpret the available information and the associated consequences in a realistic manner? The control technique for unrealistic thoughts (see section 11.8.7) contains a list of unrealistic thoughts, including the idea that life events are due to you failing as a person, that everything has to go the way you had planned, that you cannot change the way you behave, that you have to get worked up about the life event, that you cannot face life on your own, and so on.

Lazarus and Launier (1978) was the first to really focus on the way in which stress-inducing situations are being observed and interpreted, and Lazarus introduced the subjective aspect of stress in the concept of 'coping' (Lazarus, 1992). What mediating role do subjective processes play in the development of stress responses? The central question in the interpretation of bad news is how to assess information about the life event and how to deal with emotions, stress and associated consequences. What is your cognitive coping like?

Leg amputation

The client commences active rehabilitation following a leg amputation. The rehab physician refers the client to a rehab social worker to work on resolving some practical obstacles in the home situation and to work accepting his disability. The client is very down and unable to cope with his new status as a person in a wheelchair. How does the client interpret his leg amputation and the associated consequences ? To what extent does he demonstrate adequate cognitive coping?

Cognitive stress involves (1) an unrealistic interpretation of the situation and (2) an inadequate way of coping with the situation. Lazarus emphasized the manner in which the stress-inducing situation is observed and interpreted. There are two ways of interpreting a stressful situation: primary and secondary interpretation. In primary interpretation we ask ourselves: 'Is this a painful, threatening or challenging experience?' 'Am I okay or am I in trouble?' Cognitive stress occurs if a life event is interpreted as having a negative effect on our personal wellbeing: 'I am in trouble, this situation is not aligned with how I view myself, my future and so on.'

Personal failure

Cognitive stress further increases when setbacks and disappointments around the life event are seen as a form of personal failure. When faced with a setback you may have the idea (cognition) that you have failed as a person. You may also think that you should be the sacrificial lamb, thus short-changing yourself. Having unrealistic expectations poses another risk factor for developing additional stress. If your expectations of life or work are too high or too low, you run a greater risk of being disappointed.

Put in charge

A registered nurse has been given a promotion in the course of organizational change. She has been put in charge and left to do everything on her own, when in fact nothing is working well. Within a very short time, this is driving her mad, because none of the new systems she wants to put in place as the newly appointed head is functioning. After a year, her joy about being promoted has evaporated and she is home on sick leave. The social worker determines that her expectations had been at a level above what the organization was able to meet. The client blamed herself for this debacle, but eventually realized that it was her own high expectations which had led to her immense feelings of frustration, and also that the organization had ignored signs that she needed support.

Unrealistic expectations which are too high or otherwise unfounded, as illustrated in the previous example, remain unmet in practice. If you set your expectations too high, you can only get frustrated: you will never reach that level. Reducing such expectations temporarily – from the desired level – does make it possible to work towards a higher level in practice. People with strong drive and motivation, who work very hard and who are willing to sacrifice themselves, are at risk of falling victim to such unrealistically high expectations. They get into trouble because they respond to stress in the wrong way: they feel they have lost control over their work and are unable to reach their goals. If they try and persist at all costs, they get exhausted. If they take a defensive attitude, this also results in unhealthy stress levels, because tension only increases and they start to increasingly dislike the tasks they have to complete.

Inadequate knowledge and skills

Additional cognitive stress can also occur as a result of inadequate knowledge and skills. This leads to ineffective performance, thereby having a negative effect on someone's feeling of self-worth. This leads to an increased error rate in making decisions and also an increased tendency to hide those errors. When offered appropriate reading material, clients who find themselves in such situations receive information which is up to date. Through practice, such clients will acquire the current skills they need to face their problems.

The computer

The social worker notices that one of his clients is getting very frustrated in his new job because of his lack of computer skills. The client is offered help to improve his knowledge and skills in that area. An interview with his team leader is arranged to discuss a negative performance review relating to work-related errors made by the client.

When information processing is adequate, people are able to realistically deal with their problems, in spite of unhappy life events. If a difficult situation is discussed in a realistic manner, it is easier to distance yourself from problems or incidents.

When we have positive experiences it is realistic for us to give ourselves a pat on the back: 'I managed that well.' When experiences are negative, however, we have to avoid doing the opposite and not tell ourselves off.

Feelings of guilt

Feelings of guilt can develop when people feel guilty about surviving the person who died: this is what is called survivor's guilt. This often involves 'guilty thoughts' rather than feelings per se. Clients may think back to the time before the death occurred, looking for signs that they have somehow failed, in order to try and do justice to the person they lost. The tendency is to 'think ourselves guilty', guilty of neglect or lack of empathy. Small things which happened in the years leading up to the life event tend to be magnified (Lindeman, 1972, Glick et al., 1974, Degner, 1976).

If the deceased went through a long and painful illness, family members may be relieved when they die, while at the same time feeling ashamed and guilty that they feel this way. Not having any health issues may be another reason for clients to feel guilty. If clients keep viewing the life event as a form of punishment, this may be due to hidden feelings of guilt (Perez, 1982). Feelings of guilt may also be due to extreme anger associated with post-traumatic stress disorder.

People with a disability tend to view anger as morally wrong, and therefore reject their own feelings of increased hostility. They may develop feelings of guilt based on the thought that they may lose control over their anger (Krupnick & Horowitz, 1981). Feelings of guilt may be explained as a way to learn from a terrible situation and regain a certain sense of power and control (Herman, 1993).

Feelings of embarrassment

Embarrassment is strongly associated with feelings of guilt. People feel embarrassed when they are seen in a situation which does not match their self-image (Rando, 1984). Patients who are totally dependent on others or people who have been robbed of any sense of control or dignity often feel embarrassed or uncomfortable.

Feelings of embarrassment can be covered up by other emotions, such as anger or misplaced loyalty. They can also be compensated by responses such as denial or aggression. It is important to be aware of this, especially in relation to the care for patients who have been maimed and who need care for their private body parts. Young children whose brother or sister is dying often feel embarrassed because their family is now seen to be 'different'.

Dreams and hallucinations

Hallucinations, sensory delusions, frequently occur – usually in the form of brief imaginary experiences which occur within a few weeks of the life event. They usually do not reflect a complicated grief response. To some, such experiences are frightening, but others feel that they help the grieving process.

Some people start to have frequent dreams about the person who died, and these express the loss and pain associated with the life event.

Concentration problems

Concentration issues may occur and can be difficult to address. People may find themselves being forgetful, unable to focus.

The taxi driver

I told the driver where I wanted to go and leant back in my seat as he drove off. A few moments later he again asked where I wanted to go. I assumed he must be a new driver, one who was not very familiar with the city, but he told me he had a lot of things going on in his head. After a short while, he again asked me where I wanted to go, apologized and told me he was very confused. This happened again a few times and eventually I decided to ask him what was on his mind. He told me his son had died in a traffic accident the previous week.

(Worden, 1992.)

If there is no release for pain after a life event, cognitive confusion may result: the inability to think clearly or make clear decisions following the life event.

Step 3: Goal-setting: the need for helpful perspectives

Storytelling is a very human characteristic. Perhaps it is what sets us apart from other forms of life. As Brian Morton (1984) puts it:

> The world, the human world, is bound together not by protons and electrons, but by stories. Nothing has meaning in itself: all the objects in the world would be shards of bare mute blankness, spinning wildly out of orbit, if we didn't bind them together with stories.

In our stories, we frame our experience, manipulate it, give it focus and create meanings which guide us in meeting new experiences. Through the stories we create, we make meaning in and of the world. Assigning a place to life experiences, such as a loss, involves mentally integrating the story of your loss into the larger story of your life. You adapt to the new situation: you accommodate. The word 'accommodation' refers to reconsidering your assumptions about yourself, the world and the person who is no longer in your life. Accommodation is a mental function that involves symbolically finding closure for the loss: taking the time to create a new relationship with the person you lost, but also investing in a new life.

Being aware of your loss and finding a way to say goodbye – two transitional tasks clients have to engage in – are not the same as integrating the loss. The third transitional task – building memories and a new life – require both internal and external adaptation. Externally adapting to the new reality, for instance by setting the table for one rather than for two people, does not mean that you have adapted internally (accommodation).

The realization – while in the process of saying goodbye – of 'my loved one is gone, the pain is unbearable; I cannot find the words to express it' involves giving meaning to the loss in a way that makes it bearable. You learn to adapt to your new reality.

Accommodating involves adapting the internal worldview (existing schemas) from your long-term memory to the new information received. The grieving process may be seen as one where the old thinking patterns or schemas are being replaced by new ones. Both the relationship with the person who was lost and the way in which the person affected views himself and the world. The loss is being integrated into his or her future life.

In practical terms this integration is the result of clients working through explanations, ideas and meanings relating to both 'old' and 'new' information. I will take a closer look at this encryption process in Chapter 12, as it is an important mental activity to help us learn to deal with loss.

Mrs. X

A social worker is working with Mrs. X. Mrs. X continues to make a deflated impression in the assertiveness training group, in spite of the fact that her partner is very encouraging. The social worker tries to find out her thoughts about herself and the situation at home. Mrs. X admits that she has low self-esteem: 'I will never manage.'

The social worker wonders why she has such a negative view of herself and decides to use the cognitive method.

Cognitive schemas develop in response to negative events early or later on in life. Once these schemas have developed, they are consolidated and confirmed by means of *self-statements* (Jacobs, 1999). By being repeated all the time, certain views turn into a base philosophy or attitude to life; they turn into axioms, things that go without saying. They are considered to be the truth, rather than merely thoughts or opinions. Next, people start to view reality based on these 'truths', and misinterpretations may readily ensue. Many irrational thoughts may be maintained and passed on to a large extent through our upbringing and through social institutions. It is the social worker's job to encourage clients to become aware of such irrational ways of thinking, for instance by identifying potentially unrealistic thoughts and by asking clients to what extent such thoughts are realistic (the challenge technique, see section 11.8.5).

In Chapter 11 I will discuss the client's cognitive processes around making sense of things and identity transformation in more depth.

Step 4 Brainstorming around possible solutions: the need for helpful thought processes

Lazarus's primary interpretation involved the question of (Step 2): 'Is this a painful, threatening or challenging experience?' The secondary interpretation of the situation revolves around the next couple of questions:

- What can I do about it?
- What options are there to get on top of these problems?

The client evaluates various approaches – coping strategies – and their possible success rate. This process is based on previous experiences with similar situations (accessing memories), the client's self-image and the availability of the means to overcome the stressful situation.

Step 5 Decision making: the need for helpful decisions

Helpful decision making includes making decisions which results in the client's improved enjoyment of life (improved QoL). Let us think of various possible solutions. Which of these will help me the most? In the course of the decision-making process you consider solutions that would be unachievable, bizarre or unhelpful. The assumption is that clients will be cognitively capable of assessing the consequences of the various alternative options.

Step 6 Acting on the decision: the need for helpful actions

When acting on the decisions we have made, we tend to assume all manner of skills. In Chapter 13 I look at skills training, and the power of practice-makes-perfect: how can we use skills training to help clients do what is necessary to take the steps required to move forwards?

Step 7 Review by comparing the result to the goals: the need to learn from experience

Learning from experience is the last step in the problem-solving model, involving the client setting goals for himself. This step entails the client assessing whether these goals were met. If a goal has not been met, the client can consider adjusting the goals, or reflect on whether other actions are needed to achieve that goal after all. Another possibility involves a goal not having been achieved because of emotional (affective brain) or physical impediments. In such cases, we need to allow time/space for this, because learning from experience is partly a cognitive process, however it can be hampered by emotions and physical stress and so on. I will now focus on the association between cognitive learning, learning from experience and learning skills in the cycle of human learning.

11.3.2 The learning cycle: learning from experience, theoretical learning and learning by doing

We view learning as a cognitive, emotional and skills-based process which eventually results in optimal enjoyment of life. The learning process involves various stages, including receiving and interpreting information, testing new insights, reflecting on what happens to us and trying out alternative behaviours. As a psychologist, Kolb (1984) investigated the various stages in human learning, identifying four distinct phases, which can be described in terms of the needs associated with each phase:

- Concrete experience (*feeling*);
- Observation and reflection (*watching*);

- Forming abstract theories/concepts (*thinking*);
- Actively experimenting (*doing*).

The four phases follow on from each other in a logical sequence: when experiencing a certain life event (*feeling*, at the level of experiencing), it is important to reflect on such experiences (*watching*, level of reflection) and generalizing (*thinking*, forming a concept). Next you can think of an approach that will reduce stress and approach a similar event based on the learning process (*doing*, experimenting). By actually implementing the new approach/learned behaviour, you gain new experiences (concrete experience) that you can then ponder (reflection), resulting in new insights (forming concepts). This model allows us to rank the various cognitive needs. Kolb described the ideal learning model, which involves the four phases continuing to repeat themselves in this order. Kolb sees the learning process as a cyclical model (see Figure 11.2).

If you lose touch with your children (following a divorce), you can try and find a way to deal with this in a number of ways. You can try all sorts of interaction styles (experimenting) to see what works (gaining experience and presumably reflecting on this as well). You can try and recall experiences with similar life events, such as ones involving the loss of a loved one through death, because you may have had to deal with that in a similar manner (reflection), thus arriving at the most relevant interaction style (forming a concept) which you can then try out in practice (experimenting).

Another possibility is asking someone else to show you how to deal with certain life events (experience), so you can try and imagine how to deal with such life events (reflection, concept formation) and try it out in practice yourself (experimenting).

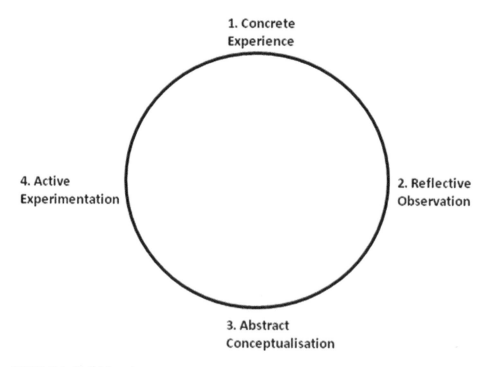

FIGURE 11.2 Kolb's learning process

If you run through all these stages, you can gain maximum benefit from the learning process. It is obvious why this is so: experience is more valuable if you reflect upon it, and any insights gained will only truly be useful if you try them out (experimenting) and test them (experience, reflection). So learning only truly starts when you move through all these stages, something that has now become widely accepted, in both education and research. Kolb (1984) describes experience as the engine driving the learning process:

> Immediate concrete experience is the basis for observation and reflection. These observations are assimilated into a theory from which new implications for action can be reduced. These implications of hypotheses then serve as guides in acting to create new experiences.

11.4 History of the cognitive method

The cognitive method is oriented towards fulfilling needs at the cognitive level, that is achieving maximizing knowledge and information processing, thought processes and internal dialogues (*self-talk*). The cognitive method contributes to constructive problem solving and information processing by positively influencing clients' unrealistic, negative and harmful thoughts about themselves and the world around them.

When psychosocial assessment (PSA) has shown that clients are affected by inadequate coping at the cognitive level, the cognitive method can be used to help them achieve adequate cognitive coping. The social worker will use cognitive techniques to inventorize, analyze and change the client's selective observations and thoughts, selective focus, memory and assessment of situations and of himself.

The cognitive method impacts the chain of thought in the situation-thought-feeling behaviour chain. Influencing this chain in a positive manner constitutes the basis for rational emotive therapy (RET).

After the initial optimism about the strength of cognitive theories and behavioural therapies – which involved the notion of people being able to learn and unlearn behaviour – it became evident that people can harbour all sorts of negative thoughts as a result of which certain tensions are maintained. This discovery about the boundaries of the learnability of behaviour was the basis for the cognitive method. Albert Ellis (1976) and Aaron Beck (1979) played a very important role in developing this method. Ellis focused on a few universal irrational thoughts which he held responsible for all sorts of neurotic psychopathology. Beck described dysfunctional mental schemas resulting in emotional disorders. Cognitive behavioural techniques are popular in clinical social work in North America: these constitute a mix of cognitive and behavioural techniques, such as the use of cognitive behavioural therapy in psychotherapy. Next, I will present in chronological order some of the psychotherapeutic concepts which underpin the cognitive method in social work.

11.4.1 How we think

According to cognitive psychologists, any knowledge we possess is organized in cognitive schemas or associative networks. Such cognitive schemas serve to help us process information, in the course of which unrealistic thoughts may develop. Such thoughts are sometimes also referred to as irrational thoughts, unreasonable thoughts, dysfunctional thoughts, incorrect thoughts, thinking errors or negative thoughts. The client may think: 'It is my fault, things will not improve, things will never get any better'. I prefer to use the term 'unrealistic thought' in my description of the cognitive method, because this makes it clear that the social worker will test a particular thought against the client's reality: 'How realistic is a particular thought?' The various terms are alternated in social work practice.

RET

When the cognitive method is applied to social work it is often referred to as rational emotive therapy (RET); in group social work, RET is synonymous with rational emotive training. Social workers often mention RET as one of the methods they apply, however it does not appear to have been described as a distinct method in social work. The method is based on the premise that there is a strong link between elements in the chain of thoughts–feelings–behaviour, like a type of three-of-a-kind. Even so, within RET the focus is mostly on the thoughts.

Jacobs (1999) views rational thoughts as being based on reality, helping people to achieve their goals, providing us with useful means to meet the requirements of daily living, and being associated with adequate emotions. Irrational thoughts, by contrast, are not aligned with reality; they can sabotage the goals the client sets himself, and can cause problems in day-to-day situations. Moreover, irrational thoughts are associated with inadequate emotions and dysfunctional behaviour. We concur with this view on the place of irrational thoughts in RET. Demanding, negative thoughts, the must-do's, are usually referred to as irrational core thoughts in RET. They form the client's core philosophies. The following are just some examples.

- Judging oneself or making statements about one's own identity: 'I am a dick,' 'I am no good,' 'He is an arsehole,' 'He is a bad one.'
- Low levels of frustration tolerance: 'I cannot stand this,' 'I am not going to survive this,' 'I cannot handle anything too difficult.'
- Doom thinking: 'It is terrible, unavoidable that . . .,' 'It is just so bad.'
- Exaggerated generalizations: 'I will never . . .,' 'People always . . .,' 'They always. . . .'

Dysfunctional thoughts

Within the field of social work, insights from cognitive therapy were also reflected in Reid's (1982) task-centred approach, through the concept of 'dysfunctional thoughts'. The way in which people view themselves and the world around them determines the way they behave. Functional thoughts, such as 'The world is round' or 'Physical violence is wrong' or 'I will be unhappy if people ignore my work' can be used as a guideline for actions and may thus result in guidelines for alleviating the current problems. Dysfunctional thoughts have the opposite effect.

Solution-focused therapy

Solution-focused therapy (Cladder, 2000), which is also known as solution-focused brief therapy (SFBT), is a new form of social work that is gaining traction in the field of social work. Solution-focused therapy assumes that clients are able to focus on how things could be done better, in a concrete and detailed manner; clients are asked to use their problem-solving skills to achieve the desired situation. The focus is on finding solutions, rather than first and foremost on the problem itself. It is important that clients identify changes in their own behaviour, whenever those changes result in improving their situation. In other words, the client's thinking is directed towards solutions rather than problems: 'So as soon as you picked up your hobby again, you started to enjoy life again? It may be good to pick up your hobby again a bit more, if that so clearly makes you feel better'.

Schema therapy

Schema therapy is gaining popularity in the field of psychotherapy. A schema is described as a fixed thought pattern that strongly influences human behaviour. Schema therapy is not part of the social work field, because it is aimed at helping people with personality disorders. Even so, it is useful for social workers to be aware of what it entails. Schema therapy was developed by the American psychologist Jeffrey Young (Young, 1999), who argues that mental health problems originate from early childhood. Children who do not receive appropriate support following traumatic experiences may develop all-pervasive negative thought patterns about themselves and their relationships with others. Such early maladaptive schemas persist and resist any form of change. Young proposes that schema therapy be used to change such maladaptive schemas through cognitive, behavioural and experience-focused techniques.

11.5 Goals

General goal

- To reduce or eliminate negative stress caused by cognitive obstacles such as unrealistic or negative thoughts and inadequate information about normal stress responses to life events and trauma and so on.

Specific goals

- The client is well-informed about a specific event, about normal responses, all relevant aspects of life which touch on his or her own life.
- The client thinks in a realistic manner.
- The client gives himself positive instructions.
- The client replaces thoughts which are harmful to himself and others by constructive thoughts.

11.6 Indications

- The client has a lack of information.
- The client has unrealistic thoughts, including doom thinking, martyrdom, *must*-urbation (feeling that you always 'have to' do things), perfectionism and disaster (catastrophic) thinking.
- The client is giving himself negative instructions.
- The client is harbouring harmful thoughts about himself or others.

11.7 Contraindications

- The client's cognitive ability is insufficient (dementia, intellectual disability, brain injury).
- The client is too confused.

11.8 Techniques

1 Education about mental health
2 Reality-check technique
3 Normalization technique
4 Diary technique
5 Challenge technique
6 Positive self-imaging technique
7 Control technique checking unrealistic thoughts
8 4G technique
9 Reframing technique
10 Setting norms technique
11 Feeling Yes – Feeling No technique
12 Solution-focused technique (exception question, 'I wonder' question)
13 Internet-related techniques.

11.8.1 Education about mental health

Educating clients about mental health is a form of cognitive support which involves informing clients about the fact that their responses are normal. Providing information in the form
of flyers, information material, bibliotherapy and education about mental health often has a
reassuring effect. Mr. Stack's story shows that we cannot take it for granted that clients will be
provided with such information.

Mr. Stack's case study

Mr. Stack was prescribed strong sleeping drugs 20 years earlier, after the stillbirth of
his first son. He was not cautioned about the possible side-effects of the medication,
nor was he told not to drink alcohol alongside these drugs. In fact, the family doctor
increased the dosage. This almost cost him his life when he wrote off his new car in
a crash. For years he suffered due to these losses and because of the inadequate social
work he had been prescribed and which only suppressed his symptoms. What had
started out as normal feelings of sadness and feeling down was treated with psychopharmaceuticals and sleeping drugs, rather than being worked through.

Providing information about normal responses to life events can provide a form of scaffolding: it is a form of cognitive control. Too often, natural responses of sadness, feeling down
or angry are medicalized and labelled as a form of illness, instead of being normalized. This is

what happened on October 10, 1997, on the occasion of the Dutch National Mental Health Day [*Landelijke Dag Psychische Gezondheid*] which focused on depression. During this day, depression was described as a mental illness which develops when someone has lost their job, or a loved one, and which as such had to be treated with psychopharmaceuticals. Never in history had antidepressants and sleeping medication been prescribed in such large amounts as what was observed at the end of the twentieth century.

These examples are sometimes referred to as forms of mental health education, where psychosocial processes are explained. The client can be offered brochures, schedules, books, audio or video material, DVDs, lectures or information about peer support or general knowledge, which are aligned to their needs, in order to normalize and ensure that clients consider their own thoughts to be normal.

11.8.2 Reality-check technique

If the client has a need for information about what happens, the nature of the suffering and any consequences – which may occur when this information has been withheld from the client – social workers can help to collect this information after the fact. In many situations, such as disasters or horrific incidents, support people may withhold the facts from clients out of concern for them. The former justify this by saying it is in the clients' best interest. In case of a death, support people may, quite understandably, say that the dead person was in no fit state to be viewed. Clients may experience this as patronizing. Where questions about the facts remain unanswered, unnecessary additional suffering may result. The social worker can take stock of what exactly the client wants to know and explore, in consultation with the client, what options exist to find the missing information, the missing pieces of the puzzle, after the fact. One example is the Photo Viewing procedure to show images of a deceased person if the client is ready to see these, usually following extensive and well-considered deliberations (see also section 25.11).

11.8.3 Normalization technique

The normalization technique is applied when educating the client about life events or traumatic experiences. The social worker will explain to the client that what he is feeling is normal, by saying, for instance, that grief is a normal response to life events, that fatigue may result when clients carry a heavy burden for a prolonged period of time, that a level of hyperarousal is normal after traumatic events, or that touch may be a very sensitive topic when someone has been physically violated. Clients will then be reassured rather than concerned about what they are feeling, because their symptoms are normalized.

Normalizing responses to life events by giving information can take away feelings of doubt and uncertainty and open the door to the process of working through the grief.

11.8.4 Diary technique

The diary technique (see also sections 5.7.9 and 13.7.1) is also referred to as 'self-monitoring'. This form of self-registration creates the foundation for changing unrealistic or negative thoughts. It creates the opportunity to formulate such thoughts more precisely and evaluate progress. The diary technique involves tallying the thoughts we wish to observe by recording them in a diary. The client uses a booklet to record how many times a particular thought crops up in practice. Example: 'When feeling tense in a social situation, go be by yourself for 10 minutes, write up your thoughts and what is making you feel tense, and what was wrong with you'.

11.8.5 Challenge technique

This involves the social worker challenging the client's thoughts: asking the client to critically reflect on his thoughts. This process is sometimes referred to as the Socratic dialogue. An example would be: 'You just said you cannot do anything (right). Is that true? What do you base that on?'

According to Geerts et al. (1999), the Socratic dialogue is the technique 'which involves developing ideas from the student's own mind, by asking him relevant questions which eventually lead to the student himself discovering the concept you are trying to teach him'. The Socratic dialogue challenges the client to think for himself.

Mr. Stack's case

Mr. Stack finds it useful to reconstruct what has happened by arranging things in 'drawers' and working through those one after the other. In the course of this reconstruction process he experiences feelings of anger, which he immediately responds to with negative instructions to himself: 'Not allowed to get angry'. The support worker discusses such negative self-instructions, with him: 'Is it realistic to tell yourself that you are not allowed to get angry? Or is anger in fact quite a normal response?' It turned out that, as a child, Mr. Stack had been very frightened on the occasion of a violent outburst of anger; and ever since had not allowed himself to ever get angry. Repeated statements by Mr. Stack, such as 'I should have done things differently' and 'it was stupid of me that I allowed those things to happen to me in the hospital' are cognitively challenged by the social worker: 'Are you sure that is right?' or 'I don't understand. Can you explain?'

When it comes to the challenge technique, the working relationship between social worker and client can be summarized as 'collaborative empiricism'. Social worker and client work as a team, and the client's thoughts are viewed as a theory about reality. The social worker gets the client to investigate to what extent the latter's theory is correct. Padesky (1993) referred to this as the process of 'guided discovery'. In the course of this process the social worker's attitude is one that is characterized by curiosity (Bögels & van Oppen, 1999). The social worker is particularly interested in the client's thought processes, wanting to know how they came to formulate a certain theory, and what experiences, information or rationale such views are based on. This attitude may be compared to that of a researcher who wants to investigate to what extent a certain theory is tenable. The cognitive method involves the social worker acting like a researcher in that he and the client look for data that are either in alignment or in contrast with the client's theory, and thinking up thought experiments to test such theories.

An example would be the client's thoughts (theory) that 'I will go mad if I allow myself to recognize the life event,' 'It is terrible that I have not managed to get over the life event yet,' 'I am a useless human being, because I did not pay attention properly,' 'My life has no meaning now that I have lost my partner.'

11.8.6 Positive self-imaging technique

Positive self-imaging is a technique which involves the social worker asking the client to name one of his or her positive traits or behaviours. Clients who think themselves 'down' (using so-called negative self-instructions) can thus be encouraged to also allow positive thoughts about themselves. An example would be: 'What do you think was positive about the way in which you contributed to this session?' Clients who harbour negative self-thoughts are usually hard-pressed to find something positive to say. The social worker can respond to this by saying: 'Take your time to see what you thought was positive about the last hour.'

Telling clients harbouring negative self-thoughts (people who keep repeating that they are useless) that they have to think positive is much too simple. The essence of cognitive restructuring is to get clients look at themselves and realize that there really are plenty of positive things to say. In this way, talking themselves down is somewhat balanced out by positive self-talk.

11.8.7 Control technique checking unrealistic thoughts

The social worker checks whether clients harbour irrational or unrealistic thoughts by going through a list of 12 irrational thoughts together with the client. Jacobs (1999) lists 12 forms of irrational thoughts, also referred to as *must*-urbations because they all include the word 'must', distinguishing three main types:

- 'I must perform well in my work and personal life [gaining the love and/or approval of others] in order to consider myself a worthwhile person [as if you are only worth something if you perform].'
- 'Other people must treat me honestly and nicely or decently, otherwise they are useless people.'
- 'Life must be pleasant and comfortable, otherwise it is useless.'

Twelve types of irrational thoughts

The 12 main types of irrational thoughts – which can obviously vary slightly from one individual to the next – are listed next:

1 'I have to be appreciated by people who are important to me,' 'I need to receive love from someone whenever I need it' (when in fact love and appreciation develop, but cannot be forced).
2 'I have to perform well, otherwise I am unprofessional/useless,' 'I have to succeed in life' (when in fact people are allowed to fail as well).
3 'People have to act in a well-considered and honest manner, otherwise they are bad people' (when in fact people do have their blind spots).

4 'Things have to go/be the way I want them to, otherwise things are terrible and horrible.'
5 'All this bad stuff had to happen to me,' 'I cannot help the way I act and feel,' 'I cannot help feeling this way.'
6 'I have to get very upset about anything that is uncertain or a threat,' 'When there is any type of danger or uncertainty it is impossible not to feel scared.'
7 'It is better to avoid any kind of trouble or responsibility, rather than face it and address it.'
8 'I have to have other people around: without them I cannot live my life,' 'I cannot handle life by myself.'
9 'I can never get away from what happened in my past, because it has had such an impact on me that that will always be the same.'
10 'When others are going through a hard time, that is terrible and I have to get upset about it.'
11 'There has to be a good solution for this problem and I cannot stand it if things cannot be resolved properly.'
12 'I always have to be in control, I cannot go crazy, it would be terrible if that happened' (when in fact everyone goes through times where they lose control, are confused or disoriented).

11.8.8 4G technique

Social workers can use the 4G schedule to map out actual problems, together with the client (Vervoort & Weiland, 2003). The 4G schedule is an extension of the ABC-schedule (*activating event–beliefs–consequences*) and involves the following elements (Note: it is called '4G' because in Dutch all the keywords start with a 'G'.)

1 Event: what situation was the cause? Example: 'I lost my job following a reorganization at my work.'
2 Thought: is the client interpreting this even based on irrational and negative thoughts? Example: 'I am a loser,' 'Why did this happen to me?,' or 'They ruined my life.'
3 Emotion: what physical and emotional responses did this result in? Example: 'I feel totally abandoned,' 'I get very easily irritated when I am home,' 'I am scared.'
4 Behaviour: what is the resulting behaviour? Example: 'I started drinking.'

The social worker challenges any unrealistic thoughts (see section 11.8.5): 'Prove to me that you are worthless,' 'Who says you need to have the ideal career?,' 'Why would everything always go your way?' and 'Who says life is fair?' Realistic thoughts will start to take over: 'Losing my job is not the end of the world,' 'I do not have to be able to cope with every kind of work,' 'I do not need to feel ashamed about who I am' and 'I can choose to try something else.' These types of thoughts also have a normalizing effect.

11.8.9 Reframing technique

Re-labelling involves providing the client's thought with a less burdensome label, thereby placing them in a less burdensome framework. An example would be: 'You say you don't understand why you feel so panicked, but if I look at everything you have been through and everything you kept bottling up, I can imagine that your emotions are ready to burst out like a volcano ready to erupt, and that may feel to you like a sense of panic.'

The sense of panic was perceived as a burden:'I am going crazy.' Re-labelling it as 'a powerful emotion that came about because you were bottling things up' has a reassuring effect.

11.8.10 Setting norms technique

Setting norms involves confronting the client with broadly accepted norms. The social worker puts boundaries in place based on such norms. Examples would be:'I want you to stop hitting your child,' or 'From now on I want you to be here at the time we had agreed,' or 'Can you let me know in advance if you are going to be a little bit late?,' or 'If drinking is your main issue and you think I can help you, I have to disappoint you and say that is not the case. You will have to go to addiction services' (see also section 13.7.12).

11.8.11 Feeling Yes – Feeling No technique

The social worker may help the client practice boundary-setting by using self-protective thinking techniques (see also section 13.7.9). In every social situation every human being has either a Yes or a No feeling. When clients have a *yes* feeling, they will say so, and likewise when they have a *no* feeling. When in doubt, they first investigate what is right and what is not before carrying on. An example would be a client who has ambivalent feelings about interacting with a certain person. Some aspects feel okay, but other aspects of the interaction do not feel okay. After some self-reflection clients may decide they do want to meet that person, but for a shorter time than requested (see also the cost–benefit technique described in section 12.9.4).

11.8.12 Solution-focused technique

The solution-focused technique poses two different questions which both need to be resolved: one relates to exceptions and the other to 'I wonder'.

Exception question

The social worker asks about situations and points in time at which the problem did not arise. Once these exceptions have been identified, the next question is how those problem-free times can be extended. One example would be:'This is a difficult issue. How have you managed to handle this in such a way that it has been manageable right up until this point in time?' or 'You passed one course but failed the rest. What did you do to successfully complete the course you passed?'

'I wonder' question

The 'I wonder' question is used to encourage the client to visualize life without the problem, just as if a 'miracle' had happened. This will encourage a client to focus more on a future without problems rather than on the past. The social worker encourages the client to describe options for a problem-free future and any steps that might be necessary to get there. An example would be:'I would like to ask you a funny question. What if a miracle were to occur tonight, while you are asleep, and that the problem you wanted help to resolve was gone.

However, since you were asleep, you were not aware that this miracle had occurred. So, how would you know, tomorrow when you wake up. What would be the difference? How could you tell that something miraculous had happened and that your problem has been resolved?' This may help clients to think of practical ways to better address their issues and thus for things to improve.

11.8.13 Internet-related techniques

Social media can be a source of support for clients. There has been increasing recognition of the strength of social media when life events occur (Westerink, 2014). The digital communities of Facebook, YouTube and other media enable people to visit online platforms almost instantly in order to ask questions, inform others and get in contact with others. Just posting a question or telling your story can be very helpful. Even face-to-face social workers can assist clients online by responding to email messages or agree on what to do in specific instances of grieving. One client experienced the murder of her twin sister, and after some searching on the internet came across the Twinlesstwins website. Private sites are created where those who have lost family members in airline disasters can interact with others in the same situation. Anything on the internet that can contribute to increased awareness, the ability to say goodbye and the opportunity to start a new life can be beneficial. Reflections on the previous session can be communicated over the internet as well.

The following website illustrates the scope of the internet when it comes to life events: http://www.remembermewheniamgone.org. This website offers a book of memories in 95 different languages which can be used by parents who do not have long to live; they can use the book to share memories of their lives together with their children, memories which will be impossible or difficult to trace once they have gone. The internet also offers the opportunity for therapeutic sessions which do not involve any face-to-face interactions between support worker/health professional and client; examples include Interapy and 113online.

It goes without saying that both the social worker and the client have to be very much aware of the dangers posed by the internet when exploring such solutions.

11.9 Social work results

- Clients are well informed.
- The client's self-assessment or assessment of the situation is more realistic.
- The client demonstrates more positive self-talk.
- The client demonstrates less harmful thoughts in relation to himself or others.

11.10 Evidence

There has been some research into the effects of the cognitive method that can also be applied to social work. Findings suggest that cognitive therapy is an effective form of treatment for several disorders, in particular anxiety-related ones; in fact, more so than other forms of therapy, especially in the long run. In a direct comparison with a waitlist condition, pharmacotherapy, relaxation therapy and non-directive therapy, Arntz & Elgersma (1999) found cognitive therapy to be a more effective treatment for anxiety disorders, both in the short and the long term.

Research has also been done into the effects of Socratic questioning, also referred to as the challenge technique (Beck & Emery, 1985). Socratic questioning ensures that:

- The client is aware of automatically occurring thoughts.
- It helps identify dysfunctional assumptions.
- It helps formulate more rational thoughts.
- It helps formulate new thinking habits.

Internet-related social work and grief therapy has been researched in relation to complicated life events such a loss (Wagner et al., 2006). Clients with complex life events such as loss ($n = 55$) were randomly assigned to either a treatment group ($n = 26$) or a waiting list control condition by way of a control group. The therapist only communicated with members of the intervention group by email. The 5-week intervention consisted of three modules: (1) exposing participants to bereavement cues, (2) cognitive re-appraisal and (3) integration and restoration.

The Impact of Event Scale (IES), a failure to adapt scale and depression and anxiety sub-scales were used to assess treatment outcomes. Participants in the treatment group showed significant improvement compared to those in the waiting condition in terms of symptoms of intrusion, avoidance, maladaptive behaviour and general psychopathology, and these effects proved to be more long term. Follow-up results showed that this improvement was maintained at the 3-month mark.

11.11 Pitfalls

- Lecturing: bombarding clients with information they have not asked for, and without introduction;
- Brainwashing: advising the client in a patronizing manner, for example by saying 'every life event either entails a benefit or a challenge';
- Asking questions without being interested in the answers (imposing your own answers).

11.12 Summary and questions

This chapter described the social worker's role in helping the client meet his primary needs: the need for adequate information and information processing. It started by describing the role and function of the rational brain when dealing with information relating to life events. It went on to describe how cognitive stress develops when the need for adequate information processing is unmet. It then described how the cognitive method can reduce cognitive stress and increase someone's cognitive strength.

Questions

1 Do you recognize examples of clients' unrealistic thoughts in yourself or other people?
2 How would you describe the difference between realistic and unrealistic thoughts?

3 What are your thoughts on the possible impact of unrealistic thoughts?

4 Why is it that clients only manage to arrive at less burdensome thoughts when challenged? Why can they not do this by themselves?

5 What are your thoughts on setting norms when it comes to the way clients think and behave?

6 What do you think is the strength of solution-focused techniques? Give an example.

12

NARRATIVE METHOD

Questions

This chapter addresses the following questions:

- What is meant by 'meaning making in grief'?
- Which are the four existential questions in grief?
- What is meant by existential stress?
- What is meant by the impact narrative and the helping narrative?
- How can the narrative method contribute to the reduction of meaning making stress and recovering one's strength?

12.1 Introduction

> My world collapsed.
> I don't know how to move on.
> You fall into this black hole.
>
> (de Mönnink, 2016)

In this chapter the role of the social worker is described in helping the client fulfil four existential needs related to meaning making.

First, the meaning of these four existential needs in grief, summed up in the acronym DUNC, is described: Dignity, Understanding of Justice, Now-in-relation-to-later and Control. Then the impact narrative (the first narrative) and helping narrative (the second narrative) in grief are defined. Afterwards we explain the functioning of the meaning making mechanism and zero-dimension of grief. Subsequently we indicate what the narrative method has to offer to reduce meaning making stress and to restore one's strength. In conclusion we give a summary of the chapter.

The case of Mr. Stack

Existential questions concern the way Mr. Stack sees life. 'Who am I?,' 'What do I want to do with my life?,' 'What is the meaning of my life?' and 'Why me?' are all examples of these types of existential questions. For years Mr. Stack carried the heavy burden of his first son's unexpected stillbirth and his second son's disability. He didn't share his sorrows with anyone, not even with his wife. Mr. Stack used misplaced gallows humour as a survival mechanism and as a means of filling up the emptiness. He fled into his bitterness and was overly critical towards social workers. This caused him not to perform the necessary grief labour, and soon his relationship with the people around him and the social workers would become problematic. Through social work sessions Mr. Stack was able to leave the chaos behind in order to get his facts straight – the impact narrative – and he was given the space to investigate the pointlessness and incomprehensibility of his losses. His psychological movie was no longer paused at the question 'Why?': he regained his grip on life. Through the narrative method he was eventually able to develop a helping narrative: 'At first I thought: why me? Now I'm thinking: it was meant to happen and I can enjoy the beautiful moments. Why not me?' Another take on his life?

12.2 DUNC: four existential needs

> In case of identity loss your life goes off-road, a landslide causes your trusted path to become impassable or to completely disappear. Your inner GPS says 'straight ahead' at the verge, but it would only lead you more astray.
>
> (de Mönnink, 2016)

The loss of existential elements can cause your identity, the entire coherence in your life's structure and meaning, to collapse. This is illustrated in the expression: 'My life was falling apart.' The meaning of life itself takes a beating. Every loss can cause severe disruptions in one's equilibrium, which causes the entire understanding of identity to be undermined. The inner cohesion or mutual coherence in the existential design becomes unsettled. This may cause a feeling of emptiness to arise: the falling apart of the involved person's existing meaning structure (Frankl, 1969). In other words: existential stress arises, there is tension between the desired condition (without loss) and the perceptible condition (with loss).

The inner DUNC guarantees your safe life-trip by continuously assessing where you came from, where you stand and where you are going. It monitors the essential meanings and assumptions you attribute to yourself and your world: 'Life is good when I'm around my mother' or 'When I play in this trusted space, with trusted people, it feels right.'

DUNC represents the four inner navigational functions in your life journey, the four existential needs that must be fulfilled for quality in life (Baumeister, 1991a):

D *Dignity*: my life structure includes a mental travelling thermometer. Loss causes me not to feel well about myself in my current life anymore; a new need for a new sense of dignity arises on my life journey.

U *Understanding of justice*: my life structure includes a mental travel guarantee. Because of loss, my sense of justice on my life path is undermined. It no longer goes the way I expected. A new need arises for new understanding and realization of justice: that I will get what I deserve.

N *Now-in-relation-to-later*: my life structure includes a mental travelling goal; loss thwarts a long-cherished dream on my life path. A renewed need for a new future perspective arises.

C *Control*: my life structure serves as a mental travel guide, gives me control. Loss causes my grip to faint, meaning that I can no longer determine who or what is reliable on my path; a new need for security, safety, grip and continuity arises.

Grief becomes manageable by creating a new personal story and a new and helping vision on reality after loss. Like Teresa Miller (2009) puts it: 'stories give messages and become road maps of our lives.' Creating structure in the chaos of experiences marks out the tragedy and renders it more bearable while doing so. The fundaments supporting your existence are fortified by reassessing core significances. By searching for the meaning of it all, for explanations and causes for the things that have happened, for your own share in it as well as your environment's share, you restore your DUNC, your navigational tools on your life journey and a helping narrative arises. How to recognize the impact narrative as a social worker: which navigational functions were put off stride? Facilitate the helping narrative: which needs are to be fulfilled? How can you help the client in getting a software upgrade for his inner GPS?

12.3 From 'impact narrative' to 'helping narrative': theory

> People use their intelligence to give meaning to the world, bit by bit. Gradually they start seeing broader, integrative patterns. The meanings they put together themselves are connected with each other. The myth that there is a bigger plan is the general belief that everything is meaningful and that everything can be understood that way.
>
> (Baumeister, 1991a, p. 73)

Making a reconstruction of the loss and turning it into a finished narrative can provide a new footing, a new grip. It can contribute to a renewed feeling of continuity between the past, present and future. How can this transformation from an unbearable loss to an acceptable destiny be completed? How can the composition of a loss narrative and the 'moving on after loss' narrative help?

Constructivism and the narrative theory cast light on this on this grief transformation process: how do you 'bring light into the darkness' with a helping narrative? Constructivism requires an active role of the person experiencing grief. From the constructivist point of view, grief processing is a process of reconstructing a world of meanings which was thrown off balance by loss. How can individuals successfully navigate through grief processing while struggling with the question how to find new perspectives after the unasked life transition which is loss?

The term 'construction' comes from the Latin word *construere*, 'to organize' or 'to structuralize'. The continuous structuring process (organization) is the conceptual heart of constructivism. Some ancestors of constructivism are Laozi (sixth century BC), Buddha (560–477 BC) and Heraclitus, the philosopher of infinite changes (540–475 BC). In Western culture, constructivist ideas are based on the theories of intellectual fathers such as Giambattista Vico (1668–1744), Immanuel Kant (1724–1804), Arthur Schopenhauer (1788–1860) and Hans Vaihinger (1852–1933).

The constructivist movement, which has been gaining popularity since the 1980s, casts light upon how people are capable of building (constructing) a new life after loss. Constructivism is an ideology based upon the idea of reality being more than what we can discover through empirical science alone. Guidance consists of creating new meanings for loss, together. From this point of view, social workers do not strive towards an objective way of thinking about the client's grief process. According to a constructivist view, the social worker helps the client in creating new meanings which help in broadening the client's possibilities in life. The emphasis on the active granting of meanings, language and culture, use of metaphors and stories as an insightful and guiding instrument are important parts of a constructive approach to grief processing (Niemeyer, 1995). One of constructivism's results is the narrative approach to grief (narrative = story).

The narrative approach presumes that the quality of the loss narrative we tell ourselves determines how we deal with our world and navigate through it. The loss narrative can help us, but can also obstruct us. It helps in putting the impact into words, but not in just leaving it at that. Otherwise it would only remain a victim narrative. The narrative model presumes that people create two different stories for life events such as loss: a first narrative or impact narrative and a second narrative or helping narrative. The impact narrative is about the bereavement itself, the crisis, the violation, the reaction, the victimization. The helping narrative is more about how to move on, how to take on your challenges in life again: 'How can I overcome this grief and how can I write a new life chapter?' or 'How can I get a breather while being on the ground?' The helping narrative is about the proactive aspect and picking up the thread in life. Reflecting upon grief and creating stories about your loss make it possible to transform your identity. By creating a second narrative and thus via helping narrative, the client's seemingly impossible inner transformation yet becomes possible. In order to accomplish this, a new rift must be introduced in the client's life (under supervision of the social worker): a rift between the loss with impact and the loss with helping.

The inner transformation process that follows may be a blockade (impact, vulnerability) but also a possible turning point (helping). The 'transformation process from blockade to turning point' in loss goes as follows (Lengelle & Meijers, 2009). From the first instance, the human response to loss can be an impact narrative: the *SOS narrative*, where SOS stands for *stuck on suffering*. This is regarded to be the first narrative, a description of the impact perception, circumstances and effects of loss. This first narrative is usually not a constructive one. It deals with the *fight–flight–freeze* mode experienced at first instance. From this perspective, the overwhelming effect of loss leads people to taking almost pre-programmed decisions – instinctive reactions – making the first narrative an impact narrative. In order to establish inner change after loss, you need to rewrite your own life path so that a new route can be started. This rewriting can be done by first creating a coherent reconstruction of the period before, during and after the loss event. For this impact narrative, answers to the following questions are needed:

- What are the precise circumstances of the loss?
- How can I experience this grief now?
- Have I lost this person or thing forever?

The second narrative or helping narrative is the result of grief labour: we look at and experience grief in another way. Our loss narrative becomes feasible; someone acknowledges (the impact of) loss and no longer reacts automatically, but searches for ways to overcome and find a new purpose for the impact of this loss. The second narrative is new, of a rather transforming nature and usually occurs in the following forms:

- Acknowledgement of the reality of grief;
- A shift in perspective;
- Discovery or construction of new meanings.

The helping narrative searches for answers to the following questions:

- What is the point of it all?
- What does this lead up to?
- How can I move on in spite of this?

The first impact narrative may be that loss is a shocking and shameful crisis experience. The second or helping narrative may imply that someone realizes his powerlessness when reliving the event, but sees it as a challenge to learn how to deal with this (coping), to reflect upon it, to invest in more suitable alternatives again – or to see loss as an opportunity to take some rest or show compassion with others who have experienced similar loss events: resignation, accepting this fate and creating a new bearable fate with it.

The case of Mr. Stack

Mr. Stack and his wife have lost their child during labour and their other child was disabled because of a shovelling accident. How can Mr. Stack and his wife come to a helping narrative? By creating an impact narrative first and then developing a helping narrative from it.

Welcome to Holland

I am often asked to describe the experience of raising a child with a disability – to try to help people who have not shared that unique experience to understand it, to imagine how it would feel. It's like this . . .

When you're going to have a baby, it's like planning a fabulous vacation trip – to Italy. You buy a bunch of guide books and make your wonderful plans. The Coliseum. The Michelangelo *David*. The gondolas in Venice. You may learn some handy phrases in Italian. It's all very exciting. After months of eager anticipation, the day finally arrives. You pack your bags and off you go. Several hours later, the plane lands. The stewardess comes in and says, 'Welcome to Holland.' 'Holland?!?' you say. 'What do you mean Holland?? I signed up for Italy! I'm supposed to be in Italy. All my life I've dreamed of going to Italy.'

But there's been a change in the flight plan. They've landed in Holland and there you must stay. The important thing is that they haven't taken you to a horrible, disgusting, filthy place, full of pestilence, famine and disease. It's just a different place. So you must go out and buy new guide books. And you must learn a whole new language. And you will meet a whole new group of people you would never have met. It's just a different place. It's slower paced than Italy, less flashy than Italy. But after you've been there for a while and you catch your breath, you look around . . . and you begin to notice that Holland has windmills . . . and Holland has tulips. Holland even has Rembrandts. But everyone you know is busy coming and going from Italy . . . and they're all bragging about what a wonderful time they had there. And for the rest of your life, you will say 'Yes, that's where I was supposed to go. That's what I had planned.'

And the pain of that will never, ever, ever, ever go away . . . because the loss of that dream is a very very significant loss. But . . . if you spend your life mourning the fact that you didn't get to Italy, you may never be free to enjoy the very special, the very lovely things . . . about Holland.

(Emily Pearl Kingsley, president of the American National Down Syndrome Congress)

In this last story, two processing narratives can be recognized: the impact narrative and the helping narrative (coping narrative). The impact narrative deals with disappointment about the fact that their child has Down syndrome. The second – helping – narrative deals with proactively overcoming this disappointment and getting it together again: being able to enjoy life again after a while, the thing that seemed impossible at first (see Table 12.1).

12.4 From impact narrative to helping narrative: a new DUNC?

12.4.1 The need for (renewed) dignity

On my life's journey my mental travelling thermometer, my dignity, my pride . . . became unsettled because of a loss.
It's not my fault, it can happen to anyone.

(de Mönnink, 2016)

TABLE 12.1 From impact narrative to helping narrative (with Welcome to Holland metaphor)

Existing life narrative	Impact narrative; transition narrative	Helping narrative
Expectations set to a mentally healthy child	Having a child with Down syndrome	Learning to love a child with Down syndrome Learning to live with the loss of expectation of a mentally healthy child
Always dreamed of a trip to . . . ITALY	The airplane lands in Holland: there has been a change in the flight plan; disappointed not being in Italy	How can I learn to love the very special and lovely things about Holland?

The first existential need is the need for dignity: 'Am I enjoying my life?,' 'Can I be proud of my life, my desires and am I happy on my life's journey?' These questions are related to the first functionality of your existential GPS: making yourself feel positive about yourself in terms of self-esteem or dignity. By attributing meanings to yourself and your world, the need for pride and respect for yourself is fulfilled as well as pride for your accomplishments, your body, parenthood, work, hearth and home. A feeling of dignity is then derived from the developed meaning structure. People with a positive feeling of dignity are people who:

> are active and successful, take the lead, stand up for their opinion, have self-confidence, are optimistic, do not overthink personal problems, have few psychosomatic complaints (headaches, insomnia).
>
> *(Keers & Wilke, 1978, p. 45).*

You experience brilliance in life thanks to your successful achievements, by what you have achieved. From your life you derive self-confidence, dignity, flow, happiness. Loss can cause you to be stuck with a negative feeling of dignity: you are convinced of your own inferiority, you feel isolated, you have no self-confidence, you do not want to stand out and worry about personal problems.

The feeling of dignity can be learned and unlearned:

> A child coming into the world has no past, no experience of how to handle himself, no standard to measure his sense of dignity up to. It must use the experiences from social contact with people around it and intercept signals they send about its worthiness or worthlessness as a human being. During the first five to six years the sense of dignity of a child is almost exclusively fed by the family surrounding it. Once the child starts going to school, other factors will come into play, but the family's influence remains most important during puberty and adolescence. Influences from the outside can amplify the child's sense of worthiness or worthlessness.
>
> *(Satir, 1978, p. 27)*

Loss events can lead to a decreased self-confidence and sense of dignity. Radical experiences of loss can cause you to think more negatively about yourself, for example thinking that 'I only have myself to thank for it' or 'it's so typical that this would happen to me now.' You feel unhappy, are vulnerable and are doubting yourself. In losing the person or thing you loved, a part of yourself was lost too, namely the part you invested in that very person or thing. Partners who were left behind appeared to have lost trust in themselves and the other person: 'So what we had was worth nothing.' Children of parents who committed suicide entirely blamed it on themselves: 'Clearly I was not worth living for.' Upon losing that other person or thing, 'self-loss' is brought about.

In sexual abuse it is a known phenomenon that victims often feel dirty and are left with a stained self-image due to violation of their physical, sexual and relational integrity. While the perpetrator obviously remains the perpetrator, the events still have a negative effect on the victim's sense of dignity.

The resilience in case of loss increases as you think more positively about yourself. When you have a positive sense of dignity, you should be more grief-proof. When you have a negative sense of dignity, you will probably wonder: 'How does a worthless human being such as myself ever get over such problems?' Or perhaps the other way around: 'I must be pretty worthless as a person, since I can't deal with my problems.'

Existentially, you are not only forced to think about the meaning and organization of the world, but also about the related topic which is personal vulnerability (Perloff, 1983). 'I am broken, sad, down, in doubt about myself . . . I feel stained by the loss.' The feeling of personal invulnerability and even personal happiness can appear to be an illusion: how to deal with this loss of dignity, how to regain grip when the existing sense of dignity about life seems to be an illusion?

Giving a meaning and explanation to loss can protect or strengthen belief in yourself (Bout, 1986). People who are severely ill help themselves in restoring the affected self-respect by attributing external causes to and giving explanations for the illness. These explanations play a clear role at the beginning of the pathological process. People create their own explanatory narrative and seem to gain more resilience by doing so.

From literary research about care in stressful situations and the environment acting as a buffer, it appeared that a sense of dignity and trust in one's own personality can be decisive elements in learning how to integrate periods of crisis into one's life (Schrameijer, 1990). When there is constant confirmation of the existent sense of dignity, a condition for growth is fulfilled. That way, putting loss into words can clear the way for a new sense of dignity (see Table 12.2).

12.4.2 The need for (renewed) understanding existential justice

> Why? Why not? Shit happens!
> This is wrong, I didn't deserve this! On my life journey, my inner travel guarantee, my understanding of justice, became unsettled because of loss.
>
> (de Mönnink, 2016)

The second existential need is the need for justice: 'Am I done with justice in my life, can I develop myself, do I get what I deserve in life, where is my inner guarantee for my life journey?' These questions are related to a second functionality of your existential GPS: believing in a righteous world. Everyone needs a righteous social work in and throughout 'life' in *events* about yourself, your accomplishments, your body, parenthood, work, hearth and home. The world is given so much meaning that the sense of justice is confirmed. 'Hard work deserves a

TABLE 12.2 The dignity narrative in having a disabled child (with Welcome to Holland metaphor)

Need for dignity	Existent dignity narrative is disrupted	New sense of dignity
I always expected delivering a healthy child. . . .	I feel bad about myself, how could I not see this coming, I am a mother of nothing?	I don't blame myself, instead I blame that one chromosome! It's only a freak of nature. . . .
Feeling yes, good feeling, proud of who I am and what I have and of my trip to Italy	My dignity took a beating. I don't feel comfortable in Holland.	Learning how to enjoy again. I feel okay about Holland, I will feel better again once I realize what I do have, and can enjoy it nevertheless

righteous reward' or 'By paying a lot of attention to X, I deserve gratitude.' There is a balance of giving and taking, the rotating account where investment means profits.

This second functionality of your existential GPS lies in giving you a sense of existential justice. By attributing meanings to the world throughout life, the need for a righteous appreciation of physical, mental, professional and relational achievements can be fulfilled. A sense of justice is derived from this developed meaning structure.

Loss can be experienced as something unfair: 'I do not deserve what I am given.' Belief in a just world – the just-world hypothesis – is one of the values which can be lost: 'This is not fair,' 'Why? Why me?' A severe loss is a violation to norms and values, the standards which you use to assess your own as well as other people's behaviour. These standards form a framework for the reference and assessment of events in everyday life: can my own or someone else's behaviour be morally accounted for? Loss events may disrupt the orientation of values because they affect the ability to judge on one's own deeds as being good or bad. Mothers who lost their children because they had killed them showed severe stress, feelings of guilt and all sorts of other problems. Their disability to consider themselves good mothers caused them to desire for a new child as quickly as possible by means of compensation for their actions (Baumeister, 1991b).

A part of the problem in loss events is the fact that values do not offer the support which they normally should. Especially now when they are needed the most, the handled values can appear to be insufficient. In that case it is very hard to use your existential GPS for matching your interpretation with your most recent loss experience. Making loss manageable does not only require understanding for the loss itself to arise, but it also requires rebuilding one's understanding of justice. One mustn't linger upon the idea of: 'This is not fair. Why? Why me?'

Why do bad things happen to good people? Belief in a 'just world' appears to be an illusion. Will you ever be capable of believing in a righteous world again? How to handle this loss of justice? How to regain your grip when the existing sense of justice in life is but an illusion?

Loss can cause belief in justice to take a severe beating: 'When did I deserve this?' 'I can't get what I deserve, because fate is unfair!' Finding a meaning, an explanation for the loss event, can recover your belief in a righteous world.

Putting injustice into words and giving explanations to loss can help you justify yourself: 'I didn't deserve this!' You can try to integrate the loss into your life by looking at yourself or at your environment when answering the question of guilt. Searching for internal and external causes and explanations doesn't just provide you with cognitive control – that is how reality works – and amplification of your dignity, but it can also grow your understanding of justice (Van den Bout, 1986). In the next example, an engine driver reports a collision on a railway level crossing and the following question of guilt.

Collision at a railway level crossing

I was approaching the level crossing and saw two ladies nicely dismounting their bicycles. A car was slowly approaching the crossing as well and I thought: that car will definitely stop as well. Except he didn't. The man was still alive – and still is, by the way – when I arrived at the wrecked car. The first thing he said to me was: 'Why didn't you whistle?' But I thought he would stop. But . . . and so on. Anyway, it kept haunting me.

> I worried and thought it over and over. I had trouble sleeping. In the end I found out where that man was hospitalized, and I went to visit him. The first thing he said when he saw me again was: 'Why didn't you whistle?' Once again, I wished the ground to open up and swallow me. My salvation was that I said to him: 'But why didn't you stop your car?' He looked at me for a while and said: 'Good gracious, why didn't I think of that. I should have stopped the car.' It was as if the world's weight was lifted from my shoulders. I came home singing and whistling. My wife thought I was drunk, but I was only relieved.
>
> (*Vrij Nederland*, June 6, 1981)

Giving meanings to loss by pointing at yourself or external causes or forces makes that you can process the loss event more easily. People who, after loss, formulated an answer to the why-questions of the situation – because! – were better off than those who didn't know how to reply (Silver et al., 1983). That way, putting injustice into words after loss can cause a renewed understanding of justice to arise (see Table 12.3).

12.4.3 The need for a (renewed) now-in-relation-to-later

> On my life journey, I lose track of my destination, my dream because of a loss.
> I don't know how to move on after loss.
> I live from day to day, enjoy life every day.
>
> (de Mönnink, 2016)

The third existential need is the need for future perspective, the now-in-relation-to-later: 'Will my dream become reality? Will I reach the destination on my life path?' These questions are related to the fourth functionality of your existential GPS: cherishing an inner dream, giving a meaning to the now-in-relation-to-later. Everyone needs goals in life. Goals in terms of your personality, achievements, your body, your parenthood, work, hearth and home. What are my ideals, how do I give my life direction, do I have a future perspective?

TABLE 12.3 The justice narrative in having a disabled child (with Welcome to Holland metaphor)

Need for justice	Injustice narrative	Developing new sense of justice
Expectations set to having a healthy child	I didn't deserve this.	I deserve proper support, get attention for this disappointment and adjust myself to my child, new understanding of justice is developed.
Mental travel guarantee: 'I expected to go to Italy, and that is what I deserve!'	We were supposed to go to Italy, that's what I signed up for, that's what I was prepared for and that's what I paid for!	I rely on fate, nothing is certain.

This third functionality of your existential GPS is giving you a sense of future, a sense of hope. Future perspective can be derived from meanings which were attributed throughout one's life. The developed meaning structure offers perspective in your physical and psychological development, the development in your relations, parenthood, work, hearth and home. In such a way the existential need for planning, ideals and life course are fulfilled.

You wish to interpret the present in relation to future events: you wish to make plans and set yourself some goals. In many types of loss, the accomplishment of long-cherished dreams for the future may be definitely obstructed and reaching the goals which were set can be blocked. This causes loss of future perspective, an important pillar in one's entire existence.

In order to understand how profound it is to lose one's future perspective, insight in the role of the 'pipe dream' in human life is of importance. Levinson (1978) calls human aspirations 'the Dream', and states that the Dream can have a powerful and far-reaching influence on one's life path. The Dream is the thread in man's life. The aforementioned is neither a daydream nor a regular dream. The Dream is more well-considered than a sheer fantasy, yet less detailed than an elaborate plan. The trials and tribulations and the fate of such a Dream are of fundamental importance for man's development.

> In its archetype, 'the Dream' is a vague notion of one's self in the adult world. It is a kind of vision, an imagined possibility which grants hope and life force. Initially this image is only a rough sketch and the connection to reality is only small, though it can include concrete imaginations such as winning the Nobel Prize or performing with a famous orchestra. It can grow to dramatic proportions in the hero's myth: the great artist, the business man or business woman, the sports hero or the famous scientist who receives extraordinary accolades for his wonderful accomplishments. It may also be of more modest proportions which, nonetheless, provide support and inspiration: becoming a skilled craftsman or -woman, a husband-father or wife-mother in a certain family, a respected member of the community.
>
> *(Levinson, 1978, p. 126)*

Loss of future perspective must be recognized in an early stage, because this type of loss can horribly scar one's life. Loss events related to migration, childbirth or resignation can unexpectedly give a dramatic plot twist to your life. The Dream can be lost causing the future to lose its significance. The challenge is not to linger in a state of: 'I am desperate, I no longer have a future, I am disoriented, I don't want to do this anymore!' Loss sometimes thwarts long-cherished dreams to come true: infertility ends one's Dream of having an own child, illness ends a period of vitality, economic depression ends a certain career, losses on the investment market make the saved pension capital disappear like snow in summer. Existential fear can be the result: awaiting the future with fear and trembling. Because of loss, one's future plans can be thwarted: the future is no longer what it used to be.

When the existing faith in a long-cherished dream does not become reality or appears to be an illusion, a bright future can turn into a dark nightmare. How can you lift yourself from the swamp? How will you take on the challenge of establishing an existential reorientation and developing a new future perspective?

Saying that life no longer makes sense after loss is not only a sign of apathy; it describes a situation where someone was robbed of his life goals and is feeling helpless. Familiar thinking and behavioural patterns no longer work. A way in which the meaning can be reconstructed is by disconnecting meanings from life and reshaping them. For example the experiences of Cuban exiles in the United States:

> The face looking back sees migration, uprooting and nostalgia and in a certain way even death, because some things die within when we are forced to leave our home country without being able to ever go back. The face looking forward sees new horizons, unknown surroundings, strangers with unknown habits and languages – in reality and in imagination – a tough challenge to survive, to adapt and to grow, and even the opportunity to create a new identity in the sudden anonymity.
>
> *(Rumbaut & Rumbaut, 1976, p. 396)*

In that way, putting the loss of old goals into words can clear one's path for looking forwards and developing new life goals (see Table 12.4).

12.4.4 The need. for (renewed) control

> How fragile we are. How fragile we are.
>
> (Sting 1987: Fragile)

> On my life journey, my mental travel guide, my grip, my control became unsettled because of loss.
>
> (de Mönnink, 2016)

The fourth existential need is the need for control over your life: do you know where you are on your life path, how much reliable information you carry about yourself and the world around you? Is the information in your inner travel guide about the world a reliable manual?

This fourth and last functionality of your existential GPS lies in providing you with grip on your life. By attributing meanings to the world – the internal and external world – throughout your life, you create grip, footing, control. The developed meaning structure about your body, psyche, relationships, parenthood, work, hearth and home fulfil the existential need for grip on the world. I live a manageable and makeable life which is organized and useful, and which provides control, safety and peace. You derive control, grip and footing from your life.

TABLE 12.4 The future narrative in having a disabled child

The need for now in relation to later	Disrupted future narrative	New future narrative?
Expectations set to having a healthy child	My dream ends in a nightmare, where is the healthy baby, our dream is disrupted?	I can develop a new future perspective, the future is not what it ought to be
My mental life goal, my escape plan, my dream of going to Italy	Disappointment, apparently Italy was not my destination: no, it was Holland!	Learning how to enjoy again and make new plans. I feel okay about Holland, I will feel better again once I realize what I do have, and can enjoy it nevertheless

By losing your job, loved ones and so forth, this control over yourself and the world can become unsettled. Loss is then experienced as an uncontrollable circumstance, endangering the grip you have acquired on the course of life events. You can no longer do things freely and are dragged down by the 'learned helplessness syndrome' (Seligman, 1975a): you feel helpless, lose your interests, are emotionally dead, afraid and so on. This pattern can jump over to other parts of your life and can have a paralyzing effect. The consequence can be a feeling of emptiness and powerlessness: the existential vacuum.

For a moment, the inner GPS has lost its way. The feeling of self-control is then undermined by your inner footing, your inner grip that is crumbling away. The meaning of life seems to (partly) go missing, causing powerlessness to arise. The illusion of control, cherished by every one of us, seems to be a disillusion: life was not the reliable interpretational structure which was makeable and controllable. Because of this loss you experience unsafety, powerlessness, commotion, insecurities . . . in short: the existent feeling of control has clearly seen better days. The question remaining: how to deal with this loss of control, how to regain grip when the existing sense of control over life seems to be an illusion?

Literally attributing a meaning to your loss can be considered an attempt of restoring control over your own existence. Whether the interpretation – cause, reason, explanation – attributed to your loss is objectively substantiated or originates from sheer subjectivity, is irrelevant; most important for those involved, is the creation of grip. By attributing causes – causal analysis – you can predict and control:

> The purpose of causal analysis – its function for our kind and the individual – is effective control. Attribution processes cannot only be interpreted as means for giving the individual a reliable view on his world, but as a way of encouraging and maintaining his effective control over the world.
>
> *(Kelley, 1971, pp. 21–22)*

Regaining grip of your life?

Your control, your grip can be regained by finding a cause or explanation for the loss event. Life is uncertain and no one has complete control over his existence. However you seem to recover more quickly after a radical event when you consider yourself to be vulnerable in a given situation (Perloff, 1983), for example by observing *how fragile we are*. A perception of unique vulnerability – the feeling that *only you* are more vulnerable than others – is less favourable for grief processing. The realization that other people are equally at risk appears to be a comforting idea. Grip on your own situation is restored by attributing comforting meanings to your reality. That way, putting the indescribable and indefinable into words, as Nicolaas Beets (1905) contends, offers you the possibility of a new grip on the same reality where grip was lost: 'What cannot be described, A description does not need. Call it by the name, . . . Only that is possible and nothing more.'

Table 12.5 illustrates the main notions of the first impact narrative and the second helping narrative. For every existential need it is pointed out which quotations belong to which type of narrative.

TABLE 12.5 The control narrative in getting a disabled child

Need for control	Impact narrative	Helping narrative
Need for grip, footing	Existing control is disrupted	Developing new grip: I must set my mind to something new and not hold on to old expectations
I experience grip by expecting a healthy child	Loss of grip due to birth of child with Down syndrome	I must adjust myself to a child with Down syndrome
I buy mental travel guides, maps, phrase books on Italy	My mind was set to Italy, I don't want to be in Holland!	I'll buy new travel guides and learn the new language

12.4.5 Meaning making

> Give sorrow words: the grief that does not speak. / Whispers the o'er-fraught heart, and bids it break.
>
> (Shakespeare, *Macbeth*)

Is Shakespeare right in saying that only giving sorrow words can prevent you from bottling everything up and getting a troubled heart? Meaning making is about our existential ability to give meaning to something that seemingly has no meaning at all.

Putting the impact of loss into words – the impact narrative – is the foundation for the development of a new and comforting perspective – the helping narrative. Our ability of meaning making makes us capable of pulling ourselves out of the swamp by our own hair. What is meant by man's 'ability to interpret' in loss?

The arisen emptiness must first be classified (impact narrative) in order to be able to continue building (a part of the) life where it came to a halt (helping narrative). In loss management, this ability is also called the meaning making competence or zero-dimension: dealing with actual, existential questions, giving zero or lack of dimension a new dimension (with words).

Loss impact may be experienced as if your world suddenly collapsed. There are no more directions and you lose complete track of everything. You are struggling with questions on the meaning of your own life. The arisen emptiness, the existential vacuum brings up questions such as: 'Why is this happening to me?' 'What is the meaning of this suffering?' 'What am I to do with this suffering?' 'What meaning is there left to life?' 'Why? Why me? Why now?' 'How do I pick myself up after loss?' You've lost track of direction in your life and don't know how to further navigate on your life journey. This may be caused by the unsettling of your navigational centre caused by loss. How do I refresh my existential GPS, so that I can start navigating again in the world that has changed after loss?' is the remaining question. Chaos, omission of perspective and the pointlessness experienced after loss are a heavy burden. Loss affects your grip. Apart from the actual loss, you also lose the lust for life. In this way, loss has an existential impact on people. Your footing in life is no longer as it used to be, before loss.

The theme of meaning making is denominated in both Western and Eastern religious and mystical movements, but also in transpersonal psychology, logotherapy and phenomenology. More and more people are also looking for answers to their life questions in a spiritual context when experiencing loss. What is the meaning of one's existence when confronted with loss, suffering and death – 'meaning' as the foundation, the source of inspiration, the significance, the motive, the eventual purpose of life? How does your faith or ideology provide you with strength, support, trust and helping?

People who experience a psychological earthquake look for new footing. When your life's home is shaking to its foundations, you try to create new footing by looking for meanings of loss on a symbolic level – through the realms of your own imagination. After all there is nothing you can change about the weight of this loss, however you can change the way you 'lift' the impact and the way you deal with this loss: loss. How can you, having arrived at an uncertain and difficult stage of loss in your life, create new footing yourself? How can you regain grip, develop new goals and feel good again? In their struggle with the feeling of uselessness and underlying existential fear, people tend to create a comforting fictional care reality, temporarily intended for grief processing. This mental activity equips us with the opportunity of developing an inner form of footing. We can derive footing from a fantasized reality, a type of personal faith which is supposed to make reality more bearable – a way of passing from the pointlessness of loss (see Figure 12.1).

12.4.6 Zero dimension

Attributing words and meanings to loss events may have a comforting effect. This comfort coming from meaning making is derived from denominating an experienced fact, putting the meaning into words and attributing it to the thing experienced as meaningless. The meaning originates from putting loss into words, in that way, as if realities are created, providing you with footing (Vaihinger, 1913).

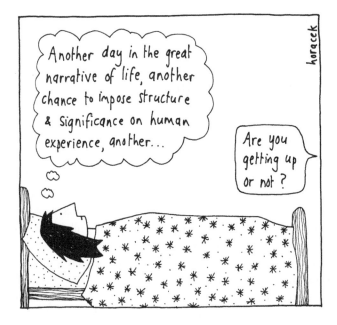

FIGURE 12.1   Another day © Judy Horacek, 1998

This illusion of footing is called the 'zero dimension' of grief processing. It literally means: by denominating 'zero' you pretend as if it may be useful giving a dimension to emptiness and lack of dimension itself.

When there is no longer a wallet in your house after it was stolen, we still talk about the stolen wallet, the thing that was lost. Strictly speaking this act of denominating: 'There is no longer a wallet in the house' is pointless, because there is no such thing as zero wallets. Zero means nothing, zero *is* nothing. However the term 'zero dimension' gives a linguistic existence to the non-existent, to the no-longer-existent: having or no longer having a wallet.

From this point of view there are many comforting words expressing the exact linguistic shortcoming in grasping this experience of emptiness, this zero experience: 'As a matter of fact, words are not enough.' The phrase: 'One word is too much, a thousand words aren't enough' was used by airline company El Al after the Bijlmer catastrophe where one of the planes crashed into the Bijlmer apartment buildings in Amsterdam. Those words tried to grasp the airline company's powerlessness, while being aware that it was their aircraft which had caused death and destruction.

You may ask: aren't you deceiving yourself when you try to describe the non-existent, speak the unspeakable, think the unthinkable, make the unreal a reality? Often it is said that talking about death is pointless: 'He's dead, you won't bring him back by talking about him!' That in itself is true, but you will miss opportunities for exchanging experiences and asking questions which may be very important for the further course of your life.

So what do you mean by 'deceiving yourself' when trying to put loss into words? Who is there to decide that your illusions, created by yourself after loss, are less real than the illusions we encounter in everyday life? Suffering, which appears to be a bearable fate, is easier to deal with than being stuck in just pointless suffering. Speaking the unspeakable can provide a certain degree of footing. In English, we speak of *coming to terms with losses*. Learning to live with losses is highly connected to the ability of giving meaning to life after loss and to the delimiting power of words, as can be seen in this enrolment text for a workshop on how to deal with losing your job:

Workshop from threat to opportunity: who am I without this job or function?

The workshop is designed for people who experience work-related losses and wish to learn how to deal with them.

You were assured of a (fixed) job, of a fixed income. You had a reliable foundation to build a life on. For a long time your job as a steady basis with steady income was self-evident.

This self-evidence has disappeared. Reorganization, cutbacks, bankruptcy . . . whatever the reason, it brought insecurity. Your function or job will disappear or has already disappeared; this means losing something you were attached to.

Dealing with this is no easy process. It causes emotions such as insecurity, anger, fear and grief to arise. Questions may arise: What is left of me? What am I still capable of? How do I move on? It may be difficult for you to accept this change, you may want to avoid emotions, which is why you enter into the fray with all your energy.

This workshop will give insight into and will let you experience how the process of dealing with loss takes place for you personally and what it means to you. From this insight and experience you will start seeing new perspectives and give meaning to a new phase in your life.

12.4.7 Constructive coping

It may be useful giving words to the reality of loss (zero dimension), but how do you build a new reality after loss? The constructive way in which you carry loss turns it from a seemingly unchangeable heavy burden into a bearable burden you can live with. Constructive coping is a process, not the end goal. When experiencing loss, you're not only continuously looking for satisfying answers to questions like: 'What happened exactly?' 'Why are they after me?' 'During the event I was thinking and feeling all sorts of things. How come?' You are looking for mutual coherence in the answers. The satisfying and mutually consistent answers to these questions may form a 'helping' narrative. You are not just looking for the truth. You are searching for a new structure in the meanings and explanations so that you can move on – moving on without always being unpleasantly reminded of the loss. How can I make loss bearable?

The individual helping narrative which arises is a coherent unity of reflections on loss. A new existential scheme (scenario) is created with the meanings from the reality before, during and after loss, integrating the old events with the new events (the loss). The helping narrative, based on a broken existence, comes into being by looking back on life (past), marking time in the present (here and now) and looking forwards (future).

Deceased daughter (10 years old)

A mother replied to the following questions: 'Are you okay?' and 'Do you still think about your daughter a lot?' with the following answers: 'That is a question to which there is no reply. Yes, always. No, never. I always carry her with me without having to think about her. Missing her is like a shirt I cannot take off, I cannot stop being the mother of a dead daughter. Deep inside I am affected. A condition. A state of being. It's the way I am. ME. That's who I am with her, without her.'

12.5 The history of the narrative method

> Giving persons in grief a breather and helping them come to a helping story.

The narrative method, originally developed by Michael White (1990), starts from the idea of man being confined but also enlightened by his story. People tell stories about each other, but also about themselves. By definition of the narrative method, a story is seen as a collection of thoughts, ideas and emotions. These stories originate in people's background, culture, ethnicity, gender and socialization among groups. These factors can also have a confining effect, apart from the creative effect. Words and stories give a certain identity to the client, people from the environment and the environment itself. The client also places himself and especially gives himself a role (victim, hero, etc., but also a leading role or only a supporting role) in his own life.

12.5.1 Conceptual definition and elucidation

The grieving person's story and recovery are at the centre of the narrative method. The narrative method clearly focuses on the narrative aspect. In order to work around existential questions, social workers have a wide array of narrative techniques at their disposal. There are three main indications for using the narrative method:

- The client's need for order and structure ('I don't know which way is up anymore');
- The need to dwell on existential questions ('Why me?');
- The need for some breathing space.

Existential questions regard someone's take on life, for example 'Who am I?,' 'What do I want to do with my life?' and 'What is the meaning of it?' The difficulty lies in the fact that 'why me' questions, which tend to arise when experiencing loss, are generally unanswerable. These are questions about how to deal with the emptiness caused by loss and how to deal with losing your grip. By using social work techniques such as mirroring and summarizing as a social worker, you offer the opportunity to create an impact narrative, to set guidelines in chaos and draw up the balance: to what degree was the client attached to the lost person or thing (past); what is the client's situation (present) and how will the client move on (future)? Making this inventory contributes to mentally preparing the client for the new situation after loss. How to recognize and acknowledge the client's current meaning making crisis, the psychological earthquake. By making it possible to share the devastating effect of loss using the narrative method and creating new meanings, you create a foundation for the helping narrative. The pointlessness is internalized and acknowledged, as seen in the case of Mr. Stack at the beginning of this chapter. As an 'exploring' method, the narrative method stimulates the client in creating an impact narrative and a helping narrative about the loss event(s).

The narrative method assumes that the client's life story, about himself or someone else, is not just a coincidental collection of facts. Individual stories reflect our culture (a pattern), not only our folklore (random frill). Stories help us in becoming aware of our history. The adage 'start where the client is' becomes clear when the social worker lets someone tell his or her story. The story is also a strong and clear foundation for a continuous dialogue in the grief counselling contact. We have already noticed that the constructivist effect of the narrative method (Whan, 1979) implies that every individual 'constructs' his own reality, creates his own stories. There are multiple versions of reality. That is what we try to show the person experiencing grief.

Australian social worker and family therapist Michael White developed an innovative and practical *storytelling* method for clients of all ages. Together with a colleague, David Epston, he investigated the power of personal stories and memories in dealing with obstacles in life, such as loss. They described their methodology in the influential book titled *Narrative Means to Therapeutic Ends* (White and Epston, 1990). Since then, their method has been known as the narrative method. For a while, White worked as a probation officer and social worker and obtained his bachelor's degree in social work. He then became a psychiatric social worker at the Adelaide Children's Hospital and afterwards started his own practice in the Dulwich Centre. In the early 1990s he applied his methodology to the New South Wales Aboriginal communities and discovered that storytelling was a useful means for tribal chiefs in dealing with the grabbing of their ancestors' lands and the forced migration that followed. The narrative method gained popularity worldwide.

12.6 Goals

General goals

- The client can give words to loss and its impact.
- The client can break from loss and its effects on his life.
- The client can rewrite his life story with the necessarily different positions.
- The client develops a valuable story around hopes, dreams, intentions for life, ethical goals, ideas and purposes.

Specific goals

- The client consciously thinks about meaning making questions.
- The client no longer coincides with his problem ('*the problem* is the problem, not *the person*').
- The client develops a clear view on problems and learns to position himself towards them based on values, intentions, ethical positions.
- The client becomes more aware of what is important or valuable to him, of his hopes, dreams, intentions in life, ethical goals, ideas and purposes.
- The clients takes initiatives in harmony with these hopes, dreams, values and intentions.
- The client notices unperceived proper initiatives and gives them meaning.
- The client reduces the influence of negative stories about himself.
- The client dares to be himself more.
- The client becomes more aware of the influence of previous and present power relations, obvious things and unspoken beliefs about what is 'normal'.
- The client unchains himself from the effects of loss.

12.7 Indications

- Perceptions for which the client has no words;
- The client makes existential statements such as: 'Why me?,' 'I can't go on' and 'I don't know anymore'.

12.8 Contraindications

- Inadequate cognitive skills (dementia, mental disability, brain damage);
- Severe confusion;

- The client is under the influence;
- Concrete informative question;
- Attributed need for assistance;
- Inadequate continuity guarantee.

12.9 Techniques

According to the narrative method, the practitioner prioritizes the stories and the knowledge and skills of clients and families, with the intention of letting them direct their own narrative. Narrative practitioners do not use a diagnosis–prescription format, a fixed agenda or formulas. Questions are used to bring up experiences, rather than to collect information. Asking questions can lead to separating the 'individual' from the 'problem', tracing desired directions and creating alternative narratives to support them. The narrative method's goal lies in acknowledging the client's personal strength and supporting relationships in order to overcome a given impact narrative. This may lead to helping narratives. The narrative method uses eight techniques to realize this:

1   Externalizing technique
2   Self-appreciation technique
3   Reframing technique
4   Cost–benefit technique
5   Metaphor technique
6   Rewriting technique
7   Re-membering technique
8   Reassessment technique.

12.9.1 Externalizing technique

'People are not problems. Problems are to be externalized. Deconstruct problems' – the social worker holds externalizing conversations with the intention of placing loss-related problems outside of the individual. *The person is not the problem. The problem is the problem.* The complaint or problem narrative is defined by a noun or sentence chosen by the person himself. Externalization causes the client to no longer coincide with the problem. Loss is externalized by summarizing it with a key word in one's personal filing cabinet (PFC), for example: 'stillbirth first son'.

People who experience loss may believe it is a reflection of their own identity, someone else's identity or the identity of their relationships. As described by the narrative method, disconnecting the person and the loss narrative has an excusing effect on the person. In the context of externalizing conversations, the problem no longer represents the 'truth' about people's identities. This causes new possibilities to arise in order to solve the 'problem', contributing to people becoming active again and really wanting to do something to actively influence their problems. Feeling depressed after loss is an example of this, and it often leaves a clear mark on people. Often the identities of these individuals coincide with their diagnosis of 'depression'. In other words, they *are* the depression. However by disconnecting it from the identity, by identifying the depression with a noun, a person is given more space and new opportunities to interpret the narratives pushed aside. The new stories have a positive influence on identity formation of the person involved.

12.9.2 Self-appreciation technique

Self-appreciation is a technique where the social worker asks the client to name a positive characteristic or positive behaviour of himself. This may encourage clients who 'think down' on themselves (the 'negative self-instructions') to allow positive thoughts about themselves as well. For example 'What was positive about your contribution to this session?' In most cases clients who think negatively about themselves cannot easily come up with an answer. A possible remark would be: 'Take your time to oversee what you thought was positive about the past hour'.

12.9.3 Reframing technique

Re-labelling consists of changing the label on the client's story, so that it becomes less negative. For example 'You say you don't understand why you can feel such panic. But when I sum it all up, the things you've been through and the emotions you held back, I can only imagine that your emotions want to erupt like a volcano. *That* feels like panic.' The 'panic' was considered a burden: 'I'm losing it.' Re-labelling it as 'a powerful emotion because you held everything back' is more comforting.

12.9.4 Cost–benefit technique

This technique allows the client to weigh up the costs and benefits of a survival strategy ('It's better to keep my emotions bottled up') or to make a choice in whatever they are facing in life ('Will I continue with this relationship or not?'). Pros and cons are listed by the client, so that they can decide. The survival strategy – for example avoidance – may no longer be needed because of the cost–benefit assessment. The social worker explains that this survival strategy 'is like an old coat that's had its time'.

12.9.5 Metaphor technique

The social worker tries to put the client's story into a more bearable perspective by using a metaphor or comparison. 'It appears that you've bottled up so many emotions that they are coming with tremendous force, as if a dam just broke. It's better to channel the emotions in an earlier stage, so that you have more control over them'. Or 'it's just like a flesh wound; if you don't take proper care, it will fester.'

The term 'metaphor' comes from the Greek word μεταφορά, 'a carrying over; a transfer': the image carries over the idea. Metaphors are illustrative expressions, pithy sayings summarizing an argumentation in a single image but saying as much as the theoretic discourse. Meaning aspects of one object (breaking dam or flesh wound) are carried over or transferred to another object (emotional discharge or behavioural problems). In the statement 'the social worker's toolbox contains 20 methods,' meaning all aspects of a toolbox are 'carried over' to the grief counselling profession. Metaphors place reality into perspective and depict a given object in the light of another object. Metaphors can improve one's knowledge with new insights. That is exactly the metaphor's narrative function.

12.9.6 Rewriting technique

The social worker uses the rewriting technique to help people:

- Experience positive things or take initiatives.
- Get more in touch with life's directions.
- Take up a strong position relative to new meanings.
- Think of new steps in a direction that feels useful.

Clients are stimulated in being the director of their own desired stories and intensifying these stories. The desired stories have a positive effect on the individual's wellbeing. This could possibly become part of the individual's identity.

The case of Mr. Stack

During the sessions, Mr. Stack finds out that he has a very creative mind but doesn't put it to use. He concludes that this was caused by his feeling of failure in his working environment because his employer subtly kept pointing out that his higher professional education degree should have been a scientific degree. This rejection of his competencies caused him to think himself unworthy and become very passive: it became part of his identity. However Mr. Stack wants to put his creativity in the limelight again.

The narrative method gives meaning to this by asking questions about the *landscape of action*. The questions are aimed at circumstances and situations, order, time and plot – in other words, questions about the behavioural factors of the narrative. In accordance with the narrative theory, the social worker also asks about the environment's reactions to let the involved person make the transition from idea towards experience.

The case of Mr. Stack

Mr. Stack calls himself a failure because all of his colleagues have a scientific degree. Most people in his life work on that same level. He was hired while having a higher professional education degree, but didn't have any luck. Within the scope of landscape-action questions, one might ask him, 'How do other people in your life see or notice that creativity means a great deal to you?'

Subsequently, the narrative method requires attention to the *landscape of identity*. A landscape-of-identity question emphasizes what colleagues or family members and the person involved find valuable in their lives, and how they would want it to be. In the narrative method it is important to amplify the desired narrative by turning descriptions of behaviour into conclusions for the identity: what does that say about who you are? After all, every story tells us something about who we are.

The case of Mr. Stack

The social worker asked Mr. Stack what he thought was important and valuable in his life. His answer was that he is actually a very creative person. When feeling creative, he feels truly alive. He is in a cheerful mood, full of energy, and feels appreciated. He concludes that he loves action and loves life. Then more attention was paid to the behaviour following from the identity conclusions: how did Mr. Stack react to this on a behavioural level? He took an advanced painting course to boost his creativity and positive feeling about himself.

12.9.7 Re-membering technique

In *re-membering* the social worker emphasizes memories of the social context and people who were of great importance to the person in grief, thus having a large influence on the life story. Apart from the literal meaning of remembering, *re-membering* also regards everyone's *membership* of a life club. Upon using this technique it is important to verify how those people contributed to making the involved person's life useful and meaningful and vice versa. Re-membering conversations do not consist of passively looking at all the persons who play or have played an important role in someone's life. The technique also aims at consciously establishing new ties with one's history of relationships with important persons, and with the identities of one's current and future life. There are many possible ways to identify persons and identities which can be reunited in people's lives. For that matter, the persons and identities do not have to be personal acquaintances for them to be important in re-membering conversations. Writers of the client's favourite books, personalities from movies and comic books are examples of this.

The woman next door

An early traumatized girl experienced lots of support coming from the woman next door. As part of re-membering, the social worker asks the girl to look at the woman next door from her point of view, but also to think about how the woman next door thought about the girl. This helped the traumatized girl in developing a story about her contribution to the woman's life. She meant a lot to the woman next door. By doing this the girl could attribute a meaning to certain aspects in her life she had neglected up to then. This conclusion cleared her way for contacting other women who were traumatized in their early childhood, because she was convinced that she can mean something to other people, the same way she meant something to the woman next door.

12.9.8 Reassessment technique

The constructive reassessment technique is about people who are important and close to the grieving person, acknowledging and revaluing this person's life. When using the constructive assessment technique, people can depict or tell their life story in front of a carefully selected audience which is not involved. These outsider witnesses react, in their turn, to the stories with retold stories. However, it is not their task to pass a value judgement on it. They only talk about the things they noticed about the story, the images the story evoked, the identification called up by their own experiences and about the way the story affected them.

This so-called reassessment indicates things that are valuable in people's lives in a very recognizable manner and with the emphasis on acceptance. Thanks to this reassessment people realize that their lives are interconnected with important common themes, causing counter-plots to arise.

Losing parents at young age

Years ago a woman was helped for losing her parents when she was young, and she was helped well. She was invited to a foster family's home where the youngest daughter had lost her parents too. First the woman listened to what the girl had to say, after which they switched positions and the woman told her story.

In this way, people's stories are influenced. Common themes being placed in a different perspective may contribute to this.

12.10 Social work result

The goals, evidence and pitfalls largely overlap with those of grief counselling, as described in Chapter 4. Next we only discuss the aspects applying specifically to the narrative method.

12.11 Evidence

In narrative therapy, clients undergo a transformation by adjusting their life story. According to White and Epston (1990) this transformation occurs by expanding the pinpricks of light or unique results – this means the development surpassing the impact narrative: the helping narrative. According to Gonçalves et al. (2009) it's the *innovative moments* or reconceptualization that cause durable changes in the client during narrative therapy. This type of innovative moments facilitates the origin of a meta-perspective regarding the transformation process itself. It also makes it possible for the person to actively position himself as the author of the helping narrative.

Narrative therapy suggests that change is caused by looking for unique results, narrative details going beyond the impact narrative (White & Epston, 1990). A pilot survey analyzed innovative moments in five successful and five failed therapy cases (Moreira et al., 2008) by using the Innovative Moments Coding System in a total of 127 sessions. Innovative moments were coded in terms of resilience and type. Sure enough, innovative moments appeared to be important for therapeutic success: two innovative moments are needed for a therapeutic transformation, two reconceptualization processes in order to experience new things.

The link between the changes in the client's narrative and the effect of therapy was investigated as well. Two groups of clients were selected for three psychotherapeutic models (cognitive, narrative and prescriptive therapy): a successful and a failed therapy group. For each client, sessions from the beginning, middle and end were investigated in terms of narrative coherence. At the end of the therapeutic process, differences in the production of narratives were found between groups. Successful therapy groups showed a significantly higher narrative change when compared to the failed therapy groups.

A pilot survey suggests that narrative therapy may be very effective in the social work of clients with traumatic experiences (Erbes et al., 2014). The survey was conducted on 14 PTSD-diagnosed veterans, 11 of whom completed the therapy. Participants were given a structured diagnostic interview and filled out a self-reporting questionnaire before narrative therapy and after 11 or 12 sessions. When the treatment was finished, 3 out of the 11 treated veterans no longer had PTSD, and 7 out of 11 showed a significant decrease of PTSD symptoms. The degree of failure was relatively low (at 21.4%) and customer satisfaction was high, so further research on the possible effect of narrative therapy as an alternative for existing PTSD treatments is obvious.

Another research showed Narrative Exposure Therapy (NET) to be effective in treating adult earthquake victims' trauma reactions (Zang et al., 2013). This randomized research with a waiting list group and a treatment group was conducted between December 2009 and March 2010 around the Chinese city Sichuan. After 2 weeks, the waiting list group was given the same treatment as the intervention group. Effect measurements were done before, directly after and 2 months after the narrative approach. In comparison to the waiting list group, the treatment group showed significant positive effects on PTSD symptoms, depression, general mental health and increased post-traumatic growth. The effects appeared to be stable after 2 months.

12.12 Pitfalls

- Missing directive indications. There is an increased need for active guidance, but the social worker does not recognize the indications.
- Continuing the non-directive method without progress. Compliance can cause the social worker to empathize with the client's stories and statements. Yet client orientation is not the same thing as automatically complying with the client: client orientation can also mean a minor confrontation with resistance to personal perception. From his client-centred attitude, the social worker searches for the thing supporting the client and establishing progression.

12.13 Summary and questions

In this chapter the role of the social worker was described in helping the grieving person fulfil four existential needs related to meaning making.

First we have described four meaning making needs that arise when experiencing loss, summed up in the acronym DUNC: the need for Dignity, Understanding of justice, Now-in-relation-to-later and Control. Meaning making stress arises when these needs are inadequately fulfilled. In conclusion we described the narrative method's contribution to reducing existential stress and restoring strength.

Questions

1   Do you recognize the following meaning making questions in situations of loss: 'Why me?' 'Why is this happening to me?'
2   What difference do you see between factual 'why' questions and existential 'why' questions?
3   Do you know people experiencing existential stress or tensions regarding their existence?
4   Do you recognize the loss of dignity in statements made by grieving persons? Give an example.
5   Do you recognize the loss of understanding of justice in statements made by grieving persons? Give an example.
6   Do you recognize the loss of now in relation to later, the loss of future perspective in statements made by grieving persons? Give an example.
7   Do you recognize the loss of control in statements made by grieving persons? Give an example.
8   Where lies the power in letting a person tell the impact narrative and the helping narrative? Give an example.
9   Which techniques of the narrative method do you find appealing? Why?

13

BEHAVIOURAL METHOD

Questions

This chapter addresses the following questions:

- How do inadequate personal skills cause behavioural stress in clients?
- By means of social skill training, what can the behavioural method's contribution be in reducing behavioural stress and restoring personal strength?

13.1 Introduction

In this chapter we describe the social worker's role in the client's effective communication: how can the client constructively turn wishes into behaviour? We use the term 'behavioural stress' to denominate insufficient assertive behaviour.

First we describe how stress is built up and maintained by clients due to the lack of skills. Then we describe what the behavioural method has to offer in order to reduce this behavioural stress and enhance social strengths.

The case of Mr. Stack

Mr. Stack finds it difficult to confront his boss with the careless way in which he brought Mr. Stack the news about his demotion (namely in passing him in the hallways). Exercises are done on how to make an appointment and how to give constructive criticism by following the four-step model (see section 13.7.11).

13.2 Behavioural stress: skill deficiency?

The client asks the social worker questions about the practical and relational consequences of the life event, such as: 'What should I do?,' 'What do you advise me to do in this case?' or 'How can I enter into this kind of conversation with. . . ?' Clearly the client cannot adequately put his finger on these practical pressure points. The imbalance between the desired circumstances ('I don't know how to talk on the phone with . . .') and the perceptible circumstances ('I don't do it because I am not capable') causes behavioural stress. The need to become more skilful can be a way of reducing this behavioural stress.

Questions for advice, such as these, are aimed at solutions and decisions (Witte, 1997). Helping in realistic decision making and behavioural actions is in order: 'What can I do about it?' 'What are the possibilities for overcoming the consequences of loss?' 'How can I achieve adequate self-confrontation and adequate avoidance?'

A pitfall for the social worker may be to immediately proceed to giving advice while only having limited client information. Preferably the social worker and the grieving person investigate the latter's current position in the problem-solving cycle (see section 6.6.3 under Advice technique).

Is the grieving person capable of taking all steps autonomously and suit the action to the word, or do they need support? Together with the client, the social worker determines what kind of support suits the circumstances. The social worker estimates the stage of the practical question in the problem-solving cycle. Advice that was given too soon may let the client down. Possibly the client doesn't need advice on the concrete problem at all, rather than advice on how to qualify in problem-solving skills. When the client asks: 'Can you help me find a new home, because I no longer want to live with either of my parents after the divorce?,' the social worker will first want to figure out more about the motives for moving out and the situation which led up to the question for support in this.

How skilled is the grieving person in adequately communicating in all social situations that occur during the grieving process? Does the grieving person know how to manage all of the social and practical affairs?

The informal carer

Take the example of the informal carer who witnesses his partner pining away and getting exhausted because of long-term illness, who can barely keep himself standing and is wondering, 'How do I keep family and friends informed?' How easily will this informal carer ask for support? Is he aware of his needs? Is this support accessibly present in his surroundings or does it need mobilizing? Is the informal carer capable of starting a newsletter and using it to communicate with the circle of most intimate friends and family about the severely ill person's current situation? Who does the informal carer allow to visit, and for how long? How assertive is the informal carer?

And when the process of dying comes to an end, the question remains: how well is the grieving person in touch with his own needs and desires in such a vulnerable situation? Does he want to plan the funeral himself? Who will support him? What about further preparations and actions for the commemoration and funeral? How can he take a worthy parting? How well is he supported? Who does he want close to him, and who doesn't he?

How well is he dealing with his children's grief, and how will he raise the children alone? What about the finances, bookkeeping, rights and obligations in terms of inheritance, insurance benefits and so forth?

For all of the abovementioned practical and material affairs, the practical-material method is without doubt the most reliable resource (see section 6.2). However, for the assertive side of the matter (How can I express my desires and emotions?) the behavioural method is indicated, because the supposition that clients communicate adequately with their environment is not realistic. Which client *does know* how to effectively share the current situation, including vulnerabilities, wishes and needs, with the outside world? This is no easy task when the necessary stress and emotion are at play at the same time.

13.2.1 Personal territories

In section 15.3.1 and 21.7.4 and in Table 15.1 all sorts of unacceptable behaviour in interpersonal traffic are described. When speaking of a grieving person's effective communication with his surroundings, the territorial theory once again provides a useful mapping. Is the grieving person capable of protecting his own territory? As seen before, there are seven human territories:

- T1 The territory of personal belongings;
- T2 The territory of your own body;
- T3 The territory of your own mind;
- T4 The territory of your own private shelter: my retirement territory;
- T5 The territory of personal space: the distance between yourself and others;
- T6 The territory of your psychological space: attention coming from others;
- T7 The territory of your field of action.

We distinguish three types of territorial skills that may be relevant for the grieving person in practicing proper skills in terms of defence, acquisition and managing own desires and territory.

13.2.2 Territorial defence skills

As a grieving person, do you effectively 'defend' your own territory against others? Questions that may arise include:

- Do you dispose of any defensive weapons?
- What is the expected result of a conflict?
- What is the importance of the disputed territory?

For example, for a widower: How close do you let other persons physically approach you (T2 and T5)? Do you determine whether or not and with whom you share your emotion (T3)? To what degree can you say 'no' when people try to come over with their best intentions and comfort you, while you would rather isolate yourself for a while (T4)? Do you dare ask for attention and visit someone while still in grief (T6)? Who decides what will happen at the memorial service (T7)? What about the division of belongings (T1)?

Territorial acquisition skills

Do you manage to acquire new territory while in grief, for example can you think about home, the workplace, friends? These acquisition skills are related to (a combination of):

- The skill of disarming the other;
- The importance of the other territories;
- The hopes you have for the acquisition.

Territorial managing skills

If the field of action (T7) is too small or too large, the following solutions may apply:

- Shrinking the territory (throwing stuff out, not wanting to see all acquaintances);
- Practicing how to manage things better (e.g. when someone takes up your time, not letting yourself be thrown off guard and keep on doing 'your own thing');
- Assistance in managing (in marking out possible contacts).

Loss may have drastically changed the client's situation. Gradually learning how to expand or shrink your territory may be an opportunity for the grieving person to take up exactly the amount of space that feels comfortable.

13.2.3 Behaviour

Practicing territorial skills may relieve stress for the grieving person. Skill training and behavioural training are possible means for achieving this. First we define the terms 'behaviour' and 'assertive behaviour' before looking at how behavioural stress arises in grieving persons and giving examples of behavioural stress.

Behaviour is the way in which you act, react, what you do. In short it is the perceptible behaviour as a reaction to a stimulus, situation or other person.

The client can learn how to behave assertively with the help of a social worker. Assertive behaviour stands for being capable of standing up for yourself without needlessly hurting another person. Assertive behaviour does not only apply to situations where others invade your personal space, for example by being dominant, but it also applies to sharing your thoughts and skills in social situations. Under the SOSKI technique (section 13.7.2), several social skills that can be interpreted as assertive behaviour are summed up.

In behavioural therapy we initially started from the aforementioned definition of behaviour, but nowadays non-perceptible behaviour is also defined as behaviour. This means that thinking and feeling are also considered to be types of behaviour. In this chapter we only focus on the first definition of behaviour because the cathartic and cognitive method already focus on the emotional and thinking aspect of the grieving person. Labelling 'emotion' and 'thinking' as types of behaviour may be rather confusing.

When clients are affected by a certain type of behaviour and label it as undesired behaviour, the social worker and the client look for ways to unlearn it and to learn new and wanted behaviour. In practice this is primarily social skill training, individually or in groups. By means of a detailed description of the client's behaviour, the social worker draws up a behaviour analysis of complaints in terms of behavioural stimuli triggering the client (e.g. points in time, people) and the behavioural consequences incited. The latter may be heart palpitations, staying at home, watching TV, drinking, getting attention from others, feeling compassionate, not having to go to work, receiving criticism, getting marital problems, losing social contacts and feeling like a failure. Then the indicated behavioural technique is deployed.

Behavioural stress in grieving persons arises due to three types of behaviour that have a pernicious influence on the subject:

1   Avoidance behaviour, for example avoiding people, public transportation, busy streets or fire; withdrawn behaviour, for example isolating oneself and not partaking in social events;
2   Unpleasant behaviour such as drawing attention and acting clingy and even verbally, non-verbally and physically aggressive behaviour;
3   Lacking behaviour, such as having inadequate skills because they are unknown or because they were unlearned.

These inadequate types of behaviour often originate from a lack of assertiveness. Clients may display sub-assertive (helpless) or aggressive behaviour. Sub-assertive behaviour is when the client does not sufficiently stand up for himself. Aggressive behaviour is when the client stands up for himself in a threatening, egoistic and demanding way. Some clients explain assertive behaviour as 'standing up for yourself', while by definition, assertiveness means 'standing up for yourself without needlessly hurting others'. Both aggressive and sub-assertive behaviour are signs of insufficient social skills.

Social skills can be subdivided into non-verbal behaviour and verbal behaviour. Examples of non-verbal skills are eye contact, shaking hands, touching, physical distance, posture, facial expressions, voice changes and timing. Examples of verbal skills are open questions, self-revelation, changing the subject, mixing into ongoing conversations, telling stories, ending conversations, expressing self-appreciation, giving and receiving compliments, speaking in first-person terms, making statements instead of asking questions, apologizing, asking for criticism and criticizing.

Avoidance and addiction behaviour

Avoiding social situations (not talking to friends about the loss or shutting down emotional subjects) is an example of avoidance behaviour. Submitting oneself to comfort drinking, comfort injections or other addictions are also forms of avoidance. A part of a directive approach may be that the social worker helps the client in overcoming certain addictions that were built on the emptiness of loss. Many clients try to escape this emptiness by never looking back or by running away. When loss is not properly dealt with, it will keep echoing in your head and in social contacts with all destructive effects that follow. Lots of energy is lost and many unnecessary side effects may be the result. Chinese philosopher Zhuangzi (fourth century BC) strikingly describes this in the shadow metaphor.

The shadow

There was once a man who didn't want to see his own footprints or shadow. He decided to escape them and ran away. As he kept running, more footprints appeared and his shadow effortlessly kept up with him. Thinking that he was moving too slowly, he kept running faster and faster, without a stop, until he finally collapsed from exhaustion and died. If he had stood still, there wouldn't have been any footprints. If he had taken a rest in the shade, his shadow would have disappeared.

(Summary from Hoff, 1989).

A non-directive and compliant approach isn't always helpful. A directive approach focuses on listing the addiction's costs and benefits. As a social worker, you talk about the unhealthy effects of *flight* reactions with the client. Flight reactions include fleeing into a drinking habit, workaholism, sex addiction and excessive drug abuse. These survival patterns probably temporarily bridge the gap made by loss and provide a certain sense of artificial anaesthesia, but loss keeps echoing restlessly. New addiction problems keep stacking up on the existent processing problem. Parallel to rehabilitation, processing problems can be dealt with. Insight in this pattern is the basis for rehabilitation. Working through it step by step and achieving small goals can have a truly encouraging effect in this.

Withdrawn behaviour

It's not unusual for people who have experienced loss to withdraw themselves from interacting with others.

> I met a young woman shortly after her mother passed away. This single woman was very sociable and loved going out to parties. Over a few months after her mother died she turned down all invitations, because it didn't feel right in this early stage of loss.
>
> *(Worden, 1992, p. 36)*

Upon losing a person, several contacts are lost as well. You may feel lonely and helpless: you don't know what to do, and your entire sense of initiative drains away. After experiencing loss, you can also visit places which remind you of the person or thing that was lost. Carrying objects with you that remind you of the person who passed away may have a comforting effect.

It appears that the generally assumed reservedness and apathy of grieving persons cannot be generalized. Many grieving persons turn in on themselves, while others turn to the outside world. Frequent sexual contact of grieving persons is reported as a desperate attempt not to succumb. Grieving persons' need for sexuality stands for the need for comforting, physical warmth and resisting the pain of loss, rejection by loss or the fear of being alone (Raphael, 1983). The increase in sexual activity is interpreted as a normal reaction to the fear that arises after death or as one's ending approaches (MacElveen-Hoehn, 1987).

Unpleasant and aggressive behaviour

Continuously drawing attention and clinging onto someone are two types of unpleasant behaviour that can have a repulsive effect in the end. This is different for aggressive behaviour. Some grieving persons are irritable and behave hostilely towards people in their surroundings. Even though anger can be a normal expression, aggressive behaviour needlessly hurts the other person. Directive techniques may help managing the anger and showing constructive behaviour: 'What do I actually wish for, what do I expect from the other, why do I let myself go and lapse into hostile behaviour?' Directive techniques work with instructions and assignments. Video home training is an example of this, giving feedback based on video recordings in the social work space or at home. This may cause a change in behaviour.

Lacking behaviour

Clients can also be so heavily affected that they react passively in a stress situation and do not look for support or ask for attention. Clearly this is not a form of assertive behaviour, and it only gives stress more room to grow.

13.3 History of the behavioural method

Practice makes perfect.

The behavioural method gained its popularity through social skill training (Goldstein, 1984) and video home training. The method focuses on practicing behaviour and skills, more specifically social skills and assertiveness. Starting from a self-conscious basic attitude, clients learn how to combine the right tone and right body language with the right assertive language. It teaches grieving persons to swap sub-assertiveness or aggression with assertiveness: standing up for yourself without needlessly hurting others. People who suffer from loss may feel entirely powerless and find new courage in behavioural progression, starting with the easiest step forwards and ending with the hardest. In behavioural therapy this is also called 'successive approximation'. Starting a conversation, calling up an authority, breaking through dilemmas, dealing with parenting and other situations differently, sharing essential emotions: all are examples of skills and assertiveness that can be practiced in the controlled environment of the social work space and afterwards in homework assignments in real life. Small successes and appreciation acknowledge the newly learned assertive behaviour. This causes the behavioural stress to decrease.

Learning new behaviour, new social skills and unlearning dysfunctional behaviour decreases personal tension caused by inadequate behaviour. The client learns a better way of standing up for himself without hurting others; he becomes more assertive.

Behavioural therapy considers the client's complaint as a form of learned (conditioned) behaviour that can also be unlearned again by using behavioural techniques. The behavioural method used in grief counselling is derived from it, but implies a smaller number of behavioural techniques. Those behavioural techniques use pressure points in perceptible behaviour as a starting point: which type of behaviour is inadequate or ineffective? Which type of behaviour is unknown to the client; which skills does he not master? In the behavioural method, a lot of these things are figured out in the social work room (*in vitro*) and are applied outside of the social work room (*in vivo*).

Within the multimethodical social work model, the behavioural method focuses on perceptible behaviour. For improvements in terms of emotions and thoughts, the cathartic method and cognitive method are applied respectively. Social skills practiced in the behavioural method can be divided into non-verbal skills and conversational skills.

- Non-verbal skills include eye contact, shaking hands, touching, physical distance, posture, facial expression, change of pitch in one's voice and timing.
- Conversational skills include: asking open questions, paying attention to voluntary information, self-revelation, changing the subject, mixing into ongoing conversations, silences, telling stories, giving non-verbal clues, ending conversations, self-appreciation, giving and receiving compliments, power bombardment, speaking in first-person terms, making statements instead of asking questions, saying the same things over and over, selective ignoring, taming anger, selecting subjects, apologizing, asking for criticism and criticizing.

Behavioural therapy is an engaging therapy, so the behavioural method is an engaging method. Because of the reciprocal inhibition principle, the behavioural method assumes that the client's reaction of anxiety decreases as the client starts adequately mastering the opposite skills (see Figure 13.1). Being more socially skilled weakens the anxiety reaction and less anxiety strengthens one's skills. This applies conversely as well: the fewer social skills, the more anxiety, the more skills are weakened and so on. In grief counselling many behavioural principles are applied without them being named as such. The point of departure in behaviour-oriented grief counselling is improvement of social functioning by learning new behaviour and unlearning disruptive behaviour. Social workers working in forensic and psychiatric sectors explicitly use behavioural techniques. In doing so, clients' possible behaviour is observed and the reward following positive behaviour is monitored. Only few books on the subject of grief counselling use the theorems as a point of departure, except for the task-oriented *casework* described by William Reid (1995). In American social work manuals, the behavioural approach is described in the *Handbook of Empirical Social Work Practice* (Thyer & Wodarski, 1998) and in *Behavioral Change in the Human Services* (Sundel & Sundel, 1999), while for

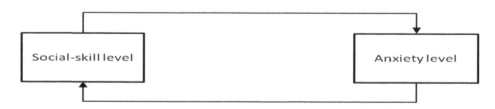

FIGURE 13.1 Reciprocal inhibition cycle between social-skill level and anxiety level: the more skills the less anxiety, and vice versa

Dutch readers there is *Taakgerichte hulpverlening en gedragsgerichte verliesbegeleiding* (Jagt & Jagt, 1990) (*Task-Oriented Assistance and Behaviour-Oriented Grief Counselling*). The latter presumes that the client undertakes pre-discussed activities to relieve or solve a problem. The tasks executed by the client almost always cause change:

- In the environment or situation; for example the client still receives a complementary allowance thanks to the arrangement that the client may still apply for it;
- In the client; for example because the client is developing assertiveness and negotiation skills;
- In the interaction between client and environment; the client now knows how to handle things and experiences the environment as less threatening.

The task-oriented approach increases the client's competence to act as much as possible, thus limiting the client's dependence on the social worker. A strong characteristic of the task-oriented approach is that it is one of the few methods in grief counselling investigating the effects of interventions.

Behavioural therapy is a subject widely written about, however only a few works mention the importance of the behavioural method in grief counselling. During the 1970s several books and articles were published on behaviour-oriented grief counselling, but did not lead to a breakthrough of behaviour-oriented practices. They described three advantages of the behavioural method (Jehu, 1973):

- The emphasis on observable reactions and the conditions preserving them;
- The usefulness with clients for whom the verbal approach is less effective due to a lack of self-insight and verbal skills;
- Specific and perceptible social work goals are used, so that the outcome is predetermined.

Behavioural therapy's origin dates from the 1950s, when the theories and behavioural therapy were developed by authors such as Wolpe, Eysenck, Pavlov, Skinner, Bandura and De Moor. The behavioural method rose from dissatisfaction with the little systematic and uncontrolled approach of psychoanalysis and later forms of conversation therapy. The externally perceptible behaviour was used as a starting point for the method, because at the time people believed that subjective perception was not a suitable starting point. For years animal experiments have defined the image of behavioural therapy as an overly simple way of symptom social work for people. Take the example of the learning process of Pavlov's dog, which produces saliva just by seeing a the light bulb flash after which its food was usually served. Or Skinner's rats that had 'learned' that food would be dropped in their cage after accidentally having flipped a switch, causing this behaviour to be encouraged or learned. According to these authors, many human complaints could be explained as being learned behaviour which can also be unlearned again. Since the 1950s this behavioural approach, behaviourism, gained a lot of popularity and behavioural therapy achieved its first successes. Over the first few decades, clients' thoughts and emotions were excluded from the problem analysis. During the years that followed, this strict limitation appeared not to be fruitful, and behavioural analysis was extended to also imply the analysis of 'learned' thoughts and emotions in the client. Around 1980 Albert Ellis introduced rational emotive therapy (RET; see section 11.4.1). Nowadays all three areas are covered in cognitive behavioural therapy: externally perceptible behaviour and learned thoughts and emotions.

13.4 Goals

General goal

- Reducing or removing negative tension caused by behavioural pressure points.

Specific goals

- The client is more socially skilled.
- The client is more assertive.
- The client communicates more adequately.
- The client recognizes impulses and boundaries (e.g. punishing behaviour towards his own child).
- The client stops the undesired (also by himself) behaviour.

13.5 Indications

- The client experiences a lack of social skills.
- The client experiences difficulties in feeling and indicating boundaries.
- The client experiences a lack of communication ('Contacts with X aren't going too smoothly').
- The social worker recognizes the client's blind spot (the client cannot properly read social situations and makes remarks such as 'Boss, you were gone for too long during your break').

13.6 Contraindications

- Verbal hindrances, such as vocal cord problems or a severe form of stuttering;
- Behavioural hindrances, as is the case for some psychic or somatic disorders;
- The client wishes not to practice his behaviour;
- The client lacks cognitive abilities (dementia, mental disability, cerebrovascular accident).

13.7 Techniques

1. Diary technique
2. SOSKI technique
3. Modelling technique
4. Shaping technique
5. Prompting technique
6. Conditioning technique
7. Task-oriented technique
8. Self-control technique
9. Feeling yes–feeling no technique
10. Nurturing technique
11. CC technique
12. Standardization technique.

13.7.1 Diary technique

Keeping a diary, also called self-monitoring, is the foundation of the behavioural method (Orlemans et al., 1995). It makes it possible to precisely define the behaviour in question and to assess progress. Monitoring is done through observation and registration of behaviour. The fact that the client keeps a diary may cause the client to become aware of his own behaviour. In self-registration, the client is literally tallying the behaviour to be observed. In a small book, the client keeps notes of how a certain type of behaviour appears in practice. For example, clients feeling tense in social situations can isolate themselves for 10 minutes and write down what makes them feel tense and what exactly was wrong with them. Using these detailed data the social worker draws up a functional analysis: he describes what happens right before the behaviour (S = stimulus) and what happens right after the behaviour (R = response). Three conclusions can be drawn from this:

- There is a surplus of behaviour which the client may want to cut back on.
- There is behaviour the client needs to replace by alternative behaviour, for example learning how to start a dialogue instead of punishing.
- There are possibilities, because the client is able to describe what he is good at.

13.7.2 SOSKI technique

Max Beekers (1982) developed the (SOSKI = Social Skills) technique based on a video-supported skill training for the poor designed by Goldstein. In this technique, the social worker practices nine social (interpersonal) skills with clients from every income category: having a chat, listening, discussing something, reacting to anger, reacting to affection and appreciation, expressing anger, expressing affection and appreciation, standing up for your opinion and opposing others (van Meer et al., 1999).

For every social skill an instruction is followed to practice the separate skills.

Having a chat

- See if you can have a chat here.
- Look at the other person.
- Greet the other person.
- Say something about what both of you can see, hear or feel.
- Pay attention to the other person's reaction.
- Pick up on it or wind up the conversation.

Listening

- Look at the other person.
- Show your interest – with or without words.
- Ask for clarification of things you do not understand.
- Briefly repeat what has been said.
- Express your opinion or feeling.
- Pay attention to the other person's reaction.

Discussing something

- Pick the right time.
- Tell the other person you wish to talk, and what you wish to talk about.
- Tell the other person what's on your mind.
- Ask what the other person thinks about it.
- Listen carefully to the other person.
- Wind up the conversation with a conclusion.

Reacting to anger

- Listen carefully to the other person.
- Show that you can see he or she is angry.
- Ask questions about things that aren't clear to you.
- Show that you understand why the other person is angry.
- If you think that now is the right time, express your opinion or describe your feeling.

Reacting to affection and appreciation

- Pay attention to the affection or appreciation the other person shows you.
- Look at the other person while doing so.
- Let it get through to you that the other person likes something about you.
- Show that you like it.
- Return the affection or appreciation if you want to.

Expressing anger

- Pay attention to your body (including your posture).
- Figure out whether something is bothering you.
- Determine who or what caused this.
- Pick a suitable moment to express it.
- Point out that you are angry and why.
- Listen to the other person's reaction.

Expressing affection and appreciation

- Figure out what you like about the other person.
- Decide whether you would like to show this.
- Pick a suitable moment to express this.
- Kindly look at the other person.
- Point out to the other person what you like about him or her.
- Pay attention to the other person's reaction.

Standing up for your opinion

- Figure out what you think about the situation.
- Decide whether you wish to stand up for your opinion.

- Clearly and fully tell the other person your opinion.
- Listen to the other person's reaction.
- If you are not satisfied with it, express your opinion once again.

Opposing others

- Listen carefully to what the other person says or asks.
- If necessary, ask questions about things that aren't clear to you.
- Figure out which are the points where you disagree.
- Clearly tell the other where you disagree and why.
- Pay attention to the other person's reaction.
- If necessary, clearly point out the things you definitely disagree with again.

13.7.3 Modelling technique

The social worker demonstrates a certain type of behaviour by modelling, so that the client can copy this behaviour. In a simulation the client can practice new behaviour in difficult social situations, in a protected environment and without the risk of 'failure'. The next steps can be taken:

1   The client describes the problematic situation and the problematic behaviour;
2   The social worker makes suggestions for a more effective approach;
3   The social worker simulates exemplary behaviour and asks the client to imitate;
4   An assessment follows where good things are appreciated and acknowledged, and attention is paid to points of possible improvement;
5   The client applies the learned behaviour in practice;
6   The social worker gives homework instructions to further practice the behaviour.

An example: the client dreads a consulting conversation and doesn't know how to behave. In the consultation room, this situation is imitated to learn the client how to behave by means of feedback on, suggestions about and appreciation for the demonstrated behaviour. The social worker gives feedback, tips and offers an alternative approach.

13.7.4 Shaping technique

The behaviour to be learned by the client is divided into small steps that are then practiced separately. Spontaneous behaviour somewhat resembling the desired behaviour is positively encouraged until it becomes part of the client's behaviour. From this new situation, behaviour which even more resembles the desired behaviour is then again positively encouraged. This process is repeated until the goal is reached.

13.7.5 Prompting technique

The social worker prompts the client in behaviour alternatives. A *prompt* can be a verbal stimulus, an instruction, a non-verbal stimulus or a physical manner of guiding the client to the desired behaviour. An example: encourage the client to state his point of view on the telephone about changing an agreement with the employer again in a self-conscious way.

13.7.6 Conditioning technique

The social worker encourages or rewards the client's behaviour: in that way he learns new behaviour. The systematic rewarding of the desired behaviour – conditioning – is used for e.g. clients with a mental disability by making a list of types of behaviour and defining the client's reward for every successful positive reaction. This systematic reward technique is also called the *token economy*. For example, the social worker encourages the client: 'How good of you to tell me this.' Or he shakes hands with the client when progress is made and says: 'How wonderful, congratulations!'

13.7.7 Task-oriented technique

The social worker proposes a task which the client will complete (upon agreement) as a homework assignment between two sessions. Examples: a man without any contacts will try to get acquainted with someone new, or a father can try to impose house rules on his children in another way.

13.7.8 Self-control technique

The social worker tries to enhance the client's self-control by means of advice. An example: every night the client 'is granted' a '15-minute scolding'. He thinks about how his day went and concentrates on all things that made him angry. The purpose being that he is 'free' from uncontrolled anger for the rest of the day.

13.7.9 Feeling yes–feeling no technique

The social worker and the client practice in defining boundaries with self-protection skills. Every person has a yes-feeling or no-feeling in every social situation. When the client feels *yes*, he states it, and the same thing goes for when he feels *no*. In case of doubt he first investigates what is and isn't right before continuing, for example when the client acts ambivalently in a contact with someone. On the one side it feels good, but on the other side something repels this contact.

13.7.10 Nurturing technique

Triple P, the Positive Pedagogical Programme, is a short, purposeful, preventive and timely skill training focusing on enhancing parents' competence and self-confidence in raising their children (Turner et al., 2007). The programme tries to strengthen the quality of a parent–child relationship and to help parents in developing effective and practical strategies for dealing with frequent behavioural and development problems, especially when the problems are directly or indirectly related to the loss situation affecting the family or certain members of it, such as death of the father, mother or child or drastic changes in the family, at school or at work. The programme uses active skill training for parents. Purposeful training and supervision from social workers using this programme is strongly advised. The four nurturing skills parents can be trained in by social workers are:

1   Developing a positive relationship with your child;
2   Stimulating desired behaviour;

3   Learning new skills and behaviour;
4   Dealing with undesired behaviour.

Per nurturing skill, Table 13.1 shows which parts it consists of and give a description, including the recommended age and goal/application.

TABLE 13.1 Nurturing skill 1: developing a positive relationship with your child

Strategy	Description	Recommended age	Goal/application
Giving time and attention to children	Frequently freeing short moments (1–2 minutes is enough) for activities the children love	All ages	Giving children the opportunity to open up and to practice their verbal skills
Talking to children	Having short conversations with children about an activity	All ages	Enhancing vocabulary, verbal skills and social skills
Show affection	Show physical affection (hugging, touching, massages, caressing)	All ages	Familiarize children with intimacy and physical affection

For other nurturing skills from Triple P: see www.triplep.net

13.7.11 Constructive Criticism (CC) technique

Constructive criticism consists of four steps which can be practiced:

1   Facts: what happened when? ('You weren't looking at me when we were just having a discussion');
2   Perception: what irritates me about it? ('It irritated me');
3   Desired behaviour: what is my wish for which type of other behaviour? ('I would like you to look at me when you are talking to me');
4   Common interest in the change in behaviour: what is constructive about this change in behaviour for our relationship? ('Eye contact makes our discussions easier').

13.7.12 Standardization technique

Some grieving people overstep limits in behaviour, for example by acting aggressively. The social worker reduces problematic behaviour by defining boundaries, for example by removing children temporarily (not as a punishment) from the room where the problematic behaviour occurred. An example: he places the upset child in a peaceful and quiet room and asks him to cool down. He does this immediately after a rule has been broken (for example the rule of not yelling) and tells what must happen now ('Show us that you are getting angry by raising your hand'). He uses, for example, 1 minute in the timeout room for every year in the child's age. When the time is up, he asks the child whether he is ready to come back and behave correctly ('Pronounce your wish, instead of immediately being angry and disappointed'). Finally he shows appreciation for the correct behaviour when it occurs.

13.8 Social work results

- The client is less tense.
- The client is socially more skilled.
- The client is more assertive.
- The client communicates more adequately.
- The client quickly recognizes impulses causing unacceptable behaviour.
- The client is capable of stopping his undesired behaviour.

13.9 Evidence

Research on the task-oriented method suggests that the basic methods of the model – task planning and task execution – have a positive effect on the problems clients are facing (Reid, 1995). This effect is substantial enough to establish essential change in the lives of many clients. There are, however, questions about the sustainability of the changes and comparison to other methods: are they equally effective?

According to research conducted on solution-oriented therapy there is an 80.4% success rate for an average of 4.6 sessions (Berg & Jong 2001). After a year and a half this success rate climbed to 86%.

Research on the effectiveness of interpersonal skill therapies showed that clients indeed become more skilled and show fewer complaints thanks to this type of therapy (Beekers, 1982). Self-appreciation levels in clients increased as well when compared to the control group. Re-measuring proved the self-appreciation to remain stable, interpersonal skills to increase and client-specific complaints to further diminish.

Behavioural techniques for children and adolescents are effective for a wide array of problem areas (Prins & Bosch, 1998). Sometimes a specific technique is perfectly suitable for a certain problem, and sometimes a combination of several behavioural techniques is even more effective (see Triple P website at www.triplep.net).

Patients suffering from non-congenital brain damage have cognitive limitations and go through changes in their personality affecting their behaviour in their social network and family. These changes often bring along disruptions between family members and make it difficult to return to work. A pilot survey was carried out to investigate the effectiveness of social skill training as part of the rehabilitation programme with an intensive schedule (3 months) full of individual and group interventions such as role play, convincing behaviour and video recordings. Participants showed significant reduction of anxious or aggressive behaviour. Progress was made in the awareness of proper limitations, in expressing opinions and emotions and in the ability of showing socially flexible behaviour in many different situations (Ojeda del Pozo et al., 2000).

Informal carers are having a hard time, also because of the loss of a healthy partner with whom they used to share life's joys and sorrows. Family members with informal carers experience a high degree of stress and strain and a reduced quality of life. A group of 354 informal carers were trained in social skills according to the COPE model. Randomized monitored research tested the use of skill training. Three types of care for informal carers were compared: (1) hospice care with social skill training; (2) hospice care with emotional support; and (3) usual hospice care. Quality of life, strain level and degree of coping were measured. It was concluded that the training was more effective than both of the other researches combined in increasing quality of life for the informal carer, reducing strain and the care tasks. Structured skill training for informal carers has shown to be very promising in the difficult hospice care environment.

The COPE model implies:

C *creativity*: keep on looking at the problems from different perspectives in order to find new solutions for the pressure points in care ('What can I do to relieve my father's pain?');

O *optimism*: being realistic yet optimistic about the problem-solving process ('I believe I can help my father with his pain').This also means communicating optimism towards the patient by showing understanding and hope and by involving the client as much as possible in the planning process;

P *planning*: defining reasonable care goals and thinking beforehand about the steps they will require ('Where can I go for help in dealing with my father's pain?');

E *expert information*: what should the informal carer know about the nature of the problem ('When can I ask for professional help, what can I do alone as an informal carer?'). Expert information also implies symptom assessment: accurate information on the characteristics and intensity of symptoms is essential in knowing when to call for professional help, but also in care planning.

13.10 Pitfall

• Teaching the client behaviour which is desired by the environment, without the client's proper consent.

13.11 Summary and questions

In this chapter we described the role of the social worker in making the grieving person more assertive, and constructively turning desires into behaviour. Lack of skills causes behavioural stress to arise, because the grieving person does not dare speak from his own desires.

First we described how grieving persons experience stress caused by lack of skills. In conclusion we described what the behavioural method has to offer in order to reduce behavioural stress in grieving persons and to enhance social strength.

Questions

1 Do you recognize examples of sub-assertive or aggressive behaviour in a situation of grief, either in yourself or in others?
2 Do you recognize that lack of skills leads to increased anxiety (reciprocal inhibition)?
3 Can you give an example of every level on which grieving persons may lack skills?
4 Which behavioural techniques do you think are useful in critical situations?
5 What are the behavioural method's results in reducing behavioural stress?

PART VI

Six systemic methods

Enhancing clients' supportive networks

Part VI deals with describing six methods that strengthen the client system to give the client situation optimal support. Reinforcing clients' social support system contributes towards optimally meeting clients' universal needs for safety, affection and self-determination. Support can be defined as 'support that is perceived as support by the client', realized in six support systems, among which are dyads (two-person relationships), family systems, support groups and the group of care professionals. Six specific social work methods are utilized to support clients most effectively.

- The social network method, for developing support in a broad social network (Chapter 14);
- The relationship-focused method, for developing support in a range of relationships – from partner relationships to relationships with neighbours (Chapter 15);
- The family method, for developing support in the core family and multi-generation support systems (Chapter 16);
- The group method, for developing support by and for fellow sufferers (Chapter 17);
- The case management method, for coordinating support for the care professionals involved (Chapter 18);
- The mediation method, for developing support in a range of relationships that have escalated to conflict situations (Chapter 19).

Positively perceived support contributes to clients' optimal enjoyment of life (optimal QoL). The six systemic interventions in social work aim at constructively affecting the support processes within the client system. The question is how to activate the supportive power of the client system to accomplish optimal fulfilment of clients' needs.

14

SOCIAL NETWORK METHOD

Questions

This chapter addresses the following questions:

- What is the significance of the social network approach?
- What is understood by one's social network and what is the function of the social network?
- What are the four support competencies that warrant client's demand for support?
- What is meant by stress buffer research and direct effect research?
- What is the social network method and what are the social network techniques?
- How does the social network contribute to meeting the actual needs for safety, affection and self-determination?

14.1 Introduction

> I'll get by with a little help from my friends.
>
> —John Lennon and Paul McCartney (1967)

Coping with life events is often perceived as a personal matter, whether it involves loss or trauma concerning a significant other, an animal, activity, object or country of origin. Still, from the PIE-ET perspective (see Chapter 2), the support factor is deemed important and not solely a personal issue. Contact with others is essential to learning how to deal with life events. As we learned from John Lennon and Paul McCartney, 'I'll get by with a little help from my friends.'

This chapter describes the social network method. Individuals' social network – social potential or social capital – can be used or activated to optimize persons' quality of life.

First, reasons are given for emphasizing the significance of the support approach in social work. Next, the difference is explained between the individual and social perspective on the quality of life (QoL). In addition, a definition is given of the term 'social network'. Next, the four support competencies are reviewed, including identifying signs, showing proximity, individually tailored support and support checks.

Furthermore, the support competencies are backed up by the research on stress buffering and direct support effects. Also, the supportive aspects of persons' social network are examined that help them cope with life events. These aspects include the size, diversity, density and availability of the social network. The next step is discussing the direct support that can be derived from the demand for support from a person's social network, which is a match between the supply and demand for support. What support can be given by neighbours, family and colleagues in times of crisis and is it really perceived as support by the receiver? In addition, the social network method is elaborated and what are the techniques involved? What is the outcome? The chapter is concluded by summing up the main points.

The case of Mr. Stack

Mr. Stack's PFC contained the following stress and empowering factors:
- (−)   great disappointment with your employer (blocking of promotion);
- (−)   tensions in the relationship with your partner (fear of divorce);
- (−)   stillbirth of your first son;
- (−)   your second son becoming disabled;
- (−)   anger with your general practitioner, lack of support (concerning incorrect dosage of sleep medication);
- (+)   support from a friend;
- (+)   support from a colleague.

In the course of eight counselling sessions Mr. Stack has learned to share the devastating impact of his losses and acknowledge the pointlessness of these life events in order to reach closure. For decades he has been struggling with the stress concerning the unexpected stillbirth of his first child and the disability of his second child. He couldn't even share his grief with his wife.

Occasionally he displayed a grim sense of humour. He found an escape in being bitter and became extremely critical of care professionals in order to fill the void and survive. Presently, Mr. Stack is no longer preoccupied with the question why all this has happened and is now getting a better grip on his own life. Despite these positive developments of stress reduction, the social worker finds that Mr. Stack is still keeping his thoughts to himself and has so far failed to share his feelings with anyone. Isn't it about time for him to share, starting with his wife, but also with his friends? After a few sessions together with the social worker and his wife, Mr. Stack is ready to brainstorm about the theme 'more sharing with others'.

From the social network analysis it emerges that Mr. Stack makes little use of his social network. He used to be friends with two of his colleagues, but lost contact with them when his situation became worse. The social worker utilizes the tree technique to work towards Mr. Stack having coffee together with his colleague. Looking at the roots of the tree reveals Mr. Stack's qualities. He appears to be very creative; he practices painting and model building, both at home and at work.

Next, the tree trunk is inspected. Are there any persons from his network that share his interests, are there opportunities for new contacts? After contacting the colleague with whom he shares an interest, the next step is to check the tree top: how to maintain contact with this colleague and how to develop this relation if the contact is enjoyable.

This approach works towards a stepwise strengthening of Mr. Stack's social network.

14.2 Focus on support enhancing quality of life

14.2.1 Why focus on the support factor?

At least four reasons can be given for focusing on the role of support for optimizing the quality of persons' lives.

The first reason is the simple fact that nobody lives on their own island. We seek each other in good times and bad times, because we are largely social animals. We are more than ourselves, both from a biological and psychological perspective. Every human being has a web of relationships, networks and dependencies.

> Everything, even individuality depends on relationships. My individuality is truly an illusion. I'm part of the bigger picture, from which I can never escape.
>
> *(D.H. Lawrence, quoted by van Ussel, 1975)*

The second reason for drawing attention to the role of support in persons' QoL is that no person is capable of coping with life events on their own. The 'social network' offers ingredients for support (Schrameijer, 1990). A third reason is that the support approach clearly reveals what the consequences of these life events are for persons' social support base. A number of life events, such as the loss of a partner, produce a double effect. Not only does the loss of a partner involve the painful experience of emotional loss, but it also entails abrupt loss of support from the loved one, and therefore we can speak of double life events.

A final reason for focusing on support is to prevent navel-gazing at a person's emotional state. From the support perspective, coping with life events becomes more than solely a personal issue. In cases of prolonged grief, the approach from the support perspective would be to examine the interrelationships of individuals and their social environment.

Instead of blaming the person concerned – you are responsible for remaining stuck in this situation – the support approach removes the blame from the person.

14.2.2 Individual versus support approach

The individual approach to a person's quality of life is also called the linear approach and focuses on the individual. The support approach to a person's quality of life is also referred to as the systemic approach and focuses on the dynamics within relationships and social systems. The linear approach examines persons' intentions underlying their behaviour after life events, the internal dynamics of a person. The systemic approach concentrates on how persons' behaviour affects other people and on the effects of the effects, the external dynamics. Central to the linear approach is what people communicate, whereas systemic thinking focuses on the interaction process.

For the linear thinking professional each separate event is essential. The systemic thinker focuses on detecting a pattern in a series of events. A linear thinking worker bases his approach on the cause-and-effect model and examines what is causing the problem. A system-oriented worker employs the circular effect model to understand the interpersonal dynamics in order to achieve stress reduction. The systemic thinking worker is not concerned with determining who is responsible or to blame for the situation. His aim is to find out how everyone is involved, whether those involved identify each other's signs and to establish any destructive or constructive circles of communication. The circular pattern arising from interactions in problematic relations is displayed in Figure 14.1.

14.2.3 Social network: definition

A person's social network is currently perceived as a whole of relationship patterns, which can be described as follows:

> the group of people with whom a person has maintained lasting relationships for the past two years to fulfil their basic human needs.

> *(Wellman, 1985)*

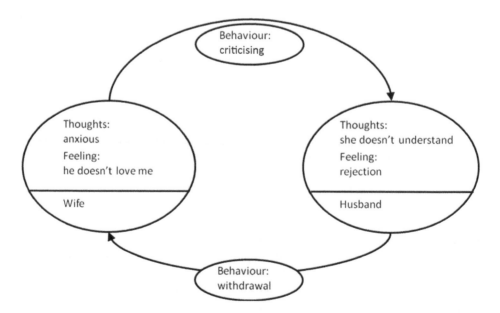

FIGURE 14.1 The circular pattern in a problematic relationship

Social support can be received from various sources, such as family, family, pets, friends and colleagues (Hogan et al., 2002, Taylor, 2011). A person's social network can be divided into two categories:

- A person's private situation: single or living together; living with partner, core family, larger family, friends and acquaintances and people from the same church.
- A person's situation outside the home, in what social organizations do they participate, such as school, work, neighbourhood, nursing home, facility for disabled persons, hospital, rehabilitation centre (Driedonks, 1993).

Professionals may find it useful to systematically map the people and services that provide support to clients. In every situation a set of circumstances determines what part of an individual's social network proves most supportive.

In the last few decades, the research tradition concerning support has seen a considerable increase due to conceptual confusion. The notion of 'support' has been defined in various ways: in some places it is considered an objective concept, in other places it is perceived as a subjective or an interactive phenomenon. Effective support to individuals experiencing life events can be defined as follows:

> Effective support from clients' social network is support that is perceived as supportive by the clients themselves.

This definition clearly points out that life event support is both a subjective and an interactive phenomenon. Although the clients themselves are key role players, there are exceptions in case of high-risk situations. Occasionally, a person's environment may be called to intervene, even if the client is opposed to such meddling and considers it harmful. Actions from others may be needed to break self-destructive patterns in increased risk situations. For instance, suicidal clients can be carefully approached to hand in their weapons or harmful objects. In cases of self-harm or alcohol abuse the clients' environment may feel the need to stop its self-destructive behaviour in spite of clients' initial resistance.

14.2.4 Why do social networks fail to offer effective support?

If the function of the social network is to buffer and channel, as the theories that will be discussed claim, what factors explain the failure of the social network to offer effective support? In other words, to what extent can social work problems be perceived as social network problems? When clients call for social work support, it reveals not only their inadequate problem-solving skills but also a failing supportive social network.

Four factors may explain the lack of adequate social network support. Each factor is then discussed in more detail.

1. Less support is provided.
2. The client doesn't ask for support or accept the support offered.
3. The professional safety net fails to identify and screen effectively.
4. The social network provides support that is ineffective.

Less support is provided

We pay a high price for the extreme individualization of our society. The crumbling of the three-generation structure, the disintegration of our neighbourhoods and the decreasing cohesion between people is increasingly resulting in persons being left to their own devices. This tendency can also be seen in large, anonymous schools. Families and neighbourhoods are providing less support because of the breakdown of three-generation families and the reduced sense of solidarity in neighbourhoods and among colleagues at work. Nowadays, the internet is more easily consulted than family or friends.

The client doesn't ask for support or accept the support offered

A determining factor in the extent of social network support is the person's threshold or (lack of) skills to ask for support or accept support. Can a client have adequate coping skills if they are unable to ask for the necessary support? People generally appeal to their family and friends for help before contacting social work. Freidson (1970) describes this phenomenon as the lay referral system, consulting lay persons. When support is indeed offered, it should be borne in mind that not all support is accepted as a matter of course. If individuals fail to take the initiative to ask for help or accept support when provided, social support will be withheld. It's essential for persons to appeal to their own social network at an early stage and maintain communication at all times.

The professional safety net fails to identify and screen effectively

When personal and work relations become more business-like, the social network's function to identify problems starts to decrease. Professional groups could take this task upon themselves to ensure timely referral to social work. Professional groups, such as doctors, nurses, physio-therapists, teachers, managers and human resource staff all come across people in problem situations. It may concern medical, nursing, physiotherapeutical, educational or work-related problems. These non-psychosocial professions could play a role in identifying and screening for personal, relational and structural problems. Due to the overall lack of professionals' formal task description concerning identifying social problems, only part of the professional group sees it as a duty to focus on social issues. On the basis of a formal task description a safety net for providing support can be developed, a stepped care system consisting of informal care (family and friends), gatekeeping (general practioners, nurses, teachers, etc.), psychosocial care (social workers) and specialist care (mental and physical health care professionals).

In the event of a life-changing situation, such as death of a loved one, the physician involved can assess whether clients are capable of coping on their own. Should they find themselves in a complex situation and need extra support, the professionals involved are in a position to identify clients' needs and refer them to the most accessible social worker. Social workers, for their part, screen clients for specialized care and may refer them to a psychologist, psychiatrist, pastor, budgeting consultant, legal advisor or another specialist. Practice shows that that a large number of clients are denied the support needed, as psychosocial care services have insufficient knowledge of each other's services and expertise.

The social network provides support that is ineffective

Even when the client's social network is providing support, the question remains whether this will prove really helpful. Theoretically speaking, people are generally well informed about how to provide adequate support. The problem is that they don't always put these ideas into practice. When outsiders are asked about ways of supporting someone who has lost their partner or child, their reactions are remarkably adequate. Only 11% of the respondents report actions that clients consider ineffective. There are reasons explaining why persons from the affected person's environment may not adequately respond to the need for support (Wortman & Lehman, 1985).

1   People from outside have many reasons for feeling negative about supporting persons in life-changing situations. The social-psychological literature on this issue reveals that people may feel threatened and exposed when confronted with others facing life-changing situations, consequently resulting in decreased effective support.
2   Very few people are experienced in dealing with others going through major life events. For this reason, a person can feel insecure about how to handle them and what to say. Realizing that the victim may become even more vulnerable if inappropriate support is given will only add to the support giver's fear.
3   Generally, persons from the social environment hold the wrong views on how individuals should cope with major life events. Beliefs about the extent of vulnerability that should be experienced and expressed as well as duration of the consequences of the life events, determine the nature of the support provided.

The questions now are: What are the characteristics of a supportive network? How can we measure if support is effective support?

14.3 Quality of support systems: four support competencies

14.3.1 Characteristics of a supportive environment

Client satisfaction is essential in measuring the support received. Research confirms that the support given isn't the key factor but rather the support perceived (Taylor, 2011).

Support can be only called support if so perceived by the receiver. Social support appears to make a valuable contribution to people's mental and physical health (see section 2.4.3).

Social support competencies

Four supportive qualities, known as social competencies, can be distinguished in providing effective support:

*   The first support competence: *cue recognition*;
*   The second support competence: *showing proximity*;
*   The third support competence: *individually tailored support*;
*   The fourth support competence: *support checks*.

These support competencies are based on a wide range of experiences with support systems, such as research on the quality of the parent–child relationship and the partner relationship. Let's explore our first support system, the parent–child relationship, to discern these four support competencies. When parents are consistent in their behaviour in meeting their baby's needs, it will develop a secure attachment bond with its parents. The baby gets fed and diapers changed when needed. What does the parent figure do when leaving the room for just a short while? When babies start crying because of this 'mini life event' (expressing distress cues), they are asking for their parents' presence: 'Stay with me'.

The question is whether parents respond to these cues in a supportive way:

- When parents identify the cues, they meet the criterion for the first support competence: 'I can hear you.'
- When parents offer proximity, they meet the criterion for the second support competence: 'Coming. . . .'
- When parents attend to the baby and fulfil baby's needs, they meet the criterion for the third support competence, a clean diaper, if needed, nutrition, if needed, or a loving presence.
- When parents check their baby's wellbeing, they meet the criterion for the fourth support competence: 'Does this specific support meet the specific needs of my child?'

The effect of these supportive actions is the gradual development of a loving, secure bond (attachment) with the first adults in the child's life. In all its helplessness, the secure bond allows the child to enjoy life. Babies feel safe and sheltered and develop a basic trust in their environment. Their self-confidence is also growing, considering the consistent responses to their inner cues: 'I'm worth responding to.' In the absence of these support competencies, babies will become anxiously attached and distrustful of relationships. This may be expressed by clinging behaviour – staying close to the attachment figure – or reckless behaviour – staying away as far as possible – and consequently overshooting their own fear. All these strategies are put in place to elicit the support that is needed. When persons experience significant life events, a similar kind of cue recognition is needed to provide support that promotes people's health and quality of life. The four support competencies can be seen as a circle of support, a support wheel whose combination of support competencies brings about effective support (see Figure 14.2).

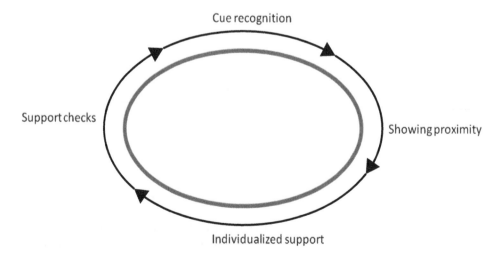

FIGURE 14.2 Support wheel for life events

These four support competencies are now further discussed as well as the findings from social science studies (also section 14.10.2). Chapters 14–19 discuss the supportive quality of the partner relationships, of family relationships of contacts with fellow suffers and with care professionals.

Chapters 20–23 look into the ways of strengthening macro support from formal provisions, such as the circle of friends, school, work, neighbourhood and care facilities.

14.3.2 Support competence 1: cue recognition in life events

A good listener needs only half the words.

Cue recognition is involved when a support provider assesses clients' cues. Clients may communicate signs that are actually a demand for indirect or direct support. In case of direct support the message can be clear: 'Help me, I can't cope on my own.' It's much more difficult to identify cues that communicate the need for indirect support.

Persons may change their behaviour in indirect ways to draw attention from other people. 'The talker' who suddenly falls silent or 'the quiet one' who, all of a sudden, starts talking incessantly. Another way of drawing attention is demonstrating 'difficult behaviour', for instance, by assuming a reproachful or negative attitude. It's rather a challenge to perceive this negative behaviour as a cry for help, considering that negative behaviour tends to create distance between individuals.

At times, the message for the supporting person may be hard to understand. Generally, it involves more than the message itself, rather how people define their relations. When someone needing support tells you: 'I'm facing this all by myself,' this is what this person is sharing with you. What they are really asking for – support, someone to talk to, active behaviour – can be indirectly inferred from what's been said, pitch of voice and gestures. This non-verbal message is also referred as the instructional, content and relationship aspect of communication.

If the direct demand for help is ignored, the support seeker will feel rejected. When support givers only meet the direct demand for support and fail to respond to the indirect demand, this may trigger feelings of rejection with those who seek help. The remarkable thing is, though, that indirect demands for attention are often discarded and disqualified as attention-seeking behaviour, which should be ignored altogether.

Fortunately, a number of professionals do respond positively to this demand for support. After all, support is also given to those experiencing major problems, without their explicit demand for help. Likewise, we tend to interfere with people with an unhealthy lifestyle, unhealthy living conditions or difficult behaviour, without being asked to do so.

The SUNA project

An example of adequate recognition of life event cues forms the successful project Suicide Aftercare (SUNA) in The Hague, focusing on supporting youth migrants following a failed suicide attempt. Instead of perceiving the failed attempt as a form of attention-seeking behaviour – which indeed occurred sometimes – the project seeks contact with these youths. Many of them are multiple problem children (abandoned by parents), who have good reasons for crying for help by seeing suicide as the only solution to their problems.

Denying the signs asking for support, which are directly or indirectly communicated, adds to the suffering: 'I'm communicating signs that I need support, which are not being acknowledged or identified.' Instead of ignoring, support givers are increasingly responding positively to the client's indirect demands. It involves having an emphatic ability to fully understand the client's whole problem situation and subsequently tuning the support to their needs.

14.3.3 Support competence 2: showing proximity

> In the most difficult times of my life so far, I have found some amazing new friends. I found them in the street where I live, during holidays and among ex-colleagues. These people did extraordinary things for me and my children, but most of all, they were there for me.
>
> (Kuiper, 2008)

A second important requirement for effective support, next to identifying cue behaviour, is 'showing proximity' – also called 'being present'. Showing proximity involves being watchful in seeking contact with clients. From the e-mail message containing the demand for support, support givers can infer how to respond appropriately, by either a reply message, phone call or personal visit.

Showing proximity does not necessarily involve physical presence, it can also be shown by a telephone call, WhatsApp, email and so forth. In other words, by giving personal attention, showing a warm heart.

> Vitamin A of attention. Attention is psychological oxygen and therefore a necessity of life. Every person contributes to another person's development or destruction.
>
> *(Laing, 1961)*

Attention

When individuals are experiencing life events, they deserve to receive attention from their environment. Should this attention be given, justice has been done. Individuals who feel they are not getting the attention they deserve may become bitter and consider the world unjust.

> Everyone knows what attention is. It is the taking possession by the mind in clear and vivid form, of one out of what seem several simultaneously possible objects or trains of thought . . . It implies withdrawal from some things in order to deal effectively with others, and is a condition which has a real opposite in the confused, dazed, scatter-brained state.
>
> *(James, 1920)*

When receiving attention, the opportunity is created to share one's life events. Persons are acknowledged in what there are going through and in the way they have been affected by the life-changing event. Acknowledgement is an affective basic need (see Chapters 8–10).

By acknowledging the suffering resulting from these life events, individuals experience a sense of justice. Ignoring is in fact denying what has happened. Denying causes people to feel that their humanity and sorrow have been denied. The absence of attention aggravates the emptiness that is experienced after life events. However painful rejection may be, it supposes limited acknowledgement of what has been rejected.

When rejection is expressed as 'I don't agree to the way you describe yourself,' the real message is, in fact, 'You don't exist.' The effects of being ignored can be devastating.

> In the worst case people's feelings are rendered worthless, their actions stripped of motives, intentions and consequences. Their situation becomes meaningless, leaving them totally bewildered and alienated.
>
> *(Laing, 1961)*

When the supply of words and gestures involving acknowledgement has reached a low level, the sustenance level, persons are more apt to accept negative attention than if the supply of attention is above the sustenance level. Humans need attention to exist, no matter how it is given. Presence is the care professionals' basic attitude in a helping relationship, which enables them to identify what support seekers need (Baart, 2001). Presence enables caregivers to provide caring support to their clients that is based on their mutual relationship. This relationship cannot be forged in a premeditated way. The caregiver tunes into what is important to the support seeker, their desires and fears. Presence forms the basis for caregivers' supportive relationship with their clients, which makes clients feel confident at key moments.

Affirmation

An acknowledging environment is a prerequisite for individuation, for becoming an individual and acquiring social skills. Affirmative reactions reinforce people's belief in their own ability to communicate, think, feel and perceive. In order to function in relationships with these inner strengths, persons need to experience received reinforcement from early childhood. The single most important factor in psychological development and stability is the affirmation of one person by the other. If the need for affirmation fails to be fulfilled or insufficiently fulfilled, this will result in lower self-esteem.

> Apart from purely exchanging information, it seems that human beings must communicate with others for the sake of their self-consciousness. This intuitive supposition is increasingly confirmed by experimental research into the deprivation of sensory impressions. It emerges that humans are unable to maintain their emotional stability over longer periods of time if they have no other persons to communicate with but themselves. In our opinion, this is the starting point for what existentialists call the encounter, and also for all other forms of a higher consciousness that form relationships with other individuals.
>
> *(Watzlawick et al., 1970)*

Affirming reactions mean accepting how persons describe themselves. Self-descriptions are seen as a series of how individuals describe themselves, which are formed, strengthened or broken down by interpersonal communication.

Definitions of self-worth are constantly present in communication. How persons communicate a message also reflects the way they think about themselves in relation to others. Affirming communication not only enhances people's self-esteem. An individual's sense of self-worth positively affects the communication during life events. If persons feel strong and confident before the life event, they will be able to cope with their lowered self-esteem. People experience limited distress when they feel convinced that they can cope with major life changes.

Rejection

Rejection results in a diminished sense of self-worth. Rejective communication makes the individual experiencing life events feel even more vulnerable than before. For instance, a woman is asking for attention because she can't comprehend that her mother is no longer alive. Her husband reacts by telling her that 'Yes, I'm afraid she has really passed away. You can sit there and keep crying but it won't do you any good. It isn't going to bring her back.' What his wife is actually trying to communicate is 'help me understand what has happened.' Her husband rejects her appeal for help and disqualifies her self-description ('I need help') by ridiculing it. What she is communicating is not accepted as valid expressions of her perceptions, thoughts and emotions. It is ineffective to remain at a distance in spite of identifying the cues. A WhatsApp message conveying the need for proximity asks for a phone call or a personal visit, rather than a reply WhatsApp message. *You Can Always Call Me* is the telling title of the book in which Kuiper (2008) criticizes caregivers' standoffish attitude:

> Don't always expect clients themselves to ask for care and support. Being a caregiver involves being present for the other person and assessing what is needed. A standoffish support only adds more to the suffering: 'You weren't there when I needed you most.'

14.3.4 Support competence 3: individually tailored support

> A friend in need is a friend indeed.

The third support competence is the individually tailored support. This means that the support given is tailored to the client's needs. For instance, practical problems ask for practical assistance and emotional distress calls for emotional support. There may be a need for a person to prepare meals or someone offering a shoulder to cry on.

Meeting clients' needs calls for a flexible attitude of the supportive social network.

Providing care from a supply-driven perspective and not focusing on clients' needs results in ineffective support. These caregivers tend to use platitudes, well-meant but ineffective words of advice, such as 'Keep your chin up, things will get better.' Person-to-person help differs from helping according to protocol. Support based on clichés tends to cause even more suffering. Encouragement may sometimes cause discouragement. This may occur when platitudes are expressed to comfort a person, such as, 'God gives, God takes,' 'The deceased is with the Lord,' 'Life events are opportunities that must be seized' and 'You have to learn to discover the positive sides of a life-changing situation'. These phrases offer false hope and do little to support individuals in times of crisis.

14.3.5 Support competence 4: support checks

Watchful waiting.

The fourth support competence is checking at regular intervals whether the support given is still tailored to the support seeker's needs. Checking is asking questions such as 'Is the support I'm giving doing enough for you or do you need something else?' This is referred to as 'watchful waiting'. When support givers focus on emotions and fail to address urgent practical problems, the support needs readjustment. Regular assessment of the client's needs is necessary. Caregivers that strictly adhere to their own care supply risk failing to identify clients' needs. This inflexible support undoubtedly leads to adding to the client's suffering.

Effective support

What forms of support are effective and not? From a study on the effectiveness of support in the loss of a partner or child (Lehman et al., 1986), it emerges that

- The majority of clients are satisfied with the support provided and are able to describe how they have been most effectively supported.
- The majority of clients can distinguish what forms of support have proved ineffective.
- There appears to be a discrepancy between how people from social networks think about giving support and how the support is actually provided.

Over 70% of the clients from the sample report having received effective support from members of their social network – support that is perceived as support. The majority of clients are able to pinpoint the most effective supportive behaviours. Effective strategies of support include 'contact with fellow-sufferers' and 'being given the opportunity to express one's thoughts and feelings'. Additionally, two more effective behaviours are considered 'being present' and 'voicing one's concerns'. Ineffective support involves 'giving advice' and 'encouraging recovery'. Furthermore, 'inappropriate remarks or behaviour' and 'trivializing' are regarded as ineffective forms of support.

Ineffective support

There are reasons why persons from an individual's environment are not able to respond adequately to a life-changing event.

(Wortman et al, 1985, p. 464)

Outsiders have many reasons for having negative feelings about supporting persons in life-changing situations. The social-psychological literature on this issue reveals that people may feel threatened and exposed when confronted with others facing life-changing situations, consequently resulting in decreased effective support.

Very few people are experienced in dealing with others going through major life events. For this reason, a person can feel insecure about how to handle and what to say. Realizing that the victim may become even more vulnerable if inappropriate support is given only adds to the support giver's fear. By and large, persons from the social environment hold the wrong views on how individuals should cope with major life events. Suppositions about the extent of vulnerability that should be experienced and expressed, as well as the duration of consequences of the life events, determine the nature of the support provided.

As a rule, people are quite knowledgeable on the subject of adequate support. The problem starts when they come to the point of putting their ideas into practice. Outsiders, who are asked how they would support a person after losing their partner or child, respond quite adequately. Theoretically speaking, they know exactly how to behave. Only 11% report saying or doing things that clients consider ineffective.

14.4 Cue recognition and proximity: the stress buffering theory

The first two competencies – cue recognition and proximity – are confirmed by studies on the stress-buffering effects of social networks. The presence of the social networks produces beneficial effects on persons' psychological and physical health – the presence of other human beings that can be counted on reduces stress levels. The social network functions as a safety net, offering strength, tranquillity and safety, without having to be actually used. These beneficial effects to people's health are based on three cohesion functions of an individual's social network.

- *Function of valuation.* Valuation and acknowledgement are derived from an individual's social network, considering that people are there in times of need.
- *Function of inclusion.* A person's network offers a sense of belonging, for instance, by sharing the same interests.
- *Function of social security.* An individual's network offers security through agreements and arrangements, among which are labour agreements, organizations and churches.

The indirect positive health effects due to the presence of one's social network are based on the fact that a sense of security in itself produces a stress-reducing effect (Krahn, 1993). Being connected with others involves relying on their presence and help, knowing that friends are there for them. The stronger the social network, the more clearly the cues (support competence 1) become identified ('they know me') and the greater the presence (support competence 2) is. Being connected makes persons feel supported by others from their environment; they feel calm and assured that support can be counted on. The supporters of the stress buffer theory argue that individuals undergo limited stress (can be controlled) by feeling secured by their environment. 'My network is there to help me when I need it'.

Rosetto, Pennsylvania

The town of Rosetto is a remarkable example of the protective presence of partners in life, fellow men, family, neighbours and a local community. Its residents were Italian Americans, who, to a large extent, had preserved the traditional Italian lifestyle.

The majority of the residents suffered from obesity because of the high percentage of fat content of their diet. Still, the death rate resulting from coronary heart diseases remained at the minimum, especially compared to other surrounding communities. Researchers investigated the characteristics of the community (Wolf, 1971). Rosetto was a patriarchal society with close social ties and relationships, involving a great deal of mutual social trust and a strong emphasis on social cohesion and tradition. In the course of time, the cultural lifestyle in Rosetto was undergoing changes towards 'the normal American lifestyle', under the influence of the media and education. Gradually, the frequency of coronary heart disease started to increase. Researchers found that this development could only be explained by the stress buffering hypothesis, the protective power of the social network. Although the power of the clan appeared strong, abandoning the three-generation structure and the increasingly individualized lifestyle had led to a weakened safety net. As a result, residents felt less supported by their traditional social network.

The stress buffering theory or social cohesion theory points out that a close social network is important for individuals' health. Social cohesion, though, can be subject to change at any given moment following a life event. In the course of time, it tends to decrease and supportive reactions fluctuate according to a certain time frame (Pennebaker, 1994). In the first couple of weeks after the life event everyone talks openly about what has happened. Social obstacles no longer exist and people get into spontaneous conversations with each other. In the 4–8 weeks that follow, the life event is no longer a topic for conversation. It's still on people's minds and they are still willing to talk about the subject but they have started to get tired of listening to these stories. Then, life goes on as usual.

Individuals who are divorced or have lost a family member, go through a similar cycle. In the first three weeks friends and family are generally very kind and understanding. There is plenty of time to talk about the life events. However, after three weeks everyone seems to have had enough of it. Friends start to avoid the bereaved person or suggest that the time has come to move on. Irritations are now likely to surface. Talking about a traumatic event for a period of three weeks is not enough per persons to really process a life changing event. Therefore, practically every culture has its topics that are preferably avoided.

(Pennebaker, 1994)

The social cohesion of a social network is enhanced by four qualities of social networks, including size, diversity, density and availability (Baars & Hosman, 1990).

14.4.1 The size of social networks

In coping with life events the size of an individual's network is of great importance. How many persons are there to rely on? It is supposed that the supporting presence of family, neighbours, friends and religious and social groups protects persons from the stressful effects associated with life events. Social networks offer families social and instrumental support, access to others and availability of information. The smaller a person's social network, the less favourable the prognosis is of successful coping behaviour when facing life events. For instance, a 39-year-single male from a farming community, living with his parents without any close friends at all, is more vulnerable after job loss, compared to a contemporary who lives independently, with family relations, contacts with colleagues and a circle of friends of his own. Individuals are at considerable risk of developing a grief disorder in our Western society, which is based on a small circle of intimates and large-scale mobility (Hobfall, 1985).

The size of a person's social network is subject to change throughout their life cycle. Some losses count as double losses, for instance, when losing a loved one who provided the most support. An individual's social network becomes more vulnerable when significant life events occur, such as death, divorce, migration and discharge. Expanding one's social network involves establishing new contacts. Another option is to deepen existing social relationships. An individual's social network produces a buffering effect on their QoL and its size is important.

14.4.2 The diversity of social networks

A diverse social network appears to be an important factor in providing optimal support (Flap & Tazelaar, 1988). Diversity can here be defined as variation in age, gender, marital status and educational training. There has been very limited research on the diversity in social networks. What we do know is that it is important for individuals to assume different roles when experiencing stressful life events. More and more varied roles offer individuals a more diverse social network. Assuming multiple roles has also a buffering effect in the loss of a loved one. Persons find it easier to adapt when they are able to fall back on the roles that need fulfilling. Researchers from various disciplines have pointed out the relationship between being active and engaged and life satisfaction. They demonstrated that common activities or activities in the presence of others have a positive effect on people's self-image.

Kinds of activities

People's activities can be classified into three groups:

- Informal activities: social interactions with family members, friends and neighbours;
- Formal activities: social participation in formal voluntary organization (associations, churches and other organizations);
- Solitary activities: watching television, reading, and hobbies of an individual nature.

The first two forms of activities mentioned here appear to contribute significantly to individuals' personal wellbeing. People's cultural background and personality traits are important factors in determining whether they are able to successfully adopt a more withdrawn lifestyle. A higher level of activities promotes elderly persons' life satisfaction. When elderly persons engage in social activities, their needs can be identified at an early stage. Not showing up for their activities may be a sign that something is wrong with them and that they need help. Elderly people living in social isolation lack the ability to communicate such behavioural cues. The next contributing factor to stress buffering in persons' QoL is the density of social networks.

14.4.3 The density of social networks

Close-knit social networks prevent people from being left to their own devices after life events. Regular contacts are maintained, customs and rituals of the community help channel the afflicted person's life event crisis. In situations where frequent contacts and rituals are lacking, there is no external support to channel people's sorrow. In case of death, close-knit social communities perform more rituals involving all members, compared to less close social networks (Rubin, 1990). Burial rituals in the Israeli kibbutz community extend far beyond the core family and encompass a wide range of social relationships. In modern American society mourning customs are limited to the core family.

Modern society

The breakdown of social networks in Western society involves risks. Western individuals can rely on only a small circle of persons and if things go wrong, support seekers are left to deal with their sorrow by themselves. Moreover, the remaining intimates will feel pressured to provide the support needed. Modern marriage is seemingly an open relationship, but is, in fact, more closed than it used to be. As a result, people may be left feeling very lonely (van den Eerenbeemt, 1993).

Families used to be larger and their interpersonal connections much stronger, allowing more mutual support. In modern society, husband and wife forge a relationship in which everything is to be resolved by the two of them. They are each other's partner, friend and lover. In modern family life, much depends on the given quality of the family relationships. Family cohesion – the extent to which family members connect with each other – plays an important supportive role when a member falls ill. The emotional ties between family members and the way they perceive their individual autonomy are key factors to assess the reactions of clients and their families to illness. Therefore, density is considered a third important factor in the buffering effect to one's quality of life.

14.4.4 The availability of social networks

> Nobody is rich enough to cope with their neighbours.
>
> (Danish saying)

A good neighbour is better than a brother far away. Modern societies no longer see family members living close to each other. Individuals therefore must depend on other relations in their environment for assistance. Their availability positively affects clients' health. Still, intimacy at a distance should not be underestimated. In the digital age the concept of 'distance' is viewed in a different light, considering the way distances can now easily be bridged by fast communication.

14.5 Individually tailored support and support checks: the direct effect theory

The effect of the third competence – individually tailored support – has been confirmed by studies on the direct effects of social support. Social networks have been proven to produce a positive effect on people's health, if the specific assistance matches clients' specific needs. From another study (Silver and Wortman, 1980), it emerges that individual-tailored support indeed positively influences persons' coping behaviour after significant life events. In addition, a longitudinal study on employees' reactions to business closure concluded that social support by partners, family members and friends contributed to reducing the level of suffering due to life-changing events.

In theory, it seems obvious that the support offered and need for support should match. How can a person be helped with something they haven't asked for? Chapter 2 pointed to a number of pitfalls concerning support providing behaviour, resulting in secondary victimization. Practice shows that there is often a mismatch or insufficient matching between the supply of and demand for support. For this reason, persons' individual needs are described on the basis of the PIE-Empowerment Theory (Chapter 2). They include survival needs, affective needs and cognitive needs, together with the methods employed by social workers to meet these needs. The survival method is suited to survival needs, the affective method is tailored to an affective need and cognitive needs call for the cognitive method. A similar train of thought can, in fact, be applied to the support given by persons' environment. Survival support goes with survival needs, affective support belongs with affective needs and cognitive support responds to cognitive needs. Every specific need and corresponding supportive action from persons' social environment is described in the next section, along with concrete illustrations, based on the work by Kuiper (2008).

14.5.1 Social support meeting survival needs

What kind of survival needs do clients have? Experiencing significant life events may cause a shortage of food, sleep, rest, safety and security (see Table 14.1). People feel the need to share their story on account of feeling threatened, unsafe and insecure or feeling unable to develop any physical activity.

TABLE 14.1 Social support meeting survival needs

Specific needs	Specific supportive action from persons' environment	Illustration
Physical need, focus on physical complaints and stress signs	Helping to acknowledge bodily symptoms and taking care of them	An activity together, for instance, cycling, dancing, preparing a monthly extra healthy meal that can be deep-frozen.
Practical-material need, providing bed, bread, bath	Helping with practical-material resources	Making arrangements: 'Would you like me to do the cooking or help you with gardening?' Offering checks that the giver can cash.
Need for trauma support, attention to coping with nightmares, reliving traumatic events	Helping normalize reactions to traumatic experiences	'This was an exceptional experience.' 'You responded in a normal way to an abnormal event.'

14.5.2 Social support meeting affective needs

Clients' affective needs have been discussed in Chapters 8–10. Experiencing stressful life events may leave clients feeling unloved and without a sense of belonging (see Table 14.2). They have the need to tell their affective story, their emotional story. 'I miss feeling close to someone, I need love and acknowledgement.' 'With whom can I share my experience?' 'I can't get my story told.'

14.5.3 Social support meeting self-determination needs

Clients' cognitive needs have been dealt with in Chapters 11–13. Due to life events clients may develop a need for more clarity, insight and sense of purpose (see Table 14.3).

TABLE 14.2 Social support meeting affective needs

Specific need	Specific supportive action from environment	Illustrations
Emotional need, focus on sorrow/anger/happiness: feeling client's emotional need	Helping release the pain, no bottling up, no 'talking about feelings' all the time	Don't try to stop crying or an outburst of anger. Listen and acknowledge, offer a shoulder to cry on.
Need for expression, attention to creativity, writing, drawing, music	Helping with creative expression	Give a CD with their favourite music, share hobbies and creativity. 'Would it help to express your thoughts and feelings in a poem?'
Need to say goodbye, attention to a respectful goodbye	Helping prepare and perform the ritual	'How would you like to say goodbye?' 'Can I help you compose the speech?'

TABLE 14.3 Social support meeting needs self-determination-needs

Specific needs	Specific supportive actions from environment	Illustrations
Cognitive needs, focus on information, realistic thinking, decision making, making plans, fully taking in the impact of the life event	Helping with fact finding, reality testing, decision making	Information: 'Take your time. It will take a while before it really sinks in.' Grieving is not a wound you can stop bleeding by applying a bandage.
Existential need, focus on dealing with existential questions. 'Why, where is this going, how can I mend my CORE?'	Listening, being acknowledging and present, person-centred attention	Attention. 'Tell me your story, what has happened?', I'm here for you: making a phone call, visit, sending a postcard, text message. 'What will your life look like 10 years from now?'
Behavioural needs, focus on communication and contact with others	Helping practicing social communicative skills	Making compliments. 'Do you know what a fine person you are?' Calling to arrange an activity together. 'Let's go shopping or see a movie.'

14.6 History of the social network method

Little can be written about the social network method from a historical perspective considering that it hasn't been known for that long. Over the last few decades we have seen an increasing need for strengthening individuals' social networks. Governments are more and more discussing the desirability to strengthen persons' social networks, for instance by means of the social network method.

The Industrial Revolution contributed towards opening up the boundaries of families (van der Hart, 1987). For instance, a son with his wife and children left their home village and moved to town because of expected job opportunities and better living conditions. Family life began to crumble and families were becoming part of persons' social network instead of being the whole social network. Social life became segmented and the family was no longer the core of individuals' social network (see the ecomap technique in section 14.10.1 and Figure 14.3). The solidarity of dense social networks is only available to families in segmented networks.

14.6.1 Social network analysis

Herman Baars et al. (1995) made an important contribution to devising the social network method. The social network analysis – developed by Baars – provides information on persons' networks. This analysis reveals the extent of individuals' social integration or isolation. After establishing the degree of clients' social isolation, social workers can focus on their social integration. The social network analysis is utilized to uncover the areas that clients need to improve.

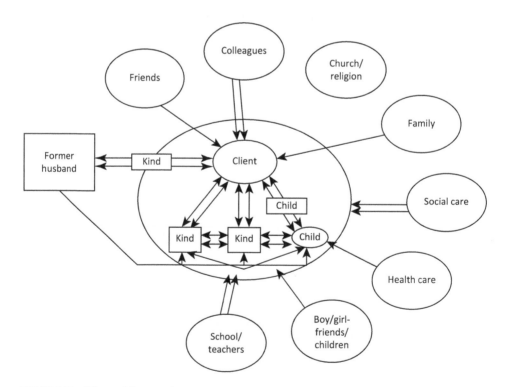

FIGURE 14.3 The social network

14.6.2 Tree technique from refugee work

Another technique has been employed in the work with refugees, known as the tree technique. Refugees are assisted in building social relations according to the tree technique (see section 14.10.3). Due to circumstances, they often live in a social vacuum or have a limited social network and therefore wish to expand their social network in the Netherlands (Logger & Martens, 2000). Although the model is mainly used for educational purposes for groups of refugees, its application in other areas of care delivery seems justified.

14.7 Goals

General goal

•   Strengthening clients' social networks.

Specific goals

•   Activating the 'sleeping' potential of clients' social network;
•   Activating clients' existing social network;
•   Enhancing clients' mutually supportive relationships with friends, colleagues, neighbours and other contacts.

14.8 Indications

•   Clients report being lonely.
•   Clients are living in social isolation.
•   Clients report having poor relationships in their social network.

14.9 Contraindications

•   Clients don't wish to activate their social network.
•   Clients that are unattractive for social contacts, for instance when producing unpleasant body odours or using strong language.

14.10 Techniques

1   Ecomap technique
2   Checklist of social support competencies
3   Tree technique
4   Network conference technique
5   Social media technique.

14.10.1 Ecomap technique

To strengthen social networks, clients' existing networks are first visualized with the use of ecomaps. This is also referred to as the social network map.

The social network map is used to establish dialogue regarding individuals' needs and sources of support, and then how the support system can meet those needs (Lewis et al., 2000).

An ecomap is a visual display of an individual's social network (see Figure 14.3). In addition, the characteristics of the individual's social network are discussed (Baars et al., 1995) as well as the size (total number of persons with whom the clients have direct, more or less lasting relationships). Attention is also paid to the social network's diversity (how homogenous or heterogeneous is the individual's social network, regarding age, gender, marital status, level of education, work situation and lifestyle), density (are the channels of communication open or not – duration of the relationship, frequency of contacts and who initiates the contacts and also the availability of the social network and the accessibility of these contacts are (see section 14.10.2).

14.10.2 Checklist of social support competencies

The social worker, client(s) and caregivers can go through the checklist together. The client validates the quality of the support provided. Additionally, social worker and client together establish which support competencies need to be improved.

Support competencies		Social support	Ineffective support
1	Cue recognition	Are behavioural cues correctly identified? 'Give attention to what I am directly or indirectly asking for.'	Insensitivity to cues by ignoring or rejecting client's need for proximity. 'Client hasn't asked for support and it is therefore not given.' Failure to recognize direct or indirect demand for support.
2	Showing proximity	Is support giver attentive and involved when contacting client? 'I need warm interest, presence.'	'I'm keeping my distance'; responding to a WhatsApp asking for emotional presence by 'You can always call me'; clichés offering nothing.
3	Individually tailored support	Does client contact involve establishing their specific needs for support? Flexible matching of supply and demand.	Supply-driven support (clichés?): Keeps supporting from their own perspective ('Chin up, things are going to work out'); offering practical support in response to emotional needs and vice versa.
4	Support checks	Regularly checking whether this support is still adequate or other support is needed. Measuring effectiveness of support.	Not following up how support is perceived. Inflexible attitude in providing support; only practical problems are addressed, emotional issues remain unresolved.

14.10.3 Tree technique

The tree technique (Logger & Martens, 2000; Figure 14.4) consists of working on expanding individuals' networks according to a systematic design of the roots, the trunk and the top of the metaphorical tree. The tree technique comprises three chronological phases.

1   *Root phase (origin, source).* In this phase the focus is on clients' autobiography. Who are they, what are their abilities, what are the good things when looking back on their lives?
2   *Trunk phase (growth, change).* This is the phase for developing a network plan. What contacts are suited to clients' wishes, how to find the persons and information needed? How will clients make these contacts, in what order and at what point in time will they start doing what?
3   *Top phase (blossoming).* This is the phase of working on consolidating contacts. How to establish contact and how are these contacts maintained?

14.10.4 Network conference technique

A Network Conference (NC), also known as Family Network Conference, for instance, Family Group Decision Making, Community Based Conference or Community Support, is a meeting with clients' family, friends and significant others, who wish to give support and help find solutions to improve clients' lives. This type of professionally led family group meeting differs from Family Group Conferencing (FGC), which is coordinated and led by volunteers of the FGC. Family network conferencing involves a wide range of client groups, including persons with psychological or psychiatric problems, somatic conditions (chronically ill) or social problems (isolation, small social network).

During the conference the client's social network members make a plan for the future. All the persons involved are responsible for this plan, in which agreements with family members and friends are formulated about how support can best be provided. The starting point is that clients and their significant others are capable of finding the most successful solutions.

For whom?

Social workers may coordinate family network conferences, not only for parents, children and youths, but also for adults and elderly persons assisted by social workers. A client may need support from their environment for parenting problems or help with leisure activities or transportation problems or help to prevent further problems. Youths, adults or elderly persons may call for a family network conference themselves to resolve problems together with their social network.

What does it involve?

The family network conference involves three steps.

Preparation

The coordinator of the family network conference is either a social worker or a person from the social network itself. They help with the preparation and support the client at the

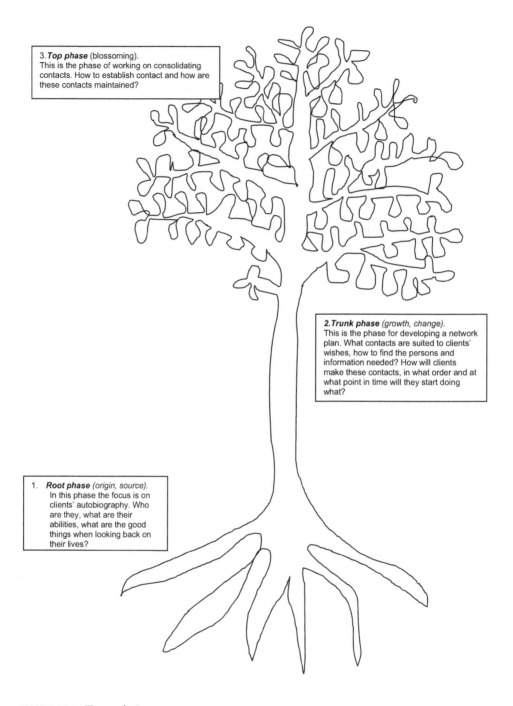

3. **Top phase** (blossoming).
This is the phase of working on consolidating contacts. How to establish contact and how are these contacts maintained?

2. **Trunk phase** *(growth, change)*.
This is the phase for developing a network plan. What contacts are suited to clients' wishes, how to find the persons and information needed? How will clients make these contacts, in what order and at what point in time will they start doing what?

1. **Root phase** *(origin, source)*.
    In this phase the focus is on clients' autobiography. Who are they, what are their abilities, what are the good things when looking back on their lives?

FIGURE 14.4   Tree technique

conference. The client composes a list of important others, including grandparents, friends, neighbours, teachers or care professionals. Then you discuss the demand for support for which a plan is needed. The next step is for the client to determine who will be invited and the date for the conference.

The family network conference

The coordinator welcomes everyone to the conference and explains the purpose of the meeting. Next, all present are given the opportunity to explain what they hope to achieve at the conference and how they can contribute to the support plan. Sometimes, it concerns specific problems. Care professionals can be asked to give more information and explain how to deal with a problem. If a family guardian is involved with the family of the client, they will explain the minimal rules and requirements for the plan. Then, all care professionals leave the room, so that everyone is able to talk freely and work on their own plan. During these private moments the coordinator remains in a separate room nearby, enabling you to ask for assistance when needed. The family network group formulates the plan and presents it to the care professionals.

Implementation team

A support plan is now ready to be implemented. Care professionals and the family network group agree on who is to keep a watch on things to ensure that everything goes according to plan. A small group from your family network forms a 'family team'. This implementation team convenes at regular intervals, about once every 6 weeks, to review what has been done and to make further arrangements. In case of long-term guidance, experience with family network conferencing shows that it may be important for social workers, acting as case managers, to monitor the implementation of the support plan.

14.10.5 Social media technique

Social media may be a source of support for clients. There is increasing recognition and acknowledgement of the power of social media in times of loss and trauma (Westerink, 2014). The digital communities of Facebook, YouTube and other media are instantly accessible for asking questions, providing information and contact. Posting a question or sharing one's story can be very supportive.

Face-to-face online counsellors support clients by responding to email messages and making arrangements about specific bereavement assignments. For instance, after some searches, a client with a murdered twin eventually found the website Twinlesstwins. Surviving relatives of air crash disasters can access secure websites to share their experiences with fellow sufferers. All internet sources that help raise individuals' awareness, help saying goodbye to a loved one, and help people rebuild their lives, form valuable contributions. Reflections on previous sessions can also be communicated online. An illustration of the scope of the internet concerning bereavement is available at the website 'Remember Me When I Am Gone' (http://www.remembermewheniamgone.org). This website includes a personal memory book that has been translated into 95 languages, designed for parents with limited life expectancy. Parents and children can use this online memory book to share their memories together, which may be difficult if not impossible for survivors to trace after their death. There are also online counselling services without face-to-face contact between professional and client, such as Interapy and 113online. Naturally, grief counsellors and clients should be aware of the risks of internet use.

14.11 Social work results

- Clients feel supported.
- Clients feel less lonely.
- Clients have improved relationships with friends, colleagues and others.

14.12 Evidence

Effective forms of support are contacts with fellow sufferers offering the opportunity for expressing feelings and thoughts. Other ways of effective support include being present and showing concern. Ineffective support forms include giving advice and encouraging persons to recover. The use of strong language, bad behaviour and downplaying client's problems are also considered ineffective ways of supporting.

Social support can have great influence on health, wellbeing, and general quality of life. To promote awareness of the social network that surrounds each transplant recipient, transplant social workers are now using the social network map as an intervention (Lewis, 1993). Because perceptions of availability and accessibility of support are key elements in the use of social network resources, awakening an individual's awareness of available resources is a significant first step in enhancing social support and, ultimately, quality of life. The social network map is used to establish dialogue regarding individuals' needs and sources of support, and then how the support system can meet those needs. Transplant social workers thus foster active use of those people in transplant recipients' networks who can meet the particular needs recipients identify.

Barman-Adhikari and Rice's (2014) findings suggest that social capital is more significant in understanding why homeless youth use employment services, relative to network structure and network influence. In particular, bonding and bridging social capital were found to have differential effects on use of employment services among this population. The results from this study provide specific directions for interventions aimed to increase use of employment services among homeless youth.

Family group conferences are usually organized in youth care settings, especially in cases of (sexual) abuse of children and domestic violence. Studies on the application of family group conferences in mental health practices are scarce, let alone in a setting even more specific, such as public mental health care. One study (de Jong & Schout, 2011) reports on an exploratory study on the applicability of family group conferencing in public mental health care. Findings suggest that there are six reasons to start family group conference pilots in public mental health care. First, care providers who work in public mental health care often need to deal with clients who are not motivated in seeking help. Family group conferences could yield support or provide a plan, even without the presence of the client. Second, conferences might complement the repertoire of treatment options between voluntary help and coercive treatment. Third, clients in public mental health care often have a limited network. Conferences promote involvement, as they expand and restore relationships and generate support. Fourth, conferences could succeed both in a crisis and in other non-critical situations. Sometimes pressure is needed for clients to accept help from their network (such as in the case of an imminent eviction), while in other situations, it is required that clients are stabilized before a conference can be organized (such as in the case of a psychotic episode). Fifth, clients who have negative experiences with care agencies and their representatives might be inclined to accept a conference because these agencies act in another (modest) role. Finally, the social network could elevate the work of professionals.

Between 1995 and 1997, the Swedish Association of Local Authorities implemented Family Group Conferences (FGC) in 10 local authorities throughout Sweden. The study of Sundell and Vinnerljung (2004) reports on client outcomes of this implementation. Ninety-seven children involved in 66 FGCs between November 1996 and October 1997 were compared with 142 children from a random sample of 104 traditional child protection investigations by the Child Protective Services (CPS). All children were followed for exactly 3 years for future child maltreatment events reported to CPS. The results suggest that the impact of the FGC was scant, accounting for 0%–7% of the statistical variance of outcome variables. Conclusion of the researchers were that the findings did not support the alleged effectiveness of the FGC model compared to traditional investigations in preventing future maltreatment cases. If these results are confirmed in future research, they serve as a reminder of the necessity to evaluate models based on untested theories or on extrapolations from other countries/cultures before these models are widely spread in a national practice context.

The trend of using social media in social work is increasing, but research which systematically reviews and evaluates their uses in actual practice is limited. Chan (2015) reviewed the social work literature to identify the uses, benefits, and limitations of social media in social work practice, and identifies current gaps in the literature to provide recommendations for future social work research. Articles in 64 social work journals published between 2000 and 2014 were screened and analyzed. The included articles ($n = 20$) were analyzed with particular reference to their level of evidence and ways of social media use. The methodological quality of the studies in this review was low, and this was consistent with the findings of recent systematic reviews of social media use in medical health care. The findings initially suggested that social media can potentially contribute to various social work processes, including: service user engagement, need assessment, intervention, and programme evaluation.

People with severe mental health problems such as psychosis have access to less social capital, defined as resources within social networks, than members of the general population. However, a lack of theoretically and empirically informed models hampers the development of social interventions which seek to enhance an individual's social networks. A paper by Webber et al. (2015) reports the findings of a qualitative study, which used ethnographic field methods in six sites in England to investigate how workers helped people recovering from psychosis to enhance their social networks. Findings are presented in four overarching themes – worker skills, attitudes and roles; connecting people processes; role of the agency; and barriers to network development. The sub-themes which were identified included worker attitudes; person-centred approach; equality of worker-individual relationship; goal setting; creating new networks and relationships; engagement through activities; practical support; existing relationships; the individual taking responsibility; identifying and overcoming barriers; and moving on. Themes were consistent with recovery models used within mental health services and will provide the basis for the development of an intervention model to enhance individuals' access to social capital within networks.

14.13 Pitfalls

- Too much emphasis on the quantity instead of quality of social work;
- Not taking sufficient account of other individual, systemic or positional indications, such as conflicts, lack of social skills and social cohesion in the neighbourhood.

14.14 Summary and questions

Individuals experiencing the loss of a loved one have to move on with their lives. Support from other people is essential to coping with this loss. After describing the elements of the social network – family, friends, neighbourhood, school and social services – the current chapter discusses the functions of the social network. The social network has the function of providing affection, connection and social security. Family, friends and social services fulfil their specific functions in providing social support.

First, it is explained why the focus on the support approach is essential to grief counselling. Then, the difference is explained between the social work perspective and the individual perspective on social work. Next, a definition is given of the concept of 'social network'. The four support competencies of the circle of support are then discussed, including cue recognition, showing proximity, individually tailored support and support checks. In addition, studies are described that have demonstrated the effect of social support on individuals' psychological and physical health.

The phenomenon of social cohesion of one's social network in dealing with loss is then discussed in more detail. Important factors include the size, diversity, density and availability of social networks. The question is then addressed of what kind of individually tailored support can be derived from an individual's social network, the match between support supply and demand.

In conclusion, the social network is explained more closely. What does it involve? What are the techniques employed? What is the outcome? The quality of one's social network is vital to the quality of life. Individuals' social networks are not strengthened if social workers concentrate only on the impact of the life event and clients' coping skills. When a client's social network proves too weak to provide the support needed, external individual help can be given on a temporary basis. It is therefore important for social workers to focus on strengthening the client's social network, by offering clients social skills practice to establish and maintain social contacts, and consequently activate and expand their social network.

Questions

1   Analyze a case study or your own situation for establishing the four support competencies of the support wheel.
2   Take a case study or your own situation as the starting point for filling out the following checklist.

TABLE 14.4 Social support checklist: what kind of support do I need from you to optimally fulfil my needs?

Human needs	Specific needs	I need your support with . . .?
Safety needs	*Physical safety* Need for oxygen, water, sleep, physical rest, warmth, food, physical movement, sex. *Materialistic safety* Need for housing, bed, bread, bath, work, money, practical problem solving. *Psychic safety* Need for psychological rest after terrifying, traumatic sensory experience.	
Affective needs	*Emotional support* Need for respect, trust, affection, care, love, inclusion, being respected, seen, heard. *Expressive support* Need for creative, musical, art, digital and drama activities for expressing inner experiences that are difficult to put into words. *Ritual support* Need for closure of unfinished experiences by a worthy say-goodbye ritual.	
Self-determination needs	*Cognitive support* Need for understanding, realistic information, overview, effective problem solving, learning, personal identification. *Narrative support – sense of purpose* Need for a sense of purpose, identity by verbal expression, by making a meaningful story, by identity transformation, and being part of a greater whole (spirituality). *Behavioural support* Need for assertive skills, competence (instead of aggression or sub assertiveness).	

15

RELATIONSHIP-FOCUSED METHOD

A relationship lasts longer, because two people make the choice to keep it, fight for it and work for it.
In a relationship crisis, it's worth it to fight for attachment.

Questions

This chapter addresses the following questions:

- Why is the relationship-focused method not meant for partner relationships?
- What is meant by relational sources of tension?
- What is seen as the relationship-focused method?
- What kind of insights does the study of human territory offer for relational bottlenecks?
- What relational techniques are there to optimize the quality of life of partners in a relationship?
- What evidence is there for the relationship-focused method?

15.1 Introduction

In life, you have to do things yourself, *but not by yourself.*

In the previous chapters, support from the social network was discussed. In this chapter, we will investigate the relationship-focused method that a social worker may utilize in order to get parties or partners to better adjust to each other's needs. First, we will highlight what the consequences are when partners don't respond to each other's signals anymore. After that, the history of the relationship-focused method will be described. Additionally, it will be discussed what light the study of territory sheds on friction in relationships and transgressional behaviour. The techniques and evidence of the relationship-focused method will be detailed. A short illustration of the relationship model will be given based on the case of Mr. Stack. We will conclude with a summary.

The case of Mr. Stack

Mr. Stack acknowledged that working on fortifying his social support network was a meaningful endeavour. This led to utilizing the relationship-focused method. The relationship-focused method was proposed to fortify the mutual support of the Stack couple: when their first son was stillborn, a lack of communication had arisen between them. The gynaecologist had taken Mr. Stack aside and forbade him to tell his wife that the child was no longer alive. From that moment on, he had decided to keep his feelings from his wife. With the relationship-focused method, they first worked on recognizing the distance between the partners. This alone brought them closer together.

15.2 Definition of concepts and elucidation

The relationship-focused method focuses on identifying, eliminating and reducing bottlenecks and blockages in the communication between two parties, such as between spouses or partners, but also between family members, between two colleagues or between employer and employee. Parties who are experiencing a crisis make the effort, under guidance of the social worker, to come to a halt and fight for attachment. In a three-way conversation the social worker talks to two members of the aforementioned relationships. The goal is for partners in a relationship to experience mutual support between each other rather than tension. In an earlier version of this method it was called the 'partner relationship-focused method'. In practice, however, social workers regularly deal with frictions of all kinds of relationships, hence the name 'relationship-focused method'. When we talk about 'partners' in this chapter, this therefore refers to two people who are in a relationship with each another.

Elucidation

A relationship can be regarded as a plant that needs to be watered regularly. A lack of water makes the plant go limp. With gentle and timely care the plant can possibly be saved. But after *a point of no return*, the plant is likely to be doomed. Apart from individual bottlenecks, bottlenecks in communication could also require some attention. Organizing relationship talks can be a good way of dealing with this. The other way around, dominant individual problems in the relationship could also come to the surface during relationship talks and could be better handled if the partner is absent. The difference between this method and the mediation method is that partners, colleagues or relatives ask for help with tensions they experience between each other, while the mediation method is deployed when a conflict is escalated and 'parties' ask a third party for an non-juridical way to reach to workable agreements.

15.3 History of the relationship-focused method

For years the relationship-focused method – as partner relationship-focused method – was a white spot in social work literature, but also in the literature of partner therapy: the method is widely used, but there is very little practice in basic education systems and there is very little literature on the subject. In the 1960s, it was a basic principle to involve the partner when the other partner had problems. It was also 'fashionable' to have a conversation with the parents when the child had learning and behavioural difficulties. Parents felt this was a double burden: they already had a child with problems and now the counsellor also said that it was their fault. This feeling was already present without the social worker actually saying it out loud. This 'fashion' had everything to do with Watzlawick's book around communications and system approach that led to a breakthrough in understanding human communication. This book – which for years was a 'must read' in social work education – analyzed a relationship in detail. The arguing spouses, named George and Martha from the film *Who's Afraid of Virginia Woolf?*, were according to the communication theory analyzed in detail as an example of how people can become involved in communication problems. Distance was taken from an individualizing stance on their relationship problems: not just the individual or the character of the person or the past could be held responsible. Watzlawick spoke in favour of communication analysis for people who have landed in a vicious circle through a power struggle. The communication approach calls this power struggle 'symmetrical escalation'. Despite Watzlawick's successful book, the theory of systemic methods of working with families remained dominant. In all reference work about systemic methods there is only a limited emphasis on the relationship-focused method. There was even a strong reasoning to work with the family system in the instance of partner relationship problems because:

1   Each topic affects every family member;
2   Each family member, in whatever way, is aware the of couple's problem;
3   Secrecy and mystification of the problem could potentially be destructive to the other family members.

There is a lot of justification for the treating of the partner relationship. Working with the two partners as subsystem together is justified because:

1   The partners have their own communication problems that require specific attention;
2   There is a need to set clear boundaries around the marriage subsystem (communication and interaction among the partners);
3   Respect needs to be shown for the privacy of the marital relationship.

In US literature, *Mirages of Marriage* (Lederer & Jackson, 1968) is considered the classic book about the partner relationship-focused method. It offers an important example of the communication approach around a partner relationship. Important Dutch authors in the field of the relationship-focused method are Marc Nevejan, Donald MacGillavry, Alfons Vansteenwegen and Cas Schaap (as psychologists). For years in systemic work, family therapy was overexposed. Nevejan, MacGillavry, Vansteenwegen and Schaap are the only ones who paid attention to partner relationship talks. In 1973 Nevejan wrote a book about partner relationship therapy called *Gezins en echtparenbehandeling* (*Family and Couples Therapy*). He is also the author of an article on a group-based approach to partner relationships. His view is that partners can get tangled up in a 'we symbiosis'. The partnership method is then directed to change the relationship into an 'I–you form'. Then, partners can choose either to continue in this new but not symbiotic 'we' form or break up. MacGillavry wrote several books on partner relationship care, such as *Buigen, barsten of bijstellen* (*Bending, Cracking or Adjusting*), *Suggesties voor echtparen* (*Suggestions for Couples*) (1979) and *Zolang de kruik te water gaat* (*As Long as the Pitcher Goes to Water*) and *Oefeningen van (echt) paren* (*Exercises for Couples*). He recognized the need for care during divorce and founded bureau Echtscheiding (The Divorce Desk) in 1985 (which failed due to lack of government support). He is now active in mediation (see Chapter 19). MacGillavry advocates for teaching partners adequate communication skills. Vansteenwegen was commended for his book *Helpen bij partnerrelatieproblemen* (*Help During Partner Relationship Problems*) (2001) by combining procedural and negotiating techniques. He also pleads for openly discussing sexual problems. Schaap was the first to develop a protocol for partner relationship therapy SRC and LSE techniques (see sections 15.7.4 and 15.7.5).

Around the turn of the century a radical change took place in the guidance of partner relationships by the new insights about partner relationships through EFT, Emotionally Focused Couple Therapy. Whether dealing with the loss of a child, a parent, a person's job or one's health, it all puts a certain pressure on family and relationships. Many partner relationships cannot cope with this type of pressure; the loss leads to removal and finally to a breakup and a (permanent) separation. Partner relationships are important for the health and personal growth of partners, but also for the welfare of the children.

The mutual support of the partners is dependent on the presence of the four support competencies in the partnership (see section 15.7.1 Relational support checklist) (de Mönnink, 2015).

EFT is very suitable to work with when improving mutual support in the partner relationship during times of distress. EFT is designed to work on, or repair the relationship between reattaching partners. The counselling helps partners to step out of destructive patterns by interrupting these so-called toxic patterns and dismantling them, and then actively building towards a more emotionally open and receiving way of interaction. EFT tries to improve relations by making use of the strong need for contact and care (need for affection that belongs to the human species) and offers many exercises to build up mutual trust (Dalgleish et al., 2014). In terms of the four support competencies, the partners in EFT work on increasing mutual signal sensitivity (first support competence), getting closer together (second support competence) and to improve intimacy in the relationship. Partners also work on effectively responding to each other's specific emotional and practical questions (third support competence) and are taught to check whether the given support is working for them, or if other support is necessary (fourth support competence). As a partner relationship therapy EFT is seen as the most effective approach in solving relational suffering (Johnson, 1999). Neuroscience and social science research shows that EFT doesn't only improve connective bonding but also has a positive effect on physical and mental health. But even at the neural level positive changes are happening in the brain because of this improved bonding (Johnson et al., 2013). When it comes to the process of change, more research has been done on the subject of EFT compared to any other therapy (Damasio, 1999, Elliott et al., 2004, Pascual & Greenberg, 2007).

One final theory that sheds light on tensions in relationships between partners, children, neighbours and so forth is the human study of territory (Bakker & Bakker 1972) (see section 15.7.8 and Appendix 5).

15.3.1 Territorial aggression

Special attention must be given to aggressive experiences in all kinds of relationships. Abuse of the elderly is an example, but that attention must be given to all ages: adults, elderly and children. With 'aggression' we do not refer to physical abuse as it is commonly understood, but rather any transgressional experience in interpersonal interaction. Insight into the study of human territories aids us in better recognizing the great variation of different forms of aggression.

The human territory, according to Bakker and Bakker (1972) and Moorter (1979), may be subdivided into differing personal territories:

- My personal property;
- My own body;
- My own mind;
- My private hideout: my retreat territory;
- My personal space: my distance to others;
- My psychological space: the attention of others;
- My action terrain.

In the study of territories, violence is understood as transgressional social interactions on (one of) the territories of the client. Every unwanted meddling in someone's territory (for example harassment but also plagiarism) is a type of aggression that brings forth alertness, flashbacks and avoidance. Experiencing violence in the territorial domain are sources of traumatic stress. It is frequently the case that these experiences fester when left untreated (see also Chapter 26).

The territory of my personal property

The first three human territories are about private domain. Private property is the jacket, the wallet, the letters, the glasses you consider yours. Someone else may not do anything to your property without your consent. Most people cannot bear that their neighbour just barges in, never mind barging into one's bedroom. Every child has toys that they consider their property.

Forms of violence include confiscating passport or ATM card, taking away of means of communication such as a phone, and destruction of property or stealing.

The territory of my own body

My body is my own territory, my private property. We can allow someone on our own body territory by means of a handshake, walking hand in hand, a pat on the shoulder, or putting an arm around someone. An unwanted touch is a territorial form of aggression, and is experienced as a violation of the body territory or assault as a very serious violation. An unwanted touch in an intimate place is seen as sexual harassment and when coupled with violence may be experienced as sexual assault or rape.

Forms of violence include smacking someone, pushing, pinching, hitting hard with the hand, pulling hair, punching with fists, kicking, strangling, hitting or stabbing with an implement (knife, screwdriver, scissors, axe), directed throwing of an object, biting, pouring hot liquid, locking up, excluding, tying up, neglect (deprive of food, care, drink, medication), circumcising a girl, manslaughter, murder, disrobing and forced sexual acts, sex without consent, forced sex, (attempted) rape or sex with someone legally incapable of giving consent.

The territory of my own mind

My mind is the domain of my feelings, thoughts, desires, dreams and intentions. Here, too, we wish to decide for ourselves if we allow someone access or not. Territorial aggression may already arise asking the question: 'What are you thinking?' Reading someone's paper may already be experienced as obtrusive. Reading of a diary without permission is seen as a strong violation of someone's territory. Also, if someone distorts our thoughts or feelings, it feels like a violation.

Forms of violence: threatening, humiliating verbally or through gestures, making it impossible to speak, abusing of threating of children or family of the victim, torturing or killing a pet that belongs to the victim, stalking or threatening.

The territory of my private hideout

The private hideout concerns the place where you feel safe – your refuge. A place that is safe enough to be yourself without having to take others into account. That place can be anywhere: you can retreat in your own house or room, behind the paper, on the toilet, or fishing. Territorial aggression can also cause irritation and conflict if the private hideout is insufficiently respected. The irritation arises for example if there is insufficient space for retreat in a hospital or at work, but also with parents that are incessantly disturbed by their kids. How much privacy someone needs differs from person to person.

Forms of violence include abuse of power, no breaks, no moment of rest or not allowing autonomy.

The territory of my personal space

The personal space is the distance you require 'in centimetres' from other people. Not everyone is allowed in the area surrounding you. That is beholden to people you love. Others are kept further at bay. The need for space differs. Territorial aggression arises when people feel threatened, when people feel like there is insufficient space around them. People from different cultures have different expectation in regards to touching and keeping distance, also between the sexes. Irritation and conflict arise when people sit too close to each other or misinterpret the distance as a sign of lack of trust or love.

Forms of violence include unwanted closeness.

The territory of my psychological space

The final two territories are about the public domain, also called the public arena.

The psychological space is the need for human attention or influence on others. At work, you do or do not ask for attention, you do or do not have the need to be the centre of attention. In a relationship there is also a distribution of psychological space: Who talks when? Who gets to talk about their day first?

Territorial aggression arises when conversational partners always put themselves and their own thoughts first and as such do not pay attention to the psychological space for the other persons. In family situations, this may lead to affective neglect.

The territory of my own action terrain

The action terrain is the human territory where you are active and where you feel entitled to act, exert control, make decisions, apply your expertise and take responsibility. What do you consider the territory that you are the boss of? At work, someone's action terrain is usually set by their job description. At home, this is usually not so well described.

Territorial aggression arises when fixed role descriptions are not present. Irritation and conflict are the consequence. Other forms of aggression are manipulation and abuse of power.

15.3.2 Transgressional behaviour

Territorial aggression and transgressional behaviour in human territories have grave consequences for identity, security and freedom. Not all territorial aggression is traumatic. The more respectful people are in learning to obtain, maintain and defend their territory, the better that is for the own identity, the own feeling of safety and freedom. In Table 15.1, a summary is given of how people may encounter violence in the seven human territories described.

TABLE 15.1 Forms of violence in the seven human territories

Invasion of human territories	Forms of violence at home, at work or in school, on the street, in public and in care institutions	Examples: the concrete behaviours that are associated with violence
My personal property (wallet, letter)	Theft, burglary, plagiarism	Confiscating passport and ATM card, taking away of means of communication such as a phone, destruction of property or stealing
My own body (control over own body, sexuality)	Physical or sexual violence, from unwanted contact to abuse, assault, rape, torture to (attempted) murder	Smacking someone, pushing, pinching, hitting hard with the hand, pulling hair, punching with fists, kicking, strangling, hitting or stabbing with an implement (knife, screwdriver, scissors, axe), directed throwing of an object, biting, pouring hot liquid, locking up, excluding, tying up, neglect (deprive of food, care, drink, medication), circumcising a girl, manslaughter, murder; disrobing and forced sexual acts, sex without consent, forced sex, (attempted) rape, or sex with someone legally incapable of giving consent
My own mind (control over own thoughts, wishes)	Psychological violence, ranging from verbal abuse, insulting, threatening, bullying, psychological terror to stalking	Threatening, humiliating verbally or through gestures, making it impossible to speak, abusing or threating of children or family of the victim, torturing or killing a pet that belongs to the victim, stalking or threatening

Invasion of human territories	Forms of violence at home, at work or in school, on the street, in public and in care institutions	Examples: the concrete behaviours that are associated with violence
My private hideout (space to retreat, to come to rest)	Insufficient/no personal space to retreat	Abuse of power, no breaks, no moment of rest, not allowing autonomy
My personal space (physical distance) between me and someone else)	Unwanted intimacy by coming too close	Unwanted closeness
My psychological space (available attention)	Insufficient/no personal attention	Affective neglect
My action terrain (control over my area of expertise)	Having little to no say about tasks at home	Manipulation or abuse of power

Social workers may endeavour to offer shelter and aftercare for people with these kinds of aggression experiences – the loss counsellor is competent in making a territorial inventory.

15.4 Goals

General goal

- Reducing or eliminating sources of tension in the relationship between partners, colleagues and others.

Specific goals

- Together clients clarify positions and viewpoints in relation to the source of tension (such as a relationship crisis, parenting problems, health issues or problems with loss).
- Clients stabilize instead of sinking deeper into the crisis.
- Clients reduce tensions between each other.
- Clients share a vision of the current state of affairs (e.g. a new start, a pause or a divorce).
- Clients transition towards a new phase in their relationship.
- Clients come to agreements together.
- Clients are less far apart from each other.
- Clients reach a new and healthy balance.

15.5 Indications

- Both partners desire to have joint sessions.
- The clients indicate that there is a relational tension, friction, a relational problem or a crisis. These problems can be in various different areas such as: communication, business, health, housing, household, financial, parenting issues or sexual intimacy.

15.6 Contraindications

- One or two clients have dominant individual problems.
- One partner does not want a relationship conversation.
- There are irreconcilable differences between the partners, for example in emotional processing or power.

- One or both partners have insufficient communication skills, for example because of brain damage.

15.7 Techniques

1 Relational support checklist
2 Communication technique
3 Attention technique
4 LSE technique
5 SRC technique
6 Blow-off-steam technique
7 Preservation technique
8 Territorial negotiation technique
9 Constructive criticism technique.

15.7.1 Relational support checklist

The social worker evaluates where the tension spans are according to the individual partners. This way, an assessment or a valuation of the existing bottlenecks can be made. To do so, 'territorial inventory' can be used (see section 15.7.8 and Appendix 5, TICL). For example, a client is traumatized and treated for this because of a false accusation by the chief of personnel (a threatening letter was sent to the board with the employee's name underneath). The employee feels strengthened enough to ask for a conversation with the chief of personnel to clear the air. The problem is that he has never been able to express his anger over the false accusations to the 'sender' of the letter. By means of valuation video recordings of the relationship talks can be used (see section 13.7.2 SOSKI technique) or the partner relationship checklist (see Table 15.2).

TABLE 15.2 Relational support checklist

Support competencies	Social support	Ineffective support
1 Signal recognition	Is signal behaviour of the partner being valued correctly? 'Give me the attention I asked for directly or indirectly!'	Signal insensitivity by ignoring or discarding the demand for closeness: 'I don't give support because he or she didn't ask.' Not recognizing direct or indirect questions.
2 Coming closer	Is contact towards the (for support asking) partner, being sought in a committed and alert way? 'I have a need for warm interest and closeness.'	Distance, not coming close: 'I stay at a distance.' A question for emotional closeness answered with: 'this is not a good time.' Offering a cliché type of closeness.
3 Customized support	Has been sorted out which specific support is needed in contact with the partner and is this support offered? Flexible matching of supply and demand.	Demand-driven aid (clichés?): continued support from your own vision of what is needed ('Cheer up, and it will all go well'); giving practical support to emotional questions and vice versa.

Support competencies	Social support	Ineffective support
4 Support checks	Is it checked regularly whether or not this support is enough or if other support is needed? Measuring the effectiveness of the support.	Not checking if help arrives: holding on to the established support that was offered, in an inflexible way. Practical bottlenecks get all the attention, emotional support stays behind.

By evaluating in what way these support competencies are sufficiently available in the partner relationship, it can be made clear where the improvement opportunities for mutual support are. This brings a reduction in partner relationship stress, but also the negative impact of that stress can be reduced for the family and the present children.

15.7.2 Communication technique

The social worker proposes to let the partners take turns to explain their story. Through the valuation technique, the first versions of the bottlenecks are put in words. During communication sessions, exchanging mutual communication about the bottleneck issues is promoted. The social worker pursues to ensure that the partners are both, substantively (facts) as well as communicatively (mutual respect), done justice. Communication rules are introduced and communication exercises are done (see Table 15.2) when communication is not adequate enough. This for example can be done, when partners interrupt each other, if one of the two partners takes a disproportionate amount of time, or if partners don't listen to each other effectively. In the example from section 15.7.1, the social worker asks the falsely accused employee and the chief of personnel to explain the bottlenecks in turns. The employee gets started, but quickly gets interrupted by the chief. The social worker asks the chief to let his colleague speak first. This is practiced with the use of the tips on proper communication (see Table 15.3).

Summary and edited text from: Lange, A. (2006). *Behavioural change in families.* Groningen: Wolters Noordhof.

15.7.3 Attention technique

The social worker suggests attention exercises if one or both partners feel they are not getting enough attention from the other. The other person is experienced as emotionally distant. There is a lack of real attention. For example, the social worker suggests that A pays attention to B and that B receives attention from A. B comes up with a personal subject and talks about it to A. When A decides to give an opinion or reacts in a judgemental way, they stop. The social worker explains that 'giving attention' means that people are listened to, without giving a personal opinion. After that A and B continue, and so on, until A has learned to pay 'free' attention to B. If desired, the social worker turns the tables on them and lets A and B repeat the exercise at home.

15.7.4 LSE technique (Schaap et al., 2000)

The social worker lets the partners effectively listen to each other by using the LSE Technique: Listening, Summarizing and Empathizing (in Dutch LSI). An example: the

TABLE 15.3 Tips on proper communication

Communication aspect	Inadequate form	Adequate form (think of an example of desired behaviour)
1 Giving criticism	Giving negative criticism: desirable, reproachful, demanding or defensive. This works destructively.	Giving constructive criticism: mutual recognition or lenient. For example: 'You're never home,' 'But I work for a living. For example: It is hard to do everything alone at home. Could you do me a favour (fighting for being right) by taking over some tasks.' 'What tasks?' This works constructively.
2 Clarity	Being vague about unfulfilled wishes, desires and needs. For example: 'I want more attention.'	Being specific about mutual desires within specific behaviours. For example: 'I would like you to ask me more often: How are you? How was your work day?'
3 A why question	Asking the 'why' question when nobody's asking for information. For example: 'Why are you nagging me?'	Asking a 'why' question when information is asked. Or otherwise, explicitly making an assertion. For example: 'I would really appreciate it if you would nag me less.'
4 Statements	Wrapped in quotation marks or formulated as questions.	Making 'un-wrapped' statements.
5 Past	Pinning someone down on earlier statements: playing upon the past.	Responding to recent communication and possibly working out the past.
6 Who are you talking for?	Talking for someone else.	Talking for yourself: saying what you want from the other person.
7 Fabrications	Linking drastic interpretations and observations: 'reading' one's thoughts.	Checking the fabrications: asking if there is something going on with the other person and asking if there is something wrong.
8 Language	Not using direct language but using words like maybe, one, someone.	Direct language: 'It's hard for me that . . .'
9 Argumentation	Debating tricks: fixating on one irrelevant point, turn-around trick, disqualifications.	Logical argumentation: 1 + 1 =

social worker practices with eye contact and a relaxed body posture and having partners say 'hmm' and nodding yes. The social worker lets the partner summarize the message of the other person. He lets one partner empathize with the other by letting the other actively say how the broadcasted message can be understood from the point of view of this person.

15.7.5 SRC technique (Schaap et al., 2000)

The social worker attempts to intervene when relational tension has built up. There are three moments to do so: during the Situation, during the Reaction, or during the Consequence (to the wrong behaviour). For example 'to intervene in the situation' is possible by agreeing that one partner leaves the other one alone for half an hour when he or she gets home. This can be done if a lot of tension arises when the partner is a still in 'work mode' when he or she gets home. 'Intervening during the reaction' means to intervene right when the unwanted behaviour occurs. The social worker for instance arranges with the client that he or she walks away when anger issues play up and to find an alternative way first. This can be done by, for example, going for a run or taking a shower. During the 'consequence intervention' a penalty is agreed upon when undesirable behaviour occurs. For example when a client, against agreements, has yelled or scolded, he or she has to bring the other client breakfast in bed 'to compensate'.

15.7.6 Blow-off-steam technique

The social worker optionally lets one or both parties 'blow off steam'. He or she can do this when a client is overwhelmed with emotion and temporarily incapable to pursue negotiations in a rational way (see also the techniques of the cathartic method in Chapter 8). A timeout for both parties could be sufficient or emotional discharge in the presence of the other party. The emotional discharge of a party in the presence of the other is not intended as leverage in the negotiations, but more as a way of increasing mutual understanding.

15.7.7 Preservation technique

The social worker allows the partners to reflect on what unites them and what they like to do together. This way, a positive spiral can be put into effect. The social worker asks the clients, for example, to make a list of things and lets the partners make clear to each other what they would like to do together. They make a commitment to put this into action between two sessions (see section 13.7.7).

15.7.8 Territorial negotiation technique

The social worker comes to the conclusion that there is a bottleneck in the relationship, which is a territorial conflict (see Table 15.1 and Appendix 6). The social worker then proposes to start negotiations about this issue. Territorial negotiations are done by working in rounds. First the social worker specifies what type territorial conflict they're dealing with. He asks questions like: 'When were you irritated, and about what?' 'What area does this irritable crossness concern?' 'What do you consider yours and what belongs to the other person?' Then the question is asked which territorial wish one partner has, and how the other partner reacts to this wish. Through back and forth conversation between partners, partners are working towards a territorial agreement. In the example from section 15.7.1, the falsely accused employee felt that his honour and reputation were negatively affected by the chief of personnel. The client wanted to have public rehabilitation by the chief within the company. He was put on inactive: his prestige and field of territory were discredited. The chief wanted to comply, but suggested to use the next work meeting on the floor to do so. The employee objected, because not everybody would be informed through this meeting. They ended up making a deal in which the chief pleaded the employee free of all blemish through a letter to all staff members as well as offering apologies for the damage made.

15.7.9 Constructive criticism technique

Constructive criticism (CC) consists of four steps that can be practiced:

1   Facts: what happened when? (Example: you did not look at me when we just discussed something);
2   Experience: what irritates me about it? (Example: it annoyed me);
3   Desirable behaviour: what type of other behaviour do I wish for? (Example: I want you to look at me when you talk to me);
4   Mutual interest for the behavioural change: how can the behavioural change be constructive for our relationship? (Example: eye contact makes our conversation much easier).

15.8 Social work results

- Clients have clarity about each other's position.
- Clients are experiencing more stability despite the crisis.
- Clients are experiencing more relaxation in the relationship.
- Clients are entering a new phase in their relationship.
- Clients have made agreements.
- Clients have a new and healthy balance.
- Clients are experiencing more feelings of closeness and mutual support to each other.
- Clients have more clarity about a new start, a break or a divorce.

15.9 Evidence

15.9.1 Relationship therapy

'Relationship Australia' regularly conducts research into various aspects of relationships. A strong connection is found between satisfaction in life and having relationships: 60% of respondents consider a good family life, having a good partner relationship and having close friends are important aspects for fulfilment in life. And 83% consider having a partner with whom to have a satisfying relationship is essential for happiness. Gurman et al. (1986) suggest that family therapy methods are investigated thoroughly and without exception proved to be effective. Earlier research by Gurman (1983) reveals the following about the couple therapy:

1   In both behavioural and non-behavioural partner relationship therapy (marital therapies) improved communication between partners is a key to a successful outcome.
2   For family problems, conjoint couples' therapy – this is the same as partner relationship therapy – is clearly preferable over individual therapy.
3   Negative results are twice as common when marital problems are treated with individual therapy than when partner relationship therapy is chosen.

Monica McGoldrick (Imber-Black, 1989) states that more partner relationship problems occur when one or more of the following 12 factors occur:

1 The couple starts seeing each other or marries shortly after a severe loss situation.
2 The desire of (one of) the partners to remain at a distance from their family of origin.
3 The family backgrounds of the partners differ greatly in terms of religion, education, social class or ethnicity, and there is a big age difference between the partners.
4 One of the partners remains too close to the original family home or stays too far away.
5 One of the partners is financially, physically or emotionally dependent on the family of origin.
6 The pair was married before the age of 20 years.
7 The pair was married after a courtship of less than six months or a courtship of more than three years.
8 The marriage was carried out in absence of family and friends.
9 The woman becomes pregnant before or during the first year of marriage.
10 One of the partners has a bad relationship with a brother or sister or parents.
11 One of the partners sees his or her childhood or adolescence as an unhappy time.
12 The marriage of the parents of one of the partners was unstable.

Proof of the effectiveness of the relationship-focused method can be found in research on EFT, Emotionally Focused Couple Therapy (see http://iceeft.com/images/PDFs/EFTResearch.pdf).

The question is: does EFT conform to any gold standard in terms of research validation and the standards set out for psychotherapy?

In terms of the gold standard set out by bodies such as the American Psychological Association for psychotherapy research, EFT epitomizes the very highest level set out by this standard. Over the last 25 years, the EFT research programme has systematically covered all the factors set out in optimal models of psychotherapy research.

The meta-analysis (Johnson et al., 1999) of the four most rigorous outcome studies conducted before the year 2000, showed a larger effect size (1.3) than any other couple intervention has achieved to date. Studies consistently show excellent follow-up results, and some studies show that significant progress continues after therapy. EFT has a body of process research showing that change does indeed occur in the way that the theory suggests. This level of linkage between in-session process and rigorous outcome measurement is unusual in the field of psychotherapy.

EFT is the only model of couple intervention that uses a systematic empirically validated theory of adult bonding as the basis for understanding and alleviating relationship problems. The generalizability of EFT across different kinds of clients and couples facing comorbidities such as depression and PTSD has been examined and results are consistently positive. Outcome and process research addressing key relationship factors, such as the forgiveness of injuries, has also been conducted with positive results. EFT studies are generally rigorous and published in the best peer reviewed journals.

In brief, EFT researchers can show that, as set out in the seminal text by Johnson (2004), *Creating Connection: The Practice of Emotionally Focused Couple Therapy*, EFT works very well, results last, we know how it works so we can train therapists to intervene efficiently, and we know it works across different populations and problems. It also links congruently to other bodies of research, such as those examining the nature of relationship distress and adult attachment processes.

Recent research involves outcome studies of couples facing trauma and stressful events (the Dalton and MacIntosh studies, and a study on EFT effects on attachment security with an FMRI component). The FMRI component shows that EFT changes the way contact with a partner mediates the effect of threat on the brain. There is an outcome study in progress of the new educational programme based on EFT (Hold Me Tight® Program: Conversations for Connection). A pilot study has also been completed at the VA in Baltimore on EFT with veteran couples dealing with PTSD.

Completed and ongoing EFT research consistently supports the efficacy of the Emotionally Focused Therapy model.

15.10 Pitfalls

- The social worker is a one-sided partisan.
- The social worker denies his or her own parallel process (as if the social worker for example, completely can separate his or her own personal relationship crisis from the relationship crisis of the clients).
- In the event of dominating individual or positional problems, the social worker stays focused too long on partner relationship therapy (only).
- The social worker locks one of the partners outside too quickly for being incapable or impaired – for example if one of the parties used violence to enforce his or her will.

15.11 Summary

In this chapter, we covered the relationship-focused method that a social worker may utilize in order to get partners to better adjust to each other's needs. First, we highlighted what the consequences are when partners don't respond to each other's signals (anymore). After that, the history of the relationship-focused method was described. Additionally, it was discussed what light the study of territory sheds on friction in relationships and transgressional behaviour. The techniques and evidence of the relationship method were detailed. A short illustration of the relationship model was given based on the case of Mr. Stack. We concluded with this summary.

Question

1   Try completing the support checklist in Table 14.4 using either a case study or one of your own personal relationships as a point of departure. What does the client/do I need from this relationship to optimally meet existing human needs?

16
FAMILY WORK METHOD

This chapter addresses the following questions:

- What is meant by 'nuclear family' and 'extended family'?
- What is meant by 'My World Triangle'?
- Why is working from the strength of the family preferable to problem-oriented working with a family?
- What is meant by horizontal and vertical stressors?
- What is meant by the Family Growth Model (FGM)?
- Which five family factors determine personal growth of family members ?
- How has the nuclear family and extended family model developed?
- Which techniques resulted from the nuclear and extended family methods?
- What evidence is there in relation to the family method?

16.1 Introduction

Your children are not your children.
They are the sons and daughters of Life's longing for itself.
They come through you but not from you,
And though they are with you yet they belong not to you.

You may give them your love but not your thoughts,
For they have their own thoughts.
You may house their bodies but not their souls,
For their souls dwell in the house of tomorrow,
which you cannot visit, not even in your dreams.
You may strive to be like them,
but seek not to make them like you.
For life goes not backward nor tarries with yesterday.

—"On Children" (Kahlil Gibran)

In social work, the nuclear and extended family methods (referred to as the family method from here on in) is focused on improving the personal growth of family members by mobilizing one's own strength to reduce sources of tension. This method aids family members in being more supportive of each other in order to meet human needs. From a PIE-ET perspective (see Chapter 2), the question surrounding the support factor within families is: how does a particular constructive or destructive influence affect personal self-esteem and the functioning of the family? The family method allows social workers to work with the family on constructive and interdependent support.

First, a definition is given of the core concepts and the dynamics between nuclear families and extended families. This is followed by a plea to move from a deficit vision to a strength vision, when working with families; and to consider any stumbling blocks/issues from a family-focused perspective as well. Next, the Growth in Family Functioning Model (GFFM) is described in detail, while the five factors of this family model are clarified: need fulfilment, communication, structure, emotional ties, and as a result the self-esteem of family members either improving or stagnating. Next, the history of the family method will be described, as well as objectives, indications, contraindications and the techniques of the family method. Following that, evidence supporting the effectiveness of the family method is detailed, as well as potential pitfalls. We conclude with a summary.

The case of Mr. Stack

Mr. Stack recognized that working on strengthening his social support system was a useful objective. That is when the family method became an option (among others). The family method was suggested in order to reduce the tension in the family surrounding the disabled son: this son required a lot of attention. History was apparently repeating itself, because Mr. Stack himself also came from a family with a disabled brother, who also required a lot of attention, which meant that Mr. Stack's needs were not met. He did not know how to handle this unsettled score in the family, because after all, he did understand. He had retained a negative self-esteem from his family, so it was a good idea to handle this unfinished business and work together on the four factors that improve QoL: constructive communication with his wife and son, clear role distribution for everyone involved, and working on emotional closeness. This caused the family to adjust and contribute to the personal growth of Mr. Stack, his wife and their son.

There were also cases of Huntington's disease in Mr. Stack's family. When Mr. Stack showed his family tree, plotted out according to a genogram, it became clear what kind of battle had raged in his family since 1880. Coincidentally, he himself had no genetic predisposition, but four of his brothers and three of his sisters did have the disease. Each time there was a funeral service for one of his brothers or sisters, there was palpable tension in the family aimed at the parents, who had this large number of offspring in spite of being aware of this genetic predisposition. Through family guidance, this mixture of sadness, resentment, jealousy and survivor's guilt can be addressed so that for the first time ever, there is some peace and quiet within the family.

16.2 Definition and elucidation

In this book the concept of 'the family' refers to the nuclear and the extended family someone is part of at this moment. The nuclear family is a term used to define a group consisting of a pair of adults (married or unmarried) or a single adult and his or her children. The nuclear family may have any number of children. The term children refers to either biological children and/or any mix of dependent children including stepchildren and adopted children. The extended family is a term used to define the constellation of family members not living under one roof.

The objective of (grand)parents should be 'getting it right for every child', thus giving all children and young people the best start in life. Like Kahlil Gibran (1923) stated in *On Children*: 'You may give children your love but not your thoughts, For they have their own thoughts.'

In the 'Getting It Right for Every Child' programme in Scotland (see Scottish government, http://www.gov.scot/Topics/People/Young-People/gettingitright/resources/girfec-diagrams), the 'My World Triangle' of children involves three questions aimed at meeting children's needs (see Figure 16.1): What do children need from the people who look after them? How do children grow and develop? How supportive is the wider world of the child? When planning and thinking about the needs of children or young persons, every social worker should think about the whole child or young person.

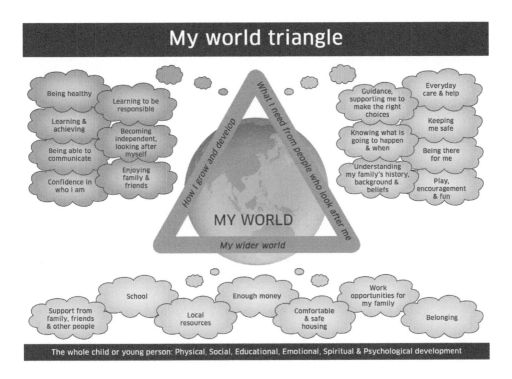

FIGURE 16.1 My World Triangle

Image courtesy of Scottish government

The family work method not only helps within the nuclear family but also in finding and reducing specific changes and frictions in the extended family context – the multi-generational line (grandparent–parent–child). The 'extended family' is defined in the following way: the client's original family and all other blood ties such as aunts, uncles, cousins and grandparents. Interventions aimed at family-related pressure points helps reducing *unfinished business* and working towards the recovery of family breakups or learning how to live with them. In the nuclear family method our basic principle was the relationship between children and parents who were still living together, whereas in the family work method we look at, for example the relationship between parents and children, while the children have already moved out. This may be the relationship between an adult and his or her father or mother (who may be 50 or even 85 years old), but also pressure points in the relationship between adult brothers and sisters, grown-up children and (beloved) uncles or aunts. Though, not all family members must necessarily participate in order to apply the family work method.

Traditionally, one's family is the place where norms and values are learned, where different generations meet and where people learn to participate in society. But what is the significance of family in the present times? Family is still family, whether you get along with them or not, which is exactly why it can be so difficult to deal with them. Problematic behaviour, for example that of a runaway, drug-addicted adolescent who has a father with a criminal history, is put into a different perspective when we see the act of running away as a type of invisible loyalty from the son towards the problematic father. In a time where everyone can be himself, the notion of blood ties seems superseded. However, it is not. How are we invisibly loyal to our parents? In the multi-generational context there is both visible and invisible loyalty through blood ties, where not only pride but also ballast, negativity and repetitive family patterns are passed on. Some examples:

16.2.1 Blood ties

Mother: 'Finish your plate, dear. If you saw the things I have seen during the war, you'd change your tune.'

Child to mother: 'After 18 years of taking crap about the war, I've had it. Get some counselling, but don't come yapping to me about your frustrations. I want my own freedom. Otherwise that war of yours was completely pointless.'

'My stepsister was conceived by a rapist. She is doing drugs and can't talk about her past.'

'My twin sister Marie died when she was 4. My grandmother Marie decided to pretend it was me, Molly, who died. That way my sister – who shared her name – would live on. She called me by her name, while she had just passed away. I still find it difficult to think back at that.'

The war-traumatized father sending his daughter a bill after doing some repair works at her house. . . . The daughter calls him a madman for doing so and no longer wants anything to do with him.

The term 'extended-family method' is not new; it bears closest resemblance to the *intergenerational method*, also called the *contextual approach*, which originated in the 1980s. The contextual approach focuses on the family context and invisible connections between family members. Ivan Nagy (1973) provided the insight that people have invisible loyalties towards their family origin. Subject matters we struggle with as individuals often originate in the family we grew up in and reveal themselves in our current relationships. Some patterns are passed on from one generation to another. Traumatized parents may cause a so-called second-generation problem. This second generation can even cause, in its turn, a third-generation problem. Intergenerational transfer of unprocessed loss experiences is the influence on parents, children and grandchildren after the loss of a beloved family member. This passing down of damages throughout generations – also called transgenerational transmission – occurs within the lines of existential loyalty, the loyalty to the person to whom you owe your life. Current problems can thus originate from all sorts of loyalty problems.

- *Subconscious loyalties* may be in the way of an adult relationship with one's current partner.
- *Split loyalty* occurs when a child is forced to choose one parent before the other.
- *Delegation* is when one child feels compelled to always be successful, while the other child is under the impression of always having to fail.
- We speak of *projective identification* when children are trapped in a forced projection of their parents, who expect their child to be the substitute child for a deceased brother or sister whose name was given to the substitute child. Resisting these forced expectations is punished, even by means of rejection or threatening to do so ('You are no longer my child'). Integration of this projection (identification) is often the result.
- *Destructive claim* is when a child feels ill-treated and, from that feeling, claims the right for himself to damage others: a parent belittles or neglects a wrongdoer, and the child believes he can treat his own partner, children, a colleague or even an innocent passer-by in the same destructive way.

In the contemporary nuclear family, economic ties to grandparents and the rest of one's family are less essential. However, on a psychological level, Nagy claims that there are still visible and invisible ties. This way, children of war-traumatized, neglected or sexually traumatized parents get a touch of their damaged parents because the latter are actively lashing out, both literally and figuratively speaking, from the pain they were dealt. This causes repetitive family routines to arise, for example breakups between parents and their children, but also amongst children alone. The family history becomes a song stuck on repeat, for generations on end. It is never an exact copy of old abusive behaviour towards the child, but rather tensions incurring unprocessed traumas (Visser, 1997).

Given the complexities of family life, family stressors can represent any of a wide range of life circumstances. Historically, social workers have worked with families affected by stressors ('problems') related to social injustice and adverse conditions (see Figure 16.2).

The stressors such families encounter today are greater than ever, fuelled by issues such as poverty, racism, substance abuse and domestic violence. These are no longer problems of the individual; they are problems deeply embedded in the family system, often over many generations. A 'family systems perspective' is needed to work effectively with the complex family stressors and strengths (see also section 16.2.3).

16.2.2 From a family deficits to a family strengths perspective?

In response to the limitations associated with a problem or deficit-oriented approach to family assessment and intervention, practitioners in social work, mental health, family services and

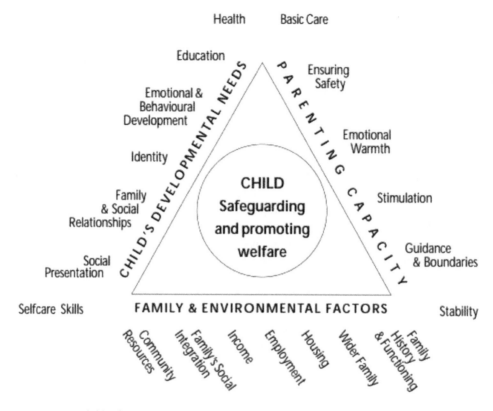

FIGURE 16.2   Child safeguarding and promoting welfare

education have expressed a heightened interest in strength-based assessment and intervention. Family strength-based practice focuses on enhancing already existing

> emotional and behavioral skills, competencies, and characteristics that create a sense of personal and family accomplishment, contribute to satisfying relationships with family members, peers, and adults, enhance one's ability to deal with adversity and stress and promote one's personal, social, and academic development.
>
> *(Epstein & Sharma, 1998)*

As such, strength-based assessment and intervention offers a strategy for empowering children and their families by building on the personal strengths and resources that are frequently overlooked or given minimal attention in more problem-oriented approaches to assessment. Important family aspects from a strength-based assessment are (Sheafor & Horejsi, 2003): members trust each other; enjoy each other; listen to and respect each other's opinions, even when they disagree; their communication is clear, positive and productive, they have clear and reasonable rules that govern behaviour and interaction; and each member's ideas, preferences, and needs are considered before making a decision that would affect the family. The family has traditions, rituals, and stories that provide a sense of history, belonging, and identity; family members share what they have and make personal sacrifices in order to help each other; members stick together and support each other in times of adversity; conflicts are acknowledged and resolved. Strengths can be identified by asking the client questions such as: can you tell about times when you successfully handled stressors similar to those you face now?

Ordinary families often worry about their own normality (Walsh, 2012): Are they doing well? Are they doing it 'right'? Differences from either average or ideal norms are often experienced as stigmatized deviance: deficient and shame-laden. The overwhelming challenges and changes in contemporary life can compound feelings of inadequacy, especially for multistressed families with limited resources. In a culture that readily blames families and touts the virtue of self-reliance, parents often feel doubly deficient: for having a problem, and for being unable to solve it on their own. Much of what is labeled as family 'resistance' to therapy stems from concerns of being judged dysfunctional and blamed for their problems. No engagement is often taken as either further evidence of their dysfunction or mistaken for insufficient caring and a lack of motivation for change. Many families have felt prejudged and blamed in interactions with schools, mental health or care providers, welfare agencies, or justice systems. Expecting a therapist to judge them negatively, they may mistake a clinician's neutral stance or well-intentioned silence as confirmation that they are somehow lacking or fail to fit a cultural ideal of the family. It can be helpful to explore families' concerns and the models and myths they hold as ideal. It is crucial to disengage assumptions of pathology from participation in therapy, taking care not to present − or imply − family deficits as the rationale for family therapy. It is essential to understand every family's challenges, affirm members' caring and efforts, and involve them as valued collaborators in therapeutic objectives.

The aim of normalizing family members' distress is to *depathologize* and *contextualize* their feelings and experience. As an example, strong emotional reactions are common and understandable in crisis situations and are normal reactions to abnormal conditions, such as war-related trauma. Normalizing is *not* intended to reduce all problems and families to a common denominator; it should neither trivialize clients' suffering, struggle or plight, nor normalize or condone harmful and destructive behaviour patterns.

16.2.3 Family life cycle perspective

The individual, coping with life cycle stressors, can only be fully understood when seen from a family life cycle perspective. This view sees the individual life cycle taking place within the family life cycle that forms the basis for human development. Although it is difficult to think of the family as a whole, as a system moving through time, because of the complexity involved, the family perspective is crucial because the family has fundamental traits which differ from all other systems. Unlike all other organizations, families incorporate new members only by birth, adoption, or marriage, and members can only leave by death, if then. No other system is subject to these constraints.

As illustrated in Figure 16.3, the flow of stress in a family can be viewed (Carter & McGoldrick, 1989a) as being both vertical and horizontal. The vertical flow in a system includes patterns of relating and functioning that are transmitted down the generations, primarily through the mechanism of emotional triangling. It includes all family attitudes, taboos, expectations, labels and loaded issues which family members grow up with. One could say that these aspects of our lives are like the one hand we are dealt, they are the given. What we do with them is the issue.

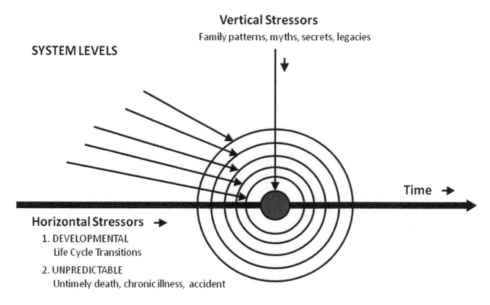

FIGURE 16.3 Horizontal and vertical stressors

The horizontal flow in the system includes the stress produced by the stressors on the family as it moves through time, coping with the changes and transitions of the family life cycle. This includes both the predictable developmental stresses and unpredictable events, 'the slings and arrows of outrageous fortune' (Shakespeare) that may disrupt the life cycle process (untimely death, birth of a disabled child, chronic illness, war, etc.). Given enough stress on the horizontal axis, any family will appear extremely dysfunctional. Even a small horizontal stress on a family in which the vertical axis is full of intense stress will create great disruption in the system.

Following Carter and McGoldrick (1989b), the degree of stress engendered by stressors on the vertical and horizontal axes at the points where they converge is the key determinant of how well the family (members) will manage through the various transitions through life. It becomes imperative, therefore, to assess not only the dimensions of the current family life cycle stress, but also their connections with extended family themes, triangles, and labels coming down in the family over historical time. Although all normative change is stressful to some degree, Carter observed that when the horizontal (developmental) stress intersects with vertical (transgenerational) stress, there is a quantum leap in stress in the family system. The transgenerational (vertical) stresses and strengths will be covered in this chapter, which will also include the extended family.

In addition to the 'stress inherited' from the past generations and that which is experienced while moving through the family cycle, there is, of course, the stress of living in this place at this moment. One cannot ignore the social, economic and political context and its impact on families moving through different phases of the life cycle at each point in history. There are huge discrepancies in social and economic circumstances between families, and this seems to be escalating in recent times.

16.3 The Growth in Family Functioning Model (GFFM)

The development of family functioning models has helped to operationalize core concepts of the process family functioning theory, further paving the way for intervention development and quantitative research (see Figure 16.4). The Growth in Family Functioning Model (GFFM) is a synthesis of the Satir Family model (1975, 1988) and the Process Model of Family Functioning (Steinhauer et al., 1984). The GFFM emphasizes family dynamics that are relevant to family health pathology.

Growth model researchers assert that 'the overriding goals of the family are to provide for the biological, psychological and social development and maintenance of family members.' Moreover, this model emphasizes how basic dimensions of family functioning are interrelated. The growth model attempts to integrate 'systems theory with theories of individual psychology' and is designed to identify areas where family structure and functioning are effective or problematic. Satir's perspective on family functioning led her to evolve a blend of a family approach with a humanistic orientation. Satir is, without a doubt, the founding mother of family therapy, which is referred to as the nuclear family method in this book: She had an enormous influence on family therapy. In 1974, Foley stated:

> Satir introduces a dimension of sentiment in the communication theory which acts as a counterweight for its intellectual basis. Satir shows warmth and care in her therapies. Of all therapists studied, she is the one who was most involved on the emotional level of the people.

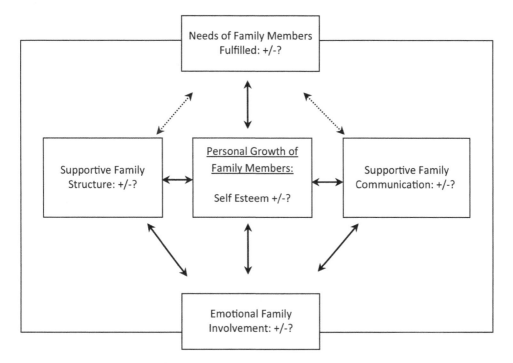

FIGURE 16.4 Growth in Family Functioning Model (GFFM): Family Factors for Personal Growth

Source: de Mönnink (2016)

TABLE 16.1 GFFM: five personal growth factors in family functioning

Family factors	Constructive family functioning	Destructive family functioning
1 Self-esteem	Strong self-esteem, growth	Weak self-esteem: stagnation
2 Needs fulfilment	Effective human needs fulfilment	Ineffective human needs fulfilment
3 Family communication	Constructive levelling	Destructive patterns: blaming, placating, computing, (super-reasoning), distracting
4 Family structure	Constructive family structure: clear, humane, overt, up-to-date, flexible	Destructive family structure: covered up, superseded, 'inhumane', rigid, unchanging
5 Emotional involvement	Positive safe involvement	Destructive anxious involvement

GFFM has its first theoretical underpinning in the model proposed by Virginia Satir. Satir, a social worker by education, proposed 'growth views' with regard to essential elements of healthy family functioning in her *Experiential Approach*. Satir's family therapy model has been referred to by various names throughout its development, including conjoint family therapy, process therapy, and the Human Validation Process Model. Satir's philosophy regarding connecting with 'inner sources' is reflected in her statement: 'I am convinced that all people can grow. It is a matter of connecting them with their inner resources. This is the therapeutic task.' The Satir model (1988) – although in revised form – is still relevant for social work today. Connecting with inner sources, Satir would have meant not only your personal inner sources but also connecting with your inner sources within the family.

The GFFM has its second theoretical underpinning in the FAM (Family Assessment Measurement) which is based on the Process Model of Family Functioning (Steinhauer et al., 1984). This model integrates different approaches in family therapy and research, and assesses seven family-related concepts (Task Accomplishment, Role Performance, Communication, Affective Expression, Involvement, Control and Values and Norms).

The five factors of GFFM

The constructive or destructive effect of the nuclear family system on the self-esteem of its members is determined by means of five factors (see Table 16.1):

1   Personal *self-esteem* of family members: how strong or weak is the self-esteem of family members?
2   Family *needs fulfilment* in different phases of the family life cycle: how effective is this?
3   Family *communication*: how direct, clear, specific, and honest is this?
4   Family *structure*: how clear, caring, and appropriate is this?
5   Family mutual *emotional involvement*: how cohesive and safe is the mutual attachment?

These factors which are described now can result in personal growth of personal stagnation of family members.

16.3.1 Personal self-esteem of family members: is it growing (+) or is it weakening (–)?

Satir theorized that persons with low self-esteem tend to marry each other and create an environment wherein their children also develop feelings of low self-esteem. She believed that low self-esteem is the foundation of individual and family mental health and that many of the problems brought in to family therapy are ultimately connected with low self-esteem. Hence raising the self-esteem of individual family members is one of the essential foci for intervention within the family approach we describe here.

Satir observed a consistent pattern in her experience with optimally functioning families – described as untroubled, vital, and nurturing. It is important for the assessment to determine how nurturing and open the nuclear family is. The central question with family function is: how constructive or destructive is the family functioning for self-esteem of its members? A constructive family system is a family characterized by strength, growth, reality, confidentiality and nurturing. The needs fulfilment is adequate. The communication is adequate (direct, clear, to the point and growth enhancing). The structure and rules are humane and thus also variable. The emotional involvement is constructive, the result is constructive, enhancing personal and family strength. There is enough room for the personal growth of the individual family members.

On the contrary, in a destructive family system there is a system characterized by stressors, with a culture of black-and-white thinking: right or wrong, life or death. The need fulfilment is inadequate. The communication in a destructive system is indirect, unclear, inconsistent, not to the point and patterned: non-growth-enhancing. The structure and rules are covered up, superseded and inhumane. The result is destructive. The self-esteem of the family members decreases (see Table 16.1).

Regardless of the specific problem of bringing a family to family therapy, Satir believed that changing those key processes relieves family pain and enhances family vitality. She regarded those aspects of family life as the basic forces operating in all families, whether an intact, one-parent, blended or institutional family, and in the growing variety and complexity of families. She was ahead of her time in attending to the spiritual dimension of healing and growth.

At the core of Satir's philosophy and central to her approach is the notion that families must respond to each other in ways that enhance each other's self-esteem. Low self-esteem can cause a person to respond to family members in unhealthy, maladaptive ways. How we choose to cope often relates to our level of self-esteem.

16.3.2 Family needs fulfilment: effective (+) or ineffective (–)?

According to this GFF-model the overriding goal of the family should be the successful fulfilment of a variety of basic, developmental, and crisis needs (needs fulfilment). Although some families do not seem to have any specific goal or orientation at all. It is through the constructive or destructive process of needs fulfilment that the family succeeds or fails to achieve objectives central to its life as a group. These functions include allowing the continued development of all family members, providing reasonable security, ensuring sufficient cohesion to maintain the family as a unit, and functioning effectively as a part of society. The process by which tasks are accomplished includes: (1) needs identification, (2) exploration of alternative satisfiers, (3) implementation of selected satisfiers, and (4) evaluation of needs fulfilments' effects. Thus needs fulfilment is the most basic activity of the family.

Evelyn Duvall's (Duvall and Miller, 1985) developmental family framework provides guidance for the examination and analysis of such basic changes and developmental needs or tasks common to most families during their life cycle (see Table 16.2). Although each family has unique characteristics, normative patterns of sequential development are common to all families.

Duvall's developmental model is an excellent guide for assessing, analyzing and planning basic family tasks in the developmental stage, however, this model does not include the family structure or physiological aspects, which should be taken into account for a comprehensive view on the family. This model is applicable for nuclear families with growing children and families who are experiencing health-related problems.

1. *Physical maintenance*: provides food, shelter, clothing, and health care to its members. It means being certain that a family can provide ample resources.
2. *Socialization of family*: involves preparation of children to live in the community and interact with people outside the family.
3. *Allocation of resources*: determines which family needs will be met and their order of priority.
4. *Maintenance of order*: needs fulfilment includes opening an effective means of communication between family members, integrating family values and enforcing common regulations for all family members.
5. *Division of labor*: who will fulfil certain roles, for example family provider, home manager, children's caregiver.
6. *Reproduction, recruitment, and release of family members.*
7. *Placement of members into larger society*: consists of selecting community activities such as church, school, politics that correlate with the family beliefs and values.
8. *Maintenance of motivation and morale*: created when members serve as supportive people for each other.

16.3.3 Family communication: constructive or destructive?

The objective of effective family communication is the achievement of mutual understanding, so that the received message is the same as the intended message. The process of communication is essential to the fulfilment of the roles, because it is important for need fulfilment.

TABLE 16.2 Stages of family development and basic family needs

Stages of development	Basic family needs: Survival/affection/self-determination
Beginning families	Physical maintenance
Early childbearing	Allocation of resources
Families with pre-schoolers	Division of labor
Families with school children	Socialization of members
Families with teenagers	Reproduction, recruitment and release of members
Launching centre families	Maintenance of order
Middle-aged families	Placement of members in larger community
Aging families	Maintenance of motivation and morale

In addition, continuous role definition is exchanged throughout this communication. Satir described five communication stands, one constructive communication stand, the leveller and four destructive communication stands: the placator, the blamer, the computer and the distractor patterns. When there is stress within the family these communication stands can have a constructive or destructive impact for family members.

Leveller: constructive communication

The first adequate form of family communication is levelling (Satir, 1988). A leveller responds to situations congruently. In this stance, our body, voice and facial expressions all match. The relationship feels easy, free, and honest. A leveller apologizes when she makes a mistake. If an error has been made, she will evaluate fairly without blaming. Sometimes she will be talking intellectually, as when she is lecturing or explaining something, but her feeling is still intact. There is no machine-like feeling when dealing with this person. When there is a problem, she will deal appropriately rather than sweeping it under the carpet. A leveller conducts life with integrity, commitment and creativity. She is able to work out problems in a real way. Satir found that when people start to level, they find their hearts, feelings, bodies and brains. As a result they find their souls and humanity. The leveller is a stress reducer and strengthens self-esteem. This form of communication leads to personal growth. Like Laura Kiser (Kiser et al., 2010) stated it: 'The language of family storytelling can become the language of family hope.'

Satir describes four destructive (dysfunctional) communication stances where family members hide the reality of one's real feelings in different ways from oneself and from others. Real feelings of low self-esteem and low self-worth are communicated to other family members as they take on various incongruent communication roles. We follow the summary of the four stress-inducing communication styles as proposed by Satir (Rasheed et al., 2011).

Placator: destructive communication

The placator hides his or her feelings of low self-worth and vulnerability by attempting to please others, not because he or she really feels like it but because his or her emotional survival depends on it. The placator engages in apologetic, tentative and self-effacing communication that is designed to please others. In attempting to please others the placator tries to avoid rejection. This person also expends enormous emotional energy in serving as a mediator between family members in family disputes. The placator's primary interest in his or her mediation attempts is to assuage his or her own feelings of low self-esteem and self-worth by gaining the acceptance of other family members – resolving family disputes is only secondary to the placator's goal of pleasing other family members. To this end the placatory may, in fact, serve to block important communication attempts between members and thus serve to inhibit open communication. Consider the example of a mother who constantly intercedes in ensuing conflict between her husband and teenage son. While on the surface it may appear that her intentions are to resolve family conflict between two warring parties, in fact the outcome is that father and son are not allowed to work through their own dyadic issues. The mother's constant interception or interference has effectively blocked communication between father and son and impeded potential problem solving between the two parties.

Blamer: destructive communication

The blamer hides his or her feelings of low self-worth and vulnerability by attempting to control others and by disagreeing indiscriminately, thus giving himself or herself a sense of importance despite his or her inner feelings of loneliness and failure. The blamer engages in fault-finding, name-calling, and criticism. It is as if the blamer cannot feel good or secure about himself or herself without placing other family members in the 'one down' position. The result is often establishing dishonest communication in which the meta-communication is 'I am better than you, and my opinion is more important than yours. I am always right.' A father rules a family (and his wife) with an iron fist, seldom yielding (or even considering) the opinions or feelings of other family members. A significant portion of his communication with other family members is criticism, and he is never wrong. Even the wife is subject to his dictatorial style of relating, and at times he even criticizes her in front of the children.

Computer (super-reasonable): destructive communication

One who takes the computer or super-reasonable stance hides his or her own feelings by attempting to anaesthetize and insulate himself or herself from his or her true feelings. His or her response to family communication, especially family conflict, is often an intellectual or overly rational one – bypassing the (emotional) inner self. This posture conveys non-involvement and control – but the reality of the super-reasonable's inner feelings is one of (emotional) vulnerability. The impact on family communication is one in which inner feelings are downplayed or avoided altogether, encouraging other family members to do the same, hence impeding open and honest communication between family members. In a family wherein there is not much positive communication and considerable open conflict, an adolescent male attempts to hide his feelings of low self-worth and contempt for his parents – even from his siblings. His responses to their attempts to create a stronger affiliation is to ignore their complaints (of which he shares the same sentiment) and to attempt to justify the dysfunctional communication and open family conflict.

Distractor (irrelevant): destructive communication

One who takes the distractor or irrelevant stance handles family conflict and stress by pretending it is not there. Internally the irrelevant stance taker feels uncared for and alienated from the family. Hence he or she attempts to refocus family communication elsewhere from the present context or topic under discussion and away from inner feelings. The irrelevant stance taker will engage in tangential or even totally irrelevant verbalizations that serve to refocus attention away from the topic at hand. The impact on family communication can be one of incomplete communication, wherein important dialogue is not fully explored. Consider this example:

A young teenage girl is a member of a very male-oriented family in which females are not very highly valued. She feels like an outsider in this family, not even aligning herself with her mother (who spends her time trying to downplay family conflict and assuage hurt feelings, never confronting or affirming the children's feelings and opinions). The teenager responds to family conflict and tension by making jokes and being sarcastic in the heat of family disputes.

Virginia Satir did not see these five communication stances as rigid and unchangeable (Satir & Baldwin, 1983). Rather any family member can take on one or all of the dysfunctional communication stances under different circumstances or contexts. It is important to note here that Satir was not naïve in her understanding of environmental factors and the role that they can play in family problems. Rather, as a social worker, Satir was very well aware of the socio-politico-economic and cultural systems and how these systems can and do have a major bearing on family distress.

16.3.4 Family structure: constructive or destructive?

Successful task accomplishment involves differentiation and performance of various roles within a family structure. Constructive family structure is clear, humane, overt, up-to-date and flexible. Destructive family structure is covered up, superseded, 'inhumane', rigid and unchanging. Role performance requires three distinctive operations: (1) the allocation or assignment of specified activities to each family member; (2) the agreement or willingness of family members to assume the assigned roles; and (3) the actual enactment or carrying out of prescribed behaviours.

Structural family therapy assumes that the individual should be treated within the context of the family system. Salvador Minuchin (1967) is considered the founder of structural family therapy as it is practiced today. He became famous for his book *Families of the Slums* (1967). The overall goal of structural family therapists is to alter the family structure in order to empower the family to move towards functional ways of conducting or transacting family business and communications. Functional families are characterized by each member's success in finding the healthy balance between belonging to a family and maintaining a separate identity. One way to find the balance between family and individual identity is to define and clarify the boundaries that exist between the subsystems. A family may have several subsystems such as a spouse, sibling, and parent–child subsystem. Each subsystem contains its own subject matter that is private and should remain within that subsystem. Boundaries between subsystems range from rigid to diffuse. Diffused boundaries can lead to over-enmeshment. Rigid boundaries allow too little interaction between family members, which may result in disengagement. Families who understand and respect differences between healthy and unhealthy subsystem boundaries and rules function successfully. Families who do not understand and respect these differences find themselves in a dysfunctional state of conflict.

Most of what Minuchin learned was by observation and in collaboration with colleagues at a school for delinquent boys. He has been praised for rescuing family therapy from intellectuality and mystery. His pragmatic approach contributed both to understanding how families function and to productive interventions for correcting malfunctions in the family system. His style was to get the family to talk briefly until he identified a central theme of concern and the leading and supporting roles in the theme. Next he examined boundaries or family rules that defined the participants, the areas of responsibility, the decision making and privacy rules. The idea was to change the immediate context of the family situation, thereby changing family members' positions. His approach was both active and directive. He would shift the family focus from the identified client to the therapist to allow the identified client to re-join the family. When treatment is completed, the therapist moves outside the family structure and leaves the family intact and connected without the loss of individual family member identities.

Central to understanding family pathology and dysfunction are Satir's concepts of *family rules and roles*. Satir saw family rules and roles as a transgenerational issue; that is, rules from one's family of origin are passed down through one or several generations to the family of procreation – either consciously or unconsciously. Family rules and family roles are an important communication factor in family pathology. Within pathological families rules are expected behaviours that get woven in the 'family fabric'. Family rules encompass all the behaviours that family members believe should or should not be performed in a given situation. Satir also described family rules as being overt, but more often it is the covert messages that are accepted among family members. Family rules and roles can influence a family in an infinite number of ways and individual behaviours, such as communication patterns and styles, sharing of information, family rituals and routines, career choices, emotional rules, family myths and secrets, how to respond to family problems and dysfunction, and behaviours for various systems and subsystems (conjugal, parent–child, and sibling). Satir describes the concept of inappropriate and unhealthy roles in *Conjoint Family Therapy* (1983). Healthy, functional and adaptive family rules and roles are those that are clear, flexible and adaptive to the environment and changing developmental needs of the family and its individual members. On the other hand, dysfunctional family rules are rigidly enforced, autocratically developed and everlasting. Satir believed that rules restricting freedom of expression are especially instrumental in decreasing self-esteem and functionality. Satir sometimes referred to family rules and family roles as 'shoulds' and 'survival beliefs' that operate as benchmarks by which one can gain approval from one's family.

Control is the process by which family members influence one another (Steinhauer et al., 1984). Critical aspects of control include whether or not the family is predictable versus inconsistent, constructive versus destructive, or responsible versus irresponsible in its management style. Based on the exertion of control, families can be typified as rigid, flexible, laissez-faire or chaotic.

How needs are defined and how the family proceeds to accomplish them may be greatly influenced by norms and values of the culture in general and the family background in particular. Important elements include whether family rules are explicit or implicit, the latitude or scope allowed for family members to determine their own attitudes and behaviour, and whether family norms are consistent with the broader cultural context. In a two-parent family, each adult brings to the family a variety of background and developmental experiences, as well as values, goals and normative beliefs. From the beginning of the relationship, the couple begins the process of negotiating which of these will be predominant in their newly created family. Although it is unlikely that a couple will become unified in every matter, in the process of relating to each other over time they will typically develop a shared system of values, goals and normative beliefs. Family systems develop and refine their own unique culture, and individual family members are encouraged to subscribe to the shared views. Some ongoing disparity between the views of family members is to be expected, and perhaps beneficial. However, the greater the disparity between family members, with respect to values, goals and normative beliefs, the more likely there will be polarization and family conflict.

16.3.5 Family emotional involvement: constructive or destructive?

The kind of emotional involvement family members have with one another can either help or hinder needs fulfilment. A vital element of the involvement process is the expression of affect (affective expression). Critical elements of affective expression include content, intensity and timing of the feelings involved. Affective expression is most likely to become blocked or distorted in times of stress and leads to reduced involvement. This has consequences for the mutual attachment and involvement between family members.

Emotional involvement refers to both the degree and quality of family members' interest in one another. Other elements include the ability of the family to meet the emotional and security needs of family members while at the same time supporting the family members' autonomy of thought and function. Family members are better able to perform role duties and interact appropriately when they feel connected, safe and secure, and when their autonomy is respected by other family members. However, in order to maintain family functions, family members must exert influence on each other to perform their duties. The quality and degree of family members' emotional *involvement* with each other is another vital aspect of family functioning. Families can range from being emotionally uninvolved to being enmeshed.

EFT (Emotionally Focused Therapy) and its application to families, EFFT (Emotionally Focused Family Therapy) are distinguished by their unique combination of attachment theory, systemic theory, humanistic experiential theory and its particular focus on emotion in sessions to produce change (Efron & Bradley, 2007). EFFT is focusing on new attachment patterns characterized by mutual accessibility and responsiveness, and a strong emotional connection between partners and family members. For social workers this includes helping parents be more emotionally accessible and responsive to their children.

The focus of EFT is to create safety and secure bonding in relationships between spouses. This creation of a safe haven and a secure base in the relationship allows individuals to regulate emotion and to 'update' their internal models of bonding. It is this change in their ability to securely attach to a partner, parent, or child which allows them to hold onto new positive behaviour patterns which are developed in the course of the therapy. Secure relationships seem evident when each partner in the relationship can reach for the other and can acknowledge distress and offer reassurance and comfort. Ultimately, EFT is successful when new bonding patterns have formed and new positive cycles of interaction are entrenched.

Emotionally focused social workers operate on the assumption that the most important conflicts in couple and family relationships are best viewed through the lens of attachment theory. Each person in the relationship is seen as having their own attachment style and attachment history. The most hurtful conflicts in relationships develop out of the systemic interaction with loved ones in which themes of accessibility and responsiveness are aroused. Attachment bonds are emotional ties, and the EFT therapist focuses on how affect is processed in these key attachment-based interactions with those closest to us. In these repeated interactional cycles family members become disconnected from their loved ones over time. They become overwhelmed with deep feelings of being alone in relation to the ones they need the most. It is the task of the EFT therapist to understand the conflict in attachment terms and help couples and families reconnect with each other in a manner which leads to safe and secure attachment.

A major systemic aspect of EFT is that the damaging cycles resulting from negative emotional interactions over time and which result in a sense of disconnection and separation distress are seen as the enemy of all family members. The damaging cycle prevents safe, warm, loving reassurance in the relationship. These destructive patterns are constantly repeated and produce self-reinforcing cycles (such as 'attack–withdraw'), poor decision making, poor problem solving and poor communication. In this model, skill building in and of itself is not regarded as likely to change the patterns. Skill building only works if basic attachment themes are addressed first.

Emotionally focused social workers use emotional processing to create new interactional cycles between family members. Typically, sessions move from an initial conflict issue ('You didn't take out the garbage after you promised to do so') to the relationship itself ('I can't ever trust you') and then to deeper feelings of personal worth and worthlessness, inadequacy, love and being unlovable (attachment views of self and others). In EFFT a typical pattern might be that when parents and their teenage children are arguing over an issue such as curfews, at a deeper level the parents feel they are bad parents and the children feel they are bad kids. Emotionally focused social workers believe that with attachment injuries, focusing mainly on 'exceptions' is not in and of itself sufficient. It is the reworking of attachment-related affect inside and in between families that restructures emotional bonds. Exceptions are often important in a way that they can lead to emotional heightening and further processing of affect from a time when family members were able to successfully connect with each other. Working it out means that they can talk about the pain and the feelings of abandonment, isolation and being overwhelmed and that the others can hear it, accept responsibility and be comforting. When important attachment issues of disconnection emerge, emotionally focused social workers actively use enactments, asking the partners to turn and directly talk to each other, not just the therapist. This is usually done after they have first shared their thoughts and emotions with the therapist before the therapist asks them to turn and risk sharing with the partner. This is often difficult for partners but is essential to the development of safe and secure relationships. Emphasis is placed on each partner watching the face of the other as they speak so that the emotion beneath the words can be seen and understood. It should be noted that EFT is not interested in catharsis or emotional ventilation for its own sake but rather sees the processing of attachment-related affect as being a powerful means for creating new relationship patterns. These new patterns are characterized by mutual accessibility and responsiveness, and a strong emotional connection between partners and family members.

Emotionally focused social workers achieve change by focusing on the present interactions which occur in the room during the therapy sessions. They are interested in deep and recent history as a way of understanding their clients' beliefs and interaction patterns, but this knowledge is used to understand and change interactions in the present. The resolution of the past is to create new relationships in the present.

16.3.6 The history of the family method

A LOT OF FAMILY AND COMMUNICATION CONCEPTS ARE KNOWN ABOUT FAMILY SINCE THE BEGINNING OF THE 1970S

1 Content level and relational level of the communication: content is what you say and relational level of the message is what you expect of the other content level of communication.
2 Homeostasis: every family system strives for preservation of the existing balance.

---

3 Family life cycle: childless phase, expansion phase, stabilization phase, empty-nest phase, possible divorce or widowhood phase.

4 Circular causality: partners can blame each other in an argument, but can well both be the cause of the endless game. Partner 1: 'I'm no longer talking because you're constantly picking.' Partner 2: 'I get agitated because you're being so quiet.'

5 The multiple problem family: not only is money a problem, but there are fights and drinking problems as well.

6 The identified patient: the family member branded 'ill'.

7 The scapegoat phenomenon: one family member is blamed for everything.

8 Parentification: children fulfil parental roles.

9 Perverse triad: one parent 'conspires' with one of the children against the other parent.

10 Tangled families: a family that lacks a clear structure and where the family members are entangled.

11 Family myths: a family pattern which is preserved but does not correspond to reality.

Over the years there have been many schools of thought in relation to nuclear family therapy, including the Milanese school and the Palo Alto school. Over the last few decades, changes in society have resulted in significant changes within families as well. There is a higher divorce rate, with the direct consequence of a corresponding number of single-parent families. The phenomenon 'stepparent' seemed to have become extinct, but re-emerged with all the corresponding and complicated family problems, as did the concept of 'step-grand-parents'. Then there are the teen parents who are very often single, and a small group of solo mothers who choose to bring up their child(ren) by themselves. The traditional family, which consists of two parents and their own children, and where the father was the breadwinner, is now a minority group. Social workers originally fulfilled a prominent role in exploring the 'systemic field', nowadays they still do a lot of family work and with specialized training become a 'family therapist'.

The term 'family method' is derived from 'family therapy'. After a period of strong focus on individual help in the social work domain, a new idea was introduced in the 1960s. It stated that the family context itself can be a source of tensions and intervention. Experience showed that an individual client, who had shown progress after an individual conversation, could relapse into the old behavioural pattern after interaction with other members of the family. In those cases, the influence of the family context was stronger than the intervention of the social worker. It was considered whether it would be better to involve the nuclear family in the problem assessment and the intervention. At the same time, during the 1970s, the (semi-)residential treatment institutions such as children's homes and family guardianship institutions also came up with questions about how the parents of the admitted children could be involved in the treatment. People started to realize that every intervention in the system of a nuclear family had an influence on all family members. Eventually, this situation brought forwards the introduction of video home training in families. Video home training is the practice of more adequate family behaviour with the help of video feedback. Social workers have been engaged in family problems ever since the very beginning in 1898. Crisis, poverty and wartime caused it to be very difficult to make ends meet, and so many families got into big trouble. At the time, the sisters of social work supported families from the hospitals (in Catholic hospitals the word 'sister' was used to mean both 'nun' and 'nurse'). Similarly, the railroad companies employed corporate social workers to assist the families of employees in need. Back then their focus was mainly on solving money and housing problems rather than on family communication.

Family therapy as a distinct professional practice within Western cultures can be argued to have had its origins in the social work movements of the nineteenth century in the United Kingdom and the United States.

Family therapy in Europe began in 1965. The Canadian family sociologist Norman Bell held a first small course on family therapy for a small number of social workers working at the Dutch Medical Educational Agencies (later integrated in Riaggs and renamed Mental Healthcare Centres).

While visiting Europe in 1970, Walter Kempler, a prominent family therapist, dropped a bombshell among proponents of conservative family therapy when he presented his own Gestalt family therapy. Gestalt therapy was very direct and confronting. Other prominent figures in the field of family therapy followed suit soon after, including Salvador Minuchin (psychiatrist), Virginia Satir (social worker), Ivan Nagy (psychiatrist) and Carl Whittaker (psychiatrist). They discussed the different frames of reference in family therapy. Some had a confusing effect, while others were very stimulating.

Ever since 1970, more and more theories on family dynamics have been emerging. These theories asked questions such as: How does communication take place within nuclear families? What rules are being set? How do the family members experience the nuclear family? They posed other questions too, such as: Is it possible that the troublesome behaviour of an individual child or parent is only a normal reaction to the pathological communication within the nuclear family?, What is the effect on the nuclear family when they lose a parent due to illness, divorce or death?

In the Netherlands, Ammy van Heusden and Else-Marie van den Eerenbeemt introduced and propagated the contextual method over the course of the 1990s. Many social workers may stumble upon the obstructing and stagnating influence of one's past and present family situation in individual contacts as well. Social workers at the nursing home often have to deal with 'psychological family inheritance' when one of the parents is about to be admitted. Social workers in hospitals may have to deal with family members who will not agree on the illness process and decision making for the admitted parent. In their work around parenting problems, social workers may notice that the influence of parents' childhood traumas is simply passed on in the family. Understanding behaviour and influences can be facilitated by making a genogram to literally map the family. No one can tell exactly what family relationships are like nowadays, hence the research conducted in 1999 to investigate *The Binding Force of Family Relationships* (Dykstra, 1999). Do people feel liberated from galling family bonds, the much regretted social pressure from the 1970s? Are we currently facing extreme individualization, going hand in hand with dissociated relationships within families? What is the role of secularization and the disappearance of local communities in it? An American research conducted in 1970 on the Italian community of Rosetto, Pennsylvania, revealed that when family structure crumbled away, so did the corresponding feeling of safety and security (see section 14.5.1, Social support). The wellbeing of younger generations dramatically decreased after the collapse of the three-generation structure, while new generations had a healthier lifestyle and no bad eating or drinking habits in comparison to the older generations. The hypothesis is that the protective and de-stressing effect of the 'family clan' was an explanation for the increase in stress-related illnesses in new generations (see section 14.4).

Around the turn of the twenty-first century, more and more so-called family constellations were used during workshops. It was Hellinger who introduced family constellations as a technique for rendering unfinished business in the family context visible without involving the actual family members (2002). A family constellation, a tableau vivant, provides profound insight into yourself, the dynamics of the family system and the power of love steering human relationships. Three basic rules are used in family constellations:

1   *Belonging.* Everyone has the right to their own place. An example: when someone is being left out, very often another family member will do something in order to repair this imbalance, for example by contacting the 'outcast'.
2   *Respect the hierarchy.* This means that those who belonged to the family first are the highest in 'ranking'. The same thing goes for stepfamilies: the biological parent is closer to the child than the adoptive parent or stepparent. It is very important for the adoptive parent or stepparent to respect the biological parents.
3   *Balance of giving and taking.* In parent–child relationships this means that the parent gives, the child takes. The child gives love in return, and the parent takes. Between partners there must be balance in giving and taking.

Members of a system can subconsciously become tangled in the fate of others. This solidarity in fate is strongest between parents and children, brothers and sisters and partners. Apart from this solidarity, there is also a strong connection between members of a previous generation who have made room for the current generation. The objective of a constellation is to visualize entanglements between the client and other member of the family system. One form of entanglement is subconscious identification with someone in the family system who is being left out or disrespected. The client then subconsciously feels, thinks and behaves like that same family member. By doing so, he takes up the parents' or grandparents' task out of loyalty to the family system. For example when parents or grandparents haven't mourned over a child that passed away, or when a family member was left out because he was 'wrong' in the war, the child yet wants to give that person a place. The whole family system is only at peace when every member has its own place.

16.4 Goals

General goal

•   Getting rid of sources of tension in the family system.

Specific goals

•   The members of the nuclear family gain more clarity about everyone's position in the family relations.
•   The members of the nuclear family share a vision on the current situation, pressure points and blockades.
•   The nuclear family stabilizes when in a crisis situation.

- Mutual tensions are relieved within the nuclear family.
- The nuclear family reaches a consensus on topical matters.
- Hierarchy is restored within the nuclear family in case of parentification of the perverse triad.
- The arisen distance is decreased between the members of the nuclear family.
- The nuclear family gains a new and healthy balance which offers the possibility to allow the self-esteem of its members to grow.

16.5 Indications

- The family actually asks for treatment.
- Pressure points or blockades within the nuclear family, such as the inadequate open acknowledgement of a loss, the inadequate structuring of chaos, the inadequate orientation in new situations, a disrupted hierarchy or lots of mutual tensions.
- A family crisis, possibly caused by an event with an enormous influence on the nuclear family system.
- Family phenomena such as one member of the nuclear family acting as a scapegoat or lightning rod. Another possibility is the projective identification (when a child is forced by his or her parents to fulfil a 'substitution role', for example as compensation for a deceased brother or sister – and is threatened to be excluded otherwise), or the perverse triad (one parent conspires against the other parent with one of the children: the natural hierarchy in the parent–child relation is disrupted).
- The referring intermediary proposes the nuclear family to be treated together because of a dominant problem within the family.

16.6 Contraindications

- It is impossible to gather all members of the nuclear family together (e.g. because of the absence of important family members).
- Relationships within the nuclear family are far too disrupted.
- There is a lack of consent and/or motivation among family members to be treated together. Family members lack the consensus or motivation to engage in joint therapy.
- There is a lack of supportive strength within the nuclear family (chaotic or crisis situation). The nuclear family lacks supportive strength (chaotic or crisis situation).
- The presence of a dominant individual issue (money problems, an overly stressed mother).
- The presence of a dominant relational issue (huge tensions between the parents).
- The presence of a dominant family issue (multiple generation line, this means that the line between the different generations within the nuclear family is the cause of tensions).
- The nuclear family lacks motivation, for example because of the forced contact with aftercare and resettlement organizations or child protection agencies.

16.7 Techniques

1 Convening technique
2 Joining technique
3 Needs assessment technique
4 Wellbeing indicators technique

5   Communication technique
6   Addressing technique
7   Genogram technique
8   Restructuring technique
9   Rules setting technique
10 Turn taking technique
11 Multifaceted partiality technique
12 Family education technique
13 Absolution technique
14 Family constellation technique
15 All techniques indicated from other systemic and individual methods.

16.7.1 Convening technique

The issue of convening a family should be taken seriously (Burnham, 1986). Motivating a family to begin family meetings is the first and most crucial intervention to initiating systemic change. The social worker should attend to who is being convened ('the minimum sufficient network'), when to conduct family sessions (fixed or flexible sessions, how many sessions), where family meetings take place (at the agency, home visits), and how people are invited to participate (by letter, telephone, personal contact). A non-blaming stance on behalf of the social worker towards family members is recommended as essential to facilitate involvement. A range of convening strategies is offered ranging from enabling (encouraging family participation) to enforcing (using a non-negotiable contract or mobilizing the referring and linking networks to exert pressure on the family by threat of prosecution, hospitalization, discharge or expulsion in cases of severe child abuse or serious addiction issues). Social workers are urged to consider their agency context, legal mandate, and the severity of the stressors as important factors in making a choice of convening strategy.

16.7.2 Joining technique

The (temporary) joining of the social worker in the nuclear family can be seen as a way to close the distance by making contact (Lange, 2002). The joining technique called *mimicry* consists of joining in the language of the family, for example: 'You say that it really turns you off, what do you mean by that?' The joining technique called *tracking* consists of really going into the matter and asking follow-up questions about personal aspects, for example: 'What does this mean to you?' The joining technique called *support* consists of accepting the problem the way it is introduced by the client and asking follow-up questions about it. The social worker should never underestimate or trivialize the problem.

16.7.3 Needs assessment technique

The social worker observes the behaviours of members of the nuclear family and asks who has a problem with what and with whom, what views the different family members hold with regard to the problem and what everyone individually thinks should be done to meet family members' needs. For a needs assessment of children, social workers use the 'My World Triangle' (see Scottish government, http://www.gov.scot/Topics/People/Young-People/getitgitright/resources/girfec-diagrams). When working with children or young people, the

'My World Triangle' is used at every stage to think about the whole world of the child or young person. Using the 'My World Triangle' allows practitioners to consider systematically:

* How the child or young person is growing and developing;
* What the child or young person needs from the people who look after him or her;
* The impact of the child or young person's wider world of family, friends and community.

It is particularly helpful to use the 'My World Triangle' to gather more information from other sources (which may include specialist sources) to identify the strengths and pressures in the child or young person's world. This may include information about health or learning, offending behaviour or information about issues affecting parenting.

For example, under 'How I grow and develop', both the Named Person or Lead Professional and the child or young person are offered prompts and statements designed to encourage them to examine their learning and development and family life.

The 'My World Triangle' supports a practice that takes into account the child or young person's needs and risks, as well as the positive features in their lives. Strengths and pressures are given equal consideration and can be structured around the triangle. Information gathered should be proportionate and relevant to the issues at hand. In many cases, it will not be necessary to explore every area of the triangle in detail but only to look at those relevant to any presenting issue. However, it is still important to keep the child's or young person's whole world in mind and provide immediate help where necessary while continuing assessment.

The following checklist for assessing the needs of children and young persons may be used (see Table 16.3).

TABLE 16.3 Needs of children checklist

Needs of children and young people	Observations
1. Everyday care & help	*Safety needs*
This is about the ability to nurture which includes day-to-day physical and emotional care, food, clothing and housing. Providing access to/facilitating health care and educational opportunities.	
Meeting the child's changing needs over time, encouraging growth of responsibility and independence. Listening to the child and being able to respond appropriately to a child's likes and dislikes. Support in meeting parenting tasks and helping carers' own needs.	
2. Keeping me safe	
Keeping the child safe within the home and exercising appropriate guidance and protection outside. Practical care though home safety such as fire-guards and stairgates, maintaining hygiene. Protecting from physical, social and emotional dangers such as bullying, anxieties about friendships. Is the caregiver able to protect the child consistently and effectively?	
Seeking help with and finding solutions to domestic problems such as mental health needs, violence, offending behaviour. Taking a responsible interest in child's friends and associates, use of internet, exposure to situations where sexual exploitation or substance misuse may present risks, staying out late or staying away from home. Are these identifiable risk factors? Is the young person being encouraged to become knowledgeable about risks and confident about keeping safe? Are the child's concerns being listened to?	

Needs of children and young people	Observations

3. Being there for me

Love, emotional warmth, attentiveness and engagement. Listening to me. Who are the people who can be relied on to recognize and respond to the child's/ young person's emotional needs? Who are the people with whom the child has particular bond? Are there issues of attachment? Who is of particular significance? Who does the child trust? Is there sufficient emotional security and responsiveness in the child's current caring environment? What is the level of stability and quality of relationships between siblings, other members of the household? Do issues between parents impact on their ability to parent? Are there issues within a family history that impinge on the family's ability to care?

Affection needs

4. Play, encouragement, fun

Stimulation and encouragement to learn and to enjoy life, responsiveness to the child or young person's unique needs and abilities. Who spends time with the child/young person, communicating, interacting, responding to the child's curiosity, providing an educationally rich environment? Is the child's/ young person's progress encouraged by sensitive responses to interests and achievements, involvement in school activities?

Is there someone to act as the child's/young person's mentor and champion and listen to their wishes?

5. Guidance, supporting me to make the right choices

Values, guidance and boundaries. Making clear to the child/young person what is expected and why. Are household roles and rules of behaviour appropriate to the age and understanding of the child/young person? Are sanctions constructive and consistent? Are responses to behaviour appropriate, modelling behaviour that represents autonomous, responsible adult expectations. Is the child/young person treated with consideration and respect, encouraged to take social responsibility within a safe and protective environment? Are there any specific aspects which may need intervention?

Self-determination needs

6. Knowing what is going to happen & when

Is the child's/young person's life stable and predictable? Are routines and expectations appropriate and helpful to age and stage of development? Are the child's/young person's needs given priority within an environment that expects mutual consideration? Who are the family members and others important to the child/young person? Is there stability and consistency within the household? Can the people who look after her or him be relied on to be open and honest about family and household relationships, about wider influences, needs, decisions and to involve the child/young person in matters which affect him or her. Transition issues must be fully explored for the child or young person during times of change.

7. Understanding my family's background & beliefs

Family and cultural history; issues of spirituality and faith. Do the child's/young person's significant carers foster and understanding of their own and the child's background – their family and extended family relationships and their origins. Is their racial, ethnic and cultural heritage given due prominence? Do those around the child/young person respect and value diversity? How well does the child understand the different relationships, for example with step-relationships and different partnerships?

16.7.4 Wellbeing indicators technique

The assessment circle in Figure 16.5 focuses on the child and young person and what is needed for their development and wellbeing. Adults who are parents or carers may have needs or problems that could affect children, and these problems should be addressed also, using the Wellbeing Indicators to identify, record and share concerns, and take action as appropriate.

Social workers will use the Wellbeing Indicators (see Scottish government, http://www.gov.scot/Topics/People/Young-People/gettingitright/resources/girfec-diagrams) to identify risks. They will need to ask:

- What are the areas of a child's wellbeing that are causing concern?
- Why do I think, on initial contact with child and family, that this child is at risk?
- What have I observed, heard or identified from the child's history that causes concern?
- Are there factors that indicate this child is at immediate risk and, in my view, are those factors severe enough to warrant immediate action?

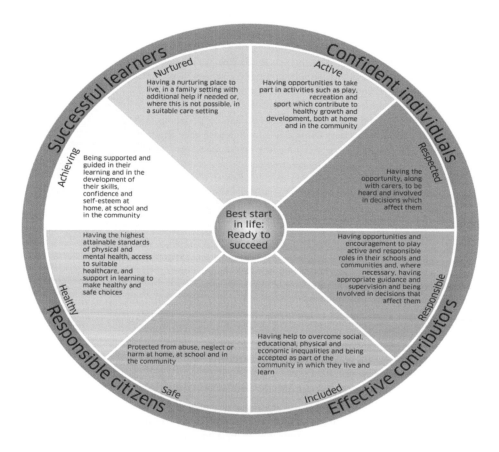

FIGURE 16.5 Wellbeing indicators

Image courtesy of the Scottish Government

Social workers should be able to identify, record and share information about concerns they have about a child at an early stage, without a situation reaching a state of crisis. If issues can be addressed when they present a low risk, it will be easier to change the situation for the better. Parents and children themselves may have worries. A concern can be an event itself, or a series of events or attributes, which affect the wellbeing or potential of a child. A concern might be an attribute or characteristic of someone associated with the child or a fact about someone associated with the child.

Social workers who have identified a concern then need to ask themselves the following five questions:

- What is getting in the way of this child's or young person's wellbeing?
- Do I have all the information I need to help this child or young person?
- What can I do now to help this child or young person?
- What can my agency do to help this child or young person?
- What additional help, if any, may be needed from others?

If the practitioner has sufficient information, help can be put in place.

16.7.5 Communication technique

The social worker pays attention to the extent of clarity and constructiveness in the actions of the sender in the communication (contact initiatives), both in the response of the receiver (confirmation of receipt) and in the interactions between the members of the nuclear family (taking turns in attention).

If the natural process of initiative and receipt is disrupted, the social worker trains the members of the nuclear family in basic communications. This basic communication contains positive family interaction, group discussions with the family and family consultation (Dekker, 1994a, 1994b). The social worker uses three communication techniques to practice this family communication:

1   The initiative/receipt technique
2   The group exchange technique
3   The consultation technique.

The *group exchange technique* (see also section 16.7.11) involves practicing in group interaction when the division of attention is out of balance. Group interaction involves natural turn taking to help every member of the nuclear family in finding his or her spot. Group interaction can be practiced using three patterns: forming a circle, turn taking and co-operation.

The *initiative/receipt technique* consists of the family practicing in being considerate to one another, looking at each other and using caring intonation, facial expression and positioning. Next up is the training in harmony (still under guidance of the social worker): the family members address one another and react in a positive way to the offering of the other family member. A part of this is the assenting identification: 'So you're saying that. . . .'

The *consultation technique* consists of practicing in the forming of an opinion, in giving content and in decision making. The forming of an opinion is the putting into words of opinions so that others can receive and understand them. Giving content means giving opinions on subjects which are of importance to family members, for example how a person looks, when he or she will be coming home, contacts with peers or conflicts which have occurred during the day. Decision making means making decisions on certain matters. Propositions are made, a consensus is reached and plans are adjusted.

16.7.6 Addressing technique

The social worker makes sure that old and present conflicts are being situated and addressed without a rift occurring, or else assists in such a way that a possible rift that occurred in the nuclear family is repaired. The 'no loss' technique is an example of this: trying to strive for win-win situations. (Gordon and Davidson, 1981). In case of reproach, accusation, fights, threats and aggression, the social worker points out the contradiction. This will cause a certain relief of tension. Letting the others finish and receiving/contrasting opinions contributes to the re-establishment of contact. If any 'old scores' emerge, the family member is encouraged to aim them at the appropriate person and to 'settle' them where they belong. One might use the example of a mother who had been terribly humiliated by her own mother, and who experienced this as an obstacle in the raising of her own children. The social worker proposes to put a few things on paper first, in the form of a letter, and to think about whether or not the client wants to communicate this to her own mother.

16.7.7 Genogram technique

When complicated relations warrant this, the social worker may propose to make a diagram or have the whole nuclear family draw it together. This so-called genogram (see Figure 16.6) shows the family structure and consists of a visual representation of relationships/relations across the multiple generations. This will show the composition of the family, who divorced whom, who is named after whom, who gave birth to which child and who is no longer alive. It also illustrates important facts in the family history, which are of direct importance for the present relationships. All this information is shown using the genogram technique. If the occasion presents itself to involve the family dynamics in the intervention, the family method is used.

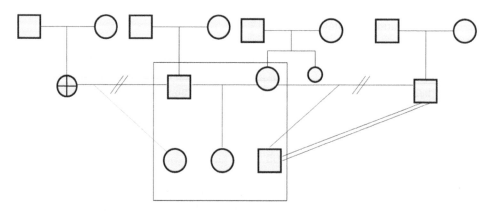

FIGURE 16.6 Example of a genogram

Source: de Mönnink (2015)

A genogram is created using simple symbols to represent gender and different styles of lines to illustrate family relationships (see Figure 16.7). Some genogram users also put circles around members who live in the same living spaces. Genograms can be prepared by using a complex word processor or a computer drawing program. There are also computer programs that are custom designed for generating genograms.

Genogram symbols will usually include the date of birth (and date of death if applicable), and the name of the individual underneath. The inside of the symbol will contain the person's current age or various codes for genetic diseases or user-defined properties: abortions, stillbirths, sudden infant death syndrome, cohabitations and so forth.

One of the advantages of a genogram is the ability to use colour-coded lines to define different types of relationships such as family relationships, emotional relationships and social relationships. Within family relationships, you can illustrate if a couple is married, divorced, living in a de facto relationship, engaged and so forth (see Figure 16.8).

Emotional relationships

Genograms may also include emotional relationships. These provide an in-depth analysis of how individuals relate to one another. Colour-coded lines represent various emotional relationships that bond individuals together (see Figure 16.9).

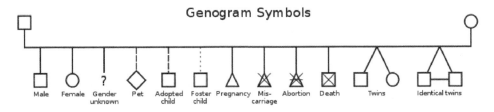

FIGURE 16.7   Genogram symbols

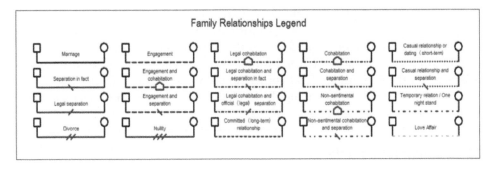

FIGURE 16.8   Family relationship legend

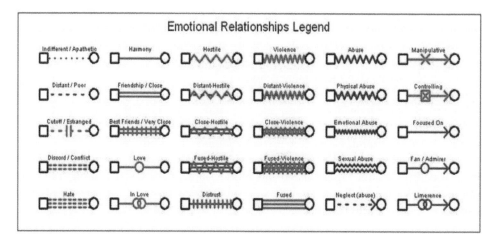

FIGURE 16.9   Emotional relationship legend

16.7.8 Restructuring technique

The social worker works on reorganizing the nuclear family structure (the family home) when one or more family members do not know their position: there is a disruption of the hierarchy, parentification, a perverse triad, a scapegoat, family myths and tangled families without a sense of structure.

Finding these unhealthy patterns and pointing them out to the nuclear family is only half of the solution. The resistance is being assessed by the social worker by thinking things over and establishing ways finding out how a positive family change can be realized. The social worker teaches the nuclear family to function as a 'system': in order to build a safe house in a step-by-step, meticulous and structured manner (van der Pas, 1992). Tangled interaction patterns are untangled and made supple again; doors that were closed are now re-opened. Destructive forces are put to an end, walls are shored up, pieces are collected and glued back together. That's how oppressive language is put to a halt, and how we fall back on the positive motives why people are together.

16.7.9 Rules setting technique

The social worker indicates the rules for constructive family communication by setting an example. For example the rule of equal participation: there are not just the talkers and the silent ones, but everyone contributes to the conversation equally. The rule of safety: everything personal that is said remains within the room. The rule of freedom: there is no obligation on the personal level, do not feel forced to do anything when someone else asks you or tells you to. Maintaining these rules is an exercise in creating a safe family environment.

16.7.10 Turn taking technique

The social worker ensures that everyone can have their say when it comes to the important themes. This can be realized by taking turns, where one nuclear family member is given the first turn and passes it randomly to another family member who has yet to speak. This keeps the conversation brisk because of the relative unpredictability of who is to speak next and it maintains the focus on who has or has not had his or her turn as yet. This ensures that absolutely everyone has a turn. Always taking turns in the same order can quickly become boring and can increase tensions.

16.7.11 Multifaceted partiality technique

The social worker must be able to focus on all family members with great flexibility. He lets them take turns in telling their stories and supports them in it. The social worker is no longer the confidential advisor of just one family member, but focuses on stimulating adequate communication between several family members. He successively takes sides for every individual family member. While doing so, the social worker acknowledges the feelings and interests of several clients. Rancour and rage can be transformed into terms of desire, trust and responsibility through the social work intervention.

16.7.12 Family education technique

In case of family tensions and feuds, the social worker can rely on '*Eerste hulp bij familievetes*' ('first aid in family feuds') (Vermeulen, 2001), which consists of the following tips:

- Even though reproaches are burning in your mouth, it's better to swallow them rather than spit them out.
- Try to keep in touch in a positive way, however minimally it may be. A birthday card can smooth out ruffled feathers, as can a gift for a new mother in the 'opposite camp' or a flower to congratulate on attaining a new job.
- It shows great class not to involve your children in the feud. 'Grandmother and I have a difference of opinion, but that doesn't mean you are no longer welcome.'
- When you take someone into your confidence, be honest, be objective and don't forget that you play a role in the conflict as well.
- Write a letter where you let it all out, read it carefully and then throw it away. Then write another letter, briefly and objectively summarizing what went wrong according to you and why you wish to change the situation. Send that letter to the other person. Even though you get no response, at least you have reached out and that provides peace of mind.
- Are you more of a spectator than a participant in the conflict? Keep it that way: impartial people are the best mediators in a later stage.
- If the other person truly doesn't want to make amends, there is nothing else to do than to accept it. Urging a reconciliation may only further escalate the conflict and nobody is waiting for that to happen.

16.7.13 Absolution technique

The social worker puts effort in making guilt-ridden subjects discussable, so that the involved family members' feelings of guilt and shame can be taken into account (Visser, 1997). It seems difficult to broach the traumatic past history without the parents experiencing it as 'getting the blame': 'You mean that I am the one who caused this?' Feelings of guilt and shame may be very close to the surface. Sometimes they are so strongly perceptible to the social worker, that the past history is preferably kept quiet. As a social worker it may be a good start to explain the possible consequences of traumatization. The social worker can link the parenthood-related behaviour and emotions to experiences from the past. Sometimes this can be done concretely and with much details, sometimes only vaguely: 'It is hard to raise children without having had a proper example yourself.' It clarifies problems in a supportive way while providing absolution, and it makes talking about the problems easier. Such a conversation can be very relieving for family members.

16.7.14 Family constellation technique

The family constellation technique (Hellinger, 2002) can only be used in groups. In this technique, the social worker asks representatives (participants from the group) to take the place of actual family members. The 'real' family members are not present. Then the representatives are positioned in the room as they are positioned in relation to each other in real life. The client determines the positioning, as he wants to figure out his own family relationships in order to break free from them. From this family constellation, the representatives are asked how they feel about having this position in the family context. Changes are proposed to determine whether stuck family patterns and corresponding frictions can be solved. The family constellation technique can also be performed with a drawing or by using dolls.

16.7.15 All techniques indicated from other systemic and individual methods

Using nuclear family techniques the social worker assesses all the time if techniques from other methods are indicated, for example *individual* methods:

- Suppressing grief/fear/anger? Indication for cathartic work method (Chapter 12);
- Denial? Insufficient insight into problem? Questioning the meaning of life? Indications for non-directive counselling method (Chapter 10);
- Information deficiency/unrealistic thinking? Indication for cognitive work method (Chapter 11);
- Financial/housing/employment stressors? Practical-material work methods (Chapter 13);
- Physical stress/vulnerability? Bodywork method (Chapter 14);
- Socially clumsy/unassertive/aggressive? Behavioural work method (Chapter 15);
- Inadequate verbal skills? Expressive work method (Chapter 16);
- Traumatic experience? Trauma-work method (Chapter 17);
- Insufficient ability to say goodbye/create distance? Ritual work method (Chapter 18).

But also *systemic* methods can be indicated, in combination with the nuclear family method:
- Stress within relationship? Relational work method (Chapter 19);
- Desire for mediation? Mediation method (Chapter 20);
- Stress within extended family? Extended-family work method (Chapter 22);
- Loneliness/isolation? Social-network method (Chapter 23) or group work method (Chapter 24);
- Am I normal?/Am I the only one? Social network method (Chapter 25);
- Insufficient case-coordination between professionals? Case management method (Chapter 25).

16.8 Social work results

- The members of the nuclear family have a clearer view of each other's position.
- The members of the nuclear family experience more stability after a crisis.
- The members of the nuclear family experience a more relaxed feeling within the family.
- The members of the family come to several agreements about tricky problems.
- The members of the nuclear family now find themselves in a new and healthy balance with one another.
- The members of the nuclear family experience more mutual proximity.
- The members of the nuclear family gain more clarity about a new start, a break or a divorce.

16.9 Evidence

Gurman et al. (1986) give a brief overview of a study which examined the process and outcome of marital and family therapy in a report titled *Research on the Process and Outcome of Marital and Family Therapy*. The 10 conclusions they draw from this meta-study of all research studies conducted in the field of marital and family therapy from 1970 until 1984 are summarized as follows:

1. Marital and relation therapy (not on a behavioural therapeutic basis) have a more favourable effect in two-thirds of the cases and the effects are better than when there is no treatment at all.
2. If both partners are involved in the treatment for relational issues, there is a larger chance of obtaining a positive result than when only one of the partners is treated.
3. The developmental stage of the identified patient (e.g. a child, adolescent or adult) does not significantly influence the results of the treatment.
4. Positive results in both marital and family therapy are obtained specifically with short-term treatments of 1–20 sessions.
5. Marital and family therapy can cause disruptions in both the individual (identified patient) and the relational sense.
6. The style of a practitioner who lacks structure during the first sessions and who confronts the patients with emotional matters has a disruptive effect on the partner or family involved. This in contrast to the healing effects of a style of treatment, which is more interaction-enhancing and supportive.
7. Family therapy is probably as effective and probably even more effective than the usual – and in most cases individual – treatments for family-related problems.
8. There is no empirical support for the superiority of treating families in co-therapy (with two therapists) in comparison to family therapy with just one family therapist.
9. An average mastery of technical skills seems to be sufficient to prevent aggravation, or to consolidate the problem level of the family for the family therapy. For real improvements in family functioning, however, more refined therapy skills are required.
10. A number of specific family variables – for example the identified patient, the quality of family interaction – cause impact studies to be unreliable.

In a follow-up study, these conclusions still seemed to be valid. There are no reasons whatsoever to presume that family interventions conducted by social workers would produce different results. After all, they use the same family techniques and disciplines as psychologists and psychotherapists within a family therapy setting.

The Family Assessment Measure (FAM III) is underpinned by a large body of research and has well-established psychometric properties (Skinner et al., 2000). It has been used to study the relationship of family functioning with regard to a number of child and family difficulties, including school phobia (Bernstein and Garfinkel, 1988; Bernstein et al., 1990), emotional disturbance (Blackman et al., 1986), and coping with disease (Cowen et al., 1985).

16.10 Pitfalls

Some of the pitfalls of FAM III include the following:

- The social worker may be unilaterally biased.
- The social worker may overlook the individual, positional or other systemic problems and continues (alone) to focus on the family for too long.
- The social worker may be too quick to exclude one of the nuclear family members and consider him or her to be deficient.
- The social worker may get too involved in the family phenomena and may therefore not keep enough critical distance.
- The social worker may underestimate the proper parallel process (counter-transfer). For example the social worker himself or herself comes from a family where there was a lot of quarrelling and is immediately irritated by the quarrelling in the family.

16.11 Summary

First, a definition was given of the core concepts and the dynamics between nuclear families and extended families. A plea was made to move from a deficit vision to a strength vision when working with families, and to consider any stumbling blocks/issues from a family-focused perspective as well. After that, the Growth in Family Functioning Model (GFFM) was detailed and the five factors of this family model were clarified: needs fulfilment, communication, structure, emotional ties, and as a result the self-esteem of family members improving or stagnating. After that, the history of the family method was detailed as well as the objectives, indications, contraindications and techniques for the family method. Following that, evidence supporting the effectiveness of the family method was detailed, as well as potential pitfalls.

Questions

1   Using either in a case study or your own personal situation, assess the status of the four support competencies of the support wheel.
2   Try completing the support checklist in Table 14.4, using either a case study or your own personal situation as a point of departure. What do I need from my family to optimally meet my human needs?

17

GROUPWORK METHOD

Questions

This chapter addresses the following questions:

- What is the importance of the group work method?
- How has the group work method developed in the history of social work?
- What is seen as alienation and what is seen as the group work method?
- Which social network techniques exist?
- How does the group work method contribute to meeting present needs on a safety, affective, and self-determination level?
- What evidence is there for the group work method?

17.1 Introduction

The empowerment formula of social workgroups:
Empowerment = contact + awareness + action.

(de Mönnink, 2016)

In this chapter, the group work method is detailed as a means to optimize clients' Quality of Life (QoL) through contact with peers.

First, a description will be given of the group work method. An in-depth look will be taken into the supporting aspects of a group of peers in meeting their human needs. This is followed by a discussion of the techniques utilized in the group work method and its results. Finally, a summary will be given.

The case of Mr. Stack

In eight social work sessions, Mr. Stack shared the disruptive effects of his loss, recognized the meaninglessness of the life events and given it a place. For decades he carried the tension surrounding his unexpectedly stillborn son and his second son becoming disabled. He did not even share the grief with his wife.

The social network analysis shows that Mr. Stack feels alone. It is therefore suggested that he join a volunteer group engaged in reducing the barriers on city provisions. This increases the possibility of him sharing his story and gives him a meaningful way to spend his time, improving access to city provisions.

17.2 Definition of concepts and elucidation

The 'group method' will, through a group approach, strengthen the client's perceived support by fellow patient contacts. If there is a lack of effective support from the client's own informal social network, then the group method is offered. Konopka (1963) defines social group work as 'a method of social work, in which the individual can be helped to improve social functioning by means of targeted group experiences, in order to deal with their personal, group or society problems in a more effective way.'

With the group method, people in similar situations are invited to meetings. They will form a group that formerly did not exist: an artificially created system where connectedness is created by means of a specific theme. The method is therefore also a systemic method, aimed to promote mutual support.

Elucidation

The group method is used by social workers in many forms: social group work, therapeutic group work as well as community work and self-help or support groups. The group method is therefore – in accordance with the wide variety of groups that social workers are engaged in – used in many different ways.

- General social work deals with grief and divorce groups with the emphasis on processing emotions and future prospects.
- Social workers in schools use parent and child groups as a way of parental counselling as well as to give support on emotional recovery after disability.
- Rehabilitation workers will offer rehabilitating patients (and partners) the opportunity to take part in groups such as partner groups for stroke patients, 'balance and recovery' groups for cancer patients, groups for patients with pain, discussion groups about rheumatism or groups where people learn how to deal with stress.
- Corporate social workers can, apart from offering group care, also give stress courses for groups after a shocking event.
- Social workers that focus on people with a disability make use of social skills groups (SSG) as well as the so-called loss groups for people who deal with a loss, for example

after the death of a partner or child. They can also make use of groups that focus on the loss of physical or sensory functions such as paralysis or loss of vision.

- Social workers in nursing homes can organize and supervise partner groups for partners of people with dementia.
- In the context of prevention, the group method is also used by social workers for various different purposes: education, training and processing emotions.

It is not remarkable that for social work in groups, the social worker leading the groups should also be well trained in working at a one-on-one basis and preferably in one-on-two situations. The idea behind it is that the group members experience a rich array of methods from the social worker's point of view (thus deepening both individual interventions as well as systemic interventions).

17.3 History of the group work method

The history of social group work has, since the last decades of the nineteenth century, always been closely linked to social work institutions that were created for the needs of the population. The group work started as a kind of idealism; it was dedicated to improve the quality of life in areas such as employment, housing shortage and leisure. After World War II the group method played an important role in promoting acceptance of democratic values within social work. Coyle (1948) saw group work as a tool for social transformation. Others saw group work as a means of participation in social change, community decision making and having a say on social issues. During the 1950s the emphasis shifted from group work towards empowerment of clients and the function of therapeutic groups. The writings of Konopka in the 1940s and 1950s (collected in 1963) formed a strong incentive to a more therapeutic approach. Vinter (social worker; Vinter & Galinski, 1967) speaks about three intervention options in his group method, focusing on individual, group and society.

1 Direct influence on the individual client in the group;
2 Indirect influences by stimulating active processes within the small group;
3 Stimulating the social environment of the participating clients.

In the 1960s and 1970s working in groups was strongly stimulated by so-called sensitivity training with encounter groups and growth groups. Growth groups are characterized by the emphasis on personal awareness. For each individual method a group variety sprung up as well, with group methods such as group psychoanalysis, behavioural therapy or Rogerian counselling. Shaffer and Galinsky (1977) provide a clear overview of the existing groups at the time: behavioural group therapy, psychoanalytic group therapy and existential-experiential group therapy. Relationship therapies were also applied in group form (Nevejan, 1985). In the 1970s and 1980s, in social-communal group work, there was a distinction between two different models: the Vinter model and Schwartz model.

The key difference between these models is that the Vinter model is a correction model while the Schwartz model is a problem-solving model. In 1967 Robert Vinter wrote the article 'Program Activities: An Analysis of Their Effects on Participant Behaviour', and is therefore seen as a representative of the 'correction model' in social group work. Vinter emphasizes with the correction model – also referred to as the 'preventive and rehabilitative' model – the remedial treatment of individual behaviour through 'small-group processes'. For participants in psychiatry and justice he continued to offer group therapy as way to effectuate socially acceptable behaviour. The social worker was playing, in his view, an active and directive role in organizing the group as well as the group meetings by introducing 'standard behaviour'. In 1971, William Schwartz wrote in his article, appropriately titled 'Social Group Work: The Interactionist-Approach' about his 'interaction model' in group social work. In this model – which is much more based on systems theory – group processes are used for many purposes, such as therapy, socialization and social ideals. The group is seen as a microcosm by Schwartz – a playground of society where group members give each other mutual assistance.

The group social worker applies his knowledge about the functioning of individuals and groups in an orderly and competent manner. He does so according to schedule: assessment, defining objectives, planning, intervention and evaluation. He assists participants in defining their issues, making sure the group theme stays the focus of attention. He guides efforts to come to a solution through, for example, role-playing and discussion. In the 1980s and 1990s, the group method focused on emancipation with women's support groups, men's groups, anti-racism groups, support groups for single women on welfare and so on. Van Riet (1987) defines emancipation as 'a process in which a subject is heading, from a situation that is regarded as negative, to a polyvalent situation'. Group social workers should focus their activities on initiating awareness-raising activities among the people they work with (Van Riet, 1987). These awareness processes are prerequisites to achieve emancipation, to get a grip on its own existence. The emancipation groups worked on freeing members of dominant social patterns that brought a sense of alienation. The following suppression formula was used in the so-called radical therapy practice groups (Wyckoff, 1979).

Alienation = oppression + lies + isolation

Time and again participants came to groups which were full of 'self-loath and self-reproach' (Wyckoff, 1979). A process of liberation was accomplished through teamwork and through group action aimed at changes and overcoming oppression. A process of awareness was needed by 'exchanging ideas to combat lies (you've done it yourself, it's your own fault) and by making contact with others for support and to eradicate isolation'.

The liberation formula was:

Liberation = contact + awareness + action

Groups work through 'radical therapy' practice groups, which liberate through the mixture of:

- Contact with others in similar positions (e.g. women);
- Awareness of personal and collective oppression (e.g. women who are stuck at home, getting less salary for doing the same work as men, the right to abort);
- Campaigning to fight injustice (e.g. walking the streets fighting for women's rights, 'boss in your own belly' and 'equal pay for equal work').

Freire and Cohn also emphasize the emancipatory objective in their group method. Freire talks about the pedagogy of liberation. According to Paolo Freire (1972, lawyer and educator) people in disadvantaged situations have a naïve consciousness (the dominant group is bigger, stronger and more powerful), and through learning by experience in groups they can come to critical consciousness and ultimately achieve emancipation. Freire uses the terms 'problematize' and 'codification', group techniques which are explained in more detail in section 17.7. The discovery of people's own history and the close relationship with one's own culture is the purpose of his method. Ruth Cohn (1979, psychoanalyst and group therapist) developed her Thematic Interactional Method (TIM, see section 17.7). The term 'living learning in groups' is hers. People can learn in a group through use of a theme, by sharing experiences and by achieving both personal and social awareness. In modern social work, the non-existence of the group method is unimaginable. On the website of BPSW (the Dutch Association of Social Workers), many different types of social group work are found.

17.4 Goals

General goal

- Reducing or taking away sources of tension with the individual client and in the group (as a microcosm for practicing social skills).

Specific goals

- Allowing the client to achieve individual progression;
- 'De-individualizing' the situation of the client by identifying with peers and learning from each other;
- Offering the client possibilities for socializing (social contacts).

17.5 Indications

- The desire of clients to participate in a group;
- The desire for contact and recognition by peers;
- Questions of clients, such as 'am I the only one?';
- Observations by the social worker noticing comparable problems with several clients;
- Observations by the social worker noticing a lack of social skills (such as assertiveness, sharing emotions, etc.).

17.6 Contraindications

- Inadequate conditions for a group: there is no second counsellor available, there is no suitable working space or there are insufficient funds;
- A group that is either not homogeneous enough or too heterogeneous;
- There are problems concerning individual dominance;
- There are problems with a dominant relationship;
- There are problems regarding dominance within a family.

17.7 Techniques

1 Scripting technique
2 Sandwich technique

3 Group crisis intervention
4 Group phase technique
5 Thematic interactional technique
6 Reflecting team technique
7 Aquarium technique
8 Task-oriented technique
9 Amusement technique
10 Role-playing technique
11 Problematizing technique
12 Codification technique
13 Individual and systemic techniques.

17.7.1 Scripting technique

For creating and starting a group in social work, a number of required preparatory and organizational activities are needed, which are recorded in a script. The scripting technique is an indirect technique (without client contact) which is essential for the success of this group method. The first steps are about setting up goals, defining the target audience and designing a layout. The next steps are about organization through recruitment (for example through leaflets and publicity); a space needs to be selected and the budget and finances need to be discussed. These components of the script for a social group work are described in a checklist.

Group work checklist

*   Defining the goals of the group. The goals for a bereavement group are, for example 'providing support for bereaved people through fellow sufferers' and 'how to prevent getting stuck in mourning'.
*   Determining the target audience. The target group can be widows or widowers of age. Decisions must be made regarding the composition of the target audience (will it be a heterogeneous or homogeneous group, or only young, only old or mixed ages?), the place of residence of the participants or the time that has elapsed since the passing (at least six months and up to three years after the death).
*   Determining the purpose. Decisions need to be made about the number of participants (6–12 participants, but the ideal is 8–10), the moderation (preferably two discussion leaders, two volunteers, or one volunteer and one professional) and the number of meetings (determine, for example if 10 meetings are satisfactory). Decisions also need to be made about the duration of each session (e.g. 2 hours or 2.5 hours), the frequency of the meetings (weekly, bi-weekly, or in the beginning weekly and then bi-weekly), and whether or not should there be a follow-up meeting to check how the participants are doing.
*   Determining the budget. Remember to include paper, envelopes, stamps, computer use, telephone use, printing leaflets, coffee, travel and videotape rental. The cost of books, rent of the accommodations, photocopying, insurance against damage of and accidents with the venue, contributions of the participants, donations and subsidies should also be included.

- Securing the venue. Think of things like rent, availability, accessibility, appropriateness, cosiness, drinks, availability of toilets and comfortable furniture.
- Taking care of recruitment and publicity. Think about things like including leaflets with the letters and publicity via the media, but also recruitment through referrals and network contacts.
- Identifying registration and admission of participants. For example, those interested can call a central point and make an appointment for an intake or will receive a guarantee for a call back.
- The intake consists of a number of elements: the introduction, a test to see what the expectations of the participant are, questions to see whether or not the person can be admitted to the group, agreements and a conclusion.
- Rejection and referral. When someone cannot be admitted to the group, it would be fair to discourage participation. The condition of that person is likely better suited for a different approach, for example, an individual contact with a fellow social worker or another professional. This requires a social card.
- Determining group moderation. The social workers who will lead the group will substantively prepare themselves by means of training. They will set dates and times for the group meetings; they will have had the necessary participation calls, and will have ordered the required materials (such as books for the reading table). They also will be taking care of the first group meeting as well as the evaluation forms.
- Establishing a task list containing the date, task and supplies. Certain elements of the task list are designing a leaflet, the execution of the design, investigating publicity channels, discussing the venue space and so on.

17.7.2 Sandwich technique

The social worker makes sure that each meeting runs in a structured, orderly fashion. One can think of the structure of a sandwich: a clear start, a clear deepening in the central part of each meeting and a clear final phase (see also section 4.7.4, Sandwich technique). In the beginning, participants are welcomed and the rules are explained (see section 4.7.3, Safeguarding confidentiality technique), a check-in is done to report everyone's presence and a topic is introduced. In the central part of the meeting the social worker will explore the topic in an in-depth manner, and in the last part the meeting finalized with a final round or a final ritual.

17.7.3 Group crisis intervention

Better check it out, then pull it out!

This checklist is used in accommodating a group of people who are involved in an impressive or traumatic experience. Requirements: an undisturbed and safe space, a circle of chairs, coffee/tea, care for the inner person, pen, paper, list of phone numbers, this group care checklist. Experience in individual and group care is required.

Sandwich structure of the group care: start → middle → completion

The start of group care

Three rules:

1 *Confidentiality*: what happens here on a personal level is confidential and stays within these walls.
2 *Equality*: everyone has an opportunity to tell his story. Each person may have many different stories, and that is OK.
3 *Ease*: there is no 'must'; do not pull things out, but check out how things are for everyone.

The central area of the group care

- *Factual reconstruction per person*: chronologically ordering the facts: Where were you just before it happened? Did you have a role in the event? What happened then? What was the first thing you saw? What did you do? How did the events evolve? Is there anything else? Finalization?
- *Map*: if desired, a picture can be drawn of the incident.
- *Reconstruction of experience per person*: we are going through the whole incident again and are going to look closely at each personal impression or impact the incident had. Did something emotionally touch you during the event? If so, what was it? Were there basic emotions that surfaced, like fear, anger or sadness? Were you able to express those emotions?
- Let each person tell their story, discharge emotions, exchange feelings, complete puzzles, ask questions, give answers, and the last question should always be: 'do you feel OK now?' Then somebody else should get a turn to say something about the incident.
- *Raising awareness*: trauma characteristics, personal filing cabinet, normal reactions, explaining how the process progresses, being vulnerable. But also multiple re-experience, avoidance and increased vigilance, prognosis.
- *Summary*: passing the red thread, including that there are individual differences, which are always there by definition and allowed to be there. Are there new questions and comments?
- Possibly a *new round*. Or otherwise closure of this round: is it OK to close this round. . . ?
- *Identify* if there are others that need more attention.

Completion of the group care

- *Final round*: I suggest doing a check-out round, where everyone can express in the end how this care ends for him or her. 'Do you want to start and pass your turn when you're done?'
- *Confidential*: after check-out round, emphasize confidentiality again and appreciation for the fact that everyone has taken the trouble to come.
- *Individual conversation*: 'If you need further information or you have other questions, you can always come and talk to me.'
- *After-effects*: be aware that you may need some time to let the incident settle. Sometimes unexpected images pop up, or emotions, or you don't want to think about it, want to go back to work like normal, or feel that you are irritable: know that these are, for a while, normal reactions to an abnormal event.

- *Follow-up:* 'Is it enough for you? Does it seem like a good idea to repeat the group care in a week? Is it wiser to put our heads together again in a few days, or a week. When should we do that?'
- *Instructions:* try to relax as much as possible but do periodically address the incident again. What can help is to talk about it to your colleagues, your spouse or a good friend. But do not keep addressing it all the time. Bodily and mental relaxation is also easily obtained through playing sport.

17.7.4 Group phase technique

The social worker takes into account the phase which the group is in at the moment. Tuckman (1965) summarized the following stages: forming, storming, norming, performing and mourning.

- *Forming* or working on group formation: the social worker provides an active introduction and aims to create safe and educational group tasks for all members so they can overcome their initial doubts, fears and so on.
- *Storming* or working on so-called group storms: as the group begins to form there will also be participants who have doubts about the benefits of the group and they might get angry about matters that annoy them (after getting questions answered such as: 'who are we?' and 'what are we looking for here?'). The social worker secures the group progress by participants who are 'stirring', not by attacking them, but by discussing the topic openly in the group. Also when roles begin to form, such as talkers and non-talkers, open communication is the device.
- *Norming* or working on norms: when the group has formed, members try to manifest their roles and values in relation to the rest of the group. If there is more commitment (engagement), the norm also becomes clearer. By having an open discussion (e.g. about arriving late to group meetings) the norms are being addressed by the social worker.
- *Performing* or working on tasks: the social worker encourages the group to work on its existing central group tasks.
- *Mourning* or working on saying goodbye: the social worker guides the process of ending the group and all related feelings of farewell that come with saying goodbye. Attempts to keep on seeing each other and reunions should be supported by the social worker, but it should also be made clear that the group was temporary and it will stop now. If members of the group want to continue seeing each other socially in real life, later on without supervision, then this continuation should be made possible by thinking along with the group members.

17.7.5 Thematic interactional technique

The thematic interactional technique (Cohn, 1979), works with the 'I-We-It' triangle (Figure 17.1). According to this triangle the theme (e.g. emotions of grief) is being deepened in an experiential way (the 'I' level: what emotions did I have?), a group-oriented way (the 'We' level: what emotions do we already know from each other as a group?), on a theoretical level (the 'It' level: what information is available in literature about emotions?) and on an environmental level (the 'global' level: what do we already know about emotions in the world through stories in the neighbourhood, or through television and radio?).

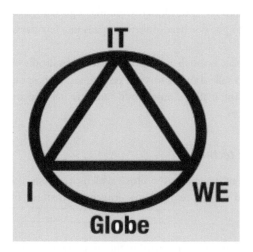

FIGURE 17.1 The I-We-It triangle

An effective group method according to Cohn consists of the balance in giving attention to these four aspects. When a social worker tends to dwell on the 'It' level in the group for too long, he will notice boredom and saturation. A social worker who dwells too long on one member in the group (the 'I' level) finds that others will detach. A social worker who lets a group discussion go on for too long (the 'We' level) will find that group members will drop out. And a social worker who stays on the subject of society in general or the direct neighbourhood (the 'global' level) will also notice that the group stops being interested.

The principles of this technique are:

- Be your own chairman (steer your own learning process).
- Speak in the first person form (instead of 'they', 'we' or 'you').
- Formulate the objective behind your question (explain why you ask a question).
- Disturbances have priority (if there is something distracting going on, give attention to it so that it disappears into the background).
- Only one person at a time can speak (let others finish talking).

With the deepening of each theme in accordance to the principles a learning process of the participants is being established.

17.7.6 Reflecting team technique

With the reflection technique the social worker gives a demonstration of a personal conversation with the group. This technique is derived from the reflection team method, which was developed by the Norwegian general practitioner and family therapist Tom Andersen. This method is adapted for working with groups by de Mönnink. Andersen (1987) asked fellow family therapists to watch his family therapy (with a family) and invited them to add additional thoughts (reflections) to it. An important principle in the reflection technique is that many roads lead to Rome, not just one. This diversity of mutually influencing minds is also the starting point for practicing the reflection technique. Now it is the participants' chance to observe an individual conversation between a social worker and one group member; they can identify with the group member or the conversation and can give their reflections. Reflections are additional thoughts. It's not about 'solving thoughts', but more about modest additions to what has already been said or come up. For example, after a demonstration of a conversation about the grieving process a member of the group can say, 'This sounded very honest and real to me, my compliments for your clarity,' or 'It made me wonder how it is possible that people respond in such a way to someone with such deep emotions.'

17.7.7 Aquarium technique

With the aquarium technique the social worker divides the group into an inner circle and an outer circle. On the inside of the group, in the inner circle, a topic is being discussed, for example the way people react to loss. Around the inner circle are the observers who can respond after the completion of a part of the discussion. The outer circle is then asked to sit in the inner circle and to give their reactions. This way, awareness is created and the difference is made clear between 'being involved in a conversation' and 'being an observer to a conversation and keeping a distance'.

17.7.8 Task-oriented technique

During the session the social worker comes to an agreement with attendees or with the entire group to do something in between the sessions or to produce something that will bring the individual learning goal closer. A participant could for example keep track of how many negative thoughts he or she has and often he or she feels down, or make a photo collage of the partner and take this to the next session, or writing down 10 energy-raising activities and actually doing two of them in the intervening period. In the group the results of these tasks are discussed (see section 13.7.7).

17.7.9 Amusement technique

The social worker introduces games to relax the atmosphere and to promote informal relations between attendees. There are a lot of different ones. An example is a clapping game where the participants go on their knees to sit in a circle, put their hands on the ground and form a circle with their hands alternating with their own hand and that of their neighbour. Then a participant gives a loud clap with a hand on the floor, followed by that of a neighbour and so on, with the goal to do this as quickly as possible around the circle. If the speed is optimal, the difficulty is increased: if a participant gives a clap on the floor twice in a row, the direction is reversed and so on. Numerous examples of games are mentioned in the book *Body and Movement* (Broich, 1994).

17.7.10 Role-playing technique

During a group session the social worker proposes to turn the situation into role-play, for example a situation at home or at the workplace. The visualization of the behaviour of the client in the particular situation is at the forefront. The group members play roles as instructed by the client. The other players give feedback on the client in a safe manner. Practicing new behaviour is also possible in role-playing.

17.7.11 Problematizing technique

The social worker approaches the group in a non-depository (oppressive) way (Freire, 1972), but in a problematizing way: such as discovering communal characteristics in people's history and present situation. For Freire problematizing is a form of self-examination, questioning the obvious in the life of the client. The social worker suggests problematizing questions such as: What is my position in society? What does my problem have to do with this social position? How have I dealt with the problem so far? What are my strengths? What is the first step I'm going to take? Who or what do I need to do so?

The participant is encouraged to problematize his or her own situation rather than that the social worker is offering a 'recipe'. According to Freire group members can come to a critical consciousness as they confront each other's problems this way.

17.7.12 Codification technique

With the codification technique the social worker makes use of an image that illustrates a specific situation of the participant, matching the theme of the meeting. The codification is a videotape, a drawing, a photograph, a song, a trip that was taken or an object that reflects the situation of each group member's life situation. When they are presented with the codification the group members can distance themselves from their own situations. The codification challenges the group to wonder about situations they are so used to that they never really think about them anymore. This way they become aware of their own situation right on the spot. In a bereavement group, members can bring the obituary, the prayer card or a photograph as a form of codification. In a women's group playing a video in which a man and a woman are arguing can be an eye-opener. Codification must meet five criteria (Freire, 1978):

1   The codification portrays a picture of the situation expressing the theme of the group meeting.
2   The codification must be immediately recognizable to other group members.
3   The content of the codification is simple.
4   The codification can be viewed in multiple ways.
5   The codification has the ability to be linked to social contexts.

When displaying the codification, the following subtechniques are used:

1   Showing inventory: let participants articulate what they see.
2   Associating: let participants express their underlying feelings.
3   Asking explicit questions: inviting participants to come up with specific experiences.
4   Thinking collectively: let participants articulate what they see as communal business and which link this has with social structures.

17.7.13 Individual and systemic techniques

The social worker is aware of the fact that all of the individual or systemic methods can be used if there is a reason for it within the group. That makes the group method attractive and instructive for it has a very rich range of practical applications of many methods and techniques. When making use of individual or systemic techniques, it also gives many possibilities to deploy members. It may also be very instructive to others struggling with similar problems if a participant works through something. When individual or systemic methods are mentioned that are useful in conjunction with the group method, the social worker refers to the relevant methodical profile for detailed information on the techniques. This way individual counselling techniques can be applied when there is uncertainty about what an individual participant has said. For example: 'You say you think this is difficult. What do you mean by that?' Or behavioural techniques to practice certain behaviour, for example an expression of something you wish for with respect to the partner: 'Can you please tell me exactly what you want from me?' After the exercise feedback is given on what was pleasant and could be improved. This is how new behaviour is conditioned. But also cognitive techniques may be helpful to explain processes or to normalize reactions. For example: 'You say you are down after the loss, but this is a pretty normal reaction for many people'. Also body techniques (relaxation or moving techniques) are used. In addition, expression techniques are used, such as drawing, making collages, working together on a painting and so on. Also ritual techniques can be used if a participant wants to make a transition to a new life stage. With the help of the group a symbolic transition can be staged. Trauma care can be carried out for a member while the others are present as silent witnesses and are able to express their appreciation. Finally, of the individual techniques, the practical techniques are available to think along about a solution to a practical problem, this way group members also can brainstorm and give advice. For example, about the question 'How do I respond to a question of a neighbour about how I am, knowing that I just lost my partner?'

Systemic methods can for example be used in a partner-relationship group. Couples set to work on a theme that they have trouble with, for example the absence of arguments in their relationship. As an example the social worker can let them talk about this subject in front of the group and stimulate reflections from other couples. The family method can also be used in, for example, a partner or family group of residents with dementia. Family relationships can be discussed and serve as a pretext for other participants to talk about family problems. A technique that is applied more and more is a technique called 'family arrangements'. The social network method can be used to make subjects like loneliness and isolation a topic of conversation. The group can act as a source of recognition but also serve as a source of possibilities for socialization. The mediation method can be used for parties who are involved in a conflict, like for instance in a team, through discussing the conflict in a group and work on constructive relationships. The method is also used in institutions that take in entire families who are in a crisis situation, and then organize joint meetings for all present families who in turn can have an example function to each other.

17.8 Social work results

- The client benefits from the group and his or her problems are improving.
- The client claims to have learned a lot.
- The client is socially more reliant.
- The client is less alone and is therefore relieved.
- The client is expanding his social contacts.

17.9 Evidence

There has been very little research into the effect of the group method in social work. Many more process evaluation studies have emerged, showing a variety of descriptions of group work, in particular by medical social workers.

17.9.1 Groups in the medical setting

Glassman (1991) describes how the humanistic values and democratic norms are fundamental to social group work and are operationalized in groups in the medical setting. Glassman delineates numerous values and norms and identifies and describes the uses of practice interventions in health care groups. The focus is on group practice that provides a healing environment of caring, empowerment, and support for members. Practitioner efforts centre on the development of group norms that enhance belonging in open-ended and closed groups, foster diversity in the group, include rather than exclude others, widen freedom of choice and open decision making, and help members question the authority of the worker as well as of the hospital system.

17.9.2 Group work for social workers themselves

Deconstruction of traditional social work departments can isolate social workers from their primary source of professional affiliation, leaving them without the support to take stands on controversial patient care issues. Sulman et al. (2004) describes an alternative: the building of a powerful social work collective based on social group work theory that potentiates professional practice while transcending management forms. The model includes group supervision, but moves beyond it to utilize the social work group as a central organizing principle. At the heart of the collective are the elements of professional accountability, support, autonomy, and collaborative decision-making within democratic peer group structures. The authors highlight current management theory, distinctions that create an authentic social work value-based practice, and outcomes.

17.9.3 Recovery groups

The recovery approach (Loumpa, 2012) has been adopted by mental health services worldwide and peer support constitutes one of the main elements of recovery-based services. Loumpa discusses the relevancy of recovery and peer support to mental health social work practice through an exploration of social work ethics and values. Furthermore, it provides an exploration of how peer support can be maximized in group work to assist the social work clinician to promote recovery and wellbeing. More specifically, Loumpa discusses how the narrative therapy concepts of 'retelling' and 'witnessing' can be used in the context of peer support to promote recovery, and also how social constructionist, dialogical, and systemic therapy approaches can assist the social work practitioner to enhance peer support in recovery-oriented group work.

17.10 Pitfalls

- There are too few opportunities for individual work within the group.
- There is insufficient eye for a client that seems to blend in with the group but doesn't work on individual questions and problems.

17.11 Summary and question

In this chapter, the group work method was detailed as a means to optimize clients' QoL through contact with peers. First, a description was given of the group work method. An in-depth look was taken into the supporting aspects of a group of peers in meeting their human needs. This was followed by a discussion of the techniques utilized in the group work method and its results. Finally, a summary was given.

Question

1   Take a case study or your own situation as the starting point for filling out the checklist in Table 14.4. What do I need from my group members to optimally meet my human needs?

18

CASE MANAGEMENT METHOD

The social worker as case manager can be compared to the contractor, who employs the right craftsmen for difficult jobs and consults with the customer to coordinate the expert services of these skilled workers.

Questions

This chapter addresses the following questions:

- What is the significance of the case management (CM) method?
- How has the CM method evolved in the history of social work?
- What techniques are employed in the CM method?
- How does the CM method contribute to fulfilling human needs?
- What is the evidence that supports the CM method?

18.1 Introduction

In life you have to do it yourself, with others to help you along.

This chapter describes the CM method as a means to improve clients' quality of life (QoL) by optimizing care coordination. First, a definition is given of the CM method. Then, the support is discussed that can be derived from adequate tuning between the professionals involved and the client system. Next, the techniques of the CM method are elaborated. After that, the results of the CM are discussed, including some successful CM projects that have been set up. Finally, a summary is presented of what has been discussed.

The case of Mr. Stack

Mr. Stack is looking for support in the chaos in which he finds himself. He can't cope by himself. The social worker first utilizes the counselling method to establish the facts of Mr. Stack's story and to assess his (un)fulfilled needs (Mr. Stack's PAC with seven drawers). The inventory leads to the following pluses (empowering factors) and minuses (stress factors) contained in

- (–) great disappointment with your employer (blocking of promotion);
- (–) tensions in the relationship with your partner (fear of divorce);
- (–) stillbirth of your first son;
- (–) your second son becoming disabled;
- (–) anger with your general practitioner, lack of support (concerning incorrect dosage of sleep medication);
- (+) support from a friend;
- (+) support from a colleague.

Considering the large number of drawers, the social worker suggests engaging a number of care professionals to successively help Mr. Stack reduce the various stress factors. The social worker proposes involving the corporate social worker to manage Mr. Stack's work-related stress. His relationship problems are best dealt with by working together with a relationship counsellor. It is suggested to involve a trauma psychologist to help Mr. Stack reduce stress related to the traumatic loss of his son. To help deal with the problems concerning his second son, the social worker proposes to contact a service that is specialized in assisting persons with a disability.

It is agreed that Mr. Stack's social worker is responsible for coordinating the care professionals involved. In doing so, progress in the problem areas can be assured.

18.2 Conceptual definition and elucidation

Case management is one of the seven systematic methods in social work. The systematic design of the case management method facilitates an efficiently working system for delivering care to a client or client system. The case management method offers optimal support in the client situation by effectively coordinating the client's care provision and consequently reducing and eliminating individual and systematic problems. The case management method constitutes a methodical approach to the demand-driven care provision for clients with needs in multiple areas, among whom are residents with complex problems, vulnerable elderly persons, persons with psychiatric complaints and all other multiple problem clients.

18.3 History of the case management method

In the history of social work, case management was first known as a form of 'indirect work'. In many areas the social practitioner worked as a 'mediator' in the client's environment. According to Mary Ellen Richmond, an American social worker in the early days of social work, adjustments were needed in the client's situation, in addition to individual direct contact with the client (Richmond, 1917). Recent empirical studies show that social workers devote 20%–25% of their time to direct client work and spend the remaining time on indirect client work. The advance of casework around 1920 – originating in the psycho-analytical body of ideas – resulted in less focus on indirect work. It is hard to understand that indirect work remained neglected, even during the economic crisis of the early twentieth century (years of poverty and depression). In reaction to this undervaluation of indirect work it was argued that indirect work was necessary. The client's life was sometimes believed to be extremely hard, not because of the client himself, but rather because of other parties beyond his influence. As there were doubts concerning the efficacy of the face-to-face contacts, renewed interest was kindled in the indirect work method. Hollis (1972) distinguishes six important roles for the social worker to fulfil in indirect work:

1   Provider of resources;
2   Facilitator of resources;
3   Referring agent to resources;
4   Interpreter of the client's needs to others;
5   The client's mediator;
6   Advocate.

Within social work there has been much debate about case management. Can it be perceived as a renewed version of 'old-fashioned social work' or is it truly a newly designed model? (Johnson, 1999). In the early days the nature of case management was rather supply-driven. In 1980 a case manager in the United States was desk-bound, directed at coordinating, evaluating and identifying problem areas in the organization of care delivery to the target group of ex-psychiatric patients (Nijenhuis-Van Weert & Nijenhuis, 2002), a kind of care provision agent. In the models of demand-driven case management the starting principle is intensive contact with the patient. Demand-driven case management gives rise to formulating different questions than before (van Doorn & Elbers, 2003):

1   Who is attentive to the client's true demand for care?
2   Who is asking for care after consulting the person in need?
3   Who is setting up the care programme without interfering?
4   What is the goal of all the efforts?
5   Who is making the results transparent?

Case management ensures adequate tuning between the supply and demand for care. A great deal of clients drop out of care due to a mismatch between person and services. Discontinuation may occur on account of the following experiences (Hoogendam & Vreenegoor, 2002):

1   Care delivery occurs on a supply-and-demand basis without the client's involvement. The client perceives himself as the ball (object) and not the player (participant).
2   As clients are facing more than a single problem area, they find themselves being sent from one organization to the other, and are thus subjected to renewed screening and assessment procedures. Coordination of care delivery and policy is often lacking and at times conflicting.
3   There is no party that monitors the process as a whole.

4   Waiting times and lists related to the nature of the problems and target group are unacceptably long.

5   Frequent changes in staff at an organization, resulting in discontinuation in the care delivery service.

6   Care delivery services mainly concentrate on their own specialism. What the target group conveys as important is overruled by what the care delivery service believes to be helpful. This may concern a present situation, or similar experiences by previous generations with care services. Parents and grandparents may have also asked for help at the time and felt let down by the care delivery services.

Case management used to be implemented by organizing and coordinating the care delivery. Van Riet and Wouters (2000) conclude that case management cannot be adequately realized by methodically focusing on emancipating clients and organizing care on the basis of the clients' needs. Intensive case management is a method of delivering care to persons experiencing multiple complex problems at the same time. It may concern problem areas of income, housing, social isolation, aggression, work, care for the living environment, relationships, broken families, health, childhood traumas and dealings with police and justice. Clients – often chronically – face material and immaterial problems that are interrelated. Both care providers and clients may lose sight of the bigger picture of all the problem areas. Typical of the intensive case management approach is client empowerment, enabling clients to make their own choices in reaching their subgoals. As a result, clients learn to get a grip on their own situation and become motivated to realize improvement. The case manager assists the clients in this process by promoting their interests. Intensive case management is supported by computerized systems.

18.4 Goals

General goal

• Reduce or remove stress factors in the multidisciplinary approach to the client.

Specific goal

• Harmonize professionals and services around a client (system).

18.5 Indications

• The demand for harmonization of the caregivers involved and/or the client;
• Uncoordinated actions of the disciplines involved.

Indication criteria often aim to identify patients with the following types of 'high risk':

• Those with catastrophic conditions;
• Those with costly injury/illness;
• Those who are non-compliant/non-adherent in following treatment plans;
• Those in the acute phase of chronic illness;
• Those in the terminal phase of illness.

All screening should include a situational analysis of the patient. Additionally, a functional screening of the patient must be conducted and include the following elements:

- Physical
- Psychosocial
- Financial
- Environmental
- Cultural/spiritual
- Vocational
- Learning potential.

18.6 Contraindications

- The client withholds consent for exchanging information between disciplines.
- The disciplines involved object to coordination for ethical reasons (for instance when client information needs to be strictly confidential due to threat of honour crimes and/or for practical reasons.
- One of the disciplines involved no longer cooperates.

18.7 Techniques

1 Assessment technique
2 Linking technique
3 Planning technique
4 Monitoring technique
5 Process evaluation technique.

18.7.1 Assessment technique

In order to draw up a needs assessment (also section 6.6.1 Inventory technique), an inventory is made of the following issues (van Riet & Wouters, 2000).

1 Unfulfilled need(s) of the client concerning income, housing, work, physical health, mental health, relationships, leisure time, ADL (Activities of Daily Living), HDL (Household Daily Life), transportation or legal matters;

2 Potential for self-care pertaining to physical, cognitive, emotional and behavioural functioning. What are this client's strengths and disabilities?

3 Potential for support and assistance from the client's own social network (also see social network method):

    a Who belongs to this person's social network?
    b In what ways do they lend support?
    c Where do they live?
    d How do they interact?
    e Are they given emotional and material support?

4   Potential for professional care supply:

    a   What are the available resources?
    b   How available are these professionals?
    c   Are these professionals available for this client?
    d   Is the care supply acceptable for the client?
    e   How accessible is the service to this client?

Psychosocial assessment forms the basis for the Social Work Case Management process and includes the following components (*Social Work Best Practice Healthcare Case Management Standards*):

1   Personal data;
2   Health status/age: Disease process.
3   Advanced directives status;
4   Emotional status;
5   Cognitive functioning: Learning ability.
6   Functional Status: Spirituality.
7   Cultural issues;
8   Patient support system;
9   Caregiver support system;
10   Financial status;
11   Vocational status/potential;
12   Community reintegration;
13   Home and community environment.

Other methodical techniques can be utilized for assessment purposes such as the biography technique (a person's life story as part of the expression method) or ecogram technique (as part of the social network method).

18.7.2 Linking technique

The linking technique is defined as the way of connecting all participants in the care delivery to a client: the client himself, persons from the social network of the client system and care professionals. Concrete agreements are made concerning the precise implementation of the collaborated effort.

18.7.3 Planning technique

By planning technique we understand: reaching consensus on a care plan by working together with all parties; client system, caregivers and case manager. Subgoals are basically formulated by the client, if necessary with the help of the case manager. In the MDC (multidisciplinary consultation) the strategy for care is developed and subsequently established in consultation with the client: what can be done by whom and what are the required resources and for what purpose?

18.7.4 Monitoring technique

The monitoring technique involves the critically monitoring and guarding of the social care programme together with the client: is the care delivery still adequate enough for the client?

18.7.5 Process evaluation technique

The process evaluation technique includes a joint and ongoing discussion on the care delivery process. How is the programme being implemented? Are there any adjustments needed? Is it the right time to conclude the care delivery programme?

18.8 Social work results

- The client is in a more relaxed state.
- The client is satisfied with the way all the parties involved have been coordinated around his own client system.

18.9 Evidence

From research it emerges that clients are more appreciative of indirect work, as in case management than of traditional social work (Johnson, 1999). Little research has been conducted on the efficacy of case management. A number of process evaluations are known on the functioning of case management projects in which social workers have participated.

The first step in scientific research has been made by studying the efficacy of case management in the three target groups that follow.

1 Neighbourhood residents with multiple problems;
2 Carers of persons with dementia;
3 Multidisciplinary collaboration around psychiatric patients.

18.9.1 Neighbourhood residents with multiple problems – community care team – case management in multiple problems in Enschede (Holland)

In the city of Enschede it is considered important that residents should be able to get by in their daily routine. The city has set up all kinds of services in the area of work, income, housing, welfare and care, and have made a combined effort and set up community care teams with community care coaches – a structure designed to facilitate support as little as possible and as intensive as needed. Situations where persons are experiencing severe problems due to insufficient solving skills and knowledge ask for increased intervention from the authorities. An indication for intensive (expensive) intervention is required to ensure accountability of government funding of this type of care. This also calls for a government body that strongly regulates the supply and 'match' of activation and support of the persons involved.

What is entailed in the project?

The community care teams mainly focus on persons that are (temporarily) unable to deal with their problems themselves. The team's motto is: 'The resident makes his own choices and the care team coach is there to support him in doing so.' The important thing is that the residents fully cooperate in finding solutions to their problems. It is an advantage that the community care team and coach are in proximity to the residents. As a consequence, more insight can be gained into their strengths and talents, into their environment and also community facilities. In the occurrence of multiple problem situations, the goal of the community care team is that families or individuals will deal with a single care professional and care plan. This will result in people having dealings with fewer care professionals.

How does the project work?

Community care teams have been set up in all five city districts, employing one community care team coach for each of the six organizations. The care team coaches operate in the care and support delivery to multiple problem families. If needed, the care team coach will ask assistance from expert partners.

What are the success factors?

The team coaches collaborate with other expert disciplines in the community care team in order to support the individuals or families that need help. The starting point is working together with the team, understanding each other's methods and expertise in order to generalize the approach as much as possible. In doing so, care delivery can be implemented more efficiently (limited duration) and more effectively (integrated approach).

18.9.2 Carers of persons with dementia – case management dementia fulfils a need

Case management is sometimes described as 'the mortar between the bricks'. Persons suffering from dementia and their families show a need for someone to help them with their problems and concerns, someone who walks beside them, who draws up a care plan, whose approach is pro-active and who is the key figure in the care and support delivery. The team coach is both coordinator and care provider, which is not an easy task in dealing with complex conditions such as dementia. The form of casework developed by the DRC team (dementia research and case management) has become increasingly popular over the years. The number of clients opting for this care provision has increased rapidly.

Positive evaluation by clients

In 2006 the first independent measurement was conducted concerning family members' and carers' satisfaction with the care and support as delivered by the DRC team and Geriant case management (http://geriant.nl). The Trimbos Institute developed a measurement instrument for this purpose. The overall rating by the clients was a score of 8.1 out of 10. In addition, 95% of the respondents advised others to apply to the DRC team.

Case management for psychiatric patients

The target group comprises a group of patients living outside the psychiatric hospital, diagnosed with a severe psychiatric disorder, often with complex problems in various aspects of life. A number of them refuse contact with care professionals.

18.9.3 Multidisciplinary collaboration around psychiatric patients – approach

FACT stands for Flexible-ACT (Assertive Community Treatment). FACT operates in an outreaching, assertive way. Care professionals approach (potential) clients through house visits, at the day-care centre or in the street – wherever the patient may be. They maintain contact with the patient, and exert pressure and coercion, if necessary. The care is delivered by a broadly assembled multidisciplinary team. A FACT community team assists approximately 180 to 220 patients in a well-defined area. In the daily follow-up a digital plan board is utilized on which the staff can register their patients' names. The FACT model operates at three levels:

1   The patient is not registered on the digital plan board. The individual care provider works with individual case management from a multidisciplinary approach, and if needed, he will consult and involve a discipline from the team.
2   The care professionals register patients on the digital plan board to gather more information or be informed by other disciplines. In the event of an impending crisis situation they will be able to notify their team and ask for more intensive care.
3   The patient is registered on the digital plan board and requires intensive care; the patient receives ACT care: home-based psychiatric care (in the community), in an active and outreaching way.

The FACT teams form part of a mental health care concern. If necessary, they realize admissions on a transmural basis, in which the FACT-teams remain responsible for the care delivery. The FACT teams work closely together with other social organizations and services and also involve the patient's family in the treatment.

Direct indications of effectiveness

Two empirical studies have been conducted on FACT. In the first study (Bak et al., 2007), on the basis of pre–post comparison, it was concluded that the introduction of FACT into daily practice may result in measured improvement of psychiatric complaints and decreased service consumption. The study demonstrated a positive effect of FACT in a number of patients with systematic remission, although the relation proved less significant after correction. In a second observational study (Drukker et al, 2008) researchers concluded that FACT receivers with unfulfilled need for care of psychiatric care were more likely to go into remission, compared to a similar group of patients given treatment as usual.

Indirect indications of effectiveness

Indirect indications of effectiveness can be derived from research into ACT. In the early years studies on ACT were mostly conducted in the United States, and later also in Britain and the

Netherlands. The research outcome in the United States and Britain cannot easily be generalized to the Dutch situation. After all, it is also difficult to compare 'care as usual' between these countries. Dutch research shows variable results.

- ACT may decrease the number of patient admission days.
- ACT results in significantly more sustained care improvement compared to care as usual.
- ACT does not show significantly better scores in comparison with care as usual as concerns admission duration, psychopathology, social functioning and quality of life.
- In early psychosis intervention ACT yields a better outcome as to psychopathology, psychosocial functioning quality of life as perceived by the patients themselves.
- ACT-treatment appears to be more cost-effective in early psychosis intervention compared to care as usual.

Summing up the effective components

- Individual case management backed by a multidisciplinary team;
- Shared caseload if needed: all team members are involved in patient work;
- Assertive outreach: an active approach to patients where they are;
- Multidisciplinary work: cure and care come together in recovery support care;
- Continuity of care: FACT teams realize patient commitment and prevent drop-out;
- Community practice workers;
- Community-based approach for the benefit of the social support system;
- Structure for guideline-based implementation of evidence-based methods;
- Switching between individual extensive support and intensive team care;
- Adequate embedding in the regional social and (transmural) health care concern.

18.10 Pitfalls

- Due to poor communication with the parties concerned, it's unclear who on the team is the case manager.
- Lack of clarity concerning the case manager's responsibilities.

18.11 Summary and question

The current chapter has discussed the CM method as a way of improving clients' QoL by optimizing care coordination. First, a definition of the CM method was given. Then, the support was discussed that can be derived from adequate tuning between the professionals involved and the client system. After that, the techniques of the CM method were elaborated. In conclusion, the results of the CM were discussed, including the description of some successful CM projects.

Question

1   Take a case study or your own situation as the starting point for filling out the checklist in Table 14.4. What do I need from my professional network to optimally meet my human needs?

19

MEDIATION METHOD

In conflicts, parties corner and fight each other, they bring each other down and destroy one another like in real wars.

—de Mönnink

Questions

This chapter addresses the following questions:

- What is meant by relational escalation?
- What is meant by the mediation method?
- How has the mediation method developed?
- Which mediation techniques are utilized to help conflicting parties to resolve areas of conflict in a dignified way?
- What evidence is known of the mediation method?

19.1 Introduction

In life you have to do it yourself, with others to help you along.

Previous chapters have focused on social support from clients' social networks, relationships, nuclear and extended family, groups of fellow sufferers and care professionals. Conflicts and conflict escalation may occur in all these relations. Therefore, this chapter discusses the mediation method, employed by social workers to help parties resolve areas of conflict. Next, an overview of history of the mediation method is presented. Then follows a discussion of the techniques and evidence of the mediation method. In addition, a brief illustration is given of the mediation method in the case of Mr. Stack. In conclusion, a summary is presented of what has been discussed in this chapter.

The case of Mr. Stack

The social worker advised Mr. Stack to contact his physician to arrange a meeting for the three parties concerned, for the purpose of taking care of unfinished business. Mr. Stack managed to successfully redress his grievances and agreed to receive a symbolic compensation of €45. For many years, Mr. Stack had paid this sum for his sleeping medication.

19.2 Definition and elucidation

The mediation method is the method where, through mediation, the social worker is trying to make arrangements with conflicting parties, who, if they both accept, will try to make agreements in the areas of conflict. Mediation may be requested by spouses who are about to separate, but also in a conflict between employees and employers, patients and doctors as well as victims and perpetrators.

19.2.1 Elucidation

Through mediation legal action can be avoided, which will minimize the escalation of conflicts. Mediation, also known as conflict mediation, is one of the most commonly used methods of conflict management because it is informal, quick, easy to apply and confidential (Dragtsma, 2000). One can speak of a conflict when opposing interests, wishes, expectations or objectives between individuals or groups are expressed. In spoken language, euphemistic terms are commonly used such as 'difference of opinion', 'friction' or 'disagreement'. In mediation, each of the parties points to an independent third party that supports them in determining their interests and finding a mutually acceptable solution. Because mediation requires that parties will agree on a solution by themselves, the outcome is entirely in their own hands. The mediator will remain neutral, will give an opinion at most, but will make no substantive statements or estimations about the outcome of the legal proceedings. If the parties reach an agreement, it will be binding.

There are two types of mediation: task oriented and process oriented. The task-oriented style gives priority to the active treatment of the conflict issue and tries to come to a solution for a problem. The process-oriented or social-emotional mediation style focuses less on the conflict issues, but more on opening up to mutual communication, clarifying and expressing mutual feelings and perceptions, as well as the facilitation of the process. It centres more on the here-and-now.

What is the role of mediation in social work? When the mediation concept made its entrance in the Netherlands almost a decade ago, there were three professional groups who dealt with it. Besides psychologists and lawyers, the social workers had to educate themselves for the benefit of parental access or visitation rights after divorce, so they were able to mediate in restorative justice (see end of this section). Based on the literature, Scholte (2002) believes that social workers have mastered basic communication skills for conflict resolution (such as between family members, tenants and housing corporations), but that the strengthening of negotiation skills around conflict management in conjunction with the relevant areas of law will still require the necessary completion. Social workers should focus on conflicts between neighbours, peer mediation among students in schools, or conflicts between tenants and landlords. When there is a request for help in the case of a conflict of a client, the question will be directed to a social worker who specializes in mediation. Another option would be that mediation can be purchased as a kind of a 'plus package' by a third party (in addition to their own clients). Not yet known is the role of social workers when it comes to restorative mediation in the rehabilitation process. Restorative mediation is targeted towards goals that are outside the areas of criminal law such as mental healing, forgiveness, reconciliation, detachment and liberation, such as could happen between victims and perpetrators. This is known as VORP, Victim-Offender Reconciliation Programs (United States); Family Group Conferences (New Zealand); and RISE, the so-called Re-integrative Shaming Experiments (Australia). Social workers are also actively involved in divorce mediation, specifically in the area of visitation rights.

19.3 History of the mediation method

In 1979 the CPR Institute for Dispute Resolution was founded in the United States. This is an institute to promote conflict resolution. The concept of mediation was born in the United States in response to, and as an alternative to, the strictly juridical treatment of divorce and parental access arrangements. After this it was used to negotiate the discussions about (centralized) labour conditions. The use of mediation became increasingly broader; it also proved successful in resolving other types of conflicts and disagreements. It was deployed in various conflicts ranging from individual labour disputes and conflicts between merging companies as well as in neighbourhood disputes and the transfer of shares between family businesses. The Netherlands has seen a similar development. In 1995 the Foundation Dutch Mediation Institute (NMI) was established. It keeps a register of qualified mediators who work according to NMI rules of conduct. There are disciplinary proceedings for mediators as well now.

19.4 Goals

General goal

- Reducing tension associated with a conflict.

Specific goals

- Enable conflicting parties to come out of the impasse they are in.
- Help conflicting parties make steps.
- Help conflicting parties steer out of the conflict situation.
- Allow conflicting parties to make (new) agreements.

19.5 Indications

- Parties are in conflict; there is an opposition of interest.
- Parties wish for mediation.
- Parties have confidence in mediation.
- Parties have confidence in mediator.

19.6 Contraindications

- One of the parties has no interest in mediation.
- One of the parties withdraws or does not hold to agreements.
- There is doubt among the parties about mediation.
- There is a power imbalance that is too complicated to be solved.
- Prior mediation with the same parties failed.
- The decision of a court (or other authority) is essential and final.
- One party is seeking a penalty.
- At least one party wants a court judgement to set a precedent.

19.7 Techniques

1   Appraisal technique
2   Contract technique
3   Territorial negotiation technique
4   Blow-off-steam technique
5   Communication technique
6   Covenant technique.

19.7.1 Appraisal technique

After a request for mediation, the social worker will define with each individual partner what the core of the conflict is. For example there is a conflict about damage claims of a social services official. This person has suffered personal, financial and psychological damage due to many years of confrontation with aggression. The officer is seeking compensation but the employer wants to reimburse only partially. Employee and employer ask for mediation.

19.7.2 Contract technique

The social worker makes sure both parties will sign up for the fact that they will abide the rules of mediation. Furthermore, the social worker makes rules such as 'do not interrupt one another' and 'do not run away'. The runaway party is responsible for a new appointment in case this happens.

19.7.3 Territorial negotiation technique

The social worker allows both parties to alternately clarify their position on the conflict. As a guide for negotiating, the territorial negotiation technique (Table 19.1) can be used. If necessary this can be alternated with the 'blow-off-steam' technique.

TABLE 19.1 Diagram for territorial negotiations

	Partner A	*Partner B*
Separately	Prepares agenda from a list of questions for B.	Prepares agenda from a list of questions for A.
Together	A reads list aloud.	B listens, repeats and makes notes.
	A listens, repeats and makes notes.	B reads list aloud.
Separately	Each assumes the false assumption: 'if I get everything I ask for, what am I willing to give towards what you are asking?'	Each assumes the false assumption: 'if I get everything I ask for, what am I willing to give towards what you are asking?'
Together	A listens, repeats and makes notes.	B reads list aloud.
	A reads list aloud.	B listens, repeats and makes notes.
Separately	Assignment: 'if I get this and this, then I want to give you that and that.'	Assignment: 'if I get this and this, then I want to give you that and that.'
Together	A reads proposal aloud.	B listens, repeats and makes notes.
	A listens, repeats and makes notes.	B reads proposal aloud.
	Each person takes turns with new proposal until solution is found.	Each person takes turns with new proposal until solution is found.

Source: Bakker & Bakker (1978)

19.7.4 Blow-off-steam technique

The social worker optionally lets one, or both parties blow off steam. He or she can do this when a client is overwhelmed with emotion and temporarily incapable to pursue negotiations in a rational way (see also the cathartic techniques in section 8.8). A timeout for both parties could be sufficient or emotional discharge in the presence of the other party. The emotional discharge of a party in the presence of the other is not intended as leverage in the negotiations, but more so as a way of increasing mutual understanding.

19.7.5 Communication technique

The social worker assumes that a part of the escalation can be based on a history of miscommunication. In the evaluation of the conflict, these communication problems are discussed or become evident. The manner in which the parties address each other during the mediation could exemplify the destructive communication. The social worker will try to 'cut through' the destructive communication by introducing constructive communication rules (see Table 19.1).

19.7.6 Covenant technique

The social worker is tries to bring the parties to an agreement. If successful, the agreements are made official into a covenant (a signed written agreement).

19.8 Social work results

- The conflicting parties are more relaxed.
- The conflicting parties are a step further into the process.
- The relationship is restored between the parties.
- The conflicting parties separate and feel they have received the help they needed.
- The conflicting parties have agreed on future steps.

19.9 Evidence

There is no research on the mediation method in social work. It appears that, within the (mostly) American and British companies where mediation is structurally applied, approximately 80% to 85% of conflicts are resolved early by both parties, which brings great satisfaction (Dragtsma, 2002).

The basic need in mediation (Weiner, 2012) is that a rigorous and intellectually honest approach to understanding 'how to mediate well' must be based on empirically verifiable information and not on untested assumptions or dogmatic beliefs about 'what makes good mediation'. Courts that sponsor mediation programmes and those that mandate the use of mediation should base their assessment of the programmes and mediators on empirically verifiable information on mediator behaviours and tactics. Mediation trainers should ground their teaching in empirically derived knowledge.

For better and for worse, though, at least in Court ADR and the cases that wind up in mediation because lawyers took them there, many, perhaps most, identify settlement as the primary objective. Given this reality and, given the relative ease of defining this result in some objective way (e.g., dismissal of litigation). I believe it makes sense to start trying to answer a simple yet perplexing question: what mediator behaviours are more likely to lead to the settlement of disputes? As of the time of this writing I have not found a comprehensive summary of empirically verifiable knowledge about what mediator behaviours are effective in moving litigants to make agreements from data collected since mediation has become institutionalized in courts and civil disputes all over the world.

19.10 Pitfalls

- The social worker overlooks individual and positional issues.
- The social worker is biased.

19.11 Summary and questions

Previous chapters focused attention on support from clients' social network, relationships, nuclear and extended family, groups of fellow sufferers and care professionals. As conflicts and conflict escalation may occur in all these relations, this chapter has dealt with the mediation method, which social workers can employ to help parties resolve areas of conflict. Furthermore, an overview of the history of the mediation method was presented. Then followed a discussion of the techniques and evidence of the mediation method. In addition, a brief illustration of the mediation method in the case of Mr. Stack was given.

Questions

1 What is your way of responding to conflict situations (for instance, parental access arrangements, property settlements or inheritance issues) or minor disagreements? What does that say about your own experience with conflict situations?
2 Picture a conflict situation and describe how you would structure the communication to reach agreement on practical and emotional obstacles to draw up a covenant.
3 How would you utilize the mediation techniques for that purpose?

PART VII

Four macro methods

Enhancing service delivery

Part VII discusses the four methods that are employed by social workers to improve structural support services for client groups in collaboration with the client system. This enhancement of service delivery is aimed at helping client groups to optimally fulfil their needs for safety, affection and self-determination.

Macro support can be defined as 'the perceived support by a group of clients', realized by a range of practical-material provisions and support by care professionals. Four specific social work methods are utilized to develop optimal support for specific client groups:

- The monitoring method, to identify structural irregularities in the services available or lack of services (Chapter 20);
- The prevention method, to develop preventive support for specific groups in various areas (Chapter 21);
- The collective advocacy method, to help client groups improve service delivery to improve their quality of life (QoL; Chapter 22);
- The research method, to develop knowledge on specific aspects of social work for the purpose of enhancing care delivery for client groups (Chapter 23).

Positively perceived macro support contributes to client groups' improved QoL. The four macro interventions aim to affect support processes by services in a constructive way. How can you, as a social worker, activate the supportive power of services so that clients' needs can be optimally met?

20

MONITORING METHOD

Besides the focus on social casework, social work should remain constantly focused on the social structure of our society. Social work should examine how to create the structure for situations in which persons feel safe. [. . .] Our support should not be limited to individual support.

(Marga Klompé, Dutch Minister of Social Work, 1959)

Questions

This chapter addresses the following questions:

- What is the importance of the monitoring method?
- What are the techniques employed in the monitoring method?

20.1 Introduction

First, the concept of monitoring is elucidated, followed by a description of the history of monitoring in social work. Next, the goals, indications, contraindications, techniques, results and evidence are discussed. After that, the pitfalls of the monitoring method are listed. In conclusion, a summary is presented with some questions.

20.2 Definition and elucidation

The goal of monitoring is to map signs of problems that help establish pathways for improvement in the quality of service delivery. Pathways for improvement may be directed to improving services and care delivery in communities by effecting changes in organizations.

Pathways for improvement in communities

Social workers may employ the four macro methods, described in the following chapters, to strengthen structural support for clients through pathways for improvement. The pathways in the level of services may be aimed at affecting community organizing and improving organizations. Rothman distinguishes three concepts of community organizing: locality development, social planning and social action. Local development involves developing a neighbourhood, town or region, to become a more democratic community and a safe and more inviting living environment, whose residents show mutual solidarity. Social planning is directed at tackling local issues, such as crime, housing problems and health care services. Improved social planning is realized by exerting influence on prominent members of society, government officials and other persons of power and influence. Social action is geared towards fighting social injustice, such as poverty, homelessness and discrimination.

Pathways for improvements in organizations

Pathways for improvement may also be targeted at organizations, making them more easily accessible to groups of service users (Sheafor & Horejsi, 2003). It depends on social workers' organizational theory to determine which pathway can be implemented to enhance social work clients in organizations. Social workers can start from one of the three organizational models.

1   The rational model
2   The natural model
3   The power politics model.

The rational model is based on the principle that employees form part of an organization – for instance, a social service agency – and that they support the aims of the organization. Social workers implement rational measures to achieve improvements, including self-evaluation, advice from consultants on dealing with clients' complaints or criticism, and training of new technologies. When social workers depart from the natural organizational model, the organization is perceived as a system, a set of individuals, roles, subsystems, formal and informal processes. People and elements of the organization may deviate from the official mission of the organization on account of 'natural' processes, such as job stress, unclear assignments and differing views on obligations and responsibilities. Changes can be effected by clarifying organizational targets, improved communication and meeting employees' social and emotional needs. When social workers base their approach on the power politics model, the organization is viewed as a political arena involving all kinds of people and elements that struggle for power, money and personal gain. According to this model, social workers should engage with powerful and influential persons to effect organizational changes. These people need convincing that a more client-oriented approach can also be to their advantage. External pressure via the media, legal supervision or court proceedings may be required to successfully achieve these improvements.

One of the key targets of social work is to achieve improvement in structural resources (Scholte, 1998). However, this core function of social work is still underdeveloped. Social workers employ the monitoring method, through data collection and analysis, to identify structural irregularities in service delivery. These are made visible so that actions for improvement can be undertaken, such as prevention (Chapter 21) and collective advocacy (Chapter 22). The moral of the fisherman's tale emphasizes that we had better focus on the cause of the problem, rather than lend support on a case-by-case basis.

The fisherman's tale

A man is walking along the river shore and sees a human body drifting downstream. A fisherman jumps into the water, pulls the body onto the shore and saves the man's life by giving him mouth-to-mouth resuscitation. The same thing happens a couple of minutes later and then again and again. Finally, one more body passes by. This time the fisherman totally ignores the drowning man and starts walking upstream along the river. The observing man asks the fisherman what he is up to. 'Why are you not trying to save the drowning man's life?' The fisherman answers: 'This time I am going upriver to find out who keeps throwing the poor devils into the water.'

Scholte (2013) defines monitoring as identifying and interpreting situations inside and outside the professional practice that may negatively affect groups of (potential) clients. Monitoring is a systematically implemented cyclical process, geared towards directly or indirectly improving client support. It involves observation and identification, decision making, analyzing decisions, taking actions and process reviewing.

20.3 History of the monitoring method

Two books have been written in Holland about monitoring in social work, *Opgelet. Systematisch signaleren* (*Watch Out. Systematic Monitoring in Social Work*) (1997), written by Margot Scholte and Peter van Splunteren; and *Signalering in het sociaal werk* (*Monitoring in Social Work*) (1996) by sociologist Siny Sluiter and colleagues. Both books claim that monitoring in social work has so far been neglected. Psychologization of social work (navel-gazing) and lack of resources and competence are considered important contributing factors. In the early days of social work, monitoring was part of the social worker's job and consisted of identifying inadequacies in social legislation.

> Helping each other is important, but only in addition to social legislation. 'Relief for the poor never forgets, it doesn't cure, it eases suffering.'
>
> *(Muller-Lulofs, 1916)*

If a social worker failed to contribute to social politics, it was perceived as a professional error. In practice it concerned left-wing politics. Directors of the first social training colleges were known as 'Progressive' and 'Red'. In Gersons's opinion (1995), social work has become alienated from its mission, which is 'solidarity with the oppressed and the deprived in a society that is defined by the gap between rich and poor, power and dependency'. Gersons is convinced that social workers should return to the crossroads of social services and that they should function as the spokespersons for people's needs and rights in local and national politics. In *Beroepsprofiel social werk* (*Professional Profile of Social Work*) by Holstvoogd (1995, chap. 28), monitoring is defined as identifying (studying) shortcomings in rules and regulations and locating dysfunctional persons and institutions. We are now seeing a growing number of social workers conducting research for the purpose of establishing successful monitoring procedures (see Chapter 23).

20.4 Goals

General goal

- Identifying stress factors in social groups due to structural obstacles.

Specific goals

- Mapping signs of structural problems in a group of clients. Problems may concern abuses, restrictive legislation, procedures, agreements, labour agreements and also unhealthy, unsafe, repressive conditions (in work environment or neighbourhood) and so forth.
- Mapping signs of structural obstacles in the care delivery process, including dissatisfaction with waiting lists, assessment procedures, consulting rooms, complaints procedures, shortcomings of the methodical toolbox, lack of quality of social work training courses and so forth.

20.5 Indications

- Dissatisfaction about structural obstacles with a number of clients;
- (Potential) deterioration in the position of a group of clients.

20.6 Contraindications

- Lack of time, finances or other resources to facilitate the monitoring process;
- Priority is given to tackling individual or systematic problems.

20.7 Techniques

1 Problem identification cards
2 Peer screening
3 Registration screening
4 Media screening
5 Checklist technique 'basic resources'
6 Other research techniques.

20.7.1 Problem identification cards

The social worker fills out special identification cards if problems arise that are structural instead of individual. It concerns evaluation forms, forms for exit interviews and complaints or registration forms. For instance, the social worker establishes that his new client is next in line of the many employees facing difficulties with functioning after a restructuring process.

20.7.2 Peer screening

Peer screening is a general or specific analysis of registration data and/or files. Social workers should brainstorm or consult with each other or with professionals from other disciplines on a regular basis – face-to-face for half an hour every 2 months – to identify potential structural irregularities and/or detrimental conditions. In this way, structural stress factors can be identified that require implementation of the prevention method or the collective advocacy method.

20.7.3 Registration screening

Registration consists of regularly reviewing (such as once every 2 months) the client registration data and of identifying signs of structural irregularities. For instance, the social worker can screen the registration data of a company, agency or region. An inventory is made of the structural signs, for which structural methods can be employed. For instance, many clients may be dealing with divorce issues, for which a group approach can be indicated within the framework of the prevention method.

20.7.4 Media screening

Media screening involves maintaining internal and external media contacts (within and outside the agency, company and region, including contacts in the corridors). In addition, it also pertains to keeping a close watch on recent developments concerning an agency, company or region and analyzing signs of structural problem areas. A number of clients may, for instance, appear to be stressed on account of corporate restructuring. A 'stress management project' can be indicated within the framework of the prevention method.

20.7.5 Checklist 'basic resources'

Social workers can make an inventory of the basic resources, accessible to groups of clients or citizens, according to a checklist derived from the FABR, the Family Access to Basic Resources. This checklist of resources, the BCL, facilitates a quick scan to establish the level of resources for a group of clients, and shows potential irregularities or shortcomings (see Table 20.1). The checklist can be completed on the basis of a single case or multiple cases in the social work team. It is determined how accessible the basic resources have been in the past year: sufficiently accessible, not sufficiently accessible or inaccessible. All resource outcomes are to be discussed.

TABLE 20.1 Basic resources checklist

Basic resource	Questions	Availability s = sufficient n = not sufficient i = inaccessible
1 Work and income	• The availability of income for work • What types of jobs are available? • Part-time or full-time? • What are the pay scales? • How is payment effected? • Do the wages cover all the living expenses? • Are there any delays in payment?	

(Continued)

TABLE 20.1 (Continued)

	• What are the bonuses?
	• What is the travel distance from home to work?
	• What training is needed for quality jobs?
	• What are the training opportunities?
	• Are there any redundancies due to closure?
	• How often does unemployment occur?
	• To what extent is unemployment structural?
2 Housing	• Ownership of housing or rental property?
	• Are there adequate facilities?
	• Are there any waiting lists for housing?
	• Is there homelessness involved?
3 Food	• What is the quality of food?
	• Is there enough variety in foods?
	• Is there enough food available?
4 Clothing	• Is there variety in clothing?
5 Health care	• What is the quality of clothing?
	• Is there enough choice?
	• Is health care available in times of crisis?
	• Are clients insured?
	• Are there any waiting lists?
6 Education	• What is the level of quality?
	• Is it available for all age groups?
	• And for people with special needs?
	• Are there options to choose from?
	• Has the client received education?
7 Child care	• How is it provided?
	• How is the allocation of child care arranged?
	• How is the child care service used?
	• What is the level of quality of child care?
	• Are there options in child care to choose from?
	• What is their policy if a child falls ill?
	• Are there any other problems involved in child care?
8 Family and parenting support	• What is the level of quality?
	• Are there options for support?
	• Is support available in times of crisis?
9 Personal care and recreation	• What are the opportunities for recreation?
	• Are they individually or family oriented?
	• What is available at walking distance?
10 Transport: which means: train, bus or car?	
	• How reliable is public transport?
	• Is it affordable?
11 Other resources	

20.7.6 Other research techniques

Chapter 23 discusses the practice research method. All the techniques described can be utilized for monitoring structural problems (see section 23.7).

20.8 Social work results

- An overview of stress factors in a number of clients in the psychosocial conditions at home, at work or in the care delivery service;
- Identifying groups at risk.

20.9 Evidence

No research has been conducted on the effectiveness of the monitoring method in social work. The process of monitoring, though, has been studied in a research by the Trimbos Institute (Arends & Hosman, 1991). Eight prevention units of mental health outpatient institutions were investigated regarding the implementation of monitoring methods. It emerged from this comparative study that the monitoring projects had two objectives:

- Collecting information about psychosocial problems and groups at risk;
- Obtaining a picture of the region and gathering information concerning the factors that may frustrate or stimulate people to function adequately.

In addition, this study employed the following methods of monitoring:

- Interviews with curative workers.;
- Interviews with key figures in primary care;
- Registration data;
- File analyses;
- Newspaper and literature search.

Furthermore, three research outcomes were established:

1   Monitoring research provided a basis for prevention measures. Well-targeted prevention policies were, for instance, directed at school drop-outs, foreign employees with multiple problem families, employees facing imminent redundancy, problem cases identified by general practitioners, families living with a dementia patient or a disabled child, at risk of becoming exhausted.
2   Monitoring research resulted in setting up prevention projects for a number of groups at risk. Target groups included, for example victims of incest, victims of acts of violence, clients with post-natal depression, clients with psychosomatic complaints, persons with relational problems, divorce problems, parenting problems, depressive complaints, bereavement problems or women living in suburban isolation.
3   Monitoring research failed to yield concrete information for prevention policies.

Policy-oriented monitoring distinguishes the following four phases:

- Formulating objectives. What decision can be reached on the basis of the research data?
- Formulating criteria. Against which criteria can this information be evaluated?
- Assessing the need for information. What information is needed to reach a decision?
- Information gathering. What is the most successful strategy to gather the required information?

20.9.1 Developing monitoring systems

As early as 1986, Coulton focused on the steps for developing monitoring systems for quality assurance and suggests key criteria and sources of data for evaluating the quality of social work services on an ongoing basis, particularly discharge planning.

20.9.2 Monitoring of psychological wellbeing

OBJECTIVE: To investigate whether *monitoring and discussing psychological wellbeing* in outpatients with diabetes improves mood, glycaemic control, and the patient's evaluation of the quality of diabetes care.

RESEARCH DESIGN AND METHODS: This study was a randomized controlled trial of 461 outpatients with diabetes who were randomly assigned to usual care or to the monitoring condition. In the latter group, the diabetes nurse specialists assessed and discussed psychological wellbeing with the patients (with an interval of 6 months) in addition to usual care. The computerized Wellbeing Questionnaire was used for this purpose. Primary outcomes were mood, HbA(1c), and the patient's evaluation of the quality of diabetes care at 1-year follow-up. The number of referrals to the psychologist was analyzed as a secondary outcome. Intention-to-treat analysis was used.

RESULTS: The monitoring group reported better mood compared with the standard care group, as indicated by significantly lower negative wellbeing and significantly higher levels of energy, higher general wellbeing, better mental health, and a more positive evaluation of the quality of the emotional support received from the diabetes nurse. The two groups did not differ for HbA(1c) or in their overall evaluation of the quality of diabetes care. In the monitoring condition, significantly more subjects were referred to the psychologist.

CONCLUSIONS: Monitoring and discussing psychological wellbeing as part of routine diabetes outpatient care had favourable effects on the mood of patients but did not affect their HbA(1c). Our results support the recommendation to monitor psychological wellbeing in patients with diabetes.

20.9.3 Proactive monitoring of sickness absence for psychosocial problems

Psychosocial problems are common in daily practice. These problems are the cause of 30% of absence from work due to sickness. Almost one-third of workers with common mental disorders experience recurrent sickness absence. Although general practitioner (GP) and occupational physician (OP) guidelines have suggested monitoring these patients, these doctors are not used to doing this. Dutch researchers (Olde Hartman & Hassink-Franke, 2014) studied a problem-solving intervention (SHARP-at work) for evaluating the effectiveness of preventing recurrent sickness absence. Although the researchers found a decrease in recurrent sickness absence, it is not clear whether this effect was caused by the intervention or by the extra contacts between doctor and employee. Support and empathy are non-specific factors which could explain these positive findings in themselves. Given the findings in this study, GPs and OPs should be more aware of the importance of *proactive monitoring* of patients with common mental disorders after they have returned to work.

20.10 Pitfalls

- Identifying problems areas but failing to take action;
- The intention to monitor in spite of a lack of resources;
- Too much of an *ad hoc* approach instead of following structural procedures;
- Too much emphasis on direct care delivery without addressing the structural problems;
- Assuming a patronizing attitude towards clients, working according to the victim triangle and attributing structural problems to the client group without their acknowledgement;
- Feeling discouraged as a social worker, believing that client work is rather pointless.

20.11 Summary and questions

The current chapter has discussed the monitoring method. First, the concept of monitoring was elucidated, followed by a description of the history of monitoring in social work. Next, the goals, indications, contraindications and techniques were described. Then, the focus was on the results and evidence of the monitoring method. Finally, a number of pitfalls were listed.

Questions

Select your own or a virtual case that shows that a group of persons are not benefitting from certain services.

1. Describe which human needs and human rights on the level of survival, affection and self-determination are not fully met.
2. Indicate which monitoring techniques can be utilized to reveal structural problem areas.
3. Draw up a plan of approach that shows how monitoring can be used to reveal how services are not fulfilling persons' needs.
4. How can you, as a social worker, avoid the pitfalls of the monitoring method?

21

PREVENTION METHOD

Prevention is concerned with keeping the vase intact, rather than trying to repair the broken pieces.

Questions

This chapter addresses the following questions:

- What risk factors are there for the worsening of the position of a group of people?
- How did the prevention method in social work start?
- Which techniques are used in the prevention method?
- What is known about the evidence of the prevention method?

21.1 Introduction

In the previous chapters, we wrote about support from the social network, support from the family system and professional support from the neighbourhood, school work and care institutions, as well as how work can be done on a macro level in signalling structural obstacles.

Like Richmond stated in 1917: 'Prevention and cure must go hand in hand'. In this chapter, we therefore will direct our attention to prevention of structural deterioration of a group of (potential) clients. First, we will show what we consider to be structural obstacles in the provision. Then we will detail the history of the prevention method and the techniques a social worker may utilize to prevent further deterioration of the quality of life of a group of people. We will conclude with a summary.

21.2 Definition and elucidation

The prevention method focuses on preventing structural problems or deterioration of an identified risk situation by setting up educational programmes and projects. It concerns a community-based approach (also see Chapter 22, promotion of collective interests method), targeted at establishing structural improvements in the collective wellbeing, safety, health and participation of social work target groups. In this respect, it differs from the practical-material method, which focuses on realizing improvements in the individual client situation.

21.3 History of the prevention method

Social work has a long history of leadership in prevention work and is well-positioned to respond to this contemporary need. Social work originally emerged as a distinct profession through primary prevention efforts in the settlement house movement. In the early days of social work much of its practice was carried out with a prevention focus. Municipal social services' records at the time describe individual support and prevention as 'repressive' and 'preventive social work', respectively. Repressive social work entailed providing 'down payments in cash or goods, affordable food supplies to the needy, employment, hygienic facilities and management of homes and shelters'. Preventive social work was defined as eliminating factors that may endanger the family's position in society by providing household education to housewives, social family care, inquiry into school absence, cooperation with consultation clinics to provide infant and child care, care for single mothers, as well as providing child protection, poverty relief, community-based social work and personal loans.

> The early 1960s saw a growing interest in welfare work or community work, which eventually became the key focus of attention. Social case work became increasingly perceived as too individually oriented.
>
> *(Engbersen & Jansen, 1991)*

Health care and prevention have long been closely linked, for instance, in fighting infectious diseases to reduce child mortality and increase life expectancy.

A wide range of measures have been taken, including well-functioning sewer systems, improved personal hygiene, improved sanitation facilities, inoculation programmes, infant screening for diseases at child consultation clinics. Prevention-focused social work is aimed at improving conditions that negatively affect client groups. Holstvoogd (1995) puts forth that preventive social work calls for more systematic development. He mentions a number of interventions, including education programmes, support groups, training groups, developing clients' social networks, engaging clients' existing social networks and taking on volunteers as educators. For decades mental health care has been focusing on preventive service delivery. Mental health professionals of a special prevention department have developed a wide range of preventive actions. First an analysis is made of the structural problems, generating the starting point for formulating the appropriate preventive activities. By reviewing the process at regular intervals (see also Chapter 23, the practice-based research method), systematic monitoring takes place of how and to what extent targets have been met. These reviews may call for adjustments to the interventions, as to starting points, targets, target groups, strategies and implementation.

21.4 Goals

General goal

- Reducing or eliminating stress-related factors in persons, reducing risk factors and enhancing persons' own strengths and protective factors.

Specific goals

- Preventing worsening of psychosocial problem areas in persons of all ages, preventing them from becoming problem clients. For instance, preventing out-of-control drug use behaviour in youths at risk or criminal behaviour or preventing stressed employees from becoming more stressed-out (i.e. primary prevention).
- Preventing further deterioration of the actual client problem situation. For instance, suicide prevention in youths or preventing stressed clients from becoming more stressed-out (i.e. secondary prevention).

21.5 Indications

- First signs of tension due to a deteriorated position of a group of residents. For instance, signs of prolonged and elevated stress in a group of employees resulting from restructuring (not yet social work clients);
- First signs of tension due to a deteriorated position of a client group, such as signs that point to diminished wellbeing in a number of clients, for example restructuring as a major cause of stress in employees.

21.6 Contraindications

- Lack of time, funding or resources to facilitate preventive activities;
- Dominant individual and/or systemic problem area would, as a result, be neglected; direct support is more urgently needed.

21.7 Techniques

1   Group educational programmes
2   Schooling
3   Preventive support groups
4   Project technique
5   Support for volunteers
6   Standardization
7   Information and consultation centres
8   Safety net technique.

21.7.1 Group education programmes

Social workers inform groups of clients about relevant subjects, such as traumatic events, health and stress, budgeting, bullying or divorce. Goal is preventing exacerbation of problems by way of educating client groups.

21.7.2 Schooling

Social workers are increasingly providing psychosocial education to disseminate knowledge and skills to prevent problems from worsening. It may concern stress management courses, but also courses such as 'Weary Heroes' (midlife crisis), 'Prospect of Retirement' (near the end of one's professional life) or 'Dealing with Unresolved Issues'. For clients with an executive function it may involve trauma relief or executive coaching courses.

21.7.3 Preventive support groups

Topics at these meetings are 'traumatic events' or 'bullying'. Preventive support groups focus on educating groups at risk of experiencing a distressing event. This group education work is aimed at avoiding unnecessary suffering. People learn what normal reactions are during a certain distressing event and learn how to deal with them. Preventive screening involves selecting persons at risk of a complication during group education meetings. As a rule, cancer patients are invited by social workers for an interview. Social workers adhere to a protocol for screening cancer patients who need more intensive psychosocial care.

21.7.4 Project technique

Specific projects can be developed to prevent problems or prevent existing problems from worsening. These include projects on stress prevention, bullying, transition management, health management and trauma relief.

Because of the high frequency that social workers have to deal with transgressional forms of violence, we will take a close look at domestic violence, child abuse and sexual abuse.

Domestic violence, sexual abuse and child abuse

Domestic violence

Situations of violence that deserve special attention are domestic violence, sexual violence and child abuse. In regards to domestic violence (violence committed by someone the victim is familiar with from home), there is a self-perpetuating cycle of violence. Domestic violence can be cyclical (see Figure 21.1). It is very important to keep children from any form of violence (see Table 21.1), and to give shelter and aftercare to those children who have come into contact with violence.

Sexual violence

Unfortunately, many children and adults are confronted with traumatic sexual abuse experiences. We speak of sexual abuse in all cases of people that are confronted with sexual or sexually charged acts against their will by a third party and where the balance of power between the parties involved or the inequality of power between the sexes plays a role.

Sexual violence, no matter the shape or form, is never without consequences. There is a wide spectrum of consequences that sexual violence have on a biopsychosocial level. Most predominant are physical, practical, emotional, social and legal consequences. Of the

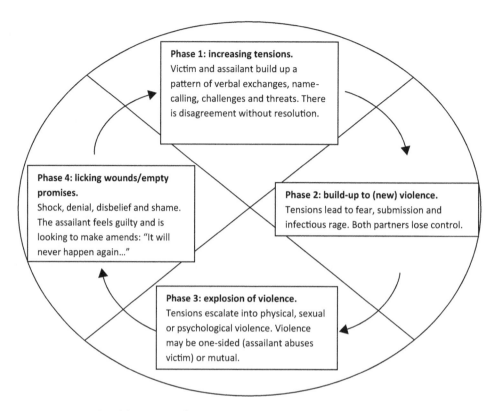

FIGURE 21.1 Cycle of domestic violence

Source: Adapted from Janssen et al. (2009)

TABLE 21.1 Types and examples of child abuse

Types of child abuse	Examples of child abuse
Physical violence/physical abuse	Varies between a hit to serious physical violence with stab wounds and burn wounds; also circumcision of girls
Sexual child abuse	Unwanted pulling in, embrace, pushing against, feeling up, up to incest and paedophilia
Psychological violence	Bullying, humiliating, threatening, psychological neglect, children witnessing domestic violence
Neglect	Physical and affective neglect, deprive of food and water
Kidnapping and lockup	Being taken against their will, kidnapping, locking up
Child murder	Killing children
Child labour	There are 250 million children worldwide between the ages of 5–17 of which 180 million perform dangerous and unhealthy labour

emotional consequences, it is know that they are far-reaching because there may be psychological trauma, post-traumatic stress disorder, dissociative issues and disorders and multiple personality disorder. Because of the many examples of (sexual) abuse, all kinds of forms of (sexual) violence are detailed.

Child abuse

(Sexual) child abuse is a glaring example of a social violence situation. In relationships, families and social networks, but also in groups and in relationships with caregivers, transgressing territorial boundaries can be an experience with far-reaching consequences, even for adults and the elderly. Transgressional experiences lead to emotions, tension and irritation that regularly result in conflicts, though not necessarily violent, and sometimes they lead to all-out domestic, local, national or international war (see Appendix 2).

THERE IS A LOT THAT KNOWLEDGEABLE PROFESSIONALS CAN DO TO PREVENT ESCALATION OF VIOLENCE

Agents hide behind a 'complex relationship', while effective instruments exist to calm partner violence. Below three preventive recommendations are described for adequate interventions.

Since the murder of nurse Linda van der Giessen (28) in the parking lot of the Twee-Steden Hospital in Waalwijk that was committed by her ex-partner, three new, similar cases have been made known. The tone of the reporting creates the impression that it is difficult for the police to respond adequately (complex relationship). It speaks for the police that that they are investigating what went wrong. Critics are very firm in finding fault and assigning blame. What remains is a string of sad incidents where police officers, out of lack of knowledge and ability, did not know what to do.

Research suggests that there are effective measures to deal with this, but it is worrisome that this knowledge hardly gets to where it needs to go. The phenomenon is not new, the recurring dismay is:

- One-third of murders and manslaughter occur as a result of domestic violence;
- One-third of violent incidents that the police are called to also occur as a result of domestic violence;
- One-fifth of all women experience domestic violence by their partner;
- 230,000 women are physically abused by their partners annually;
- 1 out of every 9 women has been raped by her partner;
- 38% of women murdered fell victim to their (ex-)partner;
- 32 female victims of partner killings per year (1996–2006);
- 7 male victims of partner killings per year (1996–2006);
- 87,323 reports of domestic violence in 2010.

One in three incidents of violence that the police is called out for concerns domestic violence. The home is the place of primary danger for women. This is where they run the biggest risk, as is shown by a comparative study by the research institute Atria. At least 1 in 5 women has been physically abused at home by their partner. That's more than 230,000 women on an annual basis. At least 1 in 9 has been raped by their partner and for younger women, this number is around 15%–20%.

Violence frequently does not only continue after separation, but can actually get worse (stalking). The World Health Organization categorizes domestic violence against women as a serious threat to public health. It is connected to stereotyping and an inequality in power and control between men and women. Even though there are a number of women that use relational violence against men, it is usually not comparable based on severity and reach. Women run a disproportionately larger risk. In spite of a steady stream of research data, these results frequently elicit disbelief and belittlement.

The UN special rapporteur on violence against women reports that of all women killed worldwide, 38% fell victim to their (ex-)partner. In the Netherlands, it appears that 1 in 3 murders and manslaughters are the result of domestic violence and women are more frequently the victim than men. Between 1996–2006, the average number of partner killings was 32 women (7 men) per year. It is precisely in the separation period, when women try to remove themselves from violent situations, when they run the biggest risk.

The death of this nurse is no exception, rather a classic example. If an intersection causes 30 deaths per year, acute measures will be taken. The scale on which partner killings occur is begging for acute action. With the recent ratification of the European Council Convention on prevention of violence against women and domestic violence (the Istanbul Convention), the Netherlands have committed to this. Some examples of what research has shown to be effective recommendations:

1   Invest in professional expertise. Pay attention to gender dynamics: men and women run different risks. A more systematic risk assessment per report is required. Article 51 of the Istanbul Convention makes assessing the risk of fatal violence mandatory. Our police already conducts a risk assessment in considering banning someone from their home. This assessment can be made broader and simpler. In the United States, more rapid response instruments have been designed to assess the risk of fatal violence and to offer adequate protection.

2   Police management must make fighting domestic violence a priority. A lot of violent crimes occur in the home, surrounded by fear and intimidation that mainly women fall victim to. The term 'complex relationship' is a misplaced euphemism. In New York, the amount of partner killings declined after the year 2000 when they demoted officers when the threat assessment of violence was insufficiently conducted.

3   Preventive legislation is also a possibility. In England, Clare's Law was introduced that allow threatened people and people in their surroundings to report threats of partner violence. The police is obligated to investigate the report. It allows for discovering and responding to (usually illegal) possession of weapons in an earlier stage. Effective intervention is definitely possible. Let's use this knowledge. There are lives at stake. Where there is a will, there is a way.

Summary of statement: Renée Römkens, former professor of Interpersonal violence and director of Atria, research institute for emancipation and women's history.

21.7.5 Support for volunteers

Social workers can ease the burden for carers (for instance, family of patients with progressive illnesses, persons with dementia and the terminally ill), by engaging volunteers and subsequently prevent carers from becoming exhausted. This project design and promotion of voluntary initiatives is called self-care support (see Chapter 27).

21.7.6 Standardization

Standardization is defining and describing what you do. Methodical standards can be employed to establish procedures and guidelines for a certain treatment. Standardization helps reduce stress and uncertainty in social work professionals by establishing clear definitions and work procedures. An example of standardization in social work is the standardization of grief support. Care facilities are increasingly seeing clients who struggle with loss resulting from death, divorce and illness. The standardization of bereavement care discloses what the tasks of the care professionals are, including the task of the social worker. An illustration of the standardization technique is the standardization of grief support (see Chapter 25).

21.7.7 Information and consultation centres

Setting up an information and consultation centre can prevent people from becoming deprived of help in extreme events, as in the Enschede fireworks disaster. Social workers have established the regional information centre 'Loss and Bereavement'. Social workers also participate in Ronald McDonald Houses, Vicki Brown Houses (for family members of cancer patients), Cancer Homes (for cancer patients, their loved ones and their care providers), Alzheimer Cafés (meeting places for those close to persons with dementia) or HIV Cafés (meeting place for HIV patients).

21.7.8 Safety net technique

Institutions with an elevated risk of trauma have set up safety networks, for example for law enforcement, firefighter services, ambulance care and hospitals. The safety net technique facilitates efficient help for persons after an extreme event. Specific procedures have been formulated for individual and group support. In doing so, preventive action is undertaken to ensure that trauma doesn't develop into trauma complication, such as PTSD (see Chapter 7).

21.8 Social work results

- Residents report that their situation has not deteriorated (primary prevention: they will not become social work clients).
- Clients report that there has not been any structural deterioration in their situation (secondary prevention: their situation has not become worse).

21.9 Evidence

Recent years have seen an increasing number of studies on prevention methods in social work.

21.9.1 Engage social workers in prevention

Hawkins et al. (2010) describe some strategies for preventing mental, emotional and behavioural disorders in young people that have been developed, tested and found to be effective in preventing the onset, persistence and severity of psychological disorders, drug abuse and delinquency. Unfortunately, tested and effective prevention policies, programmes and practices are not widely used. The authors see three strategic opportunities through which schools of social work can advance workforce development for effective prevention policies, programmes and practices. These are through general undergraduate education, pre-service training in social work at the bachelors, masters and doctoral levels, and continuing education training for workers already in practice. The advances in prevention science over the past two decades have created the need for a national workforce that is trained to move evidence-based prevention from efficacy and effectiveness trials into widespread national applications. Schools and departments in other professions and disciplines are assessing their capacity to seize this opportunity.

21.9.2 Communities That Care prevention project

Haggerty and Shapiro (2013) describe a public health orientation to drug and alcohol abuse prevention. They review the state of the science underlying a risk and protective factor approach to alcohol and drug abuse prevention. In addition, they describe Communities That Care (CTC), a community practice model that makes use of this evidence and considers how this model reflects four important principles of social work practice. The intent was to provide guidance to social workers who support the National Association of Social Work's intention to make prevention practice central to the provision of alcohol and drug abuse services by social workers. The authors provide a roadmap for social worker involvement in community-based alcohol and drug abuse prevention. CTC is being implemented in communities across the United States and in many regions of the world. Results from a multi-site community randomized trial of CTC in seven states in the United States suggest that high-quality implementations of CTC contribute to long-term, community-wide improvements in public health. Relative to control communities, CTC communities were more likely to use a risk and protective factor approach to community planning, implement a greater number of effective prevention programmes, achieve a higher degree of quality in their implementation of effective prevention programmes, and have more support for prevention among community key leaders.

21.9.3 PROSPER, community prevention teams

Greenberg et al. (2015) describes a longitudinal investigation of the Promoting School-community-university Partnerships to Enhance Resilience (PROSPER) partnership model designed to evaluate the level of sustainability funding by community prevention teams, including which factors impact teams' generation of sustainable funding. Community teams were responsible for choosing, implementing with quality, and sustaining evidence-based programmes (EBPs), intended to reduce substance abuse and promote positive youth and family development. Fourteen US rural communities and small towns were studied. Data was collected from the PROSPER community team members ($N=164$) and prevention coordinators ($N=10$) over a 5-year period. Global and specific aspects of team functioning were assessed over six waves. Outcome measures were the total funds (cash and in-kind) raised to implement prevention programmes. All 14 community teams were sustained for the first

5 years. However, there was substantial variability in the amount of funds raised, and these differences were predicted by earlier and concurrent team functioning and by team sustainability planning. Given the sufficient infrastructure and ongoing technical assistance provided by the PROSPER partnership model, local sustainability of EBPs is achievable.

21.9.4 Problematic behaviour of teenagers and the TGT project

The problematic behaviours of teenagers and the subsequent negative consequences are extensive and well-documented. Unwanted pregnancy, substance abuse, violent behaviour, depression, and social and psychological consequences of unemployment. Wodarski (2011) reviews an approach that uses cooperative learning and empirically based intervention that employs peers as teachers. This intervention of choice is Teams-Games-Tournaments (TGT), a paradigm backed by five decades of empirical support. The application of TGT in preventive health programmes incorporates elements in common with other prevention programmes. They are based on a public health orientation and constitute the essential components of health education, that is, skills training and practice in applying skills. TGT intervention supports the idea that children and adolescents from various socioeconomic classes, between the ages of 8 and 18 and in classrooms or groups ranging in size from 4 to 17 members, can work together with one another. TGT has been applied successfully in such diverse areas as adolescent development, sexual education, psychoactive substance abuse education, anger control, coping with depression and suicide, nutrition, comprehensive employment preparation, and family intervention. Extensive research on TGT is available using examples of successful projects in substance abuse, violence, and nutrition. Issues are raised that relate to the implementation of preventive health strategies for adolescents, including cognitive aspects, social and family networks, and intervention components.

21.9.5 Suicide prevention programme

For many years now, suicide has been the second leading cause of mortality in youths, following traffic accidents as the main cause of death.

The first version of the Mental Health Awareness Programme (MHAP) for adolescents − a suicide prevention programme − was initially tested in nine countries, distributed over five continents. The study showed significant improvements in attitudes and behaviours of children, parents and teachers exposed to the programme.

In 2014 suicide was responsible for 8.5% of the total mortality rate in youths between the ages of 15 and 29.

Longitudinal analyses show significant improvements in adolescent mental health by effectively reducing depression, negative emotional symptoms, conduct problems and hyperactivity and incident suicide attempts, severe suicidal ideation and suicide plans. A total of 12,395 pupils (mean age: 14.9) were recruited from 179 schools randomly selected in 11 European countries: Austria, Estonia, France, Germany, Hungary, Ireland, Israel, Italy, Romania, Slovenia and Spain, with Sweden serving as the coordinating centre.

An updated version of the programme, the Youth Aware of Mental Health (YAM) programme, was evaluated in an EU-wide Randomized Controlled Trial, namely the Saving and Empowering Young Lives in Europe (SEYLE) research project. The SEYLE-RCT research project was performed to evaluate and compare the effectiveness of different interventions for mental health promotion, suicide prevention and help-seeking behaviour among adolescents (Wasserman, D., et al., 2012, Carli et al, 2014; Wasserman, D., et al., 2015). The interventions included three different preventative approaches designed to empower key actors: Mental health professionals with the Screening by Professionals (Profscreen) programme, teachers and other school staff with Question, Persuade, Refer (QPR), a gatekeeper training programme, and the pupils themselves with Youth Aware of Mental Health (YAM).

The three interventions were compared with a control group, which, for ethical reasons, involved a minimal intervention. Structured evaluation questionnaires contained well-established psychometric scales, demographics, peer relationships, values and so forth, which were administered to pupils at baseline, and at 3-month and 12-month follow-up.

Longitudinal analyses showed significant improvements in adolescent mental health with the active YAM programme compared to the other two interventions and the control group, by effectively reducing depression and negative emotional symptoms, The most important results were the significant reductions in incident suicide attempts, severe suicidal ideation and suicide plans, which are the utmost consequences of stress and mental health problems (Wasserman, D., et al., 2015). Furthermore, the YAM programme engendered understanding between pupils, encouraged peer support and allowed the pupils to get to know each other better, helping them to understand that they were not alone with their problems and thus they were more likely to seek help when needed. It was also very well received and appreciated by the adolescents, who found it a useful and inspiring experience (Wasserman, C., et al., 2012). YAM also helped adolescents who had existing mental health problems as the programme included facilitation of clinical evaluation and help.

21.9.6 Efficacy of prevention projects

A measurement instrument has been developed for establishing the efficacy of prevention projects, called the Prevention Effect Management Instrument (Preffi). It concerns a quality instrument that aims to enhance the effectiveness of prevention projects. Preffi 2.0 was developed by NIGZ (the Dutch National Institute for Health Promotion and Illness Prevention; http://www.NIGZ.nl), consisting of eight clusters from both theory and practice (see Table 21.2). Each cluster contains a number of criteria for rating a project as weak, moderate or strong. All the scores are totalled to reach the outcome assessment of the clusters and the whole project. Actions for further improvement can be formulated on the basis of this project evaluation.

TABLE 21.2 Preffi 2.0: eight clusters from theory and practice

Development-oriented aspects	Implementation aspects
1 problem analysis	6 implementation
2 determinants	7 evaluation
3 target group	8 framework conditions and feasibility
4 goals	
5 intervention development	

21.10 Pitfall

• Perceiving failure of preventive efforts as personal failure and not realizing that some events can't be avoided.

21.11 Summary

In this chapter, we directed our attention to prevention of structural deterioration of a group of (potential) clients. First, we showed what we consider to be structural obstacles in the provision. Then we detailed the history of the prevention method and the techniques a social worker may utilize to prevent further deterioration of the quality of life of a group of people.

In the next chapter, we will address how the social worker, together with a group of people, can look after their collective interests.

Questions

Choose your own or virtual case that features an impending structural deterioration of a group of people.

1 Describe where the structural deterioration are looming: what human needs on a survival, affective, and self-determination level are insufficiently met?
2 Indicate which prevention method(s) may be applicable.
3 Make a plan of how you would proceed in a preventive fashion, in order to improve provisions and bring them in line with present needs.
4 How can a social worker prevent the pitfalls of the prevention method?

22

COLLECTIVE ADVOCACY METHOD

Questions

This chapter addresses the following questions:

- What is meant by structural stressors?
- How did the collective advocacy method develop?
- What techniques are utilized in the collective advocacy method?
- What is known about the evidence of the collective advocacy method?

22.1 Introduction

Previous chapters have discussed social support from individuals' social network, from the system of the nuclear family and extended family and professional support from neighbourhoods, schools, workplaces and care services. In addition, the focus was on identifying structural stressors and on preventive action. The current chapter concentrates on promoting the collective interests of (potential) groups of clients, who are angry because the provisions are not sufficiently meeting their human needs and human rights. Because as Martin Luther King said in 1967: 'whoever accepts evil without protesting against it, is really cooperating with it.'

First, it is explained what is meant by structural stressors in the provisions. Next, the history of the collective advocacy method is described. Then follows a discussion of the techniques available to social workers, who collaborate with a group of people for the purpose of enhancing their Quality of Life. In conclusion, a summary is presented of what has been discussed in this chapter.

22.2 Definition and elucidation

Using the collective advocacy (CA) method, the social worker supports a group of clients, who are to some extent angry and dissatisfied in their actions against the structurally wrong situation from the very beginning – in a certain degree angry and displeased in their actions against the structural stressor. Collective advocacy is where people with similar experiences or in similar situations come together, with or without external support, to pursue a common cause, provide mutual support, and get their collective voice heard. The aim of CA is to improve their social, health, legal and economic position. By carrying out actions aimed at improving the situation, by means of provisions, regulations, resolutions, settlements and laws in co-operation with social workers, tensions and frictions are reduced and the structural strengths of such social groups are enhanced. Social workers continue to carry the torch for those who need help to succeed in our society (NASW). Indeed, while only a small percentage of social workers count collective advocacy as their primary job duty, all social workers have an ethical duty to protect and empower the vulnerable and disadvantaged. Social workers do this using a range of tools, including the writing of open letters to the editor, lobbying, organizing local protests, and helping to change laws that adversely affect vulnerable and disadvantaged members of society. Today's social workers employ a full range of techniques for advocacy ranging from protests and sit-ins to harnessing the power of the internet to network with others in order to effect change. From a multimethod social work model perspective, the collective advocacy method enables the social worker to work together with advocacy groups to reduce the destructive misfit and enhance the constructive fit between environment and the person by influencing the environmental part of the PIE dynamic (the person-in-environment).

Elucidation

Social work practice is broadly defined and allows for both micro (at the level of the individual, domestic unit, or group) and macro interventions (at the level of the organization, community, or policy). Just like the other four macro methods (which includes the monitoring method expounded in Chapter 20 and the Evaluation Method expounded in Chapter 23, the collective advocacy method focuses on decreasing structural stressors such as interference, neglect, discrimination and oppression on the one hand, and on enhancing the strengths of social groups on the other hand. Tensions and frictions are usually caused by the structure or policy of a neighbourhood, company or society. By applying the social monitoring method, the social worker may want to assist social groups who have been wronged by abuse. But how? Let us start by assuming that a social group of clients is unhappy or angry about a perceived wrongdoing. Because the profession of social work is committed to seeking social and economic justice in concert with vulnerable and underserved populations, the macro practice skills of collective advocacy are necessary in confronting these inequalities (Netting et al., 2008). For example, consider a woman reported for child neglect who lives in a run-down home. The home has structural issues which she got upset about but which her landlord is refusing to fix. An individual intervention designed to strengthen her emotional coping skills might be useful, but that intervention alone would ignore the depth of the stressor facing her. It might then become apparent that she is not the only tenant suffering because of this landlord unwilling to do what is right . . . Social workers unwilling to engage in some macro practice types of activities when the need arises are not practicing social work. From a macro practice perspective, social and economic justice considerations may demand that one focuses not on individual assistance alone but on attempts to alter macro systems that fail to distribute resources in a fair manner. Often, the needs of individuals and policy overlap. Here is an example (NASW):

> A social worker works for an organization dedicated to serving homeless and low-income families. Several of her homeless clients tell her they are unable to receive emergency food stamps. When she explores why, she finds a bureaucratic glitch: because homeless families have no address they are not considered residents and are therefore ineligible for the aid.
>
> In the following weeks, the social worker meets with area service providers and state legislators, who agree to clarify the state policy and implement new regulations allowing homeless people to receive food stamps. The social worker continues her advocacy efforts at the national level, providing testimony that eventually helps to pass the federal Hunger Prevention Act of 1988 (P.L. 100–435).

Macro practice is defined as a professionally guided intervention designed to bring about change in organizational, community and policy arenas (Netting et al., 2008). *Macro* means large-scale or big. In social work, it involves the ability to see and intervene in the big picture, specifically within larger systems in the socioeconomic environment. Macro social work practice can include collaboration with consumers to strengthen and maximize opportunities for people at the organizational, community, societal, and global levels. Indeed, many social workers would argue that it is the macro level – the attention given by social workers to the big social issues of importance to consumers – that distinguishes social work from other helping professions (Glisson, 1994).

Macro practice, as all social work practice, draws from theoretical foundations while simultaneously contributing to the development of new theory. Macro practice is based on any of a number of practice approaches, and it operates within the boundaries of professional values and ethics. In today's world, macro practice is rarely the domain of one profession. Rather, it involves the skills of many disciplines and professionals in interaction.

Because codes of ethics serve as guidelines for professional practice, it is imperative that students know the content and limitations of written codes (Netting et al., 2008). For example, principle values in all national codes of ethics of social work associations include service, social justice, dignity and worth of the person, importance of human relationships, integrity and competence. The codes of ethics are intended to introduce a perspective that drives practitioners' thinking, establishes criteria for selecting goals and influences how information is interpreted and understood. Regardless of which role the social worker plays – programme coordinator, community organizer, political lobbyist or direct practitioner – these professional actions are not value-free.

Ideally, social justice is achieved when there is a fair distribution of society's resources and benefits so that every individual receives a deserved portion (Netting et al., 2008). Social work is in the business of distributing and redistributing resources, whether they are as tangible as money and jobs or as intangible as self-efficacy or a sense of self-worth. Underlying the distribution of resources in society are value considerations that influence the enactment of laws, the enforcement of regulations, and the frameworks used in making policy decisions. Jansson (2011) points out that social justice is based on equality. With the many entrenched interests one encounters in local communities, it is likely that social workers will focus their efforts on oppressed target population groups and will always be discovering new inequalities. Since so many groups face problems related to having enough financial resources, social workers often extend the principle to include economic justice, often focusing on social and economic justice concerns.

22.3 History of the collective advocacy method

The term 'collective advocacy method' originates from what was called 'consciousness movements', 'social action' or 'political action' in the 1960s. The collective advocacy method also has its roots in the emancipation movements, which took a stand for lower income groups against poverty, women's emancipation against sexism, and all other social movements such as those advocating for the rights of the physically and mentally disabled persons, gay and transgender, religious groups such as Jewish, Muslims and so on, against discrimination and racism. But the history of social work's more structural contribution to the improvement of society dates back even further.

Already in the earliest days – around 1900 – the influencing of social legislation and advocating for social reforms was seen as the core activity of social work (Waaldijk, 1996). In the history of social work, there have always been frictions between the workers who strived for the individual welfare by doing casework, and the social reformers who thought that case studies only demonstrated the necessity of social action. The founders of social work already realized that the combination of personal involvement and the analysis of structural causes should become the strength of social work rather than its weakness. Social worker Mary Richmond (1914) wrote: 'Prevention and cure must go hand in hand.'

22.3.1 To put the social back in social casework

In the United States, the National Conference of Social Work (an association for social workers) formulated the structural task of social workers as far back as 1939, when its congress stated that the aim of social work was 'to bring about and maintain the progressively more effective adjustments between social welfare resources and social welfare needs.' In other words, social workers had to develop more activities in order to make the social welfare facilities meet the apparent needs. The method of community organization (CO) was mentioned as yet another macro method, next to *social casework* and *social group work*. In Europe, CO developed further under the name 'community work'. Lippitt et al.'s (1958) book *The Dynamics of Planned Change* strongly boosted the establishment of CO theories. The rise of the Civil Rights Movement and the deadlocked Kennedy Poverty Program (a programme to tackle poverty) gave CO another impulse. The latter was an impulse in the direction of the more conflict-based strategies such as mass organization, demonstrations and marches to apply direct pressure on the structures, groups and individuals who were in the way of necessary social reforms.

The new community work developed as a branch of social work. The community work approach is different from the social casework and social group work approaches. The object of assistance is no longer the individual client, but a whole client system: a part of society. Here too, the purpose is the following: 'to guide the client system to self-responsibility and self-sufficiency in tackling problems or set-up goals through a gradually growing motivation, in a long-winded self-recognition process of the problems in the client system' (Tienen & Zwanikken, 1972). Social community work should contribute to democratization. It is a method to provide more welfare for civilians in a neighbourhood, district or city by letting the persons involved join in the thinking process, by allowing them to have a say and improving their self-sufficiency.

Political involvement of social workers can also be a way of indirect practice, influencing society by working on social justice. In 1951, just after World War II, Marga Klompé, a social worker by training, became the first and only minister of Culture, Recreation and Social Work in the Netherlands. Her political work as a minister is valued by organizations and social groups involved with the poor, also because she worked for the scientific underpinning of community social work by letting allowing for the publication of *cahiers* which contained the theory of education, methodology and methodology development.

The historiography of social work's contribution to the decrease of structural and social pressure points doesn't come to an end here, with the secession of this new branch in community work. The 'social' in social work did not disappear. During the turbulent period of the 1960s, in social work too, there was a lot of focus on social action as a method. However, the establishment of the theory on the collective advocacy method remained more ideological than practical in an ideological counter movement.

22.3.2 Disadvantaged groups

In the 1980s, conferences for socially conscious workers were organized concerning themes such as 'Social work and social discrimination'. In his book on practical experiences, Janssen (1977) questioned the method of social work in general with regard to disadvantaged groups (e.g. the unemployed, those unable to work because of sickness or disability, foreign employees, people receiving social assistance and minimum wage earners). According to Janssen, actually choosing for the underprivileged has far-reaching consequences for the political position, organizational structure and methodology of social work. In the so-called open house approach, an easily accessible walk-in facility, Janssen (1977) explains that there are many material problems such as issues of housing, insufficient clothing, no means of transportation and not being able to find an appropriate job.

There has also been a lot of criticism aimed at the psychologizing approach of social work in general. 'Social work is working on the alleviation of psychological suffering through therapeutic assistance, rather than on the reduction of these material problems. They are even working on relationships instead of working on the actual problems.' De Roeck (1977) also thought that a social worker should not focus on personal growth alone, because that would mean ignoring the social structures. 'And then, the individualizing social worker could turn societal pain into private suffering.' 'You cannot let the unhealthy society get off scot-free.'

The emancipatory approach addresses such criticisms of the individualizing character of social work. The emancipatory approach focuses on the collective awakening to oppressive circumstances and on activities that can change these circumstances. In the 1970s, social workers wrote about strategies and methodology for social action with the purpose of serving welfare workers 'who want to contribute to radical "inversions" of the social systems through study and actions' (Reckman, 1971).

At the same time the 'radical therapy' entered Europe, having originated in the United States. 'Not adjustment, but change!' was the motto of the Radical Therapist Collective (1974). In their book by the same title, antipsychiatry, women's emancipation, children's rights and gay emancipation are all discussed. *Radical social work* draws heavily upon Marxist and feminist concepts and emphasizes politics, class conflict, ideological hegemony, and socialism (Thompson, 1992). It highlights structural inequities inherent in a capitalist society and the role of culture and belief systems in perpetuating inequality. It refocuses the attention of the social worker on the environment. Radical theory creates a problem for clinical social workers in that it attributes individual difficulties to structural inequities. It would accordingly prescribe structural interventions in combination with individual, family or group work. Structural understandings should underpin social work approaches not necessarily replace them – hence the S of PCS analysis (see Figure 22.1), which is based on the idea that an adequate understanding of human experience should encompass personal, cultural and structural aspects and not rely solely on individual aspects as traditional social work does. Radical theory would thus require social workers to focus any direct practice on educating clients and empowering them to change the structures that contribute to their oppression than only helping them to cope with the status quo. Whereas more traditional individual approaches tend not to make values explicit radical social work makes those values explicit (hence the emphasis on ideology and hegemony). The danger of risk of the radical approach can be that the social worker may impose his or her values and worldviews regarding the socio-political nature of problems upon clients who are seeking help. This danger would apply to any approach. Radical social work and individual social work is in that sense more about education than indoctrination. Client self-determination is negated as the social worker educates the client on the 'real' causes of his or her problems and insists on political awareness and political action. This would be a misunderstanding. Client self-determination is enhanced by an emphasis on empowerment (gaining greater control and thus rooted in self-determination). There is no 'insisting' involved. It is a process of helping people understand the wider circumstances they find

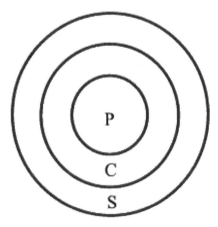

FIGURE 22.1 PCS analysis

Source: Thompson (2016)

themselves in and thus to challenge pathologizing. Radical social work can at times dehumanize the individual by solely focusing on socio-political determinants without acknowledging the role of individual choice and action.

But then radical social work is misused and misunderstood, because there is nothing inherent in the holistic approach of radical social work that means it will dehumanize people – in fact, helping people understand how their problems need to be understood more holistically is a process of humanizing. Radical social work's incorporation of a socio-political viewpoint of the environment comes at the expense of complements and contextualizes an enriched theoretical understanding of individual and subjective experiences. Subjective experiences do not happen in a vacuum – they are strongly influenced by cultural and structural factors. An approach that focuses purely on the individual relies on a partial and potentially distorted understanding of the person and their circumstances. Thompson (1992) notes, 'the oppressive social order manifests itself in a variety of significant ways – socially, psychologically and emotionally.' Thus the social worker should not neglect the individual's experience in attempting to address social issues. Some of the early radical social work texts said little about the individual as that was already the dominant thinking, so they counterbalanced this by emphasizing the wider context. However, things soon developed into a much more holistic approach that emphasized the need to understand the individual in their social context. As Thompson (2011, 2016) articulates, we are, all unique individuals, but unique individuals in a social context – to understand the person, you need to understand the individual and their social circumstances. He therefore evolved his PCS analysis in order to understand how inequalities and discrimination feature in the social circumstances of clients and in the interaction between clients and the welfare state. It could be helpful to analyze the situation in term of three levels. These three levels (personal, cultural and structural) are closely interlinked and constantly interact with one another (see Figure 22.1). If we want to develop an adequate understanding of the people we are trying to help, we need to take in account of all three dimensions: their personal perspective and life experiences to date, the cultural influences that continue to shape those life experiences (and our reactions to them) and the structural context of an uneven distribution of power and opportunities. Thus the social worker working from the PCS analysis cannot neglect the individual's experience in attempting to address social issues.

The macro task of social work also has roots in *group work* (see also Chapter 17). Since the end of the nineteenth century, the history of social group work has been closely linked to those social work institutions established to meet the needs of the population. Group work started out as a type of idealism, devoted to the improvement of the quality of social life in terms of working conditions, housing conditions and leisure activities. Around 1940 there was a remarkable shift of emphasis in the arena of social group work. The writings of Konopka dating from the 1940s and 1950s provided a strong stimulus for a more therapeutic approach. In his group method, Vinter (1967), yet another social worker, mentions three intervention possibilities entirely focused on the individual, group or society, defining direct and indirect forms of social work practice:

1   Direct influence of the individual client in the group;
2   Indirect influence by starting up small working processes in small groups;
3   Influence via the social environment of the participating clients.

Historically, another term that has been used to describe macro social work practice is *indirect work*. The concept of 'indirect practice' refers to the use of policy, advocacy, community and management methods of social work practice to bring about and manage a more humane and just social order.

Although this term is becoming less popular, the word *indirect* served for many years as a reference to social work's commitment to environmental modification and the alleviation of social problems. Whereas *direct practice* connoted face-to-face contact with clients aimed at supporting or strengthening them as individuals, *indirect practice* was the catchphrase for change efforts involving the environment and the social welfare system (Pierce, 1989). Hollis (1964) noted:

> Not since Mary Richmond's time have we given the same quality of attention to indirect as to direct work. This neglect has tended to downgrade environmental treatment in the worker's mind ... [as] something unworthy of serious analysis. ... This is an absolutely false assumption. Environmental work also takes place with people and through psychological means.

22.3.3 Social empowerment

Special attention should be given to language in national codes of ethics with reference to 'the empowerment of people'.

Empowerment is a key term for understanding and directing our efforts in terms of consumer-based 'macro' change. In a general way, *empowerment* refers to the central and direct involvement of clients in defining and determining their own struggles, strengths and future. Social workers empower others by finding ways in which clients of services can design and implement activities that accentuate their own unique assets in addressing needs (Delgado, 2000). Empowerment involves liberation. When clients exercise the ability to plan and create social change, they gain control. Frequently, politicians and policymakers make decisions 'for the sake of clients'. As well intentioned as this may seem, the net effect of such a paternalistic approach runs counter to self-determination and prevents clients from using their own capabilities to gain access to power in the social environment.

Practitioners know that when clients take charge of the change process, a fervour for finding solutions soon follows. Indeed, the entire helping relationship becomes more collaborative:

> Empowerment-based practitioners join with clients as partners and rely on clients' expertise and participation in change processes. They discern the interconnectedness between client empowerment and social change. These changes are not trivial! They redirect every phase of the practice process.
>
> *(Miley et al., 2001)*

Using an empowerment approach, clients advocate for rights, services and resources with assistance from social workers, rather than social workers acting on behalf of clients.

22.3.4 Emancipation

According to Anja Meulenbelt (1987, social worker), the three mechanisms of oppression – sexism, racism and class difference – do not function independently. Within each individual, these mechanisms are entwined, which has a very confusing effect. In her book *Fighting the Illness, Not the Patient*, she tries to give the reader a very concrete image of these oppression mechanisms. She also tries to indicate the possibility of co-operation between the oppressed and the oppressors. Meulenbelt's range of ideas had an enormous influence on social work.

During the 1960s, social workers went out on the street together with action groups to take on controversial topics such as sexism, racism and class differences, but also topics to do with wearing your hair long ('Better long-haired than short-sighted'). Today, social workers mainly work behind the scenes for groups of clients feeling structurally discriminated. Emancipation movements strived for an end to discrimination and for the acknowledgement of equality. Women felt discriminated against. They thought that they were treated unequally, just because they were women. They earned less than men, while doing the very same job, for instance. Migrants too revolted against the unequal treatment on the basis of their skin colour. When a foreign worker is rejected after a job interview because he does not have the required professional skills, for example, it is not a matter of discrimination. However, when he is rejected because of his different skin colour, it is without a doubt a matter of discrimination. This kind of abuse, where groups are being unequally treated because of irrelevant factors, can be an important sign for the social worker to take immediate action: this is where the social worker applies the collective advocacy method.

Holstvoogd (1995) describes advocacy as a form of demonstration with communicative and physical means with the purpose of bringing about collective changes, which would eventually result in the elimination of abuse. The role of the social worker in this kind of action can vary, depending on the circumstances. After all, the social worker is obligated – also according to the deontological code – to take action against abuse when it is encountered. The International Federation of Social Work (IFSW, 1997) stated that social workers do this worldwide, for example, by tackling social exclusion. This is done with the purpose of establishing an active participation in society of all citizens. In occupational social work (OSW), the O very often represents the working on structural and cultural improvements in the labour organization. Correspondingly, general social work could consider the welfare situation in her work area – district or village – as the point of departure for co-operation with residents in order to realize structural improvements (e.g. poverty programmes, safety projects, increasing the number of meeting points, improving youth services). Accreditation committees visiting social work schools suggest that social workers should improve their skills in macro practice. In 2012 Betsy Clark Executive Director of NASW declared advocacy as the cornerstone of social work:

> Advocacy is the cornerstone upon which social work is built. It is so important that it is framed in three sections of our Code of Ethics. Advocacy for individuals, communities and systems is not just a suggested activity for social workers. It's not a 'do it if you have some extra time' or a 'do it if the inequity and disparity are very great' activity. It is a requisite.

22.4 Goals

General goal

- Reducing or eliminating the structural stressors and enhancing the strengths which exceed social groups.

Specific goals

- Contributing to improvement actions of a group of upset clients concerning the structural stressors (see section 22.1);
- Supporting the structural actions of a strong, angry or unhappy group of clients that fears a worsening of its position,

22.5 Indications

- Anger and discontent in a group of clients. Social, organizational and political pressure is needed to improve the position of this group.
- Anger and discontent in a group of clients. Social, organizational and political pressure is needed to counteract the worsening of their position.

22.6 Contraindications

- Time, money or other means are not available.
- The dominant individual or systemic problem would be neglected.

22.7 Techniques

1 Force field analysis technique
2 Self-organization technique
3 Social policy technique
4 Lobbying technique
5 Action and social media techniques
6 Advocacy reports.

22.7.1 Force field analysis technique

Draw up a visual outline on paper of all the active forces and powers which are present (see Figure 22.2). If necessary, do this together with a colleague who also knows the institution,

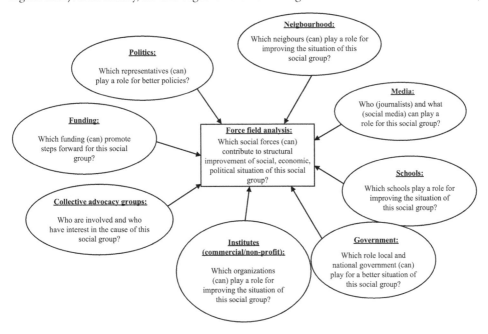

FIGURE 22.2 Force field analysis

Source: de Mönnink (2016)

company or region. As an example, imagine a situation where several colleagues want to put on the brakes because some form of reorganization is occurring far too quickly. The social worker draws up an organization chart to show which forces (e.g. board of directors, project group, works council) have an influence on the pace of reorganization. It also tries to establish whether the employees can exercise an influence on someone in order to improve their own wellbeing or that of the whole company. Also, the own terms of reference and/or the scope of practice of the company's welfare workers are assessed in this interplay of forces.

22.7.2 Self-organization technique

The company's occupational worker draws up a self-organization plan in consultation with the group of unsatisfied and frustrated employees. This plan describes how the employees can tackle the problems by working together. However, the company's welfare worker does not take up the task of a trade union, works council or organized interest group. Another example might see the company's welfare worker putting forth a proposal to the board of directors to mobilize a group of unsatisfied employees by letting them join in an assessment of their work situation (social group work approach) and letting them make proposals for the improvement of structural pressure points. Referring the employees to a trade union or works council may become necessary. The seven conditions below are presented here to enable social workers to more easily denounce abuse (Donkers, 1999):

1 The client can only be supported in trying to change things in his environment to such an extent that it is no longer a personal action of the client, and that in any case the problem concerns more than just one person.
2 The client must determine exactly how far the social worker can go.
3 It is urgently required.
4 There must be time on hand, and the worker must be able to count on the support of the institution.
5 The process must be a combined and well-coordinated action of both the social worker and the client.
6 Both the client and the social worker can autonomously take action in the environment, but the social worker cannot do so completely independently from the client.
7 The social worker must be cautious in following the client's wishes to change something in the environment. Before anything at all is done, the social worker must be fully aware of the 'why' and the 'how'.

22.7.3 Social policy technique

If an institution, company or region has an inefficient policy on making radical changes which affect many individuals, the social worker can use his influence to align the policy of the management, administration or politicians responsible with the interests of the people. This means helping in creating a 'social policy'. If the social worker applies the social policy technique in close consultation with a group of angry or dissatisfied clients, this technique also comes within the collective advocacy method. (The influencing of a social policy without consultation is considered the lobbying technique; see section 22.7.4.) Examples of radical changes which impact many people are reorganization, wholesale dismissal or the (re)construction of a railway line or airport (with the consequences of forcedly moving away and expropriation).

TABLE 22.1 Four social policy actions are described by Jansson (2005)

Policy practice activity	Definition	Examples
Policy analysis	Studying the policy to understand its goals, strategies, and potential impact	Analyzing provisions of No Child Left Behind and implications for student assessment procedures
Advocating for policy change	Interacting with policy makers in order to influence their policy decisions on particular proposals	Writing to members of Congress about changes needed in No Child Left Behind to make it more effective in meeting its goals
Building coalitions	Developing relationships with other groups to develop a coordinated advocacy message and strategy	Bringing educators, parents and child advocate groups together to work on advocating for changes in No Child Left Behind legislation
Launching a campaign	Creating an overarching strategy and message to influence not only policy makers but the public about an issue	Developing a coherent message for radio ads, flyers, a website, etc. to present arguments and rationale to support needed changes in No Child Left Behind

Jansson (2005) was one of the first social policy scholars to conceptualize policy practice as a distinct aspect of social work practice (see Table 22.1). He distinguishes between policy practice and policy advocacy in the following manner. He defines *policy practice* as efforts to change policies in legislative, agency, and community settings, whether by establishing new policies, improving existing ones, or defeating the policy initiatives of other people. People who are *skilled* in policy practice increase the odds that *their* policy preferences will be advanced.

22.7.4 Lobbying technique

Initiating interactions with key figures in decision making can contribute to the cancelling out or decrease of abuse. An example might be where active support (by means of a letter, telephone call or email) of a pending proposition for a violence, trauma or safety protocol within an institution, company or region can contribute to better violence and trauma care and to a better safety management respectively. An example would be the following statement: 'As company welfare workers, we plead for the introduction of the trauma protocol proposed by the works council, because it has a preventive effect on the employees.'

'Dos' and 'Don'ts' in lobbying by social workers are summarized (NASW) related to lobby-actions in the United States with members of Congress.

LOBBY DOs

1 Do learn members' committee assignments and where their specialties lie.
2 Do present the need for what you're asking the member of Congress to do. Use data or cases you know.

3   Do relate situations in his or her home state or district.
4   Do ask the Representative's or Senator's position and why.
5   Do – in case of voting records – ask why he or she voted a particular way.
6   Do show openness to the knowledge of counterarguments and respond to them.
7   Do admit you don't know. Offer to try to find out the answer and send information back to the office.
8   Do spend time with members whose position is against yours. You can lessen the intensity of the opposition and perhaps change it.
9   Do spend time in developing relationships with congressional staff.
10 Do thank the member for stands they have taken which you support.

LOBBY DON'Ts

1   Don't overload a congressional visit with too many issues.
2   Don't confront, threaten, pressure or beg.
3   Don't be argumentative. Speak with calmness and commitment so as not to put him or her on the defensive.
4   Don't overstate the case. Members are very busy and you're apt to lose their attention if you are too wordy.
5   Don't expect members of Congress to be specialists. Their schedules and workloads tend to make them generalists.
6   Don't be put off by smokescreens or long-winded answers. Bring the members back to the point. Maintain control of the meetings.
7   Don't make promises you can't deliver.
8   Don't be afraid to take a stand on the issues.
9   Don't shy away from meetings with legislators with known views opposite your own.
10 Don't be offended if a legislator is unable to meet and requests that you meet with his or her staff.

Lobbying is inclusive of a number of different settings in social work practice at local, state, federal and even the international levels. Though there may not be comparable bodies in each level (particularly at the international level), the settings for lobbying include citizens advocacy, grassroots-level community organizations, non-profit agencies (citizen's groups that shape policy and provide valuable community services) and the three branches of government (Jansson, 2007).

These settings across the different levels from local through international are the points of origin for the policies that affect clients and that set the parameters for the services social workers may provide. When social workers understand where the policy originated and where it needs to be changed, then they can plan effective strategies to influence that person or deliberative body. If the social worker determines that the gap in services can be resolved in the local community, he will not need to involve state or federal officials. If, however, he discovers that there are multiple gaps in service delivery due to a lack of state and federal funding, then he may need to work at those levels to advocate for increasing funding in this area to meet the needs of vulnerable people.

22.7.5 Action and social media techniques

During the 1960s and 1970s, action groups took all sorts of social and political action. They did so by means of demonstrations, blockades, occupations, mass writing or telephone calling, advertisements, a black book, media attention through advertisements, interviews on the radio and other more light-hearted forms of actions. In several cases, action groups were supported by social workers and sometimes the social workers were even a part of the action group. Nowadays, social work preventively supports an action group where there seems to be a risk of aggravation of the already existing problem situations, caused by a structural stressor. As an example, a social worker pointed out that employees who were in mourning were not allowed to have flexible working hours. The social worker supported the lobby of the Dutch Mourning Support Association by means of an expression of support for the inclusion of flexible mourning leave in the collective agreements. A second example is that of the social worker who pointed out that, after stillbirth, employees were frustrated with the official at the Registry of Births, Deaths and Marriages because he could not, by law, accept the registration of a child that had not lived (back then the law only applied for children born alive). Social work then supported the action against the Second Chamber of the Dutch Parliament in order to make them revise the Law on Disposal of the Dead, so that stillborn children could also be registered in the Registry of Births, Deaths and Marriages.

For social workers, collective advocacy represents the series of actions taken and issues highlighted to change the 'what is' of a specific disadvantaged social group into a 'what should be', considering that this 'what should be' equals a more decent and a more just society (Cohen et al., 2001). Those actions, which vary with the political, economic and social environment in which they are conducted is collaborating with the social group, have several points in common (Cohen et al., 2001). They:

- Question the way policy is administered;
- Participate in the setting of agendas, as they raise significant issues;
- Target political systems 'because those systems are not responding to people's needs';
- Are inclusive and engaging;
- Propose policy solutions;
- Open up space for public argumentation.

Action via the internet

Take action today! – Join the advocacy listserv!

In the United States, NASW's Government Relations staff is fighting hard to make the voice of professional social workers heard on Capitol Hill. It states that the most effective way to express its ideas and vision, however, is through its members. Having a network of professional social workers willing to contact their members of Congress – via letter, email or office visits regarding specific issues is essential, ensuring that NASW's legislative agenda is addressed in the Senate and House of Representatives.

The British Association of Social Workers developed a Social Media Policy (BASW, 2012). This policy states that evolution of social media has enabled social workers across the world to share knowledge and information, debate critical issues, provide support and connect with others who share interests. It helps social workers keep up-to-date with developments in policy, social work and related professions. This is contributing to the development of social workers' professional identity as an international profession based on values of human rights and social justice.

The terms 'social media' and action via 'social networking' are often used interchangeably to refer to web-based tools and technologies that support online communication and information sharing. Social media is, in effect, a publishing and broadcasting medium and includes:

- Blogs – writing a blog or commenting on people's blogs or vlogs (blog in video format);
- Micro-blogs such as Twitter;
- Social networking sites, such as Facebook, LinkedIn, Ning, and having a personal profile page on one of the social or business networking sites;
- Content-sharing services, such as Flickr, YouTube, Vimeo;
- Product or service reviews on retailer sites, or customer review sites;
- Taking part in online votes and polls;
- Taking part in conversations on public and private web forums (message boards);
- Wikis are websites developed collaboratively by a community of users, allowing any user to add and edit content;
- Podcasts;
- Social bookmarking, such as Delicious;
- Location-based services (e.g. Foursquare).

Boyd and Ellison (2007) define social networking sites as web-based services that allow individuals to construct a public (or semi-public) profile and display a list of other users with whom they share a social connection. In addition, these sites have created innovative communication channels, such as posting comments on individuals 'walls' and 'tagging' pictures, offering new ways for individuals to communicate with their online networks and make possible all forms of collective advocacy.

22.7.6 Advocacy reports

Advocacy reports are collective advocacy tools to use in all kind of structural advocacy-issues, made possible by the practical research method (Chapter 23).

One example of such a supporting report is the report by the *Advocacy Development Project* (2000). The role of the Development Project was to support National Health Service (NHS) Boards and local authorities (the Scottish Executive), along with their planning partners, to develop and implement advocacy plans in the mental health field. The Scottish Development Centre for Mental Health (SDC) was commissioned in May 2002 to undertake two research projects on collective advocacy: developing collective advocacy for people who fall within the remit of the new Mental Health (Scotland) Bill; and, developing collective advocacy for people who have long-term contact with health or social care services. The following report relates to the first project.

SUPPORTIVE REPORT: 'DEVELOPING COLLECTIVE ADVOCACY FOR PEOPLE WHO FALL WITHIN THE REMIT OF THE NEW MENTAL HEALTH (SCOTLAND) BILL'

This report is the result of a research project commissioned by the Scottish Human Services Trust that studies collective advocacy for people who fall within the remit of the new Mental Health (Scotland) Bill.

The purpose of the study was to map existing collective advocacy groups in Scotland for people with mental health problems, those with learning disabilities, people with dementia or acquired brain injury. Also, to describe the issues currently faced by collective advocacy groups and the likely challenges and opportunities presented by the proposed new legislation; and, to identify the steps that might be taken to enable collective advocacy groups to respond effectively to the new Mental Health (Scotland) Bill and other recent legislation.

A framework was developed that enabled information to be gathered on the structure and function of collective advocacy groups. Information was collected on 54 groups across Scotland. The mapping exercise showed that a wide range of different types and sizes of groups undertake collective advocacy and that a wide range of collective advocacy work is undertaken. It also became clear that the term 'collective advocacy' is not always used by groups offering a collective advocacy service.

Group interviews were then held with a sample of 16 collective advocacy groups in order to gather further information. A number of barriers to undertaking collective advocacy work were identified that focused on infrastructures and resources, capacity, awareness and attitudes, and links with others. Groups were also asked about supports and resources that they received or would like to receive. Groups also talked about issues around independence, representation and accountability and whether they felt listened to or not.

Two themes; coverage of the full age range of people, and the implications of the new Mental Health (Scotland) Bill for the development of collective advocacy were explored in further detail at two workshops.

The report concludes that it is important to take into account the breadth of collective advocacy functions. Also, that the fragility and vulnerability of much collective advocacy activity and the variable amounts of information and knowledge about legislative developments held by collective advocacy groups suggests that there is need for a considerable building of capacity.

22.8 Social work results

- The group of clients feels supported by the interventions of the social worker in their actions against the structural stressor.
- The group of clients feels supported by the interventions of the social worker in their preventive actions against the worsening of their position.

22.9 Evidence

There is no known research to date in relation to the effectiveness of the collective advocacy method.

TCC Group proposes in their paper 'What Makes an Advocacy Organization Effective?' an effort for evaluation of advocacy organizations (2009).

22.9.1 Advocacy organizational capacity: an assessment tool

TCC Group has developed an organizational assessment tool for policy and advocacy organizations – the Advocacy Core Capacity Assessment Tool (Advocacy CCAT). The Advocacy CCAT is a supplemental tool to TCC Group's more comprehensive Core Capacity Assessment Tool (CCAT), which is meant for all non-profits, including policy and advocacy organizations (information about the overall CCAT can be found at http://www.tccccat.com). Both the overall CCAT and the supplemental Advocacy CCAT assess four core capacities of successful organizations: leadership, adaptive, management and technical capacities. The Advocacy CCAT drills deeper into each of these four core capacities, adding and assessing capacities that are unique to policy and advocacy organizations; specifically those in Table 22.2.

In addition to the core capacities, organizational culture plays an important role in organizational effectiveness. Both the overall CCAT and the Advocacy CCAT also measure organizational culture. In addition to the core culture measures that are a part of the overall CCAT, TCC has added in the Advocacy CCAT culture elements that are important for policy and advocacy organizations. These include:

1   Willingness to take risks and advocate even when success is not guaranteed.
2   Overt acknowledgement of the value of partner organizations.
3   Overt acknowledgement of the value of individual staff members.
4   Celebration of success, both small- and large-scale.
5   Level of staff commitment to an issue.

TABLE 22.2 Advocacy organizational capacity: an assessment tool

Leadership	*Adaptive*
• Advocacy Board Leadership	• Strategic Partnerships
• Leadership Persuasiveness	• Measuring Policy/Advocacy Progress
• Community Credibility	• Strategic Positioning
• External Credibility	• Funding Flexibility
• Leadership Strategic Vision	
• Leadership Distribution	
Management	*Technical*
• Policy and Advocacy Staff Roles and Management	• Legal Understanding
	• General Staffing Level
• Policy and Advocacy Management Systems	• Policy Issue and Theory Knowledge
• Staff Coordination	• Stakeholder Management Skills
• Policy and Advocacy Resource Management	• Stakeholder Analysis Skills
	• Media Skills
	• Knowledge Generation Skills
	• Information Dissemination Skills

The essence of advocacy requires an organization, regardless of the advocacy strategies it adopts, to be able to adapt to rapidly changing circumstances and environments. Adaptability needs to be inherent in an organization's structure and capacity in order to encourage its advocates to be more flexible within the activist environment.

EVALUATING ADVOCACY ORGANIZATIONAL CAPACITY AND DETAILED CAPACITY LOGIC MODEL

TCC Group recommends a two-pronged approach to evaluating nonprofit advocacy organizational capacity:

1 General organizational capacities

An advocacy group should initially be evaluated as a nonprofit, using general nonprofit capacity benchmarks – such as clarity of mission, sound leadership and management practices, monitoring and evaluation activities, board composition, involvement and activity.

Over its 25 years of research and experience, TCC Group has developed a model for generally describing and understanding organizational effectiveness in the nonprofit sector. This model, specially designed for non-profits, identifies four core capacities, which are adapted in this paper for specific use by advocacy groups:

Leadership: The ability of organizational leaders to create and sustain a vision, to inspire, prioritize, make decisions, provide direction and innovate – in an effort to achieve the organizational mission.

Adaptive: The ability of a nonprofit organization to monitor, assess, and respond to internal and external changes (such as networking/collaborating, assessing organizational effectiveness, evaluating programmes and services and planning).

Management: The ability of a nonprofit to ensure the effective and efficient use of organizational resources.

Technical: The ability of a nonprofit to implement all of the key organizational and programmatic functions (such as finance, budgeting, fundraising, technology, marketing and communications).

Each of these capacities is relevant to the general nonprofit community in defining and diagnosing an organization's strengths.

2 Specific advocacy capacities

The advocacy group should then be evaluated on the unique capacities of advocacy organizations, as outlined and discussed in this paper.

The methodology for evaluating general nonprofit capacities can involve traditional approaches and tools, such as organizational assessments (e.g. TCC CCAT, EEMO, McKinsey). Further, standard information that a nonprofit collects and summarizes in the course of doing business – such as Form 990s, budgets, staffing descriptions, proposals – can also be used as evidence in assessing general organizational capacity. Appraisal of an organization's specific advocacy capacity, however, requires a more nuanced approach.

A few workbooks and checklists have been developed which rely primarily on guided self-evaluation. Such approaches to evaluating advocacy capacity can be very effective for organizations and lead them to ask and find answers to important strategic questions and should be considered as easy ways for organizations to monitor themselves on an ongoing basis. However, from an evaluation perspective, such approaches have certain limitations: Qualitative self-reflection often does not reveal 'blind' spots in the organization ('I don't know what I don't know') and because the questions are static, they do not encourage the organization to think deeper on certain issues.

For more information about the supplemental Advocacy CCAT, contact TCC Group at by email at: info@tccgrp.com.

22.9.2 Social media and collective advocacy

Can social media promote civic engagement and collective action? Advocacy organizations think so. Obar et al. (2012) surveyed 169 individuals from 53 advocacy groups of diverse interests and sizes and identified a revealing trend. All groups admitted that they use social media technologies to communicate with citizens almost every day. Respondents also believe that social media enables them to accomplish their advocacy and organizational goals across a range of specified activities. The authors note that the relationship between this and real political and ideological change is still speculative, but suggest that future studies can build on their research.

22.9.3 Health care and collective advocacy

In specific health care structural issues it was evaluated which kind of effects collective advocacy can have. Some examples have been summarized here. For effective collective advocacy for patients with inflammatory bowel disease: communication with insurance companies, school administrators, employers and other health care overseers were discussed in an article by Jaff et al. (2006). In addition to their physical challenges, children and adolescents with inflammatory bowel disease (IBD) living in the United States face a number of administrative and regulatory hurdles that affect their quality of life. This article, written by a physician, attorney/patient advocate and a social worker, discusses a number of these challenges and describes how the provider can help his or her patient overcome them. Specifically, the article discusses four areas in detail: appeals of denials of coverage from insurance companies and third-party payers; assisting children with IBD with classroom and school accommodations; assisting uninsured children in obtaining Social Security benefits; and aiding a parent to care for their child using the Family and Medical Leave Act. Although this article has a paediatric focus, adults have similar advocacy needs. Case examples and sample letters to third-party payers, schools, and employers are included in this article.

22.9.4 Health policy and collective advocacy

The collective advocacy for appropriate health policy and effective governance of the health system is discussed in another article (Mukhopadhyay, 2007). Health policies supported by sustained advocacy efforts need to continually grow and develop to respond to the increasing pressures of macro-economic policies of globalization, liberalization and privatization. Voluntary Health Association (VHA), the largest network of voluntary agencies in the health sector, is playing a critical role at both the macro- and micro-levels. Its health advocacy efforts emerge from the grassroots with an understanding of their health and development problems as well as the strategies adopted to address them. The process, of strengthening an upward mobilization of information, towards formulation of an effective health policy, is backed by serious macro research on various policy dimensions of health, done by the Independent Commission on Health and Development in India (ICDHI), set up in 1995 by VHAI. These key policy documents are both reflective and prescriptive and are presented to the highest state authorities along with a discussion at various levels with varies groups. One of the recent successes was at getting the giant tobacco companies to withdraw from cricket sponsorship with an association in the formulation of a comprehensive bill by the Union government to prevent this in future. Various well-researched policy documents have been put together by the organization based on its micro- and macro-level work and persistent advocacy. Appropriate public health and development policies with their effective implementation are the cornerstones to realize the fundamental values of Alma-Ata. The health care system needs to be removed from the current bio-medical model and closer to a socio-political and spiritual model where health care again becomes an organic part of community care as it once was in the traditional society.

22.10 Pitfall

• Taking the lead instead of working on the same level with or following the interest group.

22.11 Summary and questions

This chapter started by describing what is meant by structural stressors. Then followed an overview of the history of the collective advocacy method. Next, the techniques of the collective advocacy method were discussed that social workers utilize to optimize the Quality of Life of a group of people whose human needs and human rights have not been sufficiently met.

Questions

Select your own or virtual case that shows a group of people who may benefit from the collective advocacy method.

1   Describe which human needs at the level of survival, affection and self-determination are not being fully met?
2   Indicate which CA method can be utilized to effect improvements.
3   Draw up a plan of action that shows how provisions can more successfully satisfy the group's actual needs.
4   How can you, as a social worker, avoid the pitfalls of the CA method?

23

PRACTICAL RESEARCH METHOD

This chapter addresses the following questions:

- What is the importance of developing knowledge within the domain of social work?
- What is understood by evidence-based practice?
- What is the difference between a standard, a directive and a recommendation?
- What techniques are employed in the practical research method?
- What evidence is known to support the practical research method?

23.1 Introduction

The previous chapters focused on the macro methods that are targeted at enhancing support delivery by services. What is the importance of monitoring, prevention and collective advocacy in detecting and eliminating structural obstacles? This chapter deals with the practical research method, which is directed at developing knowledge in the field of social work and its body of knowledge, because, as Kurt Lewin stated in 1952: 'There is nothing more practical than a good theory.'

First, the concept of evidence-based social work is explained. Then, an overview is presented of the history of the practical research method. Furthermore, the techniques are described that social workers utilize to conduct research for the purpose of enhancing the quality of life (QoL) of groups of people. In conclusion, a summary is presented of what has been discussed.

23.2 Definition and elucidation

The practical research method is used in social work when knowledge about any aspect of the social work practice is lacking. In many cases there is confusion about how an issue or situation in social work is playing out: how many clients are having relationship problems? Which social work method is most frequently used? And so on. If knowledge is lacking about whatever aspect of the SW practice, the practical research method is suggested.

23.2.1 Definition

Knowledge is power. Legal recognition of the social work profession comes closer if there is more evidence of the effectiveness of social work. The practical research method can provide this evidence. This method promotes knowledge (about problems, target groups, methods and effects) of a specific field within the domain of social work. Through data collection and analysis, gaps will be filled with knowledge. There are five kinds of practical research in social work (Migchelbrink, 2001):

1   Research through inventory: to clarify everything within a field of knowledge on paper;
2   Researching requirements: to assess what needs there are;
3   Process evaluation: making the evaluation process of social work visible;
4   Evaluation of effects: making the effects of social work visible;
5   Development research: developing new methods and sub-trajectories.

23.2.2 Elucidation

When a doctor is asked, 'What exactly was he doing in the treatment room?,' and he says: 'I was just doing something,' he is likely to be called before the medical disciplinary tribunal as an unreliable doctor. A social worker who says: 'I wasn't sure what I was doing exactly. I was just doing something,' confirms the picture of the vague professional who works from the heart rather than using his brains. Every self-respecting profession will base its action on knowledge and insights are gained through research. This research with preliminary results uncovers a *body of knowledge*, which through repeated and improved research will lead to *evidence-based* knowledge. In a time of 'proven' medicine there are initiatives within the psychological and psychosocial support systems to create a better practice and to substantiate this with evidence-based protocols, guidelines and decision trees. A protocol is best compared with a script outlining how the social worker preferably deals with certain problems. How forceful this preference is (don't do this, but do that) depends on scientific evidence, 'the evidence' (Vandereycken & van Deth, 2003). 'As a consequence of the proliferation of protocols there is a real threat that one cannot see the wood for the trees anymore: also most protocols, etc. are (still) not evidence-based.' In addition to protocols, there are standards, directives and recommendations that have decreased scientifically based evidence.

•   A *standard* is a set of undisputed facts that are used as a reference norm for practice. To ignore or not respect the standard can be considered professional misconduct. Example: in every social work contact, the non-directive counselling method is embedded.
•   A *directive* is a guideline based on general practical rules that are backed by sufficient research or broad consensus. The social worker is expected that he is guided by this directive in managing his practice. For example, for restructuring debt the possibilities to repay this debt are determined and with mediation a written contract is signed between two parties.

- A *recommendation* is a proposal or option for the social worker to keep in consideration when making choices or decisions. For example with a client who uses psychotropic drugs, the social worker first needs to consider which substance is being used.

Many social workers feel resistance against the introduction of treatment protocols. This resistance is not unfounded. Working with treatment protocols has a number of fundamental and practical objections. Principled objections to treatment protocols are that some of those protocols are based on a number of myths (Vandereycken & Van Deth, 2003).

- The myth of *uniformity*: there is one specific treatment for certain psychosocial problems – the one and only appropriate treatment offered by the social worker, for one specific client.
- The myth of *specificity*: there is only one particular treatment for one specific psychosocial problem, of which the results cannot be obtained by any other treatments.
- The myth of *exclusivity*: the best treatment must be given priority above all other treatments; this is the myth that one particular treatment always belongs to one particular indication, even with different clients.

The following practical objections to treatment protocols are possible:

- They damage the therapeutic relationship between social worker and client.
- They do not meet the true needs of the client.
- They make treatment untrustworthy.
- They are not innovative.
- They threaten job satisfaction and the professional identity of social workers.
- They are not feasible in daily practice.

The social work profession is, for the aforementioned reasons, not suitable for developing and introducing treatment protocols at a session level. But the development of standards, guidelines and recommendations for clear and transparent working of social workers is surely needed. The first step towards standardization is to describe the tools (methods) of the social worker. And to determine how and when these tools are used and which knowledge this can bring to the social work practice.

23.3 History of the practical research method

In Dutch social work research tradition was missing until almost 2000. Since 1995 a number of initiatives were taken to make social workers in training more research-oriented. At the turn of the century, the Dutch social work education system took the subject into their curriculum. Towards the end of their education, students are capable to do simple research with some guidance. Another research boost in social work are the lectureships at the colleges that have a research project in the field of social work. The lecturer (a university assistant with a respectable expertise in a particular field) surrounds himself with teachers who are going to do practice-based research in a specific field. Also cooperation and mergers of colleges and universities are expected to lead to a new research impulse. Finally, the new bachelor-master system that was introduced in 2003 gives colleges more opportunities for students to do research. The bachelor-master splits the university education up in a wide-ranging 3-year bachelor's phase (undergraduate phase) and a specialized 1-, 2- or 3-year master's degree (graduate phase). In 2004, a number of master's programmes in social work started at several Dutch universities. In these courses, students are also expected to do a research for their masters.

Social workers with a master's degree are expected to be proactive in organizational and policy levels in social work and take the lead in order to monitor the quality of social work and if necessary increase it. Independently doing research is an indispensable tool.

In Canada and the United States (and several other countries) social work degree programmes have been included in the university system from the beginning of the 1900s. Therefore there is a much longer tradition of research. One who visits any American social work school is going to see bulletin boards full of questions of students asking to find cooperation with their research. In addition to their teaching obligations social work teachers also have research tasks. Teachers in universities have the usual publication obligations: every social work teacher is expected to contribute to the scientific production of knowledge in their field. This scientific production is measured by the number of publications in the form of books, articles and conference papers each teacher produces. There are many research institutes that develop social work research by making use of external funds. These research infrastructures, which facilitate more social work research, lead to knowledge through the so-called *social work research*. A social worker, who has studied at the *School of Social Work* for 3 years, will earn the title 'bachelor'. After studying for 2 more years, he gets the title 'master'. One of the components of this master is an independent practice-oriented research. Social workers with a master's degree, who go on to do a doctorate degree, can call themselves a 'doctor in social work'. A doctor in social work has done more fundamental research in the field of social work, such as validating (having a scientific foundation of) checklists. This research infrastructure in North America has contributed materials for decades which are interesting for social work at an international level. This also explains why for many years, most social workbooks in the Netherlands have been translated books and articles from North America.

23.3.1 Scientific research

There is a recurrent debate in the history of social work whether or not social work is a science in itself. It is a fact that scientifically schooled teachers originally were deployed to reinforce the profession with scientific knowledge. All kinds of supporting courses were taught such as: psychology, sociology, economics, philosophy, andragogy and law. Since these teachers only had an obligation to teach, research stayed behind. The theoretical support of the course was determined by sciences which, from many different directions, translated their own specific knowledge into practice. A coherent theoretical foundation was therefore lacking until now. In the first period that social work was expanding strongly – from 1950 – it was the scientists who were taking care of the scientific input, such as from the field of psychology and sociology. From a psychological and sociological angle they often focused on similar research topics. This brought knowledge on topics such as 'attachment behaviour of youngsters' and 'class structures of the target groups in social work'. In the last century, the Marie Kamphuis Foundation has a founded a chair in social work affiliated with the University of Utrecht. The first Dutch professor of social work is Geert van der Laan, who supports scientific promotions of social workers among other things.

As more social workers were scientifically schooled, more specialized research topics were examined. For her promotion of the effectiveness of social work intervention after stillbirth, medical social worker Christien Geerinck-Vercammen researched reduction of multiple births and termination of pregnancy (Geerinck-Vercammen, 1998). And the social worker Herman Baars did his PhD on researching the function of social network analysis in contact with psychiatric patients (Baars et al., 1995). A similar development in research is evident in the field of nursing. There are three courses in nursing science available in the Netherlands right now. Now that nurses are studying the profession themselves, much more practical knowledge around practical themes such as lifting techniques is created. Sociologists and psychologists who researched in the field of nursing, focused more on topics such as the experience of the patient and labelling processes around patients.

23.3.2 Types of research

Globally there are two types of research in social work: quantitative research and qualitative research. In quantitative research, also called evidence-based social work research, the question, 'is counselling effective when clients ask questions about the meaning of life?' is turned into measurable units. Ultimately, there is an answer to the question, with numerical data. This evidence is considered the quantitative basis of the generated knowledge. *Evidence-based social work* is the deliberate, explicit and judicious use of the best currently available knowledge when making decisions about the care of individual clients. In qualitative research, also called *practice-based social work research*, the results are not based on numbers, but for example, on judgements (subjective data) of respondents. Research into one case, the so-called N-1 trial, can provide expertise in qualitative research tradition. It's just that the scope and representativeness of the statements (the research results) are more limited. Below the developments in medicine and physiotherapy are described in relation to *evidence-based practice*. The intention is to examine what can be learned from these developments for the social work profession.

23.3.3 Evidence-based medicine

In medicine, quantitative or evidence-based research is standard for the development of knowledge (evidence-based medicine). To reduce the risk of wrong diagnosis and wrong therapy with disastrous consequences, research on what works and what does not work in medicine is widely done on a grand scale. Applying evidence-based social work means that the outcome of the most recent and best conducted scientific research is being assessed for its applicability. With that assessment the expertise that the social worker has built up over many years of practical experience plays an important role. One of the results of evidence-based medicine is the development of protocols and guidelines for the assessment, in which the latest and best scientific researches are combined with expert judgements (Noordanus, 1997). Research results within medicine have direct results on the way it is carried it out in practice. When it turns out that a particular diagnostic or therapeutic technique is preferred, this becomes a criterion for professional practice. An example is British research showing that doctors in Britain miss at least a quarter of all heart attacks, because they stick to familiar but outdated tests (electrocardiograms and so-called creatine kinase tests) to come to a diagnosis, instead of using the more reliable, so-called troponin test (NRC, 2003). According to the cardiologist Verheugt from Nijmegen, all hospitals in the Netherlands with a coronary care unit now use the troponin technique. When translated to social work it could be researched what effects social work analysis techniques and intervention techniques have. One condition is that the methods and techniques that are used in social work should be described in a manual. The multimethodical social work model lays the foundation for this kind of research, by filling the gap of an ordered description of analysis and intervention techniques.

23.3.4 Evidence-based physiotherapy

Just like in social work, in physiotherapy, a quantitative research tradition was almost completely lacking as well. This resulted in a lot of scepticism about whether physical therapy actually does help. This notion was confirmed by the Dutch Health Council in 1999 after researching devices such as lasers, electrotherapy and ultrasound and found that those devices had no added value. Within the profession a cultural change happened: physiotherapists went back to basics, by going back to exercise therapy. Now devices are rarely used in physical therapy. Instead, patients are put to work. New research in 2003 – again at the request of the Dutch Health Council – showed positive effects by exercise techniques that were recommended by physiotherapists such as: mobilizing exercises, strengthening exercises, exercises that improve endurance, coordination and relaxation techniques proved especially helpful with cystic fibrosis, chronic obstructive pulmonary disease, osteoarthritis of the knee and chronic back pain. But for many ailments no scientifically substantiated conclusions can be made on where these positive effects originate.

Philip van der Wees (see; Dutch Health Council 1999) of the Royal Dutch Society for Physiotherapy said:

> It is indicative for the change that has occurred in physiotherapy. Before, everything revolved around machines. Therapy was actually a passive affair. The pain was taken away, but within six months, you're back to square one. Now we have chosen an active approach, where the patient is put to work. This is the only way we can solve the problems beneath the surface.

According to Professor Rob Oostendorp, member of the committee that compiled the report of the Dutch Health Council, there is insufficient basis for all kinds of techniques because in physiotherapy there is no scientific tradition. Physiotherapy is a professional education and the graduates are engaged in kneading, pinching, advising and treating with devices and movement therapies. The therapists are not very involved in research. The proven effects of exercise techniques by physical therapists will play an important role in the continued discussion in whether or not insurers will reimburse physiotherapy for chronic illnesses. When translated to the profession of social work, these tendencies within the physiotherapy have the following meaning:

- The social work profession will have to explain its methods and techniques before research can be possible.
- Currently, a lot of techniques are being used of which helpfulness has not been proven.
- There is great danger that social work will suffer when cuts are being made, because the profession has not been proven to be effective: according to employers and the government other employees can easily take over tasks instead.
- It is about time that process and effect research is conducted towards the effects of techniques that social workers use during client contacts.

The development of evidence-based research in social work is still in an early stage. Research expertise and research funding is mostly lacking. Myers and Thyer (1997) are questioning in an article what the reason could be that social workers use so many unexamined, less effective methods. They name six reasons:

1   In education systems very little attention is paid to empirically tested methods.
2   Within college-courses mainly non-tested methods are used and discussed.
3   Many social workers don't read literature on research results.
4   Research results are difficult to apply in a practice situation.
5   Many social workers think that all methods are equally effective.
6   Clients are unaware of the used methods and scientific thinking behind them.

The authors do plea for prescribing on a legal and ethical basis, and for using empirically tested methods as much as possible in social work. Munroe (1998) is making an inventory on the repeated errors that were made by social workers who worked in child protection in the period between 1973 and 1994. She bases her findings on an analysis of all the research that was already carried out in the period from 1973 to 1994 (a so-called meta-analysis or meta-study). There is persistent criticism on the lack of knowledge of social workers in child protection. The quality in which social workers do research and judge practice-situations is criticized. Many problems result, according to Munroe, from the inability of the workers themselves to explain how they work. The inadequate education and training of these social workers is also criticized. The existing preference for a personal style of working of the social workers could be an important obstacle in order to integrate proven expertise and research into practice. There are national associations of social workers who have formulated a research programme for social work to do so.

23.4 Goals

General goal

*   Increasing the quality of social work by filling structural gaps in knowledge in the field of social work.

Specific goals

*   Establishing a rapport with clients, with insight into the psychosocial situation of citizens, of a client group and of methods and other aspects of social work;
*   Making the results of social work visible;
*   Validating (testing) methods and techniques and instruments in social work.

23.5 Indications

*   There is no clear picture on (the aspects of) the position of the target group of social work regarding the used intervention method(s).
*   Structural bottlenecks and blockages of the target group of social work should be viewed more closely.
*   The desire to evaluate methods should arise in order to develop new methods and to research the position of social work itself.

23.6 Contraindications

- There is no time, no money, or there are no funds for research.
- Eliminating bottlenecks at an individual or systemic level has priority.

23.7 Techniques

1   Content analysis
2   Open interview
3   Group interview
4   Questionnaire technique
5   Delphi technique
6   Nominal group technique
7   Participating observations.

23.7.1 Content analysis

With content analysis the researcher collects and processes qualitative and quantitative data from documents, from the media, from the physical and social reality: conversations, speeches, sermons, stories, poems, letters, newspapers, magazines, books, radio and TV broadcasts, recordings, video recordings, archives, records, brochures, policy plans, drawings, songs, art products and the organization of the social environment.

An example of a content analysis task: what stressors are indicated in the reports of socio-medical teams? Collect the reports. Identify what stressors you are going to look into: personal or environmental stressors? Formulate questions: what stressors in the vicinity are named in the reports on these teams? Read the reports and give a provisional answer. Create categories or classes to organize found answers. Try this way of ordering with a small selection of the chosen material. Keep checking the categories and compare them to each other. This way you can sharpen the preliminary findings and formulate the consistency.

23.7.2 Open interview

The open interview is a personal conversation with people in which information is gathered by asking open questions (also called the qualitative interview). The researcher can take three kinds of open interviews:

1   The unstructured interview
2   The semi-structured interview
3   The structured interview.

In a structured interview a set checklist is used with questions that should be addressed. In a semi-structured interview there is also room for personal views and opinions of the inter-viewee, alongside the checklist. In an unstructured interview is the 'topic' is determined, but there's no set structure for the interview.

23.7.3 Group interview

In the group interview, also called a focus interview, a number of people will be questioned at the same time. Characteristic of a group interview is that people react to each other, not just to the interviewer (see Figure 23.1). When a conversation topic is being presented to several people at the same time, a group effect will occur, which has an influence on what's being said and how it's said.

23.7.4 Questionnaire technique

The survey is a research tool in which the questions that are presented are precisely formulated in advance. These questions are exactly the same for everyone. With a questionnaire, data from a large group of people can be collected quickly. Here is an example of the phased process when creating a structured questionnaire about the expectations of a social work course:

1 Make a list of characteristics (variables – the expectations).
2 Specify characteristics (make them operational). Expectations are thoughts, desires, content requirements, methods and assessments of students.

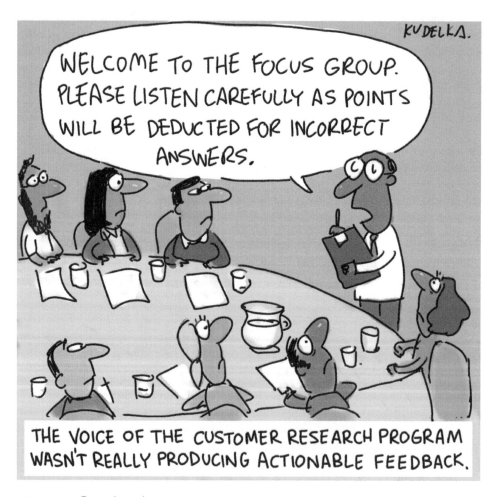

FIGURE 23.1 Group interview

3 Make a first formulation of the questions. What are your expectations of the content in this course?

4 Take these first formulations and decide about the type of questions. A question and answer, opinion, factual question or not. A choice is being made between multiple choice and open questions.

5 Set the sequence (routing) of the listed questions.

6 Think of a layout.

7 Check the questionnaire for accuracy, clarity, neutrality, acceptability, brevity and so on, by testing it on a test group or pilot group.

8 Check the questionnaire content against the actual question.

9 Try the questionnaire out on a test group or pilot group.

10 Finalize the list based on your findings from numbers 7–9 and have the desired number of questionnaires made.

23.7.5 The Delphi technique

The Delphi technique is a data collection technique for questioning general experts or experts in a particular field of knowledge. The questioning consists of multiple rounds, in which several different consecutive questionnaires are being used specially designed for this particular matter by the researcher. After each round, the responses from the participating experts are analyzed, summarized and reported back to each participant.

23.7.6 Nominal group technique

The nominal group technique is an oral technique for generating knowledge from the group in a number of rounds. The discussion rounds come to a group judgement through a voting procedure.

- The initial question is presented orally by the chairperson or the researcher.
- Without any interaction with others in the group, group members think about their answers and thoughts and submit them in writing.
- With every turn one member brings one idea of his or her list to the table.
- One by one each of the identified responses is discussed within the group.
- Each member makes a personal ranking of the scores. These scores are added for each answer, which in turn creates a group ranking. The highest scoring answer is regarded as the practical knowledge with the most support within the group.

23.7.7 Participating observations

In a participating observation, the researcher takes part in the everyday activities of the studied observations and collects data. As a researcher you spend a certain time in the 'field', to research the situation. This entails making observations as well as listening, discussing, having informal conversations, having focused conversations, interviewing and collecting documents such as reports. After a preparatory phase and description phase the researcher tries to formulate and test patterns and clusters in the thematic phase, and connects them to new observations while actively participating. The researcher presents these preliminary findings to the ones that were already researched. Based on these reflections, the examiner checks the developed knowledge of the study group within the group itself.

23.8 Social work results

- There is a report on the table which holds the intended understanding of the psychosocial situation of citizens or a client group, as well as certain aspects of client care.
- There is an availability of knowledge within the field of social work on which social workers can base their work decisions.

Building a social work research report

This index is the canvas of a social work research report. Below you can find a checklist of the elements of this report.

Title page
Resume
Preface
Index

  1   Introduction
  2   Content orientation (domain exploration)

Question and definition of concepts

    Research design
    Population/random sample respondents
    Description/justification of the research instrument
    Data collection
    Processing of data
    Analysis of data

Results
Conclusions and recommendations
Discussion and discussion propositions
Bibliography
Attachments

23.9 Evidence

23.9.1 Research on unmet needs of HIV patients

Social workers who plan or administer programmes are fundamentally concerned with meeting the needs of the clients served (Bonuck, 1996). The social work profession, while proficient at needs assessments, has paid insufficient attention to research into social bases of unmet service needs. The study of Bonuck is an examination of unmet needs of persons with HIV diagnosis. It utilizes the Health Behaviour Model (HBM) within the framework of the ecological perspective. The study of Bonuck is presented as a case example to illustrate the value of this research methodology for administration, programming and policy in the human services.

In the qualitative research synthesis (Kerson & McCoyd, 2013), interviews with 22 early health-related social workers were re-examined to identify themes that emerged when these social workers discussed the roles and goals of their work. Those interviews, with colleagues of Ida M. Cannon and those leaders in the next generation of social workers who had practiced during the first half of the twentieth century, were conducted in 1976. For this study, the themes that emerged from the original interview data as social workers' responses to perceived needs were then compared with data consisting of 80 cases, drawn from four more recent casebooks (1982, 1989, 1996, and 2010), that followed a framework of practice in context. The comparison demonstrated that themes remain consistent over time and include responses to needs created by wars, due to new and underserved populations, created by public health crises, created by technological advances, experienced by organizations, and resulting from economic and policy issues, as well as needs of clients. Analysis also suggests that caution is in order to avoid being co-opted by organizations and others in power at the cost of the profession's social justice mission and ethical imperatives.

23.9.2 Satisfaction of social work clients

There is a great satisfaction from clients about social work. This is the outcome of meta-research into the effectiveness and results of existing research such as in the Satisfaction Research of Social Work (Flikweert & Melief, 2000). To celebrate 100 years of social work, the Verwey-Jonker Institute compared 22 satisfaction surveys from 1980–1999. A meta-analysis (an analysis of the analyses of the individual studies) revealed that satisfaction in social work is great. In the studies the overall satisfaction of clients is between 73% and 91%. Individual aspects were shown to vary greatly. The benefits clients experienced can be divided into four categories:

1   Support, care, understanding and encouragement;
2   (Behavioural) changes in the psychosocial sphere;
3   Three concrete services and facilities;
4   Learning to live with the situation when the desired results are not as expected.

The criticism towards the results of the given help was much less than the positive appreciation. Nevertheless, sometimes there were reports that the results were not in line with the preferences of the client because the social worker was too hesitant, was not thorough enough, or did not choose the solutions preferred by the client. The study shows that not only the client was benefitting from the help, but also the surrounding people. The benefits for the wider environment were derived from comparing the clients own statements with priorities playing in society. For those priorities the objectives of the social policy of government were chosen as an indicator. The results of this analysis are presented in Table 23.1 (Flikweert & Melief, 2000).

23.9.3 Hospice social work and research agenda

In the United States social work is developing social work research in a systematic way, for example in the field of hospice social work. The National Association of Social Workers in the United States erected the Social Work Policy Institute (2010) and presented *Hospice Social Work: Linking Policy, Practice and Research* (Washington, DC: National Association of Social Workers). As an example of good practice for empowering international social work research strategy, we take from this publication two citations, as follows.

TABLE 23.1 Results (at client level) linked to objectives (local and national government)

Results at a client level	Linking to objectives of local and national government
Work situation improves, back to work.	Promoting social integration and participation and reducing the reliance on benefits.
Improved family situation; less stress, more attention to family members, better relationship with partner.	Reducing the appeal for and use of social benefits (welfare mothers, single-parent families as a result of divorce).
Contact with friends, family, neighbors and/or colleagues have improved. Less personal isolation.	Promoting social cohesion in the neighbourhood and the environment, promoting social relations.
Does not need help anymore, independence improves.	Reducing dependence on aid, reduce the reliance on and use of facilities.
No debts, a better grip on own finances.	Preventing arrears problems, preventing eviction, reducing dependence on aid, lessening socially relevant losses.
Fewer psychosocial problems, a better grip on own life.	Reducing the use of social services, (mental) health care and indirect secondary problems caused by mental problems (temporary work disability or early school departures).

The National Center for Social Work Research Act (S.114 – January 2009)

In the United States, Senator Daniel Inouye has introduced this legislation in each Congress since 1999. It amends the Public Health Service Act to establish the National Center for Social Work Research as an agency of the National Institutes of Health (NIH) to conduct, support and disseminate targeted research on social work methods and outcomes related to problems of significant social concern. The legislation authorizes the Director of the Center to: (1) provide research training and instruction; (2) establish research traineeships and fellowships; (3) provide stipends and allowances; and (4) make grants to nonprofit institutions to provide such training, instruction, traineeships, and fellowships. It directs the Secretary of Health and Human Services to establish an advisory council for the Center.

Agenda development for hospice research: a look to the future

Bern-Klug et al. (2005) have proposed a national social work research agenda related to palliative and end-of-life care. This agenda highlights areas for research that align with the social work professions' mission and values. The imperative to develop the agenda emerged from the 2002 and 2005 Social Work Summits on End-of-Life and Palliative Care, organized by the Social Work Leadership

Development Awards Program, sponsored by the Open Society Institute's Project on Death in America (PDIA), a project of the Soros Foundation. The Leadership Development Program supported 42 scholars and led to the creation of the Social Work Hospice and Palliative Care Network (SWHPN) (http://www.swhpn.org).

In addition to the social work research agenda, national organizations, such as the National Hospice and Palliative Care Organization (NHPCO; see http://www.nhpco.org/chipps-newsletters/may-2004) and the Hospice and Palliative Nurses Association (HPNA) have released agendas focusing on various elements of care and service administration for palliative and end-of-life care. The efforts of social work researchers contribute both to the discipline-specific and interdisciplinary research agendas. In the coming year, the effort to increase interdisciplinary research will result in the release of a collaborative research agenda from the American Academy of Hospice and Palliative Medicine (AAHPM), NHPCO, HPNA, and the Social Work Hospice and Palliative Care Network (SWHPN).

The Social Work Policy Institute from the NASW (2010) was presenting the report 'Hospice Social Work: linking policy, practice and research'. This report is a good example of empowerment of SW by a sound social work research strategy.

The Palliative End of Life Care Research Agenda in this report consists of the following themes:

Palliative and end of life care research agenda

- Continuity, gaps, fragmentation, transitions in care;
- Diversity and health care disparities;
- Financing;
- The policy/practice nexus;
- Mental health concerns and services;
- Communication;
- Individual and family care needs and experiences;
- Quality of care;
- Decision making;
- Grief and bereavement;
- Pain, symptom management;
- Curriculum development.

23.10 Pitfalls

- Not doing sufficient domain exploration. The social worker will do his or her own research rather than doing a proper inventory on existing research first: what have other researchers done, how have they done research and to what conclusions did they come?
- Trying to know too much at once. There is an initial start document missing about the research design.
- Research-technical shortcomings: unclear question (for example, two questions at once instead of one), poor operations (not sufficiently measuring what needs to be found out), weak representativeness (the conclusions are based on a small group of respondents), low reliability (measurements are not sufficiently accurate), low validity (the instruments don't measure what needs to be measured).

23.11 Summary and questions

The current chapter has dealt with the practical research method that is directed at developing knowledge in the field of social work and its body of knowledge. The concept of evidence-based social work was first elucidated. Next, the history was described of the practical research method. In addition, a description followed of the techniques utilized by social workers to conduct research that contributes to enhancing the QoL of groups of people. Finally, a number of studies in the domain of social work were discussed. In the next part of the book, Capita Selecta, some concepts, touched upon in the methods, will be described in more detail.

Questions

Select your own or a virtual case in which a group of people may benefit from social work research.

1 Describe which human needs or human rights on the level of survival, affection and self-determination were investigated for this group of people.
2 Indicate whether and which research techniques were employed to investigate this group.
3 Try to find international evidence-based social work studies that conducted randomized controlled trials. Consult international journals and PubMed. What were the conclusions? Make a strength and weakness analysis of this study.
4 Give your opinion on how social work research can contribute to enhancing the profession.

PART VIII

Capita selecta

24

HUMAN NEEDS AND HUMAN RIGHTS AS AN ETHICAL GUIDE FOR SOCIAL WORK

Start, follow and end where the needs and rights of the client are.

24.1 Introduction

Since its beginnings over a century ago, social work practice has focused on meeting human needs and developing human potential. Human rights and social justice serve as the motivation and justification for social work action.

The instrumental professionalism that is described in this book is not separate from normative professionalism: they are more like two sides of the same social work-coin (see the introduction to this book). Multimethod social work is not purely instrumental and is not devoid of value or norms. Every action, every methodical instrument of the toolbox gets its direction by being embedded in the values the social work profession stands for. It is clarified that social work, together with the client and his environment, mobilizes the strength to meet human needs and to stand for human rights, for social justice.

Within social work, people are seen as 'social beings'. They need other people. For individual development, protection, upbringing and guidance by others is needed. For their physical and psychological 'survival', human beings depend on the decisions and actions of others. It is this connectedness and dependence, and the power in social relationships that bring about that the social worker profession has given itself the assignment of improving fulfilment of needs and social justice of the individual in interacting with his environment (PIE).

This chapter offers the human needs and rights (HNR) perspective as the ethical perspective in social work (see Figure 24.1). In every client interaction, social workers help their clients address these HNR: which human needs do clients experience, how can clients be empowered to meet their own needs, which resources in the environment are available to meet these needs and which universal human rights are at stake here?

First, we will describe the classification of human needs, followed by the classification of human rights. A description will be given of what needs and rights mean, a justification will

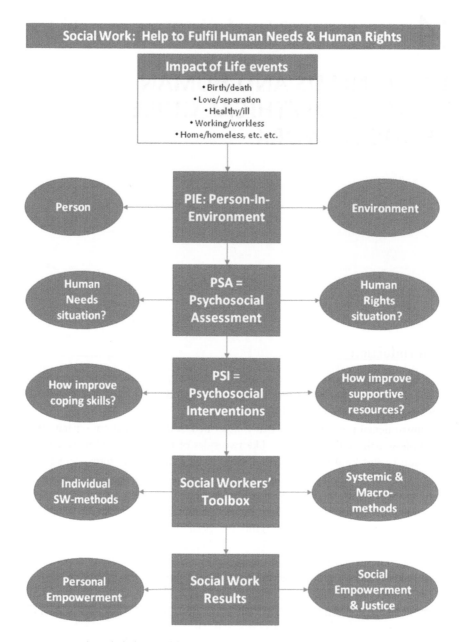

FIGURE 24.1 Social work: helping address human needs and human rights

be given of what these classifications are based on, and what historical evidence there is in social work. The described needs and human rights are illustrated by fragments from the case study of Maria (19), who, as a social work student herself, asked for help from a school social worker.

Case study Maria

Maria was a social work student who was not able to finish her grief counselling seminar, which formed part of her education as a social work student. An educator referred her to the school social worker at her college. It appeared that her unfinished emotional business was reactivated during the seminar and as a result, she found herself unable to concentrate on her studies. For a long time, Maria had been struggling with her mother's unexpected death (suicide when Maria was 5), her brother's death (overdose at the age of 14) and with the fact that her father had never been there for her during these life events. Maria remained rebellious and came close to having dealings with justice and the police. During the school social work sessions she wondered 'Why? Why do these terrible things happen in my life?' The social work sessions helped Maria sort out these troubling issues. By arranging all of the problem areas, she was able to deal with one specific area at a time and eventually got a grip back on her life.

24.2 Human needs and social work

How does a social worker measure whether a client feels that he was helped? By determining the degree in which the client receives what he needs to independently get on with things in his own life and, as much as possible, is able to give his life direction again. That is why human needs and rights is the ethical starting point for client-directed social work contact: What kind of support does the client need in order to move forwards? Which rights can the client make use of? Which approach is effective with this particular client, with these specific needs and rights, under these specific circumstances? (See also section 2.3.2, Taxonomy of universal human needs and the case study of Maria.)

Human needs are regarded as the motivating force behind human behaviour. In order to meet these needs, the universal human rights provide support. Social workers and their clients derive a mandate from these human rights, a (legal) means to actually meet these human needs. Depending on local and (inter)national (rights to) provisions, needs are either adequately met or not.

The place of the HNR perspective in social work can be clarified in Figure 24.1.

24.2.1 Needs as starting point?

HNR have a long tradition in the theory formation of social work (see also section 24.3). Increasing pressure of everyday practice for demonstrating effects of social work, in particular to show that social workers are consistently in line with the needs of their clients, necessitates using the needs concept as the central concept.

In the history of social work, objections were frequently made against the use of the term 'human needs'. This was perceived as being too 'needy' and would lead to patronizing behaviour. Reid (1978) and Saleebey (2006) both raised concerns that a focus on needs might be disempowering to clients. Yet both the strength perspective and the ecosystem perspective which are integrated are both compatible with human needs concepts (Dover, 2008). Since the ground-breaking and incisive work of Illich (1978), opposition has arisen to efforts to reduce human beings to bundles of unmet needs which are in turn defined as merely technical problems within the purview of the helping professions. Stigmatizing clients as 'needy' or as 'consumers of wants' could in turn lead to their disempowerment. However, the HNR model's combined focus on needs and rights is consistent with the strength approach within human needs theory – so, systematically working together with clients: starting, following and ending where the needs and the rights of the clients are. Ethically spoken, so social workers will not subordinate the needs or interests of people who use their services to their own needs or interests (Statement of Ethical Principles IFSW).

24.2.2 Needs and quality of life (QoL)

We defined the term 'human needs' as follows: 'the experienced wishes on a biopsychosocial terrain that, through meeting adequate satisfiers, lead to optimal QoL.'

With 'biopsychosocial' we mean that our physical condition is connected to our psychological condition, but also to the social situation in which we live and that these three components form one dynamic unit (see also section 2.5.2 and Figure 2.6). The specialist visions that disconnect the three factors mentioned have run their course, because they inevitably lead to tunnel vision. The building blocks of our lives are biopsychosocial in nature and intertwined. The damage that a human being incurs in his lifetime through loss in one part, in one building block of our life structure, has repercussions for the other building blocks with which this 'damaged' building block is intertwined.

Reasoning from this definition, the client's quality of (biopsychosocial) life decreases if and when deficiencies remain unfulfilled. And vice versa: meeting human needs raises the quality of life. In that sense, meeting human needs is a prerequisite in order to attain optimum QoL.

Of note is that the aforementioned definition speaks of an *experienced* deficiency; this presupposes an 'awareness' of the client's unmet needs. This need awareness is, however, not necessarily obvious at the start of the social work contact. Clients frequently do not come to the social worker with a well-defined request for help; they are in trouble and they don't know how to get out of it. One of the tasks of the social worker then, is to help either formulate such a request or become aware of the underlying human need (see also section 1.2.2, Needs awareness checklist). The social worker initiates the awareness-process regarding (un)met needs, using the non-directive basic method: what do you need to feel better?

Naturally, this is a topic of conversation between the client and social work, conducted among equals, in a non-patronizing manner.

24.2.3 The classification of human needs

> All you need is survival, love and helping perspectives.
> A need is something that you have to have. A want is something you would like to have.

When we talk about human needs in the sense of experienced deficiencies, then the question becomes: what types of human needs can we distinguish? In the overview of the social work

TABLE 24.1 Classification of human needs and human rights

HUMAN NEEDS	HUMAN RIGHTS
SURVIVAL NEEDS	*Corresponding SAFETY RIGHTS*
Needs for body safety in case of lack of oxygen, food, sleep, rest, health	Right to . . . physical security, basic health care, adequate food, protection from battering
Needs for social safety in case of lack of money, housing, etc.	Right to . . . social security, standard of living, adequate shelter, work
Needs for mental safety in case of traumatic experiences, violence	Right to . . . psychic security, basic psychological care, protection to inhumane treatment, to slavery
AFFECTION NEEDS	*Corresponding SOCIAL INCLUSION RIGHTS*
Needs for affection in relations	Right to . . . protection in family, social network, etc.
Needs for creative expression	Right to . . . culture, expression, play
Needs for grief and mourning	Right to . . . grief and mourning
SELF-DETERMINATION NEEDS	*Corresponding FREEDOM RIGHTS*
Needs for insights, information, rationality	Right to . . . information, education, development
Needs for identity, meaning making	Right to . . . narratives
Needs for skills and behaviour	Right to . . . education, exercise

approach (see behind the cover), three types of universal human needs and their corresponding human rights are shown: the survival, affective and self-determination needs and the safety,
social and self-determination human rights. The human needs corresponding to these human
rights form the universal legal foundation for meeting these human needs (see Table 24.1).

First we elaborate upon the scientific basis for these human needs: what neuro-scientific,
social scientific and historical bases are there for the presented needs classification of social
work? During a person's lifetime, four types of needs may emerge due to deficiencies on
awareness, survival, affective and self-determination levels. These deficiencies are further subdivided into specific needs. The question is: how does the client deal with this experienced
deficiency? We referred to this as the 'coping factor'. In meeting human needs, we also require
support from the direct environment (informal support, systemic support needs) as well as
from local and national provisions (formal support, macro support needs). We referred to this
as the 'support factor'.

24.2.4 Neuroscience and human needs

In each client, three brain parts can be active, like Arthur Koestler puts it for psychotherapy
clients: 'When a client is lying on the couch of a psychoanalyst, a horse and a crocodile are
lying next to him.' Also in social work this metaphor holds true. The crocodile signifies the
primitive and automatic survival behaviour of people that is regulated by our survival brain, also
referred to as the reptile brain (as is common in crocodiles and other reptiles); the horse signifies instinctive affective behaviour of people which is regulated by our affective brain or limbic
brain (present in all mammals); the human being on the caregiver's couch signifies the reflective
capacity that is regulated by our neocortex, the rational brain that is unique to human beings.
This metaphor of the crocodile, the horse and the human being mirrors the evolution of the

human brain to ever 'higher' brain structures, from the reptilian brain, via the limbic brain to the neocortex. We also see this kind of development from a child becoming an adult.

The neuro-scientific division of the three brain functions offers more insight into the data-processing of our brain functions and the origin of our human needs. During life events, such as loss, the signal of bad news is received in the thalamus, an area of the brain in the cognitive brain (see section 5.2, Survival brain). The thalamus is the gatekeeper of three brain functions: the crocodile, the horse and the human being, and coordinates which of the three is activated (van der Linden, 2006).

In 1990, MacLean introduced the following trinity-model of the human brain in his book *The Triune Brain in Evolution* (see Figure 24.2).

- The survival brain is approximately 500 million years old. It is the oldest part of the brain and watches over our physical survival. We have this in common with reptiles.
- The affective brain is approximately 200 million years old. It regulates our emotional connections with our surrounding world. We have this in common with all mammals.
- The unique, human, rational brain, the neocortex, is approximately 200,000 years old. It is the seat of our reflection, our thinking- and meaning-giving processes and our behaviours.

The exact location of these three brain functions as described by MacLean has since been made obsolete, but the brain functions he detailed are widely accepted. Neuroscientists researching the cognitive and affective brain have not found any exact locations for the brain functions mentioned. MacLean was a follower of the locationist school of thought, that pre-supposes that every individual emotion, such as sadness, anger or fear, is situated in a specific area of the brain. Locationists look for the exact location of emotions in the brain and assume that for numerous emotional problems, a pharmaceutical solution is principally possible. Other neuroscientists assume that emotions occur through the complex interactions of all kinds of brain functions in different locations. They form the psycho-constructionist school of thought within neuroscience. This approach presupposes that specific emotions are mental states that are made (constructed) when different brain functions work together. When

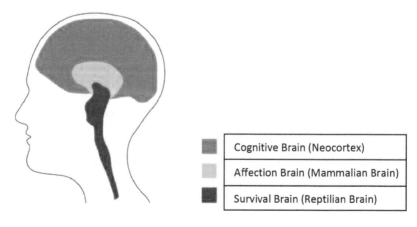

FIGURE 24.2   The 'triune brain': the brain trinity

an area of the brain dominates that cooperation, it can be life-saving but may also bring forth deviating behaviour.

The brain matrix: (im)balance between the brains?

Adequate cooperation between areas of the brain can help in adequately meeting the support needs (see Table 24.2). When the areas of the brain are balanced, it is highly likely there is an emotional calm. In the metaphor of the car driver: behind the wheel of your life-car, you make decisions about the course of your life (the rational brain with mental satellite navigation) by constantly reading the affection gauge (temperature gauge) and the survival gauge (fuel gauge/safety sensors regarding the brakes, distance to other cars) on the dashboard. You consider what is sensible and you turn the wheel in the most sensible direction. Rashly following your survival gauge (almost out of fuel) or your affection gauge (someone else is coming too close) would lead to thoughtless actions; if these gauges point to the far left or far right, that does not mean that you immediately have to turn the wheel in that direction. Fear, sadness and anger give poor advice, but the gauges need to be read, for example by parking the car and taking a moment to consider the situation. The driver of the imaginary car of life will decide a course of action after concise deliberation: every course fits best with what I need (needs).

When one of the three brains – your rationality, your feelings or your survival brain – goes offline for an extended period of time, this leads to imbalance and stress. Following only your feelings and not using your rational brain leads to impulsive actions that frequently are not in your own best interests. Sometimes it is in your own best interest, for example in extremely threatening situations, where thinking too long will lead to a bad result. Someone who is

TABLE 24.2 Brain matrix: cooperation between affective and cognitive brain

		Cognitive brain	
		Online	*Offline*
Affection brain	Online	Wise behaviour: balance between AB and CB; CB is team leader: needs are fulfilled	Emotionally focused behaviour, instinct without CB: 1 unwise decisions 2 terror of emotions 3 disproportional attention for emotions 4 disproportional anxious, angry, depressive behaviour 5 clinging/isolation, reckless behaviour
	Offline	No feelings, reasoned behaviour, cognition rules without contact with AB 1 compulsively rationalizing 2 overcontrolled type 3 no entrance to feelings	Absence of feelings, absence of reasoning, AB and CB are offline, survival brain rules 1 primitive functioning 2 fight/flight/freeze reflex

always alert or lets themselves be led by fear, sadness or anger may suffer from blind rage or panic. Imbalance may also emerge if rationality dominates feelings, as feelings will not get a chance to show how they may be of use. Some fear is so fundamental that rationality has no influence on it. Human beings as rational deciders, *homo rationalis*, as such are fictional. The multi-focus approach in social work means that the social worker recognizes and acknowledges that client behaviour is directed by these three brain functions and responds to them with his interventions by adjusting to current support needs.

24.2.5 Social science and human needs

The social-scientific foundation of the three types of needs, we base on the needs model by Maslow (1943) and current research into that area by Diener and Chan (2011). The needs model by Maslow corresponds to our arrangement of human needs based on brain functions. What Maslow refers to as basic human needs – the physiological needs and security needs – are here referred to as the survival needs. What Maslow describes as the social needs and psychological needs, are here summarized as the affective needs (affection concerns emotional ties with social and psychological aspects). What Maslow typifies as the growth or existential needs are here summarized as the autonomy needs.

For decades, the question has been whether this frequently used model of needs by Maslow can be confirmed through research and endures in modern times. In 2011, Diener and Chan gave the answer: yes, the Maslow-needs turn out to be universally human. They conducted research into the needs of human beings in 123 countries and asked questions regarding the need for money, food, shelter, security, social support, being respected, having the feeling of competence and experiencing positive or negative feelings. The researchers found that the diversity of needs as formulated by Maslow were universally human; all needs turned out to be equally important for individual happiness.

The next question was whether the hierarchy that Maslow had applied to human needs – the pyramid of needs – could also be confirmed. According to the pyramid of needs, there is an order of primary physiological needs (deficiency needs) via social and psychological to self-actualizing needs. Diener and Chen could not confirm this hierarchy: as their research shows, basic human needs do not need to be met first; the other needs – affective and autonomous – require to be met simultaneously. The order of lowest to highest level needs that must be met in succession, turned out to not be important to a person's wellbeing and pleasure in life. People are simultaneously driven by their need for good social relationships (affective needs) as well as by giving meaning (cognitive and existential needs) and by basic physiological needs.

24.2.6 History of social work and human needs

The needs concept has a recognized place within social work theory formation. As a profession, social work has long concerned itself with obtaining insight in and meeting of human needs (Dover, 2008). Many national associations for social work have, at some place in their mission statement, codified statements about the desirable match between human needs and the help offered by social workers, such as many a national association of social workers describes it in their code of ethics:

> The primary mission of the social work profession is to enhance human well-being and help meet the basic human needs of all people, with particular attention to the needs and empowerment of people who are vulnerable, oppressed, and living in poverty.

In the Global Definition of the Social Work Profession (IFSW, 2014, http://ifsw.org/get-involved/global-definition-of-social-work/), 'social work engages people and structures to address life challenges and enhance wellbeing':

> Social work is a practice-based profession and an academic discipline that promotes social change and development, social cohesion, and the empowerment and liberation of people. Principles of social justice, human rights, collective responsibility and respect for diversities are central to social work. Underpinned by theories of social work, social sciences, humanities and indigenous knowledge, social work engages people and structures to address life challenges and enhance wellbeing. The above definition may be amplified at national and/or regional levels.

As we noticed in this chapter, we assume that life events do arouse a lot of human needs; so 'addressing life challenges' includes addressing the human needs underlying these life-challenges.

Dover (2008) gives a detailed overview of the place of the human needs concept in social work. We follow Dover (2008) who summarized the use of the human needs concept through the history of social work:

- Mary Ellen Richmond, in 1922, made a distinction in her book *What Is Social Casework?* between economic needs and expressed needs of clients.
- Bertha Capen Reynolds, in 1932, supported the growing focus on client self-determination in her book *The Discovery of Need*, but worried that it could result in case-worker or societal neglect of basic human needs.
- In 1945, Charlotte Towl coined the phrase 'Common Human Needs', in the first textbook on the course *Human Behavior in the Social Environment*.
- Abraham Maslow, in his 1943 book *A Theory of Motivation*, presented his hierarchal theory of human needs – the needs pyramid – including physiological needs, safety needs, belonging/love and self-actualization.
- Erich Fromm, in 1955, argued in his book *The Sane Society* that human needs involved an idealistic striving for needs which transcends physiological needs, including relatedness, transcendence, rootedness, identity and a frame of orientation and devotion.
- In 1980, Carel B. Germain and Alex Gitterman emphasized in their book *The Life Model of Social Work Practice* the goodness-of-fit between life tasks, needs, goals, resources and stimuli.
- In 1989, Nancy Fraser proposed in her book *Struggle Over Needs: Outlines of a Socialist-Feminist Critical Theory* to stress need identification rather than need satisfaction.

- Len Doyal and Ian Gough theorized in their book from 1991, *A Theory of Human Needs*, two primary basic needs (health and autonomy) which must be met to avoid serious harm and engage in social participation. Civil, political and women's rights are prerequisites for culturally specific ways of satisfying intermediate needs, including food, water, housing, a non-hazardous environment, health, childhood security, significant primary relationships, economic security and basic education.
- Ann Robertson, in her *Critical Reflections on the Politics of Need* from 1998, stressed human needs concepts as a countervailing discourse to the domination of market principles.
- In 2008, Michael Dover explains in 'Human Needs: Overview' how human needs are realized or restricted at the intersection of the individual and the social environment. Human needs theory and research could enrich the ecosystem perspective, thus contributing to a unifying paradigm for social work practice.

In regards to human rights, an entire piece on Dutch social work will be presented next.

24.3 Human rights and social work

> Social work has, from its conception, been a human rights profession.
>
> (UN 1994)

Human rights do not replace principles of social justice, no matter how amorphous the definition of those principles seems (Reichert, 2011). Rather, the study of human rights complements and broadens the perspective of social workers when carrying out policies and practices. When they recognize the importance of human rights, social workers enhance the profession. A foundation in human rights can provide a much clearer framework and structure with which to connect the social work profession to economic, political, social and climate aims. Because then, social workers work with macro methods such as signalling, preventive, collective advocacy and research into targeted reinforcement of necessary provisions.

The case of Maria and human rights

In order to meet her needs, Maria is entitled to a number of provisions. As a university student studying social work, Maria is entitled to a guidance counsellor who guides her according to her needs. When she needed help because her studies were delayed due to force majeure, they looked into which provisions she was entitled to. When her father refused to pay the mandatory parental contribution for her studies, she was entitled to a university scholarship fund. It is then, however, required that the father officially sign a declaration of renunciation to contribute in his child's studies. If legal aid is required to facilitate in this, the social legal aid fund may be called upon. Furthermore, she is entitled to a course of action with school social work, that because it is a university provision is free of charge.

When it turned out that there were many more students than just Maria that were experiencing delays in her studies (signalling), possibilities or starting a preventive project were explored. A Dutch university started a Loss and Grief Community as a safety net for students who had an increased risk of study delays due to losing parents at a young age, suicide by fellow students or other shocking life events. Working on preventive provisions like that was an initiative taken by Maria's school social worker, who recognized acute or non-processed grief as a risk factor for study delays.

There are several reasons to add human rights to the needs-focused social worker:

- Human rights provide the legal framework for insisting that human needs must be met.
- Human rights can be viewed as the cornerstone of social justice and recognizes that human rights provide the legal mandate for meeting human needs (Wronka, 2008).
- Needs can be translated into rights the environment will support

(Hartley, 2008)

Gil (1992) clarified centrality of social needs: social justice cannot exist without first defining human needs and how satisfying them is related to achieving justice. Human rights focus on what must be given to a client, which elevates the discussion into one not simply of recognizing the needs of a client, but also satisfying those needs.

24.3.1 Definition

The term 'human rights' is defined here as follows: 'all rights bestowed upon all people based solely on their being human, that do not lean on a constitution (as constitutional rights).'

Human rights are seen as a mandate to have existing human needs met by local and national resources. Human needs are defined as the elements required for survival, affection/love and for developing helping perspectives. The proposed HNR perspective allows for a reinterpretation of the concept of poverty (Max-Neef, 2012). The traditional concept of poverty is limited and restricted, since it refers exclusively to the predicaments of people who may be classified below a certain income threshold. This concept is strictly economistic. It is suggested here that we should speak not of poverty but of poverties. In fact, any fundamental human need that is not adequately satisfied, reveals a human poverty. Some examples are:

- Poverty of survival (due to insufficient income, food, shelter, etc.), or protection (due to bad health systems, violence, arms race, etc.);
- Poverty of affection (due to authoritarianism, oppression, exploitative relations with the natural environment, etc.);

- Poverty of understanding (due to poor quality of education) or participation (due to marginalization of and discrimination against women, children and minorities);
- Poverty of identity (due to imposition of alien values upon local and regional cultures, forced migration, political exile, etc.).

But poverties are not only poverties. Much more than that, each poverty generates pathologies, destruction of human rights. This is the crux of the HNR discourse. In the context of developing countries, examples of persistent economic pathologies are unemployment, external debt and hyperinflation. Common political pathologies are fear, violence, marginalization and exile. Our challenge consists of recognizing and assessing the pathologies generated by diverse socio-economic political systems, with every system creating in its own way, obstacles to satisfying one or more needs. A further challenge is to develop and fulfil dialogue in pursuit of a constructive interpretation of needs and rights. These challenges form the basis for an ongoing programme of participatory community development since *Human Scale Development* was published (Max-Neef, 2012).

Human rights are defined to help fulfil these needs. Human rights classification follows the International Declaration of Human Rights. The classification of Human rights is used by social workers to engage with clients and structures to claim their rights.

In 1948, the United Nations recorded in the Universal Declaration of Human Rights a series of minimum requirements in how to approach humanity. One of the goals of the United Nations is protecting and improving human rights. In 1946, the United Nations set up the Human Rights Commission, with Eleanor Roosevelt as its chair. The most important task of this Commission was setting up the International Bill of Rights, consisting of a declaration and a treaty. The United Nations General Assembly (UNGA) adopted the Universal Declaration of Human Rights on December 10, 1948. In 1950, this date was proclaimed Human Rights Day. The UDHR is the first international confirmation of the universality of human rights. All human rights are universal, which means that human rights are applicable for every human in the world. Because the UDHR was adopted as a resolution in the UNGA, it is legally non-binding. Over the years, references to the UDHR have been made by other instruments, and nowadays, it is generally assumed that a large part of the contents of the UDHR is part of international common law, and as such is legally binding. The Universal Declaration of Human Rights contains 30 articles.

UN treaties

It cost considerably more effort to manifest human rights in treaties. This was partly due to tense international relations in the 1950s and 1960s. In 1966, the UNGA adopted the International Covenant on Civil and Political Rights (ICCPR) and the International Covenant on Economic, Social and Cultural Rights (ICESCR). After the 35th ratification, both treaties came into effect in 1976. For the Netherlands, the treaties have been in effect since March 11, 1979. Aside from these two general treaties, there are several treaties that devote special attention to a group of people or a specific right. Within the UN Human Rights Toolkit, there are nine core treaties:

- International Covenant on Civil and Political Rights (ICCPR);
- International Covenant on Economic, Social and Cultural Rights (ICESCR);

- International Convention on the Elimination of All Forms of Racial Discrimination (ICERD);
- Convention on the Elimination of All Forms of Discrimination Against Women (CEDAW);
- Convention Against Torture and Other Cruel, Inhuman or Degrading Treatment or Punishment (CAT);
- Convention on the Rights of the Child (CRC);
- International Convention for the Protection of All Persons From Enforced Disappearance (ICCPED);
- Convention on the Rights of Persons With Disabilities (CRPD);
- International Convention on the Protection of the Rights of All Migrant Workers and Members of Their Families (CMW).

These treaties elaborate on the different human rights in more detail. The general treaties state, for example that no one is to be tortured. The treaty against torture imposes concrete obligations on nation states and further specifies the general obligations. The treaty stipulates, for example, that nation states must regularly train their police forces in interrogation techniques so that they do not torture detainees.

The core treaties have not yet been ratified by all countries. For every one of these treaties, an independent committee of experts has been assembled that monitors adherence to the treaty. Every treaty has a reporting procedure, which means that treaty states must report regularly on their adherence to the obligations in the treaty. The committee investigates the report and adopts a final comment. Some treaties offer individuals the possibility to file a complaint regarding their government's adherence to the treaty (the so-called individual petition right). In regard to adherence to the treaties, complaints may be filed – if various requirements are met, such as following the procedures on a national level – on alleged violations of the ICCPR, ICERD, CAT and CEDAW.

24.3.2 The pursuit of social justice

Social work, as a professional group, helps ensure that people achieve self-actualization. It is with good reason then that the mission of social work, according to the professional profile of the social worker in the Netherlands is (NVMW, 2016, http://nvmw.nl/professionals/beroepsprofiel-inzien.html)

> to enhance that people in our society self-actualise, as human beings and as citizens. Social workers strive for human beings to develop themselves through interaction with their social environment, according to their own character, needs and beliefs and that they take into consideration the people with whom they live.

What does self-actualizing as a human being and as a citizen mean? Self-actualization of human beings is facilitated by the social worker through improving how they function socially. Social functioning is regarded as the competence of a person to do those things that are necessary to satisfy human needs and to fulfil social roles. In regard to satisfying needs, we noted that one might think of obtaining food, shelter and medical care, but also (self-)protection from damage, finding social acceptance and support, giving meaning and having goals in life.

In regard to fulfilling social roles, we mean fulfilling the role of family member, mother/father, partner, student, patient, employee and neighbour. The social worker enables people to self-actualize by contributing to improvements to social functioning.

Social work also stands for human beings self-actualizing as citizens. The social worker facilitates this by striving for just treatment (in their own social network) and the utilization of civil rights (through using provisions). The social worker does *not* operate from a passive position, but actively strives for social justice. Where poverty, discrimination, violence and exclusion exist, social workers act to combat them. The social worker wants to help people self-actualize as individuals, but also as family members, neighbours or professional organization. Additionally, social workers want people to self-actualize as citizens who have equal rights before the law, policy and access to provisions (Barker, 1999).

Social justice is an ideal situation in which all members of a society enjoy the same rights, the same protection, the same liberties, the same obligations and the same social advantages.

Social justice means that social institutes, such as governments, organizations and powerful groups recognize human rights. One norm directly connected to this is that society should strive for economic justice: just distribution of goods, services and money. Respecting universal human rights is the foundation upon which a safe society rests.

Application of universal human rights (Sheafor & Horejsi, 2003)

The right to food, shelter, basic medical care and essential social provisions;
The right to protection against abuse and exploitation;
The right to work and basic wage as a means of existence and dignity;
The right to marry, start a family and be united with one's family;
The right to basic education;
The right to own property;
The right to be protected against unnecessary damage and injury, for example in the workplace;
The right to pray if you want to – or not, if you don't;
The right to privacy;
The right to travel where you want to and meet who you want to;
The right to information about society, community or government;
The right to participation and influence in political decisions.

These rights go hand in hand with responsibilities. Rights and responsibilities are two sides of the same coin: the one cannot exist without the other. Unjust situations arise where people only think of their own rights and no longer feel a certain responsibility for others and society as a whole. As such, the protection of every right should go hand in hand with 'actually taking responsibility for' (Sheafor & Horejsi, 2003).

Application of universal responsibilities (Sheafor & Horejsi, 2003)

If people have the right to food, shelter, basic medical care and essential social provisions, then others are responsible for ensuring that these basic provisions are taken care of.

If people have the right to protection against abuse and exploitation, then others are responsible for ensuring that social programmes are created and action is taken in order to offer these protections.

If people have the right to work and basic wage as a means of existence and dignity, then others are responsible for ensuring that there are job opportunities and that fair wages are paid. And so on. Who are these others?

In combatting social injustice, social work is emancipatory: aimed at contributing to the assigning of equal rights, to lifting of legal, social, political, moral or intellectual restrictions. Social work contributes to the fight against sexism, racism, age discrimination, oppression of disabled people, oppression of homosexuals or other forms of oppression. Social workers do this out of the assumption that every human being has value in and of himself, and as such this intrinsic value does not need to be earned or proven. Everyday reality, however, is different: on a daily basis, people are disadvantaged based on traits such as sex, economic position, age, sexual preference, a physical or mental disability:

Sexism: women are disadvantaged, threatened and discriminated against based on prejudice; they are abused and killed based on their sex.
Age discrimination: youths (adultism) and older people (ageism) are disadvantaged.
Class discrimination: detrimental or preferential treatment of people based on their income or background.
Racism: people of another race or other nationality are disadvantaged.
Detrimental treatment based on faith: anti-Semitism towards Jewish people and anti-Islamism towards Islamic people.
Oppression of homosexuals: detrimental treatment of people with a different sexual orientation.

The list also includes oppression of people with a mental or physical disability, and all other forms of oppression based on irrelevant traits.

24.3.3 History of human rights in social work

David Androff (2016) summarized the place of the human rights concept in social work as follows:

- Jane Addams (1902) was among the first human rights pioneers of the early twentieth century. She acknowledged the human right to participation, which has the potential to free the powers of each man and connect him with the rest of life. In 1915 Jane Addams led the Women's Congress of The Hague in a protest against World War I.
- Eglantine Jebb founded Save the Children in 1919 and drafted a Convention on the Rights of the Child.
- The Association of American Social Workers (1947) proposed that 'all social workers should have a major concern, those broad human rights and collective liberties that are the birthright of every individual.'
- Ivan Illich (1978) opposed to efforts to reduce human beings to bundles of unmet needs which are in turn defined as merely technical problems within the purview of the helping professions.
- Elisabeth Reichert (2003) pointed out in her book *Social Work and Human Rights: A Foundation for Policy and Practice* that declarations of human needs were originally at the root of promulgations of international human rights.
- Joseph Wronka (1992, 2008) added that human rights provide the legal framework for insisting that human needs be met. Wronka views human rights as the cornerstone of social justice and recognized that human rights provide the legal mandate for meeting human needs.

- Onora O'Neill (1998), in the book *Necessary Goods: Our Responsibility to Meet Others' Needs,* has discussed the relationship of needs to rights and concluded that the human obligation (responsibility) to meet needs should be prioritized.
- Stanley Witkin (1998) concluded in *Human Rights and Social Work* that social work concern for human rights is linked ultimately to our commitment to the right to human need satisfaction.
- Gillian Brock (2005) stated in *Needs and Global Justice* that there is growing philosophical consensus that social justice can't be conceptualized or achieved without incorporating the concept of human needs.
- David Gil (2004) clarified in *Perspectives on Social Justice* that no conception of social justice can exist without first defining human needs and how their satisfaction is related to the achievement of justice.
- Jerome Wakefield (1988) drew upon human needs theory in his discussion of the use of the concept of distributive justice within the helping professions.
- Jeffrey Olson (2007) in *Social Work's Professional and Social Justice Projects* has conceptualized a needs-based formulation of social justice for the social work profession, one rooted in Maslow's theory of needs.

24.4 Sustainable social work: striving for green rights

> Meeting our own needs without compromising the ability of future generations to meet their needs.
>
> (UNESCO, 1997, http://www.un-documents.net/ocf-02.htm)

The term 'human development' is related to human rights, empowerment and meeting basic human needs. These three indicators are clearly related to social development as most social workers have known it. Social development approaches, also called developmental social work, have focused on building basic capacity among individuals, groups and communities through addressing basic needs (Midgley & Conley, 2010).

Four years after the World Commission on Environment, Agenda 21 of the 1992 Rio Earth Summit reiterated and added to this approach towards sustainable development.

Pillai and Grupta (2015) argued that social workers focus on both social inequality and poverty as the underlying causes of ecological degradation and poor intergenerational equity. Social workers believe that reductions in social inequality and poverty can be achieved through the use of a variety of social work methods such as social development, empowerment and advocacy for human rights. These methods enable communities to organize themselves and form partnerships within and across communities, thus enhancing social choices. Social development and improvement in social choices promote intergenerational relationships and contribute to intergenerational equity. Social workers use both the PIE- and system approaches in working with client systems.

24.5 Summary and questions

This chapter offered the human needs and rights perspective (HNR perspective) in social work as an ethical guide for social work.

First, the classification of human needs and summarily those of human rights were detailed and underpinned. A description was given of both and justifications were given regarding the basis of their classification and what historical evidence there is for them in social work. Additionally, it was detailed how *sustainable* social work is brought about aided by individual, systematic macro methods focused on social development. The human needs and human rights discussed were illustrated using fragments of Maria's (19) case study, who as a student of social work herself requested the help of a school social worker.

Questions

1   What associations do you have with the word 'needs' and what associations with the word 'human rights'? Do you work from a perspective of systematically meeting clients' needs and addressing your clients' human rights? If not, why not? If yes, how?
2   Do you recognize in your grown-up children behaviour where you see the cooperation of the three brains: the stress brain, affection brain and understanding brain?
3   Which human rights are unfulfilled by your target group? What action(s) are possible to have these human rights become more fulfilled?

25

SOCIAL WORK AND GRIEF SUPPORT

Questions

This chapter addresses the following questions:

- What is meant by the circle of loss?
- What is meant by 'all sorts and degrees of losses'?
- What are the three stages of an effective bad news interview?
- What are the social worker's tasks in specific situations involving loss?
- Which aspects of coping, social work tasks and pitfalls will you come across in those specific situations involving loss?

25.1 Introduction

> I think social workers could do with a lot more guidance in the area of grief support, as we do come across it a lot: and I mean all aspects of grief. In the mental health area, people cannot cope with even small losses, they just don't know how to deal with them.
> (Paul Tetteroo, social worker, 2016)

This chapter provides an overview of the role of social work in a diverse range of losses which may occur over the course of one's life. Social workers often interact with people who are trying to come to terms with a loss. It is evident that social work has played an important role in grief support from its very beginnings back in 1898. This chapter was written with the intent of seeing social workers embrace their role in providing grief support as a more integral part of their professional practice.

25.1.1 All sorts and degrees of losses

To this aim I will describe social work and grief support within the context of specific situations involving loss. I will start by outlining a diverse range of situations involving loss using the circle of loss and also looking at the bad news interview. I will then clarify the social worker's roles or tasks when working with these nine target groups in terms of loss: children dealing with loss, parenting a disabled child, HIV/AIDS, divorce, far-reaching changes at work, migration, dementia, death and the photo display for those whose loved ones have died in traumatic circumstances. For each situation involving a specific kind of loss, I will explain which specific aspects of coping you might come across, what tasks you have as a social worker and what pitfalls you might face. This chapter will give a number of examples specifically involving the situation in the Netherlands because it is simply not possible to describe the situation in other countries as well. These examples are merely meant to elaborate the point and are absolutely not meant to describe a standard for grief support in other countries. The reader is referred to the methodological chapters in this book for more information on the methods applied by the social worker. Internet search engines can be used to access a wealth of methodological information on the various topics involving loss as described in the following pages. It will have become clear from the preceding chapters that social work is a multilevel profession which can involve intervention and case management (coordination) at various levels, in collaboration with other relevant professional groups. This certainly also applies to losses endured over the course of our lives, involving the individual concerned, his or her caregivers and the wider network. Again the social worker needs to focus on the impact factor, the coping factor and the support factor and this focus is an integral component of grief support in order to optimize the client's quality of life or quality of death.

I will start this chapter by providing a broad definition of loss and will then use the circle of loss to describe a wide range of situations involving losses social work clients may endure over the course of their lives.

25.1.2 Circle of loss

We all experience ups and downs on our journey through life. Between the moment we are born and the moment we die, we experience times of happiness, sharing those with the ones we love, but we can also be faced with a wide range of losses (see Figure 25.1). We also gain a lot, through personal growth, promotion, good fortune, and happy times. These are the ups and downs in life. We bond with loved ones only to lose them. We experience love only to lose it again. From this perspective, loss is an inextricable part of life. Loss is like 'the headwind in life' from which trees derive their resilience. So in this example, wind is a metaphor for the setbacks and stormy weather we are faced with in life, and which are essential for us to develop and maintain our resilience. We need these to maintain the tree's/our own health and fitness. Loss can be seen as the strong gale force winds blowing or raging through our lives. And at such points in time, life will test our resilience. Once we have survived and gained wisdom from such experiences, we have learned how to deal with life's trials and tribulations. What lessons do we learn from experiencing such headwinds? Should we withdraw into ourselves and try not to get close to anyone or anything – is this the lesson you learn from life?

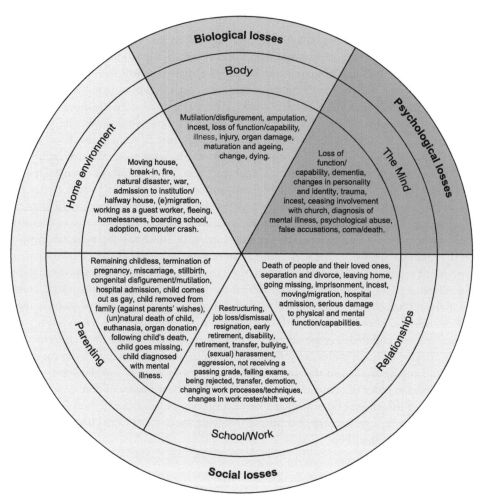

FIGURE 25.1 The circle of loss

Source: de Mönnink (2016)

Or do you see loss as the price you pay for getting involved in life: grief as the price you pay for bonding? Alfred Lord Tennyson summarized this theme of bonding and loss so well in a poem titled *In Memoriam* (1850):

'Tis better to have loved and lost, than never to have loved at all.

I will use the word 'loss' in the sense of 'the realisation that an existing close relationship with loved ones and/or other familiar elements of life has come to an end'.

The growing realization that an existing relationship has come to an end or is about to come to an end, this may be a relationship with your (grand)parents, your partner, your (grand) child, your friend, your colleague or your beloved companion animal; your physical health and your mental vitality; your job, your home, your country or a beloved object; or yourself.

This may occur for all sorts of reasons including death, illness, the maturation process, divorce, a breakup, an accident, trauma, work reorganization, job loss, age and your own death.

25.2 The bad news interview

The purpose of bad news interviews is to:

- Ensure that the recipient is able to handle the situation;
- Provide the information necessary for the recipient to be able to make decisions;
- Enhance trust in the social work relationship and in the care provided;
- Ensure that clients receive the care they need.

When conveying bad news you accept that the message recipient is entitled to respond to this as he or she sees fit.

In conveying bad news social workers have a number of tasks which may or may not be completed in an adequate manner (Keirse, 1981). Table 25.1 describes both adequate and the inadequate ways of fulfilling these social work tasks.

After conveying the bad news and supporting the recipient, social workers should evaluate the process. A careful evaluation of the bad news process includes asking ourselves the following questions:

- Were factors such as age, values and coping styles adequately taken into account?
- Were the ethical principles of the profession adequately taken into account?
- Did the social worker concerned work in collaboration with other disciplines?
- Was there a good alignment between the social worker concerned and the next of kin?

TABLE 25.1 Practice of the bad news interview

Stages of implementation	Adequate social work	Inadequate social work
1 Conveying bad news	Convey the message straightaway	Delaying the message
	Succinct	Leaving the message up in the air
	A warm and empathetic tone of voice	Sweetening the bitter pill
	Brief explanation afterwards	Justification
		Talking about oneself
2 Reducing frustration	Encourage recipient to put their feelings into words	Counter-aggression
	Non-directive attitude	Information that goes against the individual concerned
	Quietly supportive presence	Suppressing anger
	Succinctly provide clarification	Contradicting denial too soon
3 Resolving problems	Listen to find out in what direction the recipient is looking for a solution	Suggesting solutions so as to reduce frustration
	Suggest points of advice	Defend/sell one's points of advice
	Address underlying emotions	

- Was a cost–benefit analysis carried out for each of the 'truth options' (complete, incomplete, misleading or delayed information)?
- Were timing and language use adequate for the client?
- Was the client appropriately supported?

The way in which news is conveyed and social work provided are of great importance for the way in which a loss can be processed.

25.3   Social work involving children and young people after a loss

Children are entitled to mourn and grief when such situations occur. We shortchange them when we act on the assumption that we should keep them at a distance when it comes to saying goodbye, without allowing them to feel the loss. With adults, only grief that has been 'lived' can turn into something beneficial, and the same applies to children.

Children may be confronted with loss at a young age. Every adult who is involved with children going through grieving, struggles with questions such as: 'How do I tell children the truth about their loss?' 'Should I tell the child the truth?' 'What will be the consequence if I confront the child with the loss?' 'Will the child not needlessly lose its innocence before its time?'

It is indisputably true that we need to create a space for loss at home, at school and in health care institutions. The more we treat loss as a normal part of life, the better children will be able to process loss. Caregivers are advised to teach their children to deal with loss by paying attention to what is going on for them in terms of their feelings. Learning to cope with small losses is good practice for learning to assimilate the more significant losses in our lives.

25.3.1 Specific aspects of coping

Children do not mourn 24 hours per day. Sometimes they go straight back to playing after the funeral. However, they may also feel acutely overwhelmed by loss at times. Sometimes children develop problems after a few months or even years. This may take the form of bedwetting, problems focusing or sleeping, stuttering or aggressive behaviour. It is important that we recognize such delayed reactions and realize that children are different from adults in terms of their response patterns; they may be subject to more sudden mood changes than adults. After a loss, children may show the following behaviours signalling loss responses, listed here in order from lesser to greater degree of seriousness (Ligthart & de Keyser, 1993):

- Appearing sad and unhappy;
- Acting helpless;
- Wanting attention;
- Being overactive;
- Crying a lot;
- Physical symptoms;
- Being grumpy, curt;
- Bad school reports;
- Problems sleeping;
- Not being able to get on with grown-ups;
- Aggressive behaviour;
- Not being able to get on with age-group peers;

- Eating disorders;
- Being destructive; vandalism;
- Problems with toilet training.

Children who have suffered a significant loss may feel unsafe: 'If my sister can be taken from me just like that, then how can I be sure about anything else?' Their trust in other people may have been affected after such a loss. The child has to learn to trust again (and learn who can be trusted). Trust exercises can be beneficial here. One option involves using the circle of loss and using masks (Hemming, 1995). Anger can also reflect a response to feelings of abandonment, despair, hurt and rejection. Parents do not always appreciate anger and may see it as a problem.

> My 5-year-old son has become impossible ever since my Dad, his grandfather died. He did not attend the funeral and his behaviour has been unreasonable and troublesome ever since. Eventually, we discovered that he wanted to ride in the ambulance to go and see Granddad, because that was the car which had taken Granddad's bed, so he thought that that car would be able to take him to Granddad.

Anger is a normal response to a loss which is incomprehensible to the child. Games have been developed to help children deal with such losses, one example being the *All About Me* game devised by Hemming (1995).

Children may also resort to magical thinking to try and resolve the loss. They may think that there are very personal reasons for the loss. Children may develop feelings of guilt or may feel responsible, particularly when they have absolutely no reason to feel that way.

25.3.2 Social work tasks

Open communication, honesty and concrete preparations at the level of the child are essential for children who have to work through a loss. If you are providing the support, it is your role to take the child's level of psychological development into account. Always consider the level of abstraction children can deal with at a certain age and what they have to deal with and got through in certain situations involving loss.

Saying goodbye

If you are providing the support, it is your role to allow the child to say goodbye in his or her own way and own time. You should not only talk to the child, but also draw, engage in games, play music or tell the child stories – all of these can give the child something to hold on to.

Keeping a diary can make it easier to express feelings. This can provide a sense of peace. The child may think: 'I don't have to try and hold on to all of this in my head, because it is down on paper,' just like the 14-year-old who wrote about the loss of Tinus, the cat:

> My (lovely) pussy cat
> You died when I was eight years old and before that
> You could no longer use your left hind leg.
> You could be sweet and mean as well.
> Sometimes you even hurt me
> But I have been missing you of late

You were my lovely little mate
I was not there when you passed away
I had gone to see Santa Claus that day
You died in Daddy's arms without much pain
But now I think I would have wanted to be there.
And this is what I wanted to tell you
I want to put some flowers on your grave
In my heart you will always be my (lovely) pussycat
Even though you were sometimes a bit of a prat

When providing support, it is your role to prepare children for what awaits them after a loss and to do so in very concrete terms. If there is to be a funeral or cremation service, you tell them what to expect. When one of their parents loses their job, you tell them what that entails and what that will be like for the parent, depending on the child's developmental age.

If the child is developing depressions or phobias, it is your task to ensure he or she receives support in the early stages (Heuves, 1991).

Educating about loss

Another part of your role involves making schools aware of the importance of educating children about loss. Talking about loss in a relaxed and creative manner can help inform children and serve as preparation for social work support relating to all manner of loss. Play therapy, including playing with dolls, is a commonly used technique to facilitate the coping process in children and to help convey information. Children often communicate their needs symbolically. Playing with dolls can be a useful means to encourage questions and help express feelings.

Group-based support

When providing support, it is your role to make the link between loss and any behavioural changes. You need to be able to assess when group-based support may be needed. Children may appreciate being able to talk about their loss with their peers. The grown-up's overly protective attitude may do more harm than good: trying to safeguard children from hurt may result in children getting worried and confused. Such an overly protective approach may come at a high cost. Without anyone realizing it, children's hidden concerns can turn into problems involving their growth and development, behaviour and learning. Children can be taught to say goodbye and deal with concerns: we can learn to say farewell and deal with worries from a young age: what's learned in the cradle lasts till the tomb.

Offering suggestions

In your role as support worker you must also offer suggestions to grown-ups as to how they can support children after a loss. Some of these suggestions are listed below.

- 'There is more than one truth when it comes to dealing with loss.' (Adults should be aware of their own experiences of loss, and not confuse these with what is going on for the child: what is it this child needs now and from whom?)
- 'Give the child the opportunity to express itself in its own way and in its own good time.'

- 'Provide relevant information about loss and possible responses to a death.'
- 'Use appropriate language and imagery, aligned with the child's level of development and previous experiences.'
- 'Encourage creative expression: drawing, working with clay or playdough, play and so on.'
- 'Create a safe environment for the child following a shocking loss, such as when someone has suddenly died in an accident.'
- 'Take the initiative and keep interacting with the child, also by touch, and also if you feel that there does not appear to be any response to the loss.'
- 'Give the child the opportunity to create memories.'
- 'Be a role model, not a hero.'
- 'Keep things light-hearted and allow the child to discover whatever it wants to.'
- 'Keep listening and listening.'

25.3.3 Pitfalls

The first pitfall to avoid when providing social work to children is to keep the truth from them. As an example, when a loved one is terminally ill and does not have long to live, withholding the truth may result in children developing imagined ideas which are far from the truth, such as: 'Daddy doesn't love me anymore, because he doesn't play with me anymore':

> In the past there was a tendency to protect children from death, so as not to burden them with all that sadness. But in reality, children feel abandoned when this happens. They will often feel excluded, because they don't know what is going on. Children's imagined ideas are often worse than the truth.
>
> *(Oderkerk, 1995)*

A second pitfall involves the social worker feeling that too much emphasis is being placed on the loss. When adults feel uneasy and unsure what to do, this may be because many of us have had to suppress our own feelings about a number of losses in our lives.

The third pitfall is thinking that all situations involving loss are the same: 'Children deal with this in such and such a way, and this is what you should do'.

Losing someone who has meant a lot to them, or losing an important item can be a terrible experience for children, but it does not necessarily need to be a harmful experience. The quality of social work provided to children in the first few months or years following a loss can make all the difference. Children whose feelings and thoughts are treated sensitively and with respect will feel encouraged and supported in the coping process.

25.4 Social work relating to the birth of a disabled child

25.4.1 Specific aspects of coping

Parents may find it very hard to cope with infertility problems, terminations of pregnancy, miscarriage, stillbirths or cot death. Like Metz stated in 1994 in 'Stillborn Expectations': 'things went wrong when it turned out that our son had Down syndrome: my husband wanted nothing to do with him'. Parents expected a healthy child and that expectation is now squashed resulting in severe disappointment. Parents may go through similar emotions when they have a disabled child. Emily Pearl Kingsley, chairperson of the American National Down

Syndrome Congress, described such feelings in *Welkom in Nederland* (Welcome to Holland; see also Chapter 12).

Mothers, fathers and siblings of a disabled child may struggle with all kinds of personal and emotional problems. There may be feelings of incredulity, depression, deep sadness, fear for the future and envy of families with healthy children; in addition, parents may feel guilty. Feelings of anger and aggression are still not fully accepted as a normal aspect of coping. Aggression against fate, the outside world which does not offer any assistance, against the messengers conveying the bad news, or those providing support to the child. The most difficult aspect is anger directed at the child itself: 'Look what you have done to us by being like that.' When providing support, you need to allow space for people to express these contradictory emotions.

25.4.2 Social work tasks

Parents will find it difficult to accept their lot. When providing support, working towards normalizing such feelings – telling parents, when the time is right, that feelings of envy, aggression and so forth are normal when parents have a disabled child – is a prerequisite to enhancing bonding with the child. Encouraging parents to name both positive and negative aspects will allow them to view the child objectively. Providing social work to the parents of a disabled child is a bit like the art of judo: on the one hand, going along with the way the parents and older siblings tell their story, and express themselves, on the one hand, but also confronting them with reality when necessary. Sometimes an intervention is needed whereby everything is structured: the previous reality involving wonderful expectations and the new reality involving the disabled child are expressed and named.

25.4.3 Pitfalls

The first pitfall occurs when those providing support fail to identify the hurt of previously experienced grief: past wounds which have not healed properly will open up when it turns out that the child has an intellectual disability. You should never assume that the grieving process is complete at a certain point in time. When children become ill or are removed from the home the entire process of letting go and bonding often starts all over again.

The second pitfall involves parents receiving technical support and support with household chores, but no support in terms of the feelings of pain and shame and the socially undesirable feelings they often develop. It is essential that you seek to align yourself with the parents. If their feelings of loyalty to the child mean they can cope with a lot of the demands placed upon them, the resulting ties will outweigh any well-intentioned external reflection. Some situations may appear unhealthy to you, but are no reason to intervene. In such cases it is better that contact with the family is maintained, rather than risking a confrontation involving the significant likelihood that there will be no further contact.

The third pitfall occurs when your own norms start to take over to the extent that your attitude becomes akin to moralizing. When parents express themselves in a socially undesirable manner, this may be hard for you to take, in your support role. One example would be parents endlessly referring to their child as 'a child like that', or considering or deciding to adopt their child out. Or if their attitude does not show any love whatsoever. It is better to take a more humble approach. Who are you to say 'that isn't allowed' or 'you have to do such and such'? The parents will have to carry on by themselves.

The final pitfall involves losing sight of a balanced distribution of attention within the nuclear family. If you keep focusing on the parents' concerns about their disabled child, you will not be doing any favours to the other children, who do not have a disability.

25.5 Social work relating to HIV/AIDS

> AIDS may not appear that significant if viewed only from a quantitative perspective – fortunately – but qualitative terms it is a condition which can be devastating for both the patient and for those providing support
>
> (Roscam Abbing, 1994)

25.5.1 Specific aspects of coping

In 2013 there were 45 million people living with AIDS around the world (by comparison, the number of people with cancer was 12.1 million). The biggest problem with AIDS is not so much the infection itself, but the social isolation which results (and we can see this phenomenon even more strongly with regard to those infected with Ebola). On January 1, 2014, there were 19,065 individuals in the Netherlands who were HIV-positive. An overwhelming majority (77%) were male, 2% used intravenous drugs while 1% were haemophiliacs; 44% were either homosexual or bisexual, while 44% had been infected through heterosexual sex. The virus is transferred through blood–blood contact, including by way of blood transfusions, dirty needles or transfer between mother and child, or via blood–sperm contact due to unsafe sex. Women form the largest growing group of HIV-positive people.

When people are told that they are seropositive, this usually comes as an enormous shock. Resistance, denial, anger and feelings of guilt are stronger than fear: the fear of being excluded and the fear of dying within the short term. This is why those affected often choose to keep this as their 'big secret', and this goes for gay men, haemophiliacs and intravenous drug users.

The future starts to take on a whole new perspective, because there is an incubation time of approximately nine years: 'We all die a bit day by day, but in my case those little bits amount to rather a lot.'

People develop a mindset which is focused more on enjoying the moment: 'What am I going to do with my time if I only have a limited number of years left?' Relationships come to be under a lot of pressure.

The success rate of the current combination therapy appears to herald the advent of a better outlook for people who are HIV-positive.

25.5.2 Social work tasks

Social work to people with AIDS requires a careful approach, a constructive attitude and expert knowledge. Bad news should be conveyed with the necessary care. When conveying bad news to gay people with a diagnosis of AIDS, you have to first think about what it means to be gay, think how they are socialized and consider the possible resistance from within society.

When providing support, you should have the knowledge required, not just in terms of what the condition entails, but also when it comes to arrangements before and after death. Knowing that all arrangements before and after their passing have been taken care of, will be a load off the client's mind.

Finally, part of your role will be to try and bring family and friends of the person with HIV closer together.

25.5.3 Pitfalls

When providing social work to HIV carriers, you should not wait and wait before they ask for help, but be proactive in approaching them with an offer of social work support.

It is also important to be mindful of your own responses as the person providing support. It is totally understandable if you are afraid of being infected, especially if your interactions with AIDS patients are of a long-term and intensive nature. This fear is often the result of ignorance about the risk of infection.

The third social work pitfall involves underestimating the emotional work stress involved in care and treatment: the risk of burnout is very much present (see also Chapter 27). Because many patients are so young, overly identifying with them can lead to emotional tensions, especially when those providing support are gay themselves.

Finally it is essential to observe the confidential character of support interactions. One pitfall could involve overlooking confidentiality due to a sense of duty of care towards the community/society at large. In the Netherlands, absolute confidentiality is maintained and the individual is given absolute responsibility for preventing the infection of other people.

25.6 Social work relating to divorce

25.6.1 Specific aspects of coping

Separation and divorce cause suffering, in an emotional, physical, legal, financial and material and social sense. Every divorce is different, if only because different people are involved. If we look at marriage as a plant, we will realize that sooner or later such a plant will inevitably die if we do not water it. Relationships need our attention: we can have times of strife alternated by times of enjoyment, however it is very clear that bonding and closeness sometimes involve a fight: fighting for the relationship, fighting to be seen and heard. Sometimes there is a gap which cannot be bridged resulting in divorce.

To provide social work, we need to have an insight in the divorce process: what force field and what dynamics are involved in divorce. When two people divorce, it is not the partners who die, but the relationship between them.

A divorce is usually preceded by a process of emotional distancing, which started much earlier. According to some researchers, this starts 2 years before the actual divorce.

Former partners can be present larger than life even when they are not physically there. For the divorce process to be able to move forwards, people need to have an outlet, but more importantly they need the skills to share the pain of the divorce with others.

Inadequate communication patterns

Certain communication patterns may hamper this process (Satir, 1975): the computer style, the placator style, the blamer style and the distracter style.

- *Computer*: the man who always dealt with any tensions in a rational, computer-like manner now faces having to change his way of coping.

- *Placator*: the woman who always blamed herself for any problems and who tries to maintain harmony no matter what is unable to express her anger.
- *Blamer*: the man who always responds to tensions by blaming others may discover that blaming only serves to escalate the issues.
- *Distracter*: the woman who tries to hide everything away, looking for distractions, will need to face herself and the consequences of the divorce sooner or later.

Children can find the divorce almost impossible to cope with: the Mum and Dad who gave you life are splitting up.

> My little girl came to see me. 'I wish I had never been born,' she said, 'I just sat and cried and cried.'
> 'What makes you say that?' I asked.
> 'Mum and you have to stay together.'
> I tried to explain to her why that was not possible. But she just didn't understand. The only thing she understood was that parents should be together.

When children go through a divorce, they can feel torn up inside, and this can only get better when the parents get back together or when they show that they will remain in touch, albeit at a different level.

> One of the things Chrysta found the hardest, was sending a card to her Dad after our divorce. I think she was about 7 years of age. I think the holidays were coming up. She just wanted all of us to be around the table together one more time. It was a beautiful card. She wrote that she didn't remember what it was like to have a Dad. It was hard for me, because he showed me the card, so I knew that whatever I did, I could never be Mum and Dad at the same time. I already knew that. A child needs both parents. No matter how hard you try, you cannot replace the other parent. Children go through a lot of hurt and confusion after a divorce.

Divorce can have a significant impact on children in terms of their own relationships down the track. The impact can be positive when parents demonstrate being able to separate their own emotions from their care for the child. In that case, the divorce shows that partners do not have to remain together forever in a relationship which will never improve and that divorce may be a necessary solution. However, divorce may also have a negative impact on the children's relationships down the line. This is especially true when parents draw their children into a power struggle. In such cases, the divorce may come as a relief for the children involved. According to the World Health Organization divorce can be the second most impactful life event for children; with the death of their parents being the most impactful event. How children respond will depend on their age. Appendix 1 contains a list of children's possible age-specific responses to divorce. Appendix 2 contains a list of tips for parents and grandparents.

25.6.2 Social work tasks

Which social workers are likely to work with couples going through a divorce and in what capacity? You may work as a social worker in a community centre and an older woman may ask you for advice, saying she is worried her husband may leave her. You may be a community police officer called to a domestic dispute, where a man will not accept that his wife wants to leave him, and engages in domestic violence or even threatens to kill her for that reason. You may be a primary care physician or family doctor, or pastoral care worker, and be confronted with stories about a man whose wife has left him, or a woman who has become depressed because her ex is stopping her from seeing her children. No matter what situation social workers are in when they are faced with divorce, they should always assess the situation and what opportunities there are for support. It is important that we facilitate a healthy divorce process, especially when there are children involved.

Divorce-related social work tasks can involve supporting both partners during this relationship crisis. In your role as support worker, you have the knowledge and skills to assist the partners when it comes to the emotional, legal, economic, social and mental health aspects of a divorce: you can provide information, ensure issues can be discussed, liaise when it comes to negotiating financial matters and help the partners with deciding on shared parenting. Through your support, couples going through a divorce can remain or become more willing to talk to each other, if only in the interest of the children. Specialists in liaising between parties in a divorce do a good job, using *mediation* techniques.

25.6.3 Pitfalls

The first pitfall in a divorce is for social workers to avoid being drawn into a power struggle.

Support workers also run the risk of going along with patterns introduced into social work interactions by one of the parties, for instance when he blames the other party for the trouble he is in. Your job is to show this person the way he or she is transferring the blame and get him or her to stop doing this. You are doing the client a service by getting him to stop this habit, so as not to burden new relationships with these behaviours.

The third pitfall is that you are drowning in the chaos of marital disputes. You can become the target of anger and dissatisfaction in the confusion of little games, intrigues and incidents.

The fourth pitfall may be you working harder than the two partners in your support role: *don't push the river too hard*. You may realize that one of the parties concerned may have seen his parents gone through a divorce and may not have processed all that old hurt. It is not your job to keep working on that, but the client's.

Finally, it is important that the children are not forgotten about in the midst of all this, and that enough attention is paid to care for the children after the divorce process. Research has shown that the idea that children are alright after a divorce is incorrect (Wallerstein, 1991). The Moving Past Divorce website (http://www.movingpastdivorce.com) describes the so-called sleeper effect: teenage girls in particular are confronted with themselves when entering into intimate relationships, going through a delayed response to the hurt caused by the divorce: they become aware of the consequences of the divorce. Apparently suppressed negative emotions show up as a fear of allowing someone to get close. Wallerstein discovered the sleeper effect after following a group of children whose parents had gone through a divorce 40 years previously, after they had become grown-ups themselves.

25.7 Social work relating to impactful changes at work

When people live to work, their life falls apart when they lose their job. When your life revolves around your work, your life really does fall apart when faced with a job loss. There are a lot of similarities between job loss or a loss at work and other losses. When a man ends up on the street just before retirement, he not only loses his job, but also his trust in other people, his interactions with age-group peers and his income.

No job change, retirement or job loss situation is the same. Every job loss is different, and in turn we cannot compare job loss to demotion (going down to a lower-level position with a reduction in wages) or with a forced transfer, either in terms of position or geographical location. Employees, entrepreneurs and those running small businesses can feel badly affected following a business takeover, merger or receivership. Painful decisions are inevitable when managing a situation responsibly, and it is essential that we do not lose sight of the human aspect. Staff members of the personnel and organization or human resource department often become involved, as well as outplacement organizations and company social workers. Affected staff may also be offered themed courses such as 'Leaving Work' and 'Close to Retirement'. Labour organizations are increasingly aware of the 'grief at work' topic: how to deal with employees who are grieving the death of a colleague or a loved one? This is also referred to as grief management when it is offered by the human resource department.

25.7.1 Specific aspects of coping

Far-reaching changes at work may impact on people in a lot of different ways. Aside from financial consequences, there may be consequences in terms of accommodation, family life, leisure time activities and social status. Dealing with loss can be like a game of dominoes: knocking over one tile can impact on the relationship between the partners, children, enjoyment of life, regularity, time and expenses.

People will not readily ask for help with problems around job loss; if losing one's job is considered shameful, asking for help will only serve to increase those feelings of shame. And this is even more true when considering that the majority of the many jobless are men, who do not find it easy to ask for help at the best of times.

Impactful changes in life affect people in four different ways. Figure 25.2 shows the types of meaning we derive from work. Work provides a sense of control, a meaningful way to spend one's time, it regulates time thereby giving us a sense of control over reality. Jobs provide status, a sense of self-esteem. They also provide a source of income. When someone loses his or her job, this affects that person to the DUNC (see section 12.2). If we want to provide social work to those who have been through impactful changes at work, it is essential that we understand what work means to them.

25.7.2 Social work tasks

From the perspective of pre- and aftercare, it is the role of the human resource employee, the staffing consultant, the training facilitator, the outplacement support worker to give shape to social work at the individual level. Staff members employed by the organization provide a listening ear to employees who feel rejected and excluded. It is important that the organization, 'the bad guy', the source of all this misery, shows a human face when giving staff the bad news and when providing after care. Provision of initial support and assistance by psychosocial support workers – no matter how well intentioned – is not aligned with what many of those involved want. This is why hardly anyone takes up the support offered in instances of mass job losses and reorganizations (if such support is offered at all). It would appear more appropriate to have initiatives which are directly linked to the company: company social work offered by services external to the organization and company chaplains.

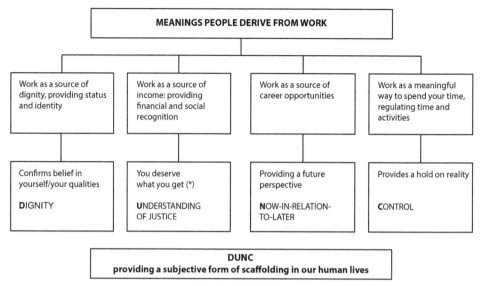

(*) and you get what you deserve?

FIGURE 25.2 What work means to people: DUNC

Source: de Mönnink (2016)

Exit process

It is very important to the employees concerned for the managers responsible to be open to the hurt and tragedy caused at individual level, and equally important that they listen to what is going on for people by providing an exit process. This can help prevent a situation where both those who have lost their job and those who stay look at the company and society with lingering resentment. Social work aims to help people let go of their previous relationship with work and the company and to look at the new situation with fresh eyes. In your role as support worker you can indicate where someone sits in terms of the exit process, where can you have some impact, where can you have a say, can you lodge any objections. In this way, you can help clarify the status, (im)possibilities and structure of options for appeal and social work. You can also make it clear that there are no 'must dos' in social work and that everything can be discussed.

In terms of helping clients regain their sense of self-esteem, it is important that support workers show an interest in the human aspect of the situation: 'How are you?,' 'reading between the lines I think I can tell that things are not easy for you?,' 'Or is it a relief, in a way?'

You can also tell the individual concerned about the many different responses and emotions he may experience, and emphasize that it is important to list important points in his career as well as the way in which he became steadily more involved with the company.

Sense of fairness and future perspective

In helping restore a sense of justice, your role in providing support is to do justice to the employee's wishes, choices and worldview, after this impactful change in employment. The staff member is entitled to having information which is as open as possible as to decide on a change in status or redeployment – for this reason, based on these considerations, based on those criteria. People are entitled to either know the reason why, or to being told why an explanation cannot be made available. Finally, it is your job to help the person develop some sense of future perspective. You show empathy for employees to whom the change in status or redeployment comes as a shock.

You communicate in a clear and careful manner with the employee concerned, so that he or she can be encouraged to enter into a new psychological contract with the new organization.

25.7.3 Pitfalls

Incorrect timing is the first pitfall in relation to social work following a job loss. If you start to talk about the role the employee himself may have played, in order to try and get him to get on top of things again, you may be told, and justifiably so: 'Not you as well: you make it sound as if it is all down to me.' It is not always immediately clear to employees that *they* also have to work on processing their grief. If someone is struggling to deal with the fact that he has lost his job, the suggestion that he has to work on things himself may feel like an additional kick in the guts.

The moment the person starts to realize that things cannot carry on the way they are, that the effects of the job loss have reached a certain point, the time may be ripe to not only consider how the job loss affected him, but also what he himself can do to cope with the loss.

The second pitfall consists in promising the person the earth. The support worker needs to remind himself of the reality of structural unemployment. It would be more appropriate to encourage the person in a realistic manner. The best thing to do is to work with what the client indicates he wants and to build up a relationship of trust, so that you can explore the issues together and start to work on building a new life.

The third pitfall consists in setting your sights too high or in being so flexible that you become infected by the client's powerlessness, depression and sense of hopelessness.

Once the social worker is also filled with a sense of dread, it will be impossible for him or her to provide any kind of support.

The fourth pitfall consists in forgetting about those who remain following a reorganization. Research has shown that things can be extremely hard for these people, even though they have kept their jobs; Scandinavian research has shown that employees who remain following restructuring showed much increased levels of sick leave and a cardiovascular death risk twice that of the total population when compared to sectors of the industry that had not been subjected to reorganizations (Vahtera et al., 2004). It is therefore great that in 2016 one of the Netherlands trade union organizations has taken the initiative to not only represent employees' material rights, but also their social and emotional interests around such impactful processes. The FNV, or Dutch Federation of Labor unions, has commenced a project on Dealing with Loss, to provide social and emotional assistance to those who lost their jobs, as well as those who remain and those looking for work, all of this in collaboration with social workers.

25.8 Social work relating to migration

> In migration each step is like having a stroke. You have to learn to walk, learn and move in the world again.
>
> (Rakoff, 1985, p. 34)

A migrant is 'someone who has left his country'. This includes the category of 'refugee', a concept defined at the 1951 United Nations Convention as:

> someone who owing to a well-founded fear of being persecuted, for reasons of race, religion, nationality, membership of a particular social group or political opinion, is outside the country of his nationality, and is unable to, or owing to such fear, is unwilling to avail himself of the protection of that country.

Mass migrations are not uncommon in the history of the world. Towards the end of 2006, the UNHCR, the UN High Commission for Refugees, announced that 34 million people were either displaced or refugees. A much larger number of people migrates for economic and other reasons. Many countries have been melting pots of different cultures and nationalities through the centuries. Examples of such melting pot situations can be provided for every country, if we look at immigration waves through history. See Table 25.2 for an example of immigration waves into the Netherlands.

Obviously, generalizing and stereotyping should be avoided at all cost when providing social work to migrants. When providing support to migrants, we really need to be aware of this, because the latter are often affected by discrimination based on biases and stereotypes.

25.8.1 Specific aspects of coping

Migration undeniably involves elements of people being uprooted, of loss, letting go and leaving behind. Migrants miss their loved ones, the social network and all that was familiar, and this can be reflected in many different ways. This unavoidable uprooting involves more than leaving behind their home, it also means leaving behind family, friends, their country of origin and their culture. In this sense, migrants experience many different kinds of loss: they lose people they were close to, as reflected in the statement that: 'Distant friendship is so distant'; they lose a sense of identity: 'Am I still the person I was proud to be?'; they lose their language: 'Anything I think, no matter how subtle and nuanced, sounds so awkward when I try and express it.' There is loss of status: 'I was held in respect over there, but that disappeared like snow before the sun'; and a loss of goals: 'It is as if I have lost my direction in life.'

Consequences for identity development

Migration can have far-reaching consequences on identity development (Graafsma & Tieken, 1987). The first generation of migrants resolves the identity issue by trying to identify with the recipient society as much as possible and by cutting old ties; this process is sometimes referred to as assimilation. Others try to avoid interaction with the recipient society as much as they can, maintaining a silo which offers a sense of secure isolation. In a sense assimilation is premature: cutting old ties being akin to suppressing a part of one's own identity. Secure silos are not a good solution either, as in time, living in isolation will result in stagnated development. In other words, rejecting one's new environment and rejecting the old one are both due to the psychological conflict which results from migration. It is better for migrants to gradually start to feel a part of their new environment, while maintaining warm and close ties to where they came from. Developing a new culture which is somewhere in between the old

TABLE 25.2 Waves of immigration into the Netherlands from the sixteenth century onwards

Era	Waves of immigration
Late sixteenth century	Around 100,000 Flemish migrants (from present-day Belgium and Northern France) migrated to cities such as Amsterdam, Haarlem, Leiden, Middelburg and Gouda
Seventeenth to nineteenth centuries	Tens of thousands 'migrating workers' move to the coastal area of the Netherlands for seasonal work
Early seventeenth century	A few thousand relatively wealthy Sephardic Jews flee Portugal, with the majority ending up in Amsterdam
1635–1800	20,000 Ashkenazi Jews flee to the Netherlands from Central and Eastern Europe
After 1685	Around 50,000 Huguenots flee to the Netherlands from France, where they are persecuted. Around 12,000 of these end up in Amsterdam
From 1900 onwards	18,000 labourers are attracted from Germany, Belgium, Poland, Italy Czechoslovakia and Slovenia to work in the coal mines in the Dutch province of Limburg
1920–1930	Approx. 10,000 Jews flee to the Netherlands from Eastern Europe with another 20,000 fleeing from Germany
1949	When Indonesia becomes an independent republic, 20,000 expats return to the Netherlands, including around 12,000 people from the Moluccas (an island group in Indonesia)
1950	170,000 Dutch passport holders/nationals move to the Netherlands from the Netherlands Antilles
1965–1973	225,000 guest workers are recruited to work in the Netherlands as guest workers from Italy, Spain, Yugoslavia, Greece, Turkey, Morocco and Tunisia
1974–1991	Around 100,000 people arrive in the Netherlands from Suriname, around a third of the population of Suriname
From 1980 onwards	In 1994, the Netherlands receive around 90,000 requests for asylum from countries such as the former Yugoslavia, Somalia, Iran, Iraq, Romania, Zaire and Sri Lanka
From 2007 onwards	By 2007 the number of requests for asylum has reduced to 9,700 (of which 7,100 relate to first-time requests); the majority from Iraqi and Somali asylum seekers
From 2012 onwards	The number of requests for asylum has increased exponentially, due to the influx of large numbers of refugees from Syria and other war-torn areas or areas affected by famine

and the new is sometimes referred to as the *condición migrante*, the migrant condition. Together migrants form the culture of 'permanent temporary residence'.

A number of factors can make it more likely that migrants get stuck somewhere along the migration process. The more negative factors there are, the greater likelihood that migrants will get stuck (see Table 25.3). A great many signs may flag migrants' issues with grief. Home-sickness and emotional outbursts may be seen as a direct reflection of feelings of loss. Indirectly, migrants may display a large range of symptoms and issues (see Table 25.4).

TABLE 25.3 Risk factors before, during and following migration

	Risk factors	Description
Pre-migration factors		
1	Social status	What status did the migrant leave behind?
2	Individual/family history	Any impactful events in the past?
3	Reason for migration	Did the migrant choose to leave or were you forced to leave?
4	Trauma	Any trauma due to executions, rape, isolation, being forcibly deprived of food and sleep, intimidation?
5	Abruptness	How abruptly or how gradually did migration occur?
6	Way migrant said goodbye to country of origin	Was the migrant able to say goodbye in/to country of origin?
Transmigration factors		
7	Manner of move/transport	How did migrant move/by what means of transport and under what circumstances?
8	Nature of initial reception in the recipient society	Was the initial reception perceived to be hospitable?
Post-migration factors		
9	Reception following arrival	How were migrants received following initial reception?
10	Possibilities for integration, accommodation, work	How was reception when migrants moved into first house, learned the language, were first employed, experienced health problems?
11	Type and scale of discrimination	What was the level of discrimination in the receiving country, in terms of avoidance, name-calling or people being physically aggressive?
12	Individual or family events	Which events in the individual's life/family life are stressful/impactful?

In 1982 migrant/foreign born clients made up less than 0.5% of the total number of clients from regional institutions of ambulatory mental health services (referred to as RIAGG in the Netherlands). Twenty-five years later, this had increased to 6.8%. Obviously, we need to take into account the fact that the number of foreign-born Netherlands residents had increased in the meantime. Foreign-born residents have different needs for care than native-born residents.

Aside from mental health issues, they often also suffer psychosocial and material problems. They are more likely to have psychotic disorders and more likely to be addicted to substances (drugs). The increased number of foreign-born residents in the Netherlands will undoubtedly

TABLE 25.4 Coping problems related to migration

Coping problems	Description	Examples
Physical	Physical problems	Headaches, dizziness, muscle aches (neck/shoulders), joint aches, fatigue, intestinal complaints (stomach, bowels)
Social	Social isolation, loneliness	Communication diminishes both in a quantitative and qualitative sense. Choosing to be independent results in loss of protection by own system/environment
	Negative identity/image: outcast, criminal, drop-out	Internalizing suppression due to previous experiences, discrimination
	School dropout, unemployed	Barriers to entering the job market
Psychological	Depressed	Loyalty to what is old and familiar by rejecting all that is new and not familiar
	Divided loyalties	Enjoying the new and unfamiliar is perceived as betrayal of the old and familiar
	Problems with aggression	Aggressiveness direct at oneself and others; reliving fear of trauma, being discriminated in violent dreams, dreaming of angry spirits, suicidal thoughts and behaviour.
	Attention or memory problems	Aggressiveness directed at oneself and others; reliving fear of trauma, being discriminated in violent dreams, dreaming of angry spirits, suicidal thoughts and suicidal behaviour
Existential	Emptiness, hopelessness	No outlook, feeling lost and abandoned, also by God, Allah, etc.

involve an increased incidence of issues related to psychosis and substance abuse. The problems of foreign-born residents are often complex and often involve several different areas (physical health care, accommodation, income, how they spend their days). There is a role here for mental health services, but for other agencies as well.

25.8.2 Social work tasks

Those who support migrants often work with families affected by multiple issues. For this reason, social work tasks around losses will cover a wide range of assistance and support, and communication plays an important role in all this.

The language of misery

It is your task to understand the migrant's language of misery. Every culture or cultural group has its own way of expressing this 'language of misery'; and this mode of expression is clearly understood by everyone within such groups (de Kuiper, 1994). Whether and in what way such pain is addressed therefore strongly depends on the support worker's cultural background. Attention and empathetic understanding will be optimal if the 'pain-related' behaviour corresponds to what is expected from someone who is in pain. If you are confronted with pain when providing support, you will need to be aware of the type of pain-related behaviour observed and you will need to ask yourself whether this 'fits'; you will have to be aware of different upbringings and of the types of pain considered either 'normal' or 'abnormal' and how these are expected to be treated. It is also your role to identify any generational gaps and get the different generations to talk to each other, if need be. Culture shock can cause the gap between first-, second- and even third-generation migrants to grow. In some cases you can detect a certain amount of distancing and can then try to (re)establish contact or rapprochement.

The social context

It is also your role to place mental health issues in the context in which they developed. Placing a psychological label on migrant issues only serves to increase their feelings of guilt. The fact that many migrants belong to the bottom rungs of society, with limited opportunities to escape, means it is desirable that we avoid causing any feelings of guilt and blame.

When providing support in situations of loss, it is also your role to be actively aware of certain signals, because most migrants are not accustomed to asking for support and voicing what support it is they need. You need to be aware of possible loneliness, the need for interaction and any trauma which individuals may struggle with all by themselves.

Social workers providing grief support also need to address age specific problems. Young migrants need to be removed from no man's land and provided with a new outlook. An increasing number of town and city councils are trying to reduce criminal behaviour by young people through implementing projects based on the philosophy that 'Young people should be at school or at work, and that's it, end of story' (Braams, 1994).

The communicative approach: TOPOI

When providing social work to migrants clear communication is of the essence. If misunderstandings occur, we need to identify possible reasons for these. It is better to use a communicative approach such as LOPOI, rather than a culture-specific approach involving stereotyping and generalizations. LOPOI stands for Language, Ordering, Perspectives, Organization and Influence/Effort, five areas in which misunderstandings may arise (Arts 1994). In Dutch this is abbreviated as TOPOI, reminding us of the Greek word τόποι, which means 'places/locations' (as in 'topography').

L   *Language* involves thinking about the consequences of differences in language (use): ensure an open-ended conversation by asking questions such as: 'What happened?,' 'Who is involved?' or 'Why is it that we are talking about. . . ?'

O   *Ordering* involves respect for differences in the way each party views the truth. Avoid conflict and avoid the question as to who is telling the truth, the other-ness can open people's eyes to things they themselves took for granted.

P   *Perspectives* involves taking into account people's personal perspective, for instance the fact that certain words and rules can be 'loaded'; also taking into account the social perspective, including discrimination and resistance within society.

O   *Organization* involves considering the formal organization and concrete setting in which the parties find themselves, such as the fact that it may be busy at the counter and the fact that migrants are dependent.

I   *Influence* and *effort* involve looking at people's intentions and their efforts to plead their case. There may be a difference between intentions and effects.

25.8.3 Pitfalls

The first pitfall involves the grief support worker drawing up a sort of recipe for interacting with each different group of foreign-born migrants. As a result the client is not approached as an individual with specific needs, but as a representative of a particular group of the population. This is folkloristic in a way – summarizing someone's customs in a number of typically folkloristic examples – as well as being ethnocentric: the support worker's culture is central and superior to the other culture.

It is easy to underestimate the number of communicative misunderstandings which may arise from language differences. You may unintentionally use words or concepts which are not aligned with the migrant's knowledge or lexicon. There is a difference between hearing and recalling information and understanding it.

The third pitfall involves the support worker overestimating the migrant's level of assertiveness. Some migrants may keep quiet, because of rules of politeness, or because they do not want to impose on others, even if you expressly invite them to ask you any questions they may have.

You may also go about asking questions the wrong way. If you ask concrete questions, you are likely to receive concrete answers. When asking open questions such as: 'How are you?' and: 'Do you have any questions?,' you may not really get any response. Out of politeness, migrants may say: 'I'm fine' and: 'Everything is clear'.

A fifth pitfall may involve failing to detect and correctly identify symptoms of post-traumatic stress (see Table 7.2). If migrants have some unresolved trauma, they may re-experience the trauma, and show avoidance and hyperalertness. Information and training through multicultural agencies and organizations such as the Stichting Pharos (an agency focusing on reducing health inequalities among migrants and refugees) and Steunpunt Gezondheidszorg Vluchtelingen (an agency that advocates on behalf of refugees) in the Netherlands, reduce barriers to the Dutch health care system for refugees in terms of symptoms affecting their physical, mental and social functioning.

Support workers may be very hesitant to intervene or be directive, out of a fear of failure, or because they do not want to be labelled racist or accused of discrimination. Where social workers might encourage Dutch clients to take the initiative, and to be less dependent, we accept more from migrants than we should and in doing so we do not do them any favours. Fear of doing the wrong thing makes social workers put up with clients complaining or blaming more than they should.

The final pitfall involves thinking that you should be like a rock when providing support to migrants. Confronted as you are with all those feelings of hopelessness in the face of structural unemployment, waiting for years to be granted refugee status, an overwhelming history of trauma, boredom, negativity and emotional outbursts all impact on you as the support worker, and mean that you are at high risk of burnout.

25.9 Social work in relation to dementia

Dementia has been referred to as the epidemic of the coming years. Aging involves loss in many different areas. Older people do not just have to cope with loss of physical abilities and deteriorating health, they also lose family members, friends and acquaintances as they die. Retiring and moving into a home all have an impact. Old trees do not like being uprooted and replanted. The more unexpected and the more forced the admission or transfer to another place of residence, the more difficult older people will find the move. And because people are surviving longer, the incidence of dementia has gone up.

Primary dementia

We distinguish between two different syndromes: primary and secondary dementia. Primary dementia involves a brain condition where dementia is the core complex. Alzheimer's disease is the most well-known and most common form of dementia (50% to 60% of all patients affected by dementia), while other forms of dementia include Fronto-Temporal Dementia (FTD), Huntington's Chorea, dementia due to Parkinson's Disease and Creutzfeldt-Jakob's Disease. Dementia starts unnoticeably and follows a gradual, progressively worsening course.

Secondary dementia

Secondary dementia develops as a consequence of a primary illness. This category includes vascular dementias and dementia as a result of alcohol abuse, carbon monoxide or prescription drug poisoning, brain injury, AIDS or a thyroid disorder.

Multi-infarct dementia is a form of vascular dementia and the second most important cause of dementia (20% of all patients). Bleeds or clots result in a loss of function and an incremental memory loss, bit by bit.

Symptoms

All those affected by dementia suffer confusion. Some lose almost all of their memory, others get lost in their past, while others again cannot find the right words or start to wet the bed. All of these signs and symptoms are due to the mind falling apart, the disruption of thinking, feeling and doing, both separately and in relation to each other (van Dam, 1992). The process of dementia can progress from amnesia (memory loss) towards global dementia syndrome (more extensive memory loss) finishing up in agnostic, aphasic and apraxic dementia syndrome, with more and more capabilities affected (see Table 25.5). 'Agnosia' refers to a disruption of visual recognition, 'aphasia' to a speech disorder, and 'apraxia' to a disruption of the ability to carry out certain actions.

It is impossible to predict exactly how dementia will progress. There may be periods where there is some improvement. We do not have a consistent diagnosis of dementia. Two-thirds of those with dementia are cared for at home. In the Netherlands this involves over 120,000 people. Most of these live in their own homes and are cared for by their spouse or other members of the family, usually daughters (in-law). Others live with other members of the family, usually with one of the children. Some family members bear a relatively heavy burden with relative ease, while others struggle with what would objectively seem to be a relatively light load.

TABLE 25.5 Loss of function in progressive dementia

Functions/capabilities	Amnestic dementia	Global dementia	Aphasic, apraxic, agnostic dementia
Short-term memory	Affected	Affected	Affected
Long-term memory	Affected	Affected	Affected
Orientation in time	Affected	Affected	Affected
Orientation to new environment	Affected	Affected	Affected
Orientation to new faces	Affected	Affected	Affected
Orientation to old familiar environment		Affected	Affected
Orientation to familiar faces		Affected	Affected
Speech			Affected
Actions			Affected
Visual recognition			Affected
Intellectual skills		Affected	Affected
Physical functions/capabilities			Affected
Ability to learn	Affected	Affected	Affected

25.9.1 Specific aspects of coping

> Are you ever scared?
> Yes, scared of going crazy: I cannot hold it together anymore, life is slipping through my fingers like sand.

Dementia affects the mind itself, and its regulatory powers. In other words dementia involves a process of disintegration for the individuals concerned: they have no control over the process itself. Knowing that the human spirit, being human, is linked to our consciousness, and that dementia affects our conscious self, we could say that dementia robs us of the essence of 'being human'. Losing our mind, means losing our identity and personality. For loved ones, including partners, siblings, parents and children, seeing dementia take over can involve a poignant farewelling of a proud man, father or mother. 'You lose your husband and you gain a child in return'. And: 'He's there but at the same time he's not'.

The process of progressively developing dementia involves five types of loss (see Table 25.6). We can add the loss of decorum to the losses listed below. Individuals lose their ability to look after themselves and look groomed, resulting in them looking unkempt, and behaving oddly.

Initially the person concerned may try and cover up what is happening, and this is a natural response to a painful reality. The individual tries to hide his or her embarrassment and loss of face with regard to the growing loss of abilities. Anger and fear are distinctive and familiar expressions of memory loss and the associated loss of identity.

> Something is not quite right in my head.

A gentleman who used to be well-spoken now states, in response to some simple questions:

> I'm sorry, I'm at a loss for words now.

TABLE 25.6 Losses related to dementia

Losses involved	Description
Physical losses	Aging, illness, brain
Loss of conscious self and self-control	No longer a clear sense of identity; literally losing themselves
Social losses	Social stimuli derived from loved ones, job, role
Intellectual losses	Diminished ability to think rationally; loss of this ability
Personal losses	Ability to internalize things is diminished or lost: as does the ability to incorporate weaknesses and deal with losses; loss of balance between the old and the new

Source: Feil (1991).

Not setting the bar too high and providing care and social work at the level someone is at in the process can do the person some justice.

Marriages in which one spouse suffers from dementia come under pressure. The balance in the relationship between the partners, relationships within the nuclear and extended families are disrupted and require intervention. Individuals may be admitted to a home and visits from the partner, and visits to Mum or Dad by the adult children may involve an ongoing confrontation with the past and with the loss of a loved one, as people affected by dementia are often perceived as having 'passed on' even though they are physically still alive.

25.9.2 Social work tasks

Primary care providers including family doctors, nurses and social workers, are all faced with the consequences of dementia, as are team leaders, nurse aides and care assistants, and occupational and recreational therapists working at the level of secondary care. Family doctors focus on obvious behavioural changes. People affected by dementia may have a significant need for support, empathy and understanding. Initially they will be aware of the fact that they are mentally deteriorating. Social workers and other professionals have to have conversations with loved ones as to the nature of the loss and what this means to each person. Going along with the narratives of the person affected by dementia is the appropriate approach, as explained below (*validation* approach).

ROT

For many years, people working in the field of psychogeriatrics approached people with dementia based on the principles of the reality orientation approach, or Reality Orientation Training (ROT). ROT is based on the principle of 'use it or lose it'. The idea is that memory will remain intact for longer if we undertake memory training. This is combined with sensory stimuli and with approaches with appeal to the person's social skills. While ROT did appear to have some stimulating effects when carried out with groups of people with dementia, it became apparent time and time again that participants did not respond to memory training at

all. In many cases this even resulted in a fear of failure: 'I am not a very smart guy,' or participants trying to leave the group: 'I have to go home because my daughter is waiting for me' or
denial: 'My eyesight is so bad that I cannot read numbers anymore'.

Validation

Observations of the effects of the ROT approach, resulted in a different approach, one which
was based on communication at the emotional level. The question was asked as to why we
should try and orient residents with dementia towards 'reality'. And whether it was not in fact
arrogant of social workers to pretend that their reality was the only 'reality'. Another question
was why social workers felt so disappointed to see people with dementia stubbornly holding
on to their own sense of reality. These questions resulted in new insights at two different levels:
people affected by dementia live in their own little world, *and* they appreciate someone being
able to find a way into that world, or even being prepared to join them in that world.

The willingness to enter the 'world' of people affected by dementia requires us to overcome our own fear of aging, dementia and social isolation, affecting either ourselves or older
people close to us (partner, siblings, parents and grandparents). It requires the willingness to
accept others as they are, in their confusion, anxiety, sadness; aggressive and deteriorating. It
becomes clear that what therapists and health care providers refer to as 'reality' is in fact a
much diminished form of reality, which values facts over feelings. The most important aspect
of the validation approach is the fact that it appeals to lived experiences and *universal feelings.*

Loved ones affected by symptoms of depression

The next of kin of people affected by dementia can develop symptoms of depression. There
are various options for treating such symptoms. Cognitive and relationship therapies offer
ways to address unrealistic thoughts and tensions within relationships. Antidepressants can be
prescribed. The next of kin may find the process whereby their loved ones are increasingly
affected by dementia exhausting. The balance between coping ability and mental burden may
be significantly disrupted: individual and group therapy approaches are options for supporting family members who are farewelling loved ones. Coping with losses of such a significant
nature is not an automatic process, but one which requires attention. Saying goodbye can be
problematic, especially when the relationship between the spouses, parents and children was
ambivalent. The process of coping may also be delayed when those involved find it difficult
to express their feelings.

Taking stock

Social work in relation to people saying goodbye to a long-term relationship is focused on
farewelling what it is the partners shared in that relationship. You need to work on drawing
up a profit-and-loss account together with the partner. Questions will include: 'How did we
meet, what were the positive things we shared, what did this partner mean to me?' 'How come
it is all over now?'

Once you have assisted in taking stock, there will be questions about the new relationship:
'What can I be to him and what can he be to me?' 'If he is no longer someone and if he does
not give me anything in return, if he no longer knows who I am, then maybe it is better if he

does not live here anymore, maybe he is better off dead?' Significant others struggle with these types of questions and they need the social workers' attention in the process.

It is harrowing for the next of kin to lower their expectations of the person affected by dementia. Significant others will not be able to cope with the loss of a significant relationship just like that. Time and time again, significant others whose expectations are too high will be disappointed in what remains of their loved ones. This may result in outbursts of anger and acute rejection.

25.9.3 Pitfalls

One pitfall in the care of those affected by dementia is the constrictive nature of treatment plans: the care for these people cannot be tied up in fixed schedules. The burden people carry is determined by multiple factors, and cannot therefore be tied down in regulations, but requires an individual approach. Those who fail to comprehend the unpredictable nature of dementia, can do more harm than good: such miscomprehensions include the idea that dementia starts with slight memory loss, when it is increasingly clear that subtle changes in personality and odd decisions are often the first sign that something is amiss.

A second pitfall involves the assumption that everyone is very aware of information around dementia. A great number of primary caregivers do not understand the reasons underlying a family member's behaviour due to a lack of information. Once they have been made aware, primary caregivers understand the reason for the odd behaviour. A lot of issues in interacting with people affected by dementia are due to a lack of awareness of what happens when someone is affected by dementia.

It would also be wrong to generalize family members' responses, as these can vary a lot and can be as unpredictable as dementia itself (Duijnstee, 1992). Daughters may be furious when their mother dies, because they feel abandoned, while others see this as a form of grief which is part of life: 'Because of her, I am experiencing things which help me become more mature, and help me grow up'. Older people should not be confronted with their failings, their inability to remember, or mistakes. We need to communicate with people affected by dementia at their level.

Some social workers and some who find dementia a fearful perspective, may find it difficult to imagine what the world of the person with dementia looks like: 'They can shoot me if I ever get to that stage'. The last thing people with dementia need is your misplaced sense of pity or distant attitude.

When people suffer memory loss, this need not always be perceived as a sign of incipient dementia. On the other hand, social workers need to ensure that they do pick up on the relevant signs in a timely manner when someone does have dementia.

25.10 Palliative social work

In life we can be sure of one thing: we are all going to die. Social work for the dying has been commonplace since 1990. Professional programmes of study and training courses focus on this aspect of support and many standard texts include a section on social work for the dying. Initially some were hesitant to embrace the concept of 'social work for the dying' due to a fear of standardized approaches and 'mass-produced' social work, and this hesitance is still justified. Dying is such a personal process that it does not allow any kind of 'standardization'. Caring social workers get a sense of the type of support that is needed and intuitively go about things the right way. The important thing is to take the time.

25.10.1 Specific aspects of coping

Five stages model

Kübler-Ross's (1969) model of the five stages of dying arose from an attempt to provide some scaffolding to social workers as to what happens in the last stages of life, thus enabling social workers to address these with sensitivity. These stages were referred to as: denial, anger, bargaining, depression and acceptance. The model has been much criticized for its unintentional effects, including the risk that vulnerable people risk being approached with a number of stereotypes in their last stage of life.

Task model

For this reason the 'Five stages model' is being increasingly abandoned by professional training programmes, and replaced by a task model (Corr, 1992). Just like someone may decide to mow the grass one day, to get rid of grass clippings another day, and on the third day decide that he only wants to mow the front lawn, a dying person may want to be surrounded by loved ones one day, be left alone the second day, and may only want to be with one particular person on the third day. When using a task-oriented model we have a client-oriented approach to the person who is dying, and we let him carry out his tasks how he chooses. The four tasks of dying people have been listed in Table 25.7.

Social work for the dying and their next of kin, does not just extend to the psychological, but also to the physical and spiritual areas, and especially to the social area. What are the caregivers' needs. What is it they need within this emotional process of saying goodbye? How to deal with conflicts and broken relationships within families? There may be practical ways of helping the client system, for instance help with last wills, powers of attorney, getting important paperwork organized as well as arrangements regarding (care for) the children. Social workers should never assume that anything is set in concrete when providing support to the dying: it would be unrealistic to do so. Patients who indicated at some point in time that they would not be prepared to carry on if their condition were to deteriorate to a certain level,

TABLE 25.7 Task-oriented approach to dying

Dimensions	Tasks
Physical dimensions	Satisfying physical needs and minimizing physical suffering, in ways which are in line with other values
Psychological dimensions	Maximizing psychological safety, autonomy and satisfaction
Social dimensions	Maintaining and intensifying interpersonal relationships which are important to the dying person, and attending to the social consequences of dying
Spiritual dimensions	Recognizing, developing or reconfirming sources of spiritual energy and deriving hope from the same

may well have a completely different view once they have reached that point. And people who appeared to be vibrant and able to keep going until the end, may be overwhelmed when their condition deteriorates significantly and may then give up. People can show enormous flexibility in the last stages of their lives, so it can be sad to observe next of kin being unable to demonstrate equal levels of flexibility.

25.10.2 Social work tasks

Task-oriented models are based on the assumption that people who are dying have tasks to fulfil in four different areas: the physical, psychological, social and spiritual areas. The task-oriented model offers those who provide support guidance in four different ways:

- It provides us with the foundation we need to understand every need of each individual involved in the process of dying.
- It encourages people who are dying to live through all available options during a stage of life, which is not at all easy.
- It emphasizes the importance of participation and sharing when coping with the process of dying – aspects which involve people in small communities getting together and supporting each other within social networks.
- It provides guidance to those caring for the dying.

A task-oriented model provides guidance to all those involved in caring for the dying. When it has become clear which tasks the dying has to fulfil, those providing support need to take the responsibility to decide whether and how they can make themselves useful in carrying out such tasks. Helping the dying and their next of kin to carry out such tasks allows for the autonomy of the client system to remain intact.

> What people need most when they are dying is relief from the distressing symptoms of disease, the security of a caring environment, sustained expert care and the assurance that they and their families won't be abandoned.
>
> *(Craven & Wald, 1975)*

This one sentence sums up the needs of the dying and those close to them. When people are dying they are first and foremost alive, and that is why we need to focus on the person rather than on the disease.

Hospice programme

Acknowledging the psychosocial dimensions of people, both living or dying, is a big step forwards, and this is the case in hospice care. Hospice care is based on the principles outlined in Table 25.8. Care that is based on the hospice philosophy, can be provided in hospitals, nursing homes or hospices, special homes for the dying. In *Palliative Social Work*, Altilio and Otis Green, provide an overview, describe the beginnings of hospice care as follows:

> Care Dame Cicely Saunders who was trained as a nurse, medical social worker and finally as a physician founded St. Christophers' Hospice in 1967 as the first research and

TABLE 25.8 The philosophy and principles underpinning hospice care

	Principles	Description
1	The hospice is a starting point, not a facility	The emphasis is on the approach and the attitude, not on creating a separate facility
2	The hospice philosophy is life-affirming, not death-affirming	Hospice care means care to people who may be dying but who are still alive
3	The hospice philosophy promotes optimal quality of life	Hospice care means a type of palliative, symptom-oriented care which minimizes discomfort
4	The hospice philosophy takes care of the patient system	In the hospice philosophy, it is not just the dying who count, but all those who are significant to the dying person
5	Hospice care is holistic care	The focus is on the whole person with all his or her physical, psychological, social and spiritual dimensions
6	Hospices provide continuity of care and continued care for the next of kin	Care continues after death
7	The hospice approach seeks an appropriate combination of professional skills and human presence through interdisciplinary collaboration	Expertise in providing terminal care and symptom management go hand in hand with human companionship through the collaboration between social workers and volunteers
8	Hospices provide care 24/7	If terminal care by the social network is missing or is insufficient, the hospice provides comprehensive care
9	Hospice programmes support their own staff	Terminal care is satisfying, but can also cause stress: hospices take good care of their own staff

Source: Adapted from Corr (1994)

teaching hospice linked with clinical care. This has been a pioneer in the field of palliative medicine, which has now been established worldwide.

Social workers and health practitioners may experience a sense of personal failure when faced with death. Social workers may feel that they were unable to heal the part of the body which caused the problem. Present-day hospitals are establishments providing acute and short-term care, their main purpose being the treatment of specific health care conditions.

Aside from hospitals, we now have nursing homes, which are intended for those affected by disability or chronic disease. Terminal care has traditionally been the focus of nursing homes, because they are increasingly the final stop for a growing number of nursing home residents.

Hospice-type terminal homecare originated from the idea that the dying require *care* rather than *cure* and there are now hospices in many countries, special facilities for the dying. Internationally, the International Association of Palliative Medicine, which was established in 1990, has provided a strong impetus to the hospice philosophy within the field of palliative medicine, nursing and nursing home care. Many social workers consider the provision of support to the dying and their next of kin a very satisfying aspect of their work. When people are dying, they no longer need to pretend. They can be more open than ever before and this may result in some very meaningful and in-depth conversations. People of all ages find support in carrying out rituals or expressing themselves creatively. They need to be given the opportunity to express their loss in a creative manner, with the aid of art, music or creative writing (Bailey, 1995).

25.10.3 Pitfalls

When providing social work for the dying, the first pitfall involves misinterpreting people's request to be allowed to die. Rather than interpreting such statements as: 'I don't want this life, this misery anymore', you may interpret this as an actual death wish (the wish to die).

Conversely, you may interpret such a death wish as a call for attention, rather than the actual wish to die.

You should also take care not to take sides in situations which are marred by conflict. In such situations it becomes even more important that the social worker is alert to any possible signals, so as he can consider how these could perhaps be discussed. Sometimes it is appropriate to involve a colleague who has the trust of all parties, to act as a mediator. Conflict situations may involve there being not just a wife, but also a girlfriend present, or situations where family members are adamantly opposed to the dying person's request for euthanasia, even though the patient just wants to die.

Finally, support workers should not dig around too much in someone's past, but they do need to show an interest in a past history that may involve a lot of complicated matters. Dying people are often open and honest, and this adds to their vulnerability. It is essential that we create an environment in which they can relate their story.

25.11 Photo viewing following a traumatic loss

> Seeing is believing.
>> (next of kin of a victim of the plane crash in Libya, June 2010)

> Sometimes what you imagine is worse than reality in its worst form.

A display of photos involves next of kin who have suffered a traumatic loss – and who have expressly requested this – to view drawings, followed by photos of the body of their loved one. The aim of this photo display is to help next of kin develop a better sense of the death of a loved one. All too often, next of kin are denied the opportunity to face the bodies of their deceased loved ones after traumatic events such as murder, suicide and disasters (see also Chapter 7 and Appendix 4). Professionals may advise this for a range of reasons. This may be due to a paternalistic attitude on the part of such professionals, who have often not seen the effects of the violent event on the victim themselves, but who immediately state: 'It is better if you do not have a look'. Social workers who offer a photo viewing when the grieving loved ones come with questions, do not display a patronizing attitude but are facilitating a conscious and careful process of decision making by the next of kin, by providing information about whether to use the available sensory evidence. When disasters strike, such as the plane crash at Tripoli which occurred on May 12, 2010, and which claimed the lives of 70 Dutch passengers – next of kin were mostly advised against viewing the victims' bodies. As a result, a large group of loved ones felt serious doubt as to whether their next of kin had actually died. Reports on technical identification were not or only poorly understood by a number of relatives and a number of them imagined the absolute worst. The advice they were given (not to view the bodies) was diagonally opposed to the wish of many of the next of kin to view the bodies. Social workers employed by the Dutch Victim Support agency were trained to prepare and provide a therapeutic photo viewing in collaboration with the next of kin.

CHECKLIST FOR THERAPEUTIC VIEWING OF PHOTOS

	Preparation	
1	The grief therapist keeps a record/file of steps taken and what was agreed with the client	This is important for you, but also in case of a handover, or for possible research. The official request for a photo viewing for therapeutic reasons is signed by the next of kin and added to the file.
2	Contact the next of kin, requesting a second opinion therapeutic record photo viewing and record what the next of kin remembers as to what was said about the 'viewability' of the body and by whom	Note down what the next of kin is trying to get out of the photo viewing. Also ask for photos of deceased loved ones by way of comparison with the photos of the bodies of the deceased loved ones.
3	The grief therapist arranges the first photo viewing (views all available photos)	Draft proposal for complete, partial or non-photo viewing and for an alternative display (drawing?). Possibly brainstorm with the pathologist as to whether the appearance of the body yields any information as to the cause of death, the deceased's last moments and duration of any suffering.
4	Preparing photo viewing	Photo viewing is completely arranged as per the grief therapist's own preferences: starting by informing the next of kin as to what is going to be viewed, followed by photos, and finally by the actual photos.
5	The definitive proposal with regard to the display/photos is put to the family in a face-to-face interview	The next of kin are asked for an initial response. They may be given time to consider the proposal and this may be passed on by telephone. If there is going to be a display, or if photos are going to be viewed, a date is agreed upon, including who will be present.
	Executive stage	
6	The grief therapist is present at the time and on the date agreed, with the photos	This can also be done directly, when you are with the family.

(*Continued*)

(Continued)

	Preparation	
7	The therapist starts by asking how everyone now feels about the photo display	The next of kin are allowed to change their minds at any time: they remain in control at all times.
8	Photo viewing proper	Next the grief therapist goes ahead with the photo viewing in accordance with the procedure planned.
9	Request for a second opinion	The Disaster Identification Team, National Forensic Investigation Team, or Public Prosecutor may ask the next of kin for a second opinion if desired.
10	Agreements/arrangements about handing over and return of material	The grief therapist comes to an arrangement with the Disaster Identification Team, National Forensic Investigation Team, or Public Prosecutor as how and when photos and other material will be handed over and returned.
11	Recording any responses	Distinctive or striking responses (both positive and negative) are recorded retrospectively.
12	Conclusion	Concluding the photo display and agreeing on a time and date for a follow-up interview with relation aftercare.
	Aftercare stage	
13	Looking back	The aftercare interview allows reflection on how the next of kin responded/felt after the photo display. Which objectives were achieved? Which objectives remain? What steps are appropriate to achieve those aims? Involve volunteer/others
14	Checks and experts	When concluding the display, agree on possible later checks and the involvement of other experts if need be.
15	Self-care/aftercare	Personal aftercare for yourself.
16	Buddy	Have you managed to catch up with your buddy in the interim, to find closure and let off some steam?
17	Results of second opinion: effect on anxiety level	Baseline measurement (at start of interaction)
	Baseline agitation scale: (not agitated) 0–1–2–3–4–5–6–7–8–9–10 (hyper agitated)	
		Allow the client to indicate what causes him or her to feel agitated
		Agitation = psychological, physical or relational disquiet
	Interim measurement (second interaction) agitation scale: (not agitated) 0–1–2–3–4–5–6–7–8–9–10 (hyper agitated)	
		Allow the client to indicate what causes him or her to feel greater, lesser or same level of agitation in interactions with you
	Final measurement (final interaction) agitation scale: (not agitated) 0–1–2–3–4–5–6–7–8–9–10 (hyper agitated)	
		Allow the client to indicate what causes him or her to feel greater, lesser or same level of agitation in interactions with you
	Scoring	Indicate the scores in a graph, together with areas causing feelings of agitation; enabling you to visualize level of stress reduction resulting from your interventions.

Next of kin must be given the opportunity to see the (mutilated/disfigured) body of their loved ones when they want to, even following a traumatic death. Giving them time to make up their minds and good social work support are of the essence in these cases. Research into the train disaster in Granville (Australia) has shown that people who can view the body of accident victims recover better psychologically speaking, while research into the 1987 ferry disaster near Zeebrugge (Belgium) has shown that viewing the bodies may cause fear and stress in the short run, but results in less stress in the long term. However, these studies do not provide social workers with clear advice as to how to deal with such situations.

Chapple and Ziebland interviewed 80 people in the United Kingdom: all people who had lost a loved one through suicide or through a serious accident (Chapple & Ziebland, 2010). There were various reasons why interviewees wanted to view the body. Some had been asked by police to identify the body, while others (incorrectly) thought that they were supposed to do so. Some wanted to make sure there had not been a mistake, while others wanted to care for the deceased, do something, see what state their family member was in, or say goodbye.

Expectations and responses differed between families and causes of death. People were upset in various ways, but rarely regretted their decisions, even when they had seen wounds, bruising or signs of decomposition. Seeing deceased persons whose bodies have been completely burned, or who had been knifed to death or killed by bullets did lead to doubt as to whether the decision to view the body was the right one. Some, particularly those who had lost their loved ones through suicide, were relieved to see them look so peaceful after all the stress and unhappiness they had gone through before death. Viewing the body also helped them to accept the death.

Some had no choice. A body hadn't been found, or they were not allowed to have a look for legal reasons. In one instance – the Bali bombing – the body had been completely destroyed.

The next of kin may need some time and they need to know that they do not *have* to see the body and that they are always allowed to change their minds. When bodies have to be identified, DNA or dental records are always another option. The researchers did not find any evidence of family members being harmed through seeing a mutilated body. What stood out were the positive responses of next of kin who had gone through with viewing carefully prepared photo displays, and who made statements such as: 'I feel I have a bit of my daughter back.' Or: 'I am very happy I did this, I had already lost my husband, but his body had also disappeared without a trace. I can get on with my life now.'

25.12 Summary and questions

This chapter discussed social work support to people in specific situations involving loss, summarized in the circle of loss. I started by discussing the bad news interviews social workers may become involved in. Next I clarified the social worker's tasks in eight situations involving loss: children going through loss, parenting a disabled child, HIV, divorce, impactful changes at work, migration, dementia, death and the next of kin of people who have died a traumatic death. For each situation I clarified what specific aspects of coping social workers may come across, the social work tasks involved in this type of loss as well as the possible pitfalls. I showed that caution is also advised when providing social work support to people in specific situations involving loss, because generalizations, stereotyping or 'mass-produced' social work does not do justice to the tailor-made social work approach that is in fact needed. We have also seen how importance it is that social workers remain clear about what they are doing and do not allow themselves to be negatively influenced by the emotions and struggles of the people concerned. Finally, it is important to consider working under supervision or utilizing a team-based approach in complicated cases.

Questions

1　Have you ever had to convey bad news? Can you relate to the different stages?
2　Which situations involving loss do you come across in practice? Do you recognize the various aspects of coping, social work tasks and pitfalls described?
3　Do you think you could organize a photo viewing in your role as a social worker? What do you think you would need to help put together such a display, in spite of the fact that there may be an initial fear for images which are difficult to take and a fear of very strong emotions?

26

UNFINISHED BUSINESS SYNDROME (UBS)

The risks of the smouldering peat fires

I told a client that his complaints could be related to a number of unfinished matters he had also mentioned; he confirmed this and said: Indeed, I was thinking myself that it is time for me to take stock, which issues do I still need to address and which ones should I draw to a close, because I don't want to carry this around with me any longer.

Questions

This chapter addresses the following questions:

- What does 'unfinished-business syndrome' mean?
- What are unexplained symptoms?
- What are sensory triggers?
- What are unfinished life experiences?
- What are the elements of complaint maintaining coping with loss and grief support?
- What is the difference between UBS type 1 and UBS type 2?
- Why is the unaddressed loss of a parent at a young age an example of UBS?

26.1 Introduction

Heal the past, live the present, dream the future.

This chapter advocates for renewed and focused attention to old pain. UBS is presented here as a phenomenon whereby old pain maintains various *current unexplained* symptoms (caused and maintained).

New in UBS is the way it explicitly names the gestalt of unaddressed life events (1), unexplained complaints (2), trigger-effect (3) and multiplier-effect (4). UBS becomes thereby an explanatory system for a widespread phenomenon, many people are suffering from and often not are helped properly. UBS is not seen as a medical syndrome, but more a description of the experience of people who suffer from old pain, some decades later. Also new is the difference between the type 1 UBS and type 2 UBS. People who experience type 1 UBS complaints also called the stress type of UBS, can be treated by social work. People who experience type 2 UBS – also called the complicated type of UBS – can be better treated by specialists. At last, new is the UBS treatment including cleansing and finishing the old unfinished business, to create perspective in cases sometimes were stuck.

Early recognition of the *unfinished business syndrome* could offer perspective to a group of people who for some time have experienced suffering as a result of unexplained symptoms.

This perspective develops when they are still bringing closure to unfinished life events. professionals, who wish to pay attention to UBS, will find a theoretical foundation and support for their caring and professional role.

26.1.1 A combination approach to unexplained complaints

The current solution-focused short-term approach to problems within the biopsychosocial domain often works on solutions in a refreshing way. Attention to unfinished issues from the past is not always necessary. In our pragmatically established articulation of time, in which many people have found their way into support services, attention to the past has escaped notice to the point where it is almost 'not done'. Attention to the past has even been described as long and futile 'digging into the past'. Nevertheless, a combination approach focused on current as well as old pain can be useful and necessary, especially for the client group with unexplained complaints.

It is estimated there are some 500,000 patients with unexplained *medical* complaints such as unexplained pain and lethargy, backache, headache, pain in arms or legs, chest pain, stomach/bowel complaints, joint aches and dizziness. In addition, there is an unknown number of people suffering unexplained *psychological* symptoms such as anxieties, depressions and aggression. Finally, there are an unknown number of people with unexplained social complaints such as family and relationship problems and employment related problems, none of which is understood.

26.1.2 Secondary victimization

The media sometimes have a tendency to portray people with unexplained complaints as people with vague complaints or reproach them as weak. They are also perceived as people who simulate. This results in secondary victimization. (Unnecessary additional pain, see also Chapter 1). Secondary victimization often occurs, because this group of people feel their caseworker has not adequately listened to them. Possible reasons for this are:

- Mono-disciplinary thinking of the caseworker: 'Stick to what you know' and being afraid to make the wrong diagnosis.
- Treatment shyness of the caseworker: he did not know what to do with old pain.

- Overload of old pain: the caseworker like the client could not see the wood for the trees; the problems did not have a beginning or end.
- Short-term approach: the caseworker considered digging in the past to be futile, he preferred to focus on symptom-maintaining elements, 'the past is the past and the present is the present'.

26.1.3 Signs

It is not always easy to recognize UBS. In a client situation, it is therefore wise to pay attention to the following signs that could indicate UBS.

- *Medical shopping history*: did the client visit many professionals without adequate results?
- *Multiple problem situation*: are problems reported on many levels?
- *Slow treatment progress*: does focusing on current complaints provide relatively little progress?
- *Disproportionate responses from the client*: does doubt or intensity of the current responses and complaints match a current *life event*?
- *Direct signals* from the client: is there more, or anything else that occurred in the past?
- *Incomprehensible signals*: it is incomprehensible how something from the past can still demand so much attention now.
- *Inadequate support*: negative attitude in regard to support, including professionals: secondary victimization because of a lack of recognition in the past?
- *Inadequate coping*: withdrawal, isolation?

In order to be able to value the signals, an anamnesis/first consultation is of great importance: are there four UBS characteristics (see section 26.2)? A UBS approach needs to be considered when there is old pain. The metaphor of the smouldering volcano appeals to the imagination: tackling the original and inner core pressures (the pain of the unfinished life experience) could in some cases prevent and stop the smouldering peat fires from burning again and again. The UBS-combination approach focuses itself on a reduction of the current complaints as well as bringing closure to the previously unfinished life experience.

This chapter will first further define the concept of UBS after which the four UBS characteristics are clarified. Following this explanation, a distinction is then made between two types of UBS.

The chapter elaborates on the unprocessed loss of a parent at a young age which is considered to be a *risk factor* of UBS. At the end, there will be a summary of a number of sources who use unfinished business as a concept. In order to illustrate UBS, examples of case studies are systematically spread out across the chapter.

26.2 Definition of UBS and case study example: the four characteristics of UBS

UBS is the combined presence of four characteristics in the client situation:

1   Current *unexplained complaints* on a biopsychosocial level, that is medical (bio), personal (psycho), relation, family or employment related (social);

2   One or more sensory *triggers* causing an increase in complaints/symptoms; triggers are specific sensory stimuli that reactivate old pain from previously unfinished life experiences in the here and now;

3   Previous *unfinished life events* in the client's biography, such as previously unaddressed experiences of loss, unprocessed traumatic experiences, unfinished conflicts ad unfinished life periods;

4   Complaint maintaining avoidance problem *coping* and negative support.

The unfinished-business syndrome (UBS) is the cohesive phenomenon of these four characteristics. UBS is best described as an interaction between these characteristics. It is important to recognize the client's current complaints/symptoms. Subsequently, the three other characteristics that could potentially maintain the actual complaint are mapped out together with the client. Within the multimethodical approach, these factors are managed systematically. This occurs using non-directive counselling combined with more directive methods, aimed at breaking the vicious circle of complaints and their consequences (see Chapter 4). Treatment perspective could appear to be developing when the current unexplained complaints are set against a background of unfinished life experiences.

There could be an indirect connection between the *current* unexplained complaints and *previous* incomplete life experiences (unfinished business). Specific sensory triggers in the here and now that evoke old pain, could be the connecting elements between current complaints and old pain (*trigger*-effect), maintain the current complaints and even aggravate those (*multiplier*-effect). The old pain that is triggered will sometimes bring on negative coping and negative support which in turn maintains the complaint (see Figure 26.1).

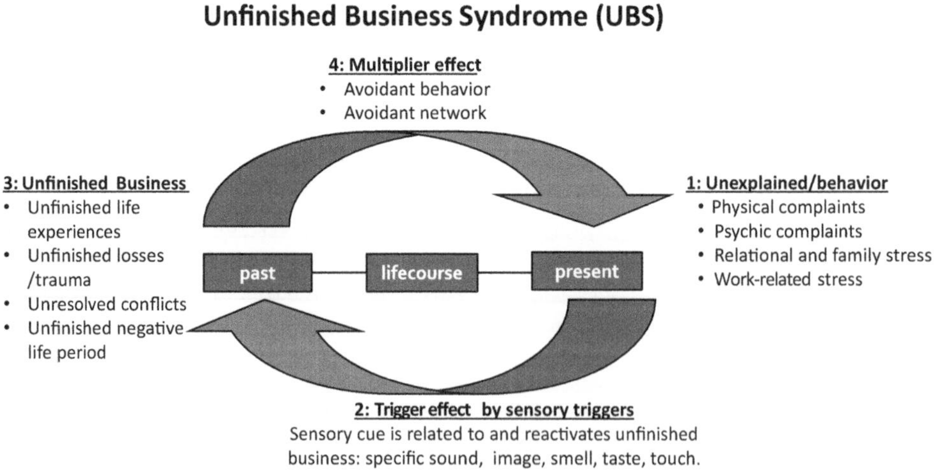

Unfinished Business Syndrome (UBS)

4: Multiplier effect
- Avoidant behavior
- Avoidant network

3: Unfinished Business
- Unfinished life experiences
- Unfinished losses /trauma
- Unresolved conflicts
- Unfinished negative life period

past — lifecourse — present

1: Unexplained/behavior
- Physical complaints
- Psychic complaints
- Relational and family stress
- Work-related stress

2: Trigger effect by sensory triggers
Sensory cue is related to and reactivates unfinished business: specific sound, image, smell, taste, touch.

FIGURE 26.1   The negative UBS spiral with trigger effect and multiplier effect: triggered old pain works as a 'multiplier' for current and existing unexplained complaints/behaviour

Source: de Mönnink 2016

CASE 26.1 MRS. FEAR

During an intervention at the hospital, Mrs. Fatigue responds to the insertion of a drip with a strong unexpected reaction of fear (upset, crying) [1. unexplained complaints/behaviour, Figure 26.1]. Seeing the needle evokes strong memories of her little daughter who died 5 years ago in another hospital [2. reactivating old pain and 3. no proper goodbye from her daughter]. The visual perception of the needle – coupled with the death following an accident – appears to be the 'trigger' for old unprocessed pain [3]. So far, the patient has managed to avoid any discussion in relation to the loss [4. avoidant coping] but also received insufficient support [4. ineffective support]. She has unexplained anxieties and fears various medical interventions, that worsen by avoidance and the UBS-circle is complete.

The Hospital Social Worker together with the patient can begin to unravel the UBS-dynamic and start a brief support intervention.

Because of inner rest being established, the drip can be inserted without any problems at future hospital visits.

CASE 26.2 MRS. FATIGUE (69), UNEXPLAINED FATIGUE, MOOD COMPLAINTS AND RELATIONSHIP PROBLEMS

UBS characteristics	Case
1 Unexplained complaints	*Unexplained* fatigue, tension symptoms, dejected, relationship problems with partner because he has a higher sex drive
2 Sensory triggers	Touch trigger: any physical/sexual advance evokes aversion: the therapist's proposal to use massage first instead of sex causes an aversive reaction
3 Unfinished life experiences	Unaddressed rape by boy in neighbourhood when a young girl (9 years)
4 Coping avoidance and inadequate support maintaining the complaints	*Negative coping*: would rather not talk to partner, avoids conversation, by pretending to be asleep for example
	Positive coping: Motivated to undergo treatment
	Negative support: told mother at the time about the rape, but she did not wish to cause problems with the neighbours and kept quiet; currently no support from partner as partner 'is the problem'; no one else to talk to
	Positive support: general practitioner is supportive, through specific referral.
	UBS-approach: combined approach aimed at current complaints, and previously unfinished experiences:
	1 manage current complaints with relaxation approach and energy exercises, relationship sessions;
	2 manage old pain by bringing closure to the unfinished sexually violent experience, the key issue through treatment.

UBS characteristics	**Case**

Th(erapist)   First of all let's reconstruct the aversive response, when did you become so aversive to sex and touching?

Cl(ient)   My experiences are of an unrestricted and happy childhood up until the rape when 9 years old.

After this the little girl was scared, showing withdrawn-like behaviour; always on her own; no development of a normal relationship; for 60 years experiencing aversion to physical touching, on sexual and social level and as an extension of this, experience relationship tensions and mood problems.

Th   Proposal therapist to still bring closure to unfinished experience of rape. In vitro (in the treatment room) return to the past in a symbolical format, alternately working out the fantasy about the desired reaction of mother back then and own response at that time: what do you need from your mother and what do you need from the perpetrator?

Cl   Together with mother, visit the home of the perpetrator and make him take responsibility; father on the doorstep, perpetrator on the doorstep. She verbalizes what her mother would say, and what she would want her to say and to do.

Th   Is his response satisfactory? Still went ahead and verbalized the incident with powerful release of grief and rising anger. Finally, are you able to leave this incident behind you and move on?

Cl   No.

Th   In conclusion, what do you need still?

Cl   I would like to kick him between the legs. Expressed in a symbolical way through a kick aimed at the perpetrator's door.

Tension complaint level decreased from level 8 to 2; complaints mood level increased from 2 to 6; relationship tensions reduced from 8 to 3: satisfactory period of sex life followed.

26.2.1 Characteristic 1: unexplained complaints/behaviour

With UBS there could be a single or multiple presence of the following unexplained complaints on a physical, psychological and social (relationship, family and work) level.

- *Physical complaints/behaviour* such as unexplainable (serious) medical complaints, for example unexplained pain complaints, (chronic) complaints relating physical tension, for example headache, abdominal pain, and psychosomatic, for example skin rash, fatigue;
- *Psychological complaints/behaviour* such as acting out or anti-social behaviour that is not understood, motion unrest, negative behaviour against others, dejection or depression with withdrawing behaviour, (chronic) psychological complaints, identity problems, insecurity, uncontrolled fear, uncontrolled anger or psychopathology such as adjustment disorder, anxiety/panic attacks, personality disorders;
- *Relationship and family* complaints/behaviour such as unexplained (chronic) tensions privately and in the work environment in terms of quality of work/life balance, unexplained tensions in mutual relationships, recurring relationship and family tensions, parenting problems, intimacy, sexuality, for example (chronic) communication problems and (persisting) conflicts;
- *Work-related complaints/behaviour* such as unexplained workaholic pattern, concentration problems at work, not being able to find employment.

Elucidation

Unexplained complaints are evident when those complaints are referred to as such by the involved caseworker and tells the client that there is no known cause for these medical, psychological or relationship/work related complaints. Another common expression used is 'essential' complaints. For example, high blood pressure with an unknown cause is referred to as essential or primary hypertension.

'Incubation period'

Unexplained complaints are a latent form of UBS, old pain is invisibly present. The time frame between recognizing the old complaints and the occurrence of the life event is called the incubation period of UBS, named after medical analogy. The *incubation period* or *incubation time* of a medical condition is the time that elapses between contamination and the first clinical symptoms of the condition.

The UBS incubation period is the time that expires between the moment of the life event (loss, trauma, unresolved conflict, negative life episodes) and the moment of recognition as old pain complaints. In the incubation period, there are a number of complaints not yet recognized as old pain complaints.

The UBS incubation period can vary from a couple of months to a couple of decades. Unexplained complaints could already be apparent a couple of months after the experience of loss, trauma, conflict or the negative life episode, *if the caseworker after all is unable to establish a cause.* Examples of the incubation periods are as follows.

- *Three months*, in the case of a young man of 19 years old suffering anxiety complaints that became apparent 2 months after the sudden suicide of his cousin aged 19. After 3 months, the support worker told him he was experiencing an anxiety disorder unrelated to the suicide of his cousin (no cause could be established here either). After 4 months, another support worker established that the anxious response had been a normal reaction to extraordinary loss, so that the processing of this loss could begin.
- *Six years*, in the case of a veteran who, 6 years after discharge from the army presented with unexplained complaints resulting in the support services establishing old pain. This predated a 6-year period in which the veteran carried with him unexplained tension complaints and anger management problems.
- *Ten years*, a woman who after 10 years became conscious of her incestuous past when entering into an adult relationship and the first sexual steps as part of the relationship. This followed a period of unexplained head- and stomach ache and identity issues.
- *Fifteen years*, an abused woman who once again became conscious of her loveless childhood period, when after 15 years – at age 30 – she had children herself and did not know how to love them.

26.2.2 Characteristic 2: sensory triggers

A trigger is a mechanism which brings about pain that has gone unaddressed and has not been brought to rest adequately. Triggers are sensory stimuli linked to unfinished life experiences. Those moments in which the initial pain flares up are described as trigger moments. At the stage when the person in question is confronted with triggers that are connected to the original loss or trauma, the old emotional burden resurfaces. During these moments the unfinished life experience is re-activated hereby causing the involved to experience unrest: the flare effect. The complaints will become more intense or present themselves for the first time.

Elucidation

Trigger zones

Trigger zones are named after the sensory zones they are related to; they can present as combined:

- *Visual triggers*, for example seeing a deceased aunt in a coffin triggers grief in relation to own mother, the unaddressed loss of a parent at a young age;
- *Sound triggers*, for example hearing new and bad news (partner says: 'I want a divorce') triggers sadness and anger with the man who has often been deserted in his life;
- *Touch triggers*, for example touching triggers anxiety in a woman who experienced sexual violence however has not dealt with this yet;
- *Smell triggers*, for example the odour of rotten meat triggers fear in a road accident victim who suffers from unaddressed burn experiences;
- *Taste triggers*, for example the taste of a particular dessert triggers sadness in someone with unaddressed and family feuds (the memory of happily eating dessert).

Triggers reflect painful details of a previously impressive life experience. A former neutral sensory stimulant was charged through sensory branding. From that moment onwards, specific sensory stimuli are charged through the impressive life experience.

Trigger generalization

Specific sensory triggers can be generalized in relation to much more aspects of life than the original trigger can. For example, the burn victim triggered when seeing or smelling fire, could already be stimulated when seeing matches, or watching flames on TV. Original triggers, through generalization, can be 'contagious' or' infectious' to more connected stimuli. This process of the spreading out of original stimuli over more stimuli is called trigger generalization. The spreading could involve stimuli that initially existed as an obvious response to the radical life event, however gradually as a cause was lost sight of.

26.2.3 Characteristic 3: previous unfinished life experiences

Unfinished business (UB) is the collective principle of unfinished life experiences requiring closure, such as unaddressed experiences of loss, trauma-experiences, conflicts and negative life periods (see Table 26.1).

The four mentioned unaddressed life experiences are often found in combination, such as when there is war and sexual violence whereby there are issues of loss as well as traumatic circumstances, with unresolved conflicts and unaddressed life periods.

TABLE 26.1 Four types of unaddressed life experiences

	Unaddressed loss	Unaddressed trauma	Unresolved conflict	Negative life period
Definition	Not allowing sufficient time to reflect and consider the impact of losing a loved one or otherwise valuable part of life	Paying insufficient attention to one or more exceptional consideration branded sensory experiences	Insufficient resolution of conflict of interest	Not giving sufficient attention to negative life period
Examples	Loss of parent at a young age, unaddressed young divorce, unaddressed dismissal	War, disaster, road accidents sexual abuse	Arguments, feuds, honour revenge, genocide	Affective neglect, incest, bully, negative boarding school, prison, discrimination and oppression on the grounds of sex, race, beliefs to genocide

Explanation

An unfinished life experience is a painful life experience from the distant or near past with the pain continuing to force itself upon the present. At that time, the life event was not closed. Issues were never fully discussed or sorted out, emotions not sufficiently expressed, facts not explored, etc. Old pain is re-activated because of new life events. For all four types of UB mentioned above, similar experiences function as a here-and-now trigger. Unaddressed bereavement (losing a parent when young), a new loss in the here and now will not only cause new pain, but also evoke the old pain connected to the loss of a mother or father at a young age.

With previously unaddressed traumas (car accident), the experience of another accident would again be painful, but the old pain of the previous accident is evoked once again.

This also applies to unaddressed conflicts from the past that are triggered by new conflicts. Finally, this also applies to negative life periods (affected child neglect). Not taking any notice in one's personal or work situation can lead to new pain, but also evoke old pain.

26.2.4 Characteristic 4: avoidance coping and avoidance support

The fourth UB characteristic involves the continuous negative own association with the previous unaddressed experience (avoidance coping) and receiving inadequate support from the environment (avoidance support). Coping and support have a negative impact on the closure tasks being carried out and the life event remains unaddressed (see Figure 26.2).

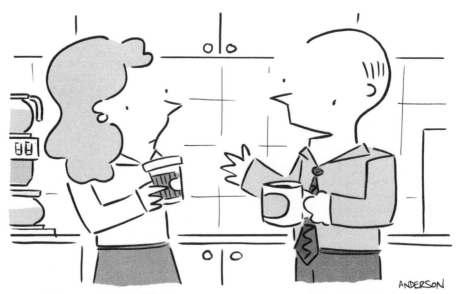

"Things have gotten a lot easier since I moved everything from my to-do list to my it-is-what-it-is list."

FIGURE 26.2 Avoidance of grief work

Source: Figure courtesy of Mark Anderson

Elucidation

When a new life experience evokes an old experience of loss (trigger effect), the accompanying coping-and support reactions are also activated. These coping-and support reactions are not adequate, as is apparent from the unaddressed past. The loss is avoided, because it was considered too painful (avoidance coping). The support was apparently not adequate either. Either support was not offered or offered badly and inappropriately.

Maintaining of complaint

Not only were the negative coping and negative support complaint-causing factors, but also became complaint-maintaining factors. The pain triggered in relation to unaddressed life experiences is maintained through the imbedded coping reaction and support reactions. If the coping and support remain negative, an increase in complaints and chronicity of complaints are to be expected. By working on positive coping and positive support, it becomes possible to fulfil the closure tasks (acceptance-cleansing-transfer). Peace and calm is created which eventually contributes to wellbeing. When inadequate coping of loss takes place, the client is unable to manage the problem situation realistically, but rather avoids this.

Internal and external coping

Negative coping can be outlined twofold: internalization (inward) and externalization (outward) (see Table 26.2). When support is inadequate, the environment does not positively support the person concerned. The individual's own coping, which was considered inadequate at the time, can also cause complaints when no support is offered from the environment. However, even the current reaction from the environment can still have a negative impact: how do parents, family, teachers, professionals react?

26.2.5 UBS type 1 (stress causing) and UBS type 2 (damage)

A distinction is made between two types of UBS: UBS type 1 involves UBS with stressful effects (without damage) and UBS type 2 involves UBS with damaging effects. They vary in degree. Type 1: the complaints are a burden to the environment and/or a burden to the individual involved. Type 2: disorders that could be considered as forms of self-harm, self-neglect reaching to suicidal tendencies and behaviour. The disorders could also lead to the damage to others, neglect of others, acting-out behaviour and aggression against other people up to (attempted) murder.

26.3 Physical disorders through old pain

Loss not dealt with, unaddressed trauma, unresolved conflict and unaddressed negative life periods: all of these situations cause long-lasting stress. What are the long-term consequences?

26.3.1 Immune weakness and chronic stress

It would appear that the long-lasting stress situation – also described as chronic stress – has a delaying impact on the physical immune system (*immune* response, a term used in the psychoneuro-immunology). The immune response weakens in people who have been dealing with unresolved issue for some time. These people appear to be more susceptible to ailments, psychosomatic symptoms and illnesses.

TABLE 26.2 Ineffective coping in UBS type 1 and UBS type 2

	UBS type 1: stressful UBS	UBS type 2: damaging UBS
Internalizing coping	• Be burden to oneself • Isolation • Self neglect	• Hard drug abuse/addiction • Auto mutilation • Self harm • Suicide fantasy, attempted suicide (AS), suicide
Externalizing coping	• Neglect of environment • Burden for environment	• Damaging for environment • Extremely threatening • Aggressive • Abusive • Killing fantasy • Manslaughter/murder

How does this happen? Research into stress discovered mechanisms that explained why chronic stress could lead to health damage. When the stress persists, or in other words becomes chronic, damage to one's health has to be taken into account.

Chronic stress occurs when:

- Unfavourable elements continue to exist within the environment, such as high workload, insecurity and substantial burden within the private situation.
- Consequences of unhealthy stress persist (months, years).
- There is a process whereby the psychological and biological disturbances culminate.

There are no adverse consequences for a person's functioning and health as long as they have the opportunity to fully recover before they start to take part in life again – regardless of the severity of a particular burden (work pressure, conflicts, fatigue) (Krahn, 1993). Studies have without exception, indicated that effective support – meaning support experienced as support by the individual concerned – has a positive impact on for example processing of loss (Silver & Wortman, 1980). It would appear that from a long study into reactions to dismissal after organizational closure, social support from partner, relatives and friends confined the pain connected to the loss (Cobb & Kasl, 1977).

26.3.2 Consequences of persisting stress

The golden rule in stress processing reads as: effort is alternated with sufficient relaxation. A persistent breach of this rule will not remain without consequence. When there is insufficient recovery time, one's functioning and health will experience damage from the persistent and unhealthy stress. A dramatic event, such as the A-bomb on Hiroshima led to the survivors suffering from deep and long-lasting emotional disorders. (Lifton, 1969).

The consequence of chronic stress is a higher risk of become ill: when someone suffers from unhealthy stress that continues to be chronic, a downward spiral will develop. That person will encounter a keepnet from which it is difficult to escape. The psycho-biological balance becomes more and more disrupted. This leads to the creation of psychological and psycho-somatic complaints and patho-physiological (illness-inducing) processes.

26.3.3 Psychological complaints

Problems in the psychological sense develop in relation to:

- Concentration: easily distracted, no energy;
- Own behaviour; over containment by pacing up and down, fiddling, fidgeting, quickly irritated, increase in smoking, drinking, eating disorders;
- Own thoughts: over containment by worrying, brooding, fretting;
- Own body: over containment resulting in headache, dizziness, stomach problems, hyperventilation, nervous tics, stutter, shaking hands, sleeping problems.

26.3.4 Physical complaints

From a physical perspective, chronic, unhealthy stress has two consequences.

- Chronic stimuli: this is apparent when the person is unable to adequately manage the cause of stress. The increase of cortisol and testosterone in the body continues to persist. There is insufficient recovery and the increased activity remains in place, because the control mechanisms responsible for de-activation are put out of action by higher mechanisms in the central nervous system. Through the continuous pressure of a particular organ, changes occur that are difficult to reverse when the pressure or threat is removed. This causes tissue damage: among other things reduced elasticity of the vessel wall and arthritis.
- Disruption of the physiological control circuits: by chronic exposure to unhealthy stress, the inset levels of the control circuits are reduced. This means that the blood pressure never or quite possibly ever returns to its original level. This leads to people in demanding and threatening situations reacting even more intensely compared to their previous reactions and experience much more difficulty recovering. This explains why the blood pressure remains at chronic and increased level, even though the actual reason is no longer present.

The chronic processes of unhealthy stress are clarified well through the use of the thermostat process in a central heating system (Gaillard, 2003). The thermostat is a sensor that sends a signal to the boiler: the temperature in the living room is lower than the minimum allowed. The boiler will burn until the desired temperature is reached in the living room. This closed control circuit is being broken when someone opens the window. The boiler continues to work 'desperately' until the desired temperature is reached. A disruption of the regulation of various unconscious physical processes, such as blood pressure and heartbeat, occurs in a similar way. When the sensor assumes a level that is too high, the control centre will do anything to try and reduce the pressure. This will happen unless our emotions or our thinking *overrule* these actions. Chronic stress leads to a reduced sensitivity of the baroreceptors in the aortic artery. Consequently, the control system continues to tune itself to different values, which leads to higher rest values (for example during sleep and at the start of a working day). This eventually leads to a chronically increased blood pressure (hypertension). A high blood pressure developed in this way is difficult to treat with medication, because the issue is actually a control problem. Administering medication could be regarded as the opening of a window to reduce the temperature in the living room. As long as the core processes concern themselves with regulation (for example someone who feels threatened), treatment will not be successful. Therefore, treatment has to focus on removing negative feelings and emotions, combined with relaxation, however also learning coping strategies to offer a solution to the problems.

26.4 UBS-treatment

26.4.1 Social workers versus specialists

In cases of type 1 UBS social workers can be effective. In cases of type 2 UBS specialists like psychologists and psychotherapists can be helpful.

In any case of UBS, there is work to be done. The actual processing can still be taken to hand in order to bring closure to the past and to learn to enjoy the present. Closure of the incomplete life experience is desired. What do we mean by closure?

> The conscious 'cleansing' of something that was incomplete in relation to a previously negative life experience, in order for this experience to exist as a memory only instead

of old pain. By having brought closure, eventually physical, emotional and social rest is established.

One or more closure tasks belonging to the life event are not adequately fulfilled when managing unfinished life experiences (see Table 26.3).

Closure is achieved when closing tasks are once again carried out and completed.

Closure suggests there is an overview of unfinished aspects of the previous life experience. Together with the client, these unfinished aspects are traced. By using the checklist in Table 26.1, it will be possible to check which life levels contain one or more unfinished aspects of previously unaddressed life experiences. Each unfinished aspect will offer an indication as to which method could be used in order to achieve closure, if so desired.

Not medicalizing but seeing the symptoms in the right UBS-context grief counsellors and grief therapists can contribute to people with UBS. UBS needs not a simple approach but a multimethod approach (see Table 26.4). A eclective approach could be less effective because with working eclected is more throwing methods in a pot, without enough logic behind it, so coherence of approach is missing.

TABLE 26.3 Closure tasks: finished and unfinished business

Closure tasks loss	Explanation of closure tasks	Examples of unaddressed
1 Awareness task (cognitive level) and reconstruct facts of life event(s) about life event	Re-acknowledging, facing up to insufficient information	Not present at final goodbye
2 Cleansing task (emotionally, practical-material, physical expressive, trauma, support level stress, re-expressing and once again seeking support, etc.)	Conscious cleaning of life event[s] by again off-loading emotional pain, re-taking practical steps, re-occupying oneself with physical	Bottling up or blocking out grief/anger/fear/ (absence of pain offload/ discharge)
3 Transfer task	The inner and external transfer from the old to the new situation by undertaking a closure ritual	Inability to say goodbye in own time and way (finishing touch was missing)

TABLE 26.4 Checklist: levels of unfinished business indicating for specific social work methods

Life levels	Possible unfinished aspects	Indicated method
Existential level	Giving insufficient consideration to meaningful questions such as: Why? Why me?	1 Non-directive core method
Cognitive level	Insufficient information about seriousness of the situation at that time and factual nature. Insufficient sensory evidence sought for serious life event (sensory and physical level)	2 Cognitive method
Emotional level	Presence of grief, anger, fear, insufficient discharge/ offloading	3 cathartic method

Life levels	Possible unfinished aspects	Indicated method
Practical-material level	Insufficient practical-material closure	4 Practical-material method
Physical level	Insufficient stress reduction	5 Bodywork method
Behavioural level	Insufficiently skilled in managing social and communication issues	6 Behavioural method
Creative level	Insufficiently expressive	7 Expression method
Trauma level	Insufficient reconstruction of experience and fact	8 Trauma care method
Parting level	Insufficient ritual goodbye	9 Ritual work method
Support level life experience	Insufficient support with	• Relationship-focused method
		• Mediation method
		• Family method
		• Social networking method
		• Group method
		• Case management method

26.5 Practical example: unaddressed loss of a parent at a young age

An example of people that run the risk of UBS is the group of adults that experienced unaddressed loss of a parent at a young age (UPY). Here, UBS will be clarified using UPY: how does one recognize the four symptoms of UBS in adults who lost one or both parents at a young age? About 10% of the adult Dutch population lost one or both parents by age 20. This means that there are 1.6 million adults who lost a parent at a young age. If 20% of those people experience issues based on UPY, this is a group of 300,000 adults. In this section, I will look at how UPY leads to many unaddressed issues, how certain sensory triggers may open up old wounds (trigger effect), and how issues may get worse (multiplier effect). Of course, there are also people who cope adequately with losing a parent at a young age.

26.5.1 UBS by UPY

As a response to UPY, a number of children respond in a depressed, fearful and aggressive way later in life (in adolescence and adulthood). Symptomatic is that they do not always connect their issues to UPY; this makes them examples of UBS. These people may experience a lot of physical, psychological or relational unrest, frequently for years, ever since the loss of their parent. Caregivers not familiar with UPY will refer to these issues as 'poorly understood': no cause is known. Caregivers who are familiar with UPY will see that these people are not at peace because they may not have been allowed to see their parents to say goodbye, were too young or have become stuck in processing the loss of the parent at a young age.

Poorly understood issues

Survey research (de Mönnink, 2006) shows that adults with unaddressed experiences of parental loss at a young age may experience issues on several levels (multilevel issues). These are the issues addressed in section 26.2: poorly understood physical psychological, relationship and family issues as well as poorly understood work-related issues.

Trigger moment

Another finding that emerged from the interviews with UPY-respondents is that people often experience a breakdown moment, a stagnation in their functioning. after functioning reasonably well for years. This stagnation may, for example, be triggered by a new loss situation, a photo or another trigger that reminds them of the loss of a parent at a young age.

At the breakdown moment, the respondent becomes aware of the cramped and constricted way in which he lived and worked. He cannot continue because the avoiding coping mechanism of the original unaddressed loss or trauma can no longer endure. This breakdown moment may, if it remains misunderstood, lead to further complications. But if the breakdown moment is seen as a part of UBS, it can become a breakthrough moment. This is the case if the appropriate therapy is offered. In that case, the UPY can still be treated therapeutically, allowing the client to let go of the existing negative patterns of behaviour.

The impact of parent loss at a young age

A combination of the great loss, the eventual issues, the trigger, avoidant grief support and negative coping with loss causes children to experience significant impediments in their quality of life, later in life. It is for good reason that one UPY-expert, Harris (1997) gave her book the title *Een verlies voor altijd* (A loss forever).

Case 26.3 The case of Maria (case study in other chapters): Poorly understood study-related problems

1: Poorly understood issues. A 19-year-old student, living by herself, harbours a poorly understood fear of failure. She is depressed, confused and unable to focus; she has a bad relationship with her mother and spells of aggression.

2: Sensory triggers. A visual trigger is that she repeatedly fails the test on dealing with loss. The book *Dealing With Loss?* opens up old wounds.

3: Incomplete life experience. She has an unaddressed experience of loss, the loss of her mother through suicide when she was 7 months old. Her father had three different partners afterwards. The student lost her father because he was absent; her older brother died due to a cocaine overdose.

4: Avoidance coping/inadequate support. The student prefers not to talk about it, has remained silent and kept it to herself (*avoidance coping*). She gets no support from home: the mother has passed away, the father is absent figuratively, stepmothers are not supportive (*avoidance support*). She is, however, becoming optimistic and, after a lot of caregiver support, is very motivated to work on it (*positive coping*); her boyfriend is very supportive (*positive support*).

Type UBS: this is a Type 1 UBS: emptiness, self-neglect, tendency to live 'all out', lots of stress, no damage. The therapist elects to proceed with the UBS-combination approach:

- Tackling the actual issues through the cognitive method and activation through fitness; this provides calmness but the other issues remain;
- Dealing with old wounds by bringing the incomplete loss experiences to a close, this being the main theme of the treatment.

Th: 'Is has become clear that present issues did not improve by the way in which they were being handled. The *Coping With Loss?* test may be a trigger for something else; let's first do a reconstruction of the test experience: What causes you to experience fear of failure, depression, confusion and lack of focus; what causes you to repeatedly not pass the test?'

Cl: 'The issues began when I started reading the book *Grief Counseling*; a lot surfaced there. I couldn't concentrate. I have never made the link between my issues and my unhappy childhood, but my mother committed suicide when I was 7 months old; after that I had three stepfathers who all thought their own kids were more important. As a girl I became more and more aggressive; I was taken to the police station more than once. My brother started doing soft and hard drugs which eventually killed him. I had many relationship problems and friendships never seemed to last very long, but now I finally have a boyfriend and we've been together for 6 months. In actual fact, I lost both my mother and my father'.

Th: 'I suggest bringing your incomplete experience of loss to a close nonetheless. Back to then, changing between dealing with losing your mother through a creative approach utilizing drawing and drama (on a children's level). We will bring up and go through the loss of your mother and the emotions attached to that. And then we will say goodbye in a farewell ceremony'.

Cl: 'I went to her grave yesterday. I lay down on her grave and smoked a joint. I felt like I got in touch with her. I managed to say goodbye: "Too bad you were in so much trouble, that you didn't see how much I needed you, but I see now that there was no other way."'

Th: 'Is it okay like this?'

Cl: 'Yeah'.

Th: 'Same approach for your father. Would you like to have a three-way conversation with your father present?'

Cl: 'I'd appreciate that, talk things out. And so on and so forth'.

Th: (at the end of the three-way conversation): 'How are things now?'

Cl: 'I feel like I got a bit of both of my parents back and that I can bring the unfinished period to a close.'

During the treatment, the level of tension went from 6 to 2; Maria passed the social work test in grief support with a B.

The impact of losing a parent at a young age is extensive. Even though an inheritance is usually something positive, it can be very negative in UPY. Losing a parent when parents are still necessary, leaves an inheritance of sadness, anger and emptiness in UPY; this is an undesired inheritance, but an inheritance nonetheless. This inheritance can become an impediment throughout someone's life. When growing up, the proverbial 'young flower' requires the strength of the roots of the parents. If one or both roots are severed through death, divorce, loss, a term in prison or a psychiatric disorder, this causes a deep life crisis for the child. Positive grief support from the remaining parent, family or friend is essential for good coping with loss. Is the child involved in the funeral? Is the child's developmental stage taken into consideration? If the child experiences closeness and support, it can say its goodbyes in a dignified way (positive coping with loss) and bring this life chapter to a close.

26.5.2 Avoidant grief support

Grief support and coping with loss may fall short for different reasons. Harris (1997) lists four negative support patterns of remaining parents that are counterproductive in children dealing with loss. This is a case of avoidant grief support:

- The broken-down parent;
- The absent parent;
- The violent parent;
- The parent looking for love and friendship in the child.

Children that had to make do with this kind of avoidant grief support have very painful memories of the remaining parent, who failed in their parental role. Some remember that the remaining parent was completely worn out by their own emotional response to the loss. These children remember the parent as depressed (the broken down parent), not capable of action (the absent parent) or angry (the violent parent).

The remaining parent

The broken down parent does not give at home, because the disbelief is so predominant that a child becomes scared and insecure. Due to mourning the partner, the remaining parent has no energy to give guidance and support to the family.

The absent parent gives no support, because he is – literally or figuratively – not there. Sometimes, children are sent to stay with family temporarily. Many children experience disinterest and neglect when the remaining parent remarries and chooses for a new life and the new family. The remaining parent is thus emotionally unavailable to the children,

The violent parent may change into a tyrant or torturous parent instead of being supportive, because of the stress of the loss.

The parent that is looking for love and friendship in the child, causes the child to no longer be able to be a child but a peer and partner. Through subtle, implicit demands, the child's status becomes that of an adult. The child may be thrust into one of two role patterns: that of the friend and that of the surrogate partner. The friendship is obviously a pseudo-friendship. With children older than 10, a pseudo-marriage may arise, where the child assumes the responsibilities of the man or woman of the house to the detriment of his or her own development.

Friends and family

If the grief support by the remaining partner is insufficient, or if both parents were lost, support from outside the family may be a solution. Mourning families may also form closed systems: family and friends do not know how to deal with the pain of the death and the emptiness of loss. They frequently do not show up; sometimes out of respect, but mostly because they feel uneasy. As such, the child does not receive support other than from the remaining parent. This does not amount to a lot of positive grief support and may cause the coping and dealing with loss to be blocked even more.

26.5.3 Avoidant coping with loss

Because of the desperation of losing a parent at a young age, children are faced with the task of making life bearable. Coping with loss may develop negatively: initially, the child will deal with the given life situation adequately. Just like adults, children do look for solutions in any given problem situation.

Case 26.4 The case of Mr. Ojo: an employee with poorly understood chronic pain issues

1: *Poorly understood issues*. Mr. Ojo, age 49 years, reports poorly understood chronic pain issues. In loss situation of close family members, he feels nothing; he finds this odd.

2: *Triggers*. One visual trigger is that when attending a workshop on 'parental loss at a young age', Mr. Ojo sees others crying while he himself experiences pain issues. In traffic, he is easily incensed and sometimes angry at others for displaying high risk behaviour in traffic.

3: *Incomplete life experience*. The client lost both parents in a car crash at the age of 16.

4: *Negative coping/negative support*. The client does not feel, is a workaholic, standing beside himself. His parents are gone, he gets no support from his environment and has been through medical care, has received caregiver support and alternative medical care for years (*negative support*). His partner supports him through thick and thin (*positive support*).

Type UBS: UBS type 1: chronic pain immobilizing the client.
   UBS-combination approach:

- Dealing with present issues via the cognitive approach and physical awareness through fitness training, increased self-awareness but other issues remained;
- Dealing with old wounds by completing incomplete loss experiences, general theme of the treatment.

   Th:'It has become clear that your present issues did not improve by addressing them. Pain issues may represent something else; let's do a reconstruction of the pain issues; when and since when do you experience pain issues?'

Cl: 'The issues became stronger when I participated in a "parental loss at a young age" workshop; everyone is emotional, I felt nothing at the time, but I later experienced pain in my limbs; I recall experiencing this since high school; prior to the accident I had no pain issues. I played high level volleyball, but since I lost my parents in a car crash at the age of 16, I quit sports. I never talked about the loss or the accident, my parents were not there and support from others was not available.'

Th: 'Parental loss at a young age workshop is apparently a trigger for the pain surrounding the double parent loss.'

Cl: 'Does nothing to me anymore. . . .'

Th: 'Pain issues may be conversion of emotional pain into physical pain. Proposal: shall we look into how the pain issues developed in the first place?'

Cl: 'First a lot of headaches; muscle soreness that I attributed to quitting sports; after that more and more pain in my limbs and joints; consulted loads of medical specialists, psychologists, alternative healers; no improvement.'

Th: 'Proposal: continue focusing on physical pain and let's see how you deal with it: what do you do when you're in pain, what do you feel, etc.?'

Cl: 'Afraid of being touched, because that causes more pain; I won't let my wife touch me.'

Th: 'Proposal: see what touching does to you?'

Cl: 'Scares me.'

Th: 'Explore fear further; maybe hold hands when you feel fear?'

Cl: 'That really scares me. . . .'

Th: 'Further exploration of fear and let fear catharsis happen; maybe other emotions will surface after that. . . .'

Cl: 'OK, but steady on please.'

Th: 'Holding hands provides security and closeness. . . .'

Cl: 'A lot is happening (trembles with fear, crying . . .) I feel so abandoned, but it's not their fault.'

Th: 'Proposal to finally bring the incomplete experience of loss to an end. Did you manage to say your goodbyes?'

Cl: 'No, didn't say goodbye at all.'

Th: 'How might you still accomplish this?' (Think about it and write down in detail.)

Cl: (after some thought): 'Go to the place of the accident and say something that symbolizes a farewell and what it has done to me. Perform a farewell ritual to say goodbye to my mother and father.' (Ritual performed with partner present.)

Th: 'Is it okay like this?'

Cl: 'Yes.'

Pain issue level down from 6 to 2; anger in traffic reduced from 7 to 3.

Myths

Children with UPY apparently select magical solutions that provide support in youth, but become an impediment later in life: turning into negative coping. By selecting magical solutions, children create order in chaos; the alternative is living in constant despair. This survival coping with loss of children, according to Harris (1997) is composed of several magical solutions, sometimes called myths, that relate to several components of the life of the child which lost its parent(s), for example:

- Myths about the lost parent;
- Myths about itself;
- Myths about the bond that could have existed;
- Personal myths about all kinds of things.

The lost parent may be idealized as the fantastic parent, generous, funny, sensitive and unique, fixed in time. This myth about the lost parent may be responsible for many disappointments in later life. This happens when a child, as an adult, starts looking for friends and partners that live up to that same ideal. The child may also build up a collection of misconceptions about itself: fantasies about who the child actually is, usually connected to a certain idea of misfortune responsible for the death of the parent, and fantasies about who the child might have grown up to be had it not lost its parent. Children may develop the idea that they were bad and therefore abandoned. In most children, the imagined bond with the lost parent stems from its own feeling of loss and desire for something that could have been. Sometimes, the myth is fed by family members. The myth may also take a negative form: he never loved me anyway, so there is no need to mourn. The last type of myth that children with UPY may develop are personal myths based on the remnants of their despair to create order in the world. Frequently, these personal myths form the basis for a feeling of personal identity and of connectedness with others. There are personal myths, such as: 'I am always perfect' or 'I take care of the remaining parent,' 'Always be pleasant and never show your dark side' in order to find favour with others. The life motto may also become: 'Always be prepared' or 'Never be prepared for anything' or 'Never get upset.' But also myths like 'Never be too happy' or 'Lightning never strikes the same place twice' may provide some security. It is not strange that children construct illogical explanation systems, but it is remarkable that people who lost parents at a young age often stick to these views.

UPY may cause all manner of poorly understood issues, such as in the case of the man who lost both parents in a car crash and developed chronic pain issues as a result. The UPY-approach – just like UBS in general – consists of client directed multimethodical grief support in three steps as described in Chapter 1: PFC–PSA–PSI. By creating a personal filing cabinet (PFC) it becomes clear that there are at least two drawers in that cabinet that require attention: the present pain and the unfinished business. Subsequently, the psychosocial assessment (PSA) shows how the impact of the loss is, how someone is coping with the loss and the amount of support surrounding the loss (the grief support) is dealt with. When the pluses and minuses in the client situation have become clear, psycho social stress interventions (PSI) are utilized to strengthen the pluses and reduce the minuses. Finally, by bringing the incomplete life experiences to a close and calming the present issues, peace can emerge in the client situation. The difference in approach of present unaddressed loss and the approach of UBS, is that in UBS a combined approach is required to address not only the present sources of tension but also any previous incomplete experiences.

26.6 Summary and questions

There is a natural tendency to finish 'unfinished business'. When people are not given the opportunity to do so, or deal with the matter in a wrong way, all kinds of poorly understood issues may result. The four characteristics of UBS were described, as well as which two types of UBS occur. Subsequently, UBS was explained using the group of adults with unaddressed loss of parents at a young age. Finally, it was detailed where 'incomplete life experiences' stand in the literature. In the following chapters, it will be detailed what is understood as grief support.

Questions

1   What is the importance of renewed attention to old wounds?
2   What signals are there for the possible presence of UBS?
3   What is the importance of making a timeline?
4   What are the four characteristics of UBS?
5   What is type 1 UBS and what is type 2 UBS?
6   Which three tasks are there for finalizing UB?
7   What characteristics of UBS are pertinent in unaddressed parental loss at a young age?

27

JOB STRESS AMONG SOCIAL WORKERS

The stress matrix

Questions

This chapter addresses the following questions:

- How can emotional situations lead to exhaustion (burnout)?
- How can emotional situations lead to psychological traumas, such as PTSD?
- What signs, behaviours and risk factors are involved in burnout syndrome and PTSD?
- How to deal with burnout and PTSD and how can they be prevented?
- What is the role of coping styles?
- What is the role of support from the home and work situation?

27.1 Introduction

It seems odd, but it is day-to-day practice of social workers in the Neurology Department. A stroke, Parkinson's disease, a brain tumour or aneurism has far-reaching consequences for both patient and family. As a consequence, social workers may feel the extra pressure and at times, be overwhelmed by these experiences. At the same time, the job can be enormously fulfilling.

(Social Worker University Hospital Utrecht, De Volkskrant, 23 March 1993)

It's not always easy to be exposed to other peoples' suffering. Even though social workers are selected on the basis of their resilience and ability to manage stress, it doesn't mean they have to be able to cope with every situation.

This chapter explores work-related stress that is caused by emotional situations. The first question is to find out how chronic work-related stress can lead to burnout syndrome, a state of total exhaustion. The signs are described that point to burnout, the burnout syndrome is explained as well as the risk factors for developing burnout. Next, it is discussed how emotional job stress can develop into post-traumatic stress disorder (PTSD). In addition, a number of stress reduction methods are discussed, including coping styles, the importance of physical and emotional release and of realistic thinking. Attention is also given to the support-ive role of the work and home situation. In conclusion, recommendations are given for organ-izing educational training courses in the area of grief counselling and traumatic job stress.

Stress is a complex phenomenon. The concept of 'stress' is sometimes used to describe a source of tension and sometimes even to indicate the consequences of that tension. Modern theories define stress as the tension that arises from the interaction between individuals and their environment (see Figure 27.1). Some of the theories on stress have been discussed in

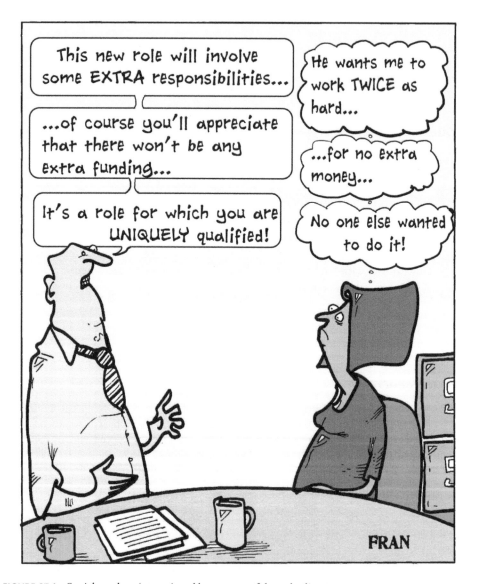

FIGURE 27.1   Social workers 'sometimes' have a stressful work climate ......

Source: Image courtesy of Fran Orford

Chapter 5. In the stress matrix the theories of job stress and job support are summarized (see Table 27.1).

Job stress is increasingly the cause of sickness absence. It costs a great deal of money and in the worst case it can lead to what the Japanese call 'karoshi' or 'occupational sudden death'. According to the UN International Labour Organization, ILO, stress is the number one illness of the century (DPA, 1993). Much has been written about stress and policy makers are becoming more and more concerned about the number of employees that report sick for psychological reasons. Emotional job stress is linked with other factors concerning work-related stress, such as, a heavy workload, tensions in the workplace and personal circumstances. Emotional job stress can be defined as the tension that arises from being professionally exposed to certain situations, possibly leading to burnout or psychological trauma. Two types of emotional job stress can be distinguished, exhausting stress and traumatic stress (see Table 27.2).

27.1.1 Exhausting job stress

Health care professionals may find it emotionally upsetting to be confronted with human suffering. Other people's suffering may elicit feelings of sadness, fear and anger. These emotions may lead to exhaustion and psychological traumas, exhausting and traumatizing job stress. Exhausting job stress is a state of exhaustion that follows prolonged occupational exposure to emotional situations.

TABLE 27.1 Types of emotional job stress

Type	Description	Example
Exhausting job stress	Prolonged exposure to suffering in the workplace	Many deaths, relapse in healing process, powerlessness
Traumatic job stress	Acute exposure to abnormal situations deviating from normal work practice	Physical/psychological threat, injury, suicide, murder, loss of blood

TABLE 27.2 The stress matrix: job stress levels, support needed, risks in social work

Work stress level in social work (combined with personal stress)	Needed form of support	Risk with insufficient support
7–10 (extreme stress)	Direct support is needed by trained colleagues (UST) - Stress debriefing team - Possibly therapy	Traumatic work stress - Damaging sensory inburned experiences - PTSD risk
5–7 (high stress) 3–5 (medium stress)	Stress management by direct colleagues -Support during daytime -Structural support on a regular base	Exhaustive work stress - Stack stress (last drip effect) - Exhaustion risk - Burnout risk
0–3 (low stress)	No special support needed	No risks (sometimes professionals can suffer from under stress)

UST = unit support team; PTSD = post-traumatic stress disorder

If you, as a social worker, are continually exposed to distressing experiences and fail to get it out of your system, you will eventually become exhausted:

> Looking back, I realize that my sickness didn't come out of the blue. For years I had been submerged by other people's losses and traumas. At a certain point I felt I was low on energy. Even though I was feeling considerably tired, I was still able to help people cope with their distressing situations and move on afterwards. Over the years I found myself becoming more and more exhausted.

In section 27.2 we elucidate the burnout syndrome.

27.1.2 Traumatic job stress

Job stress can become traumatic when it involves acute exposure to traumatic experiences. Traumatic work stress is defined as the tension that arises from sudden exposure to shocking events, which are violent by nature, such as physical and psychological violence, suicide or traffic violence. Exhausting and traumatic work stress also occurs in combination. Highly stressed professionals may feel overwhelmed when being exposed to a traumatic event, such as seeing the mutilated bodily remains of a young person after throwing himself under a train. Confrontations in situations like this may profoundly impact social workers and leave them in a state of shock. Also, the threat or actual confrontation with physical violence or gun violence can make a deep impression.

Whether or not job stress is going to develop into exhaustion or trauma can't be predicted. Anyone can become exhausted or develop psychological trauma. It's not a trait that belongs to 'vulnerable employees', who have themselves to blame. However, much can be done to reduce the chance of developing exhaustion or psychological trauma.

Preventive action can be taken by developing healthy coping styles and offering active and timely social support from inside the organization. In addition, both employees and companies or services should be proactive and attentive to identifying the risk factors for burnout and psychological trauma.

In section 27.3.1 we elucidate PTSD.

27.2 Exhausting job stress: burnout syndrome

Higher rates of work incapacity indicate that increasingly more health care professionals are facing emotional problems at work and are subsequently becoming stressed and burned out. The estimated number of nursing staff, teachers, social workers and psychotherapists suffering from burnout syndrome vary between 10% and 25% (Tinnemans, 1993).

The last few decades have seen a shift from physical to mental workload and there is no sign that this epidemic of psychological work incapacity is coming to an end. Burnout is especially prevalent among workers who work intensively with others for long stretches of time. The symptoms – which are later discussed in more detail – include feeling emotionally exhausted, reduced sense of involvement and poor performance (Baart, 1995).

Health care and rescue workers regularly face situations involving human suffering. It appears that an increasing number of them are sooner or later paying the price for providing acute and intensive care. You, as a care worker, are concerned for your clients or patients, you feel for them, you are affected by the disappointments and traumas they are experiencing. A policeman put it like this:

> When I was leaving the scene of the incident, I really started feeling the emotions of the parents of the child that had just died. That's when it hit me.

A nurse described the frustration in the workplace as follows:

> You expect to able to do much more, but your contribution is often marginal. It has made me feel somewhat disillusioned and at the same time it has kept me grounded.

Burnout can be summed up as:

> an upset balance between psychological strain and psychological coping ability result- ing from changes in the individual coping ability and/or psychological burden. Consequently, the affected individual develops a reduced ability to function socially, accompanied by physical complaints, mood and/or behavioural problems.

> *(Schröer, 1991)*

In the care profession, burnout can be defined as the loss of feeling involved with the people you work for. A clinical burnout is characterized by three groups of symptoms:

* Prolonged fatigue (physical or mental);
* Cynicism (the care profession no longer genuinely cares for people);
* Reduced competence (lack of concentration, making more mistakes).

27.2.1 Signs of burnout

Signs that may point to burnout are identified in psychological, behavioural and physiological areas, including fatigue, irritability, headaches, insomnia, reduced concentration, anxiety, light-headedness and diminished sense of wellbeing (see Appendix 3).

27.2.2 The burnout syndrome

When the relationship between coping ability and burden becomes too distorted, workers reach the point where they can no longer function and then call in sick to work. There's no longer a balance between workload and a person's coping ability. The relationship between burden and coping ability, the stress quotient, indicates an individual's state of actual pressure and coping ability (see Table 27.3).

TABLE 27.3 Forms of stress: under stress, positive stress, overstress

	Under stress	No stress	Positive stress	Over stress
Burden: Coping ability	4:5	5:5	6:5	10:5

Over-burdening and under-burdening are both causes of stress. Although, to a certain extent, stress can also be stimulating and challenging. If the relationship between burden and coping ability is 6 to 5, an individual may still experience positive stress. If the relationship is expressed as 8 to 5, the person is overloaded and experiencing negative stress. If a person's coping ability in relation to the pressure is 5 to 10, this indicates a state of acute overload and high risk of PTSD.

On our way to a condition of burn out we can recognize different phases (see Table 27.4).

In the care profession a number of changes in workers' attitude may point to burnout. Care professionals may develop a tendency to treat clients in a non-involved, mechanical way. You become cynical and rigid, which is referred to as psychological containment. It's as if you are building a wall around you to protect you from experiencing the work pressure. Your dissatisfaction with your own situation, the loss of idealism and involvement elicit feelings of guilt may lead you to take it out on the people around you. There are several questionnaires that can be utilized as a measure and an indication of the level of burnout (see internet: Maslach burnout inventory test online).

27.2.3 Risk factors

The following 12 factors increase the risk of burnout (see Table 27.5).

TABLE 27.4 Phases in developing burnout

Phase	Description
Alarm	You become more easily annoyed, get tired sooner, and have more doubts about decisions than before.
Feverish activity level	You are extremely active, the sky is the limit and you work with unbridled energy, especially when dealing with minor issues.
Depression and apathy	You show complaining behaviour, are often detached and complacent, and very much in doubt of your own abilities.
Total burnout	Mentally and physically totally exhausted, vitally exhausted, and presenting a range of complaints in physical, psychological and behavioural areas.

TABLE 27.5 Risk factors for burnout

External factors	Personal factors
1 Undervaluation of achievements	8 Perceiving failure as personal failure
2 Workload too high/low	9 Not recognizing signs of burnout
3 Not recognizing signs of burnout	10 Unrealistic expectations
4 Stress provoking role structure	11 Change of job
5 Lack of autonomy	12 Lack of knowledge/skills
6 Stressful work climate	
7 Lack of growth opportunities	

External factors

Undervaluation

The nature of the caring professions and rescue jobs, such as nursing staff, doctors, social workers, police officers and firefighters, involves an increased risk of burnout. These professions involve support seekers and support givers who are emotionally involved with the former (Tinnemans, 1993). The support giver's own person is the main instrument. Without this strong engagement the job can't be done. However, at the same time, this engagement poses a risk to the care worker. In the longer run, an individual's emotional investment may exceed what is given in return.

Doctors, nurses and prison guards, whose balance between investment and proceeds is upset, are more likely to develop burnout. When employees' commitment is not acknowledged or insufficiently acknowledged, they feel underappreciated. In the nursing profession, emotional engagement is not always appreciated by senior staff, depending on the unit concerned. Senior staff on nursing wards and intensive care units appeared to vary greatly in their valuation of nurses' emotional engagement with their patients. Nursing staff on units who reported feeling emotionally engaged with their patients, received more positive evaluations from their head than colleagues who found that they were not being that involved.

The opposite relationship was found for nurses working in operating theatres and on intensive care units. Nurses who reported not being emotionally engaged with their patients scored higher on their evaluation reports than those who did report being emotionally engaged. (Roelens, 1983)

Workload

Many care professionals face a heavy load. They attend to many people at same time and are regularly exposed to human suffering, sorrow, despair, aggression and violence. Care workers who often face difficult, emotional situations are more at risk of developing burnout than colleagues who deal with relatively less emotional cases.

Youth care workers working with problem families show the highest burnout ratings. The phenomenon of burnout in psychotherapists can be linked to the emergence of Rogerian therapy. Since the 1960s the client has played a key role in the support delivery. Care workers have become clients' counsellor and are expected to be understanding and supportive. Subsequently, care professionals have not learned how to deal with their feelings resulting from intensive client contact. A low or strongly variable workload can also be included as a risk factor.

External parties' failure to recognize signs

Care professionals deserve to have colleagues and managers who identify their signs. An important aspect is how close managers are to employees. Due to organizational changes many managers hardly know their employees, making them inattentive to their employees' signs. Care professionals' feelings are insufficiently acknowledged by their colleagues and staff managers. Colleagues tend to neglect their own needs and focus only on those of their clients. As a result, employees' first signs of burnout often go unrecognized or are not taken seriously, increasing the risk of developing burnout. An individual's stress level is raised if one or more principals are giving contradictory assignments. The situation becomes even worse if there is a lack of sufficient information concerning the tasks that need to be performed.

Lack of autonomy

The lack of autonomy that is created within the organization creates a sense of helplessness and powerlessness in the individual employee. Lack of control over what is going on appears to be an important stress factor. When humans and animals become repeatedly exposed to stressful situations beyond their control, this results in learned helplessness and depression (Seligman, 1975a, 1975b). Being exposed to uncontrollable events leads to demotivation and mental deterioration. Care professionals who have limited autonomy, may end up feeling numb and detached. It emerges from a Swedish study – quoted in the ILO study on work stress (DPA, 1993) – that employees suffer less from depression and heart disease, when their job involves bearing responsibility and having a say in the decision-making process. They show half the sickness rate of other groups of employees.

Stressful work climate

An unhealthy work climate produces increased stress levels (see Figure 27.2). Poor relationships between colleagues and inadequate staff management lead to vicious circles of escalating differences of opinions, feelings of resignation and poor job performance.

Burnout in care professionals not only impacts the workers, the quality of care is also affected. This occurred at a psychiatric hospital where staff members were experiencing less job satisfaction and were gradually becoming burned out. At the same time, patients relapsed into previous stages of treatment, were demonstrating more acting-out behaviour and the number of suicide attempts increased. (Roelens, 1991). Sometimes less involvement can be a way for people to protect themselves. Particularly when it concerns a group of staff members suffering from burnout, a kind of burnout subculture emerges, which may further impact the quality of work. 'Our talking like this is bringing us all down' or 'I'm doing what being asked, nothing more.' Workers can find it hard to concentrate:

> I used to be an emotional sponge that could suck up everything; at a certain point the sponge becomes saturated, it can't take up much more.

A work climate where commitment is taken for granted, may increase workers' stress. If an employee gets feedback exclusively on things that go wrong, this can have a demotivating effect. Support, on the other hand, should be provided in a climate with an emphasis on positive reinforcement, as in performance management. Learning from mistakes is valued instead of focusing only on the mistakes themselves. Management is about setting clear objectives and giving compliments when certain goals have been reached (Vonk, 1995).

Lack of growth opportunities

Lack of variation in work tasks, lack of clarity concerning employees' job effectiveness and insufficient feedback on persons' functioning, may, at a certain point, cause workers to fall into a work routine, leaving them dissatisfied with their job. Setting up a mobility plan, laying down employees' internal and external mobility opportunities are less of a concern for the employees.

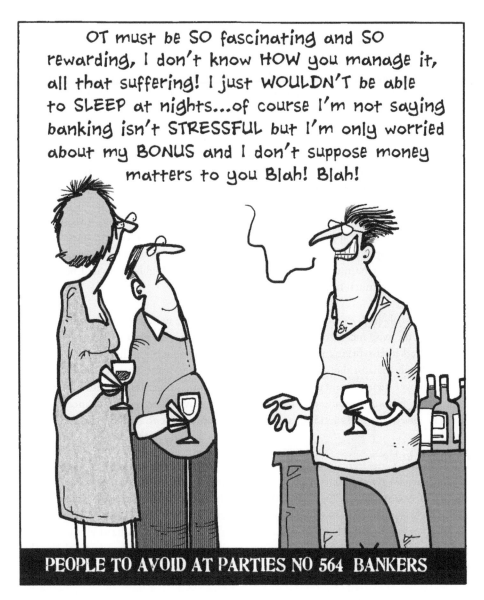

FIGURE 27.2 Social work must be so fascinating

Source: Image courtesy of Fran Orford

Personal factors

Failures

Care professionals are in a caring relationship with their clients. As a consequence, failures in the professional support delivery may also be perceived as personal failures. This can make them feel inadequate as a person. The high prevalence of burnout in care professionals has everything to do with the entangled relationship between worker and person.

Not recognizing the signs

Care professionals' feelings are insufficiently acknowledged, not only by colleagues, but also by the professionals themselves. Because of the nature of the care profession, workers tend to sacrifice themselves. The client-centred orientation distracts attention away from care workers' personal responses. As a result, the first signs of burnout are not recognized, let alone taken seriously.

Unrealistic expectations

Another risk factor for developing burnout is cherishing unrealistic expectations. If workers' job expectations are too low or too high, it increases the risk of burnout. An employee used these words to describe his experience:

> I was promoted after organizational restructuring and my job was to manage company business. As newly appointed supervisor I soon found that a lot of things that weren't working properly, which was rather upsetting. My expectations had been too high and could not be met by the organization. I became highly frustrated because I had expected too much from the organization.

Care professionals' high expectations play an important role in developing burnout. Unrealistic, high or otherwise incorrect expectations don't come true in practice. Particularly strongly motivated and hard-working people who are prepared to sacrifice themselves are at risk of burnout. People exhaust themselves by reacting wrongly to stress. They feel that they are losing control over their job and that their objectives can no longer be realized. If they keep on pushing, they become exhausted. If they become defensive, there is equal chance of burnout. This only adds to the stress and they will more and more come to dislike their clients and job.

Transitions in life

Burnout particularly manifests itself at the start and middle phase of a person's career. The majority of victims are aged between 30 and 40, although the syndrome may also occur later in life. The higher the level of education, the higher the burnout rate. Singles are more at risk than married employees. Male victims more often develop depersonalization, they behave in an impersonal way, are aloof and indifferent towards their clients and consider them objects instead of persons. Women are more often emotionally exhausted.

Lack of knowledge and skills

A lack of up-to-date knowledge and skills leads to ineffectiveness and has a negative impact on a person's self-esteem. The percentage of mistakes increases as well as the tendency to conceal them. Adequate training policies are geared towards training employees to update their knowledge and skills.

27.3 Post-traumatic job stress

Major life events, such as robbery, murder, suicide, physical threat, care accident or fire may cause a high sense of powerlessness and disruption in the persons involved. The Dutch Labour Organization (Arbowet) obliges organizations to conduct policies concerning aggression and violence towards employees. For that reason, as of 1991, coaching teams have been set up for police officers, fire fighters, army personnel, and also for nursing staff, bus drivers and ambulance workers. These workers' prolonged exposure to powerlessness and violence (in the sense of criminal violence, natural disaster, physical and sexual violence) convinced organizational management that they needed to take responsibility for their employees.

Around 1900, psychiatrists Janet and Freud were the first to write about psychological traumas. The numerous wars that were fought during the century that followed generated much human suffering for psychologists and psychiatrists to deal with. World Wars I and II, the Vietnam War, the Falklands War, the Gulf War and the Balkan Conflict led to extensive documentation on human reactions to distressing events. A large number of veterans from World Wars I and II had to be hospitalized on account of severe psychiatric symptoms. In the Vietnam War, with a death toll of 53,000 American soldiers, the shocking fact is that as many as 120,000 veterans committed suicide in the years that followed.

Since the 1990s, increasing attention has been given to psychological trauma, considering the vast body of articles, programmes and books. After 1994, the following reports were published, not long after each other: *Niemand is van steen* (*Nobody Is Made of Stone*) (distressing experiences in the fire department), *Ingrijpende gebeurtenissen in politiewerk* (*Distressing Events in Police Work*), *Traumatische ervaringen van verpleegkundigen* (*Traumatic Experiences by Nursing Staff*), and *Omgaan met schokkende gebeurtenissen, onderzoek naar de behoefte aan traumapreventie en behandeling onder ambulancehulpverleners in Nederland* (*Dealing With Shocking Events, Study on the Need for Trauma Prevention and Treatment of Ambulance Workers in the Netherlands*).

Specific treatment methods for psychological trauma are gradually being developed. We are also seeing an increasing number of scientific studies on psychological traumas in the police force and fire department. Police officers deal with 42 types of incidents that may potentially produce a traumatic effect (Carter & McGoldrick, 1989a). These incidents can be grouped into two categories, as being either very violent or very depressing incidents.

27.3.1 Post-traumatic stress disorder

The three categories of signs in trauma processing have been discussed in Chapter 7 (see Table 7.1). As it is very important to recognize the signs of distress in occupational practice, they are now mentioned as well: re-experiencing, avoidance and hypervigilance (see section 7.2.3). Feelings of shock are normal reactions to abnormal situations. After a distressing event – involving traumatic loss – a post-traumatic stress response (PTSR) may occur. The psychiatric classification system DSM distinguishes 17 symptoms of PTSR (see Table 7.2).

Shortly after the event these responses are considered normal reactions to abnormal events. After a period of time – some say 3 months, others 6 months or longer – persistence of six of the symptoms across the three categories indicate that the individual has developed PTSD. We speak of fully developed PTSD if symptoms occur in a certain combination of the three categories:

*   Re-experiencing: minimally one symptom;
*   Avoidance: minimally three symptoms;
*   Hypervigilance: minimally two symptoms.

If symptoms do occur, but not in the above combination, we speak of partial PTSD. If a distressing incident involving powerlessness and disruption, results in persistent symptoms over

TABLE 27.6 Risk factors for PTSD

External factors	Personal factors
1 Type of incident; emotional exhaustion, severity of latest trauma, severity of previous traumas	8 Social introversion (bottling up)
	9 Finding it hard to express feelings
	10 No hobbies
2 Lack of time to process grief	11 Sleeping problems
3 Dissatisfaction with support	12 Concentration problems
4 Dissatisfaction with job	13 Feelings of guilt
5 Worrying about job	14 Intense sadness when remembering trauma
6 Discussing trauma with parents	15 Being emotionally unstable, plus introversion
7 Lack of collegiality	16 Masculinity

a longer period of time, we speak of complicated grief, which can be successfully treated (see Chapter 25 on grief counselling).

It's a well-known fact that the pressure can't be on all the time. Chronic overburdening is a risk factor. If personal and work situations change dramatically, as in the case of restructuring and employees are becoming increasingly dissatisfied, these factors may contribute to an increased risk of PTSD. Another contributing factor to PTSD is poor communication between colleagues. For instance, there is a lot of complaining but nothing is done, criticism is given in an indirect or tactless way or inappropriate joking by those who weren't present at the scene. Last but not least, the nature of the incident experienced may increase the risk of burnout.

Psychologically speaking, a number of personal risk factors include unrealistic work attitude, bottling things up, no hobbies, sleeping problems, concentration problems, feelings of guilt, intense sadness when remembering the trauma, being emotionally unstable and showing masculinity.

An inventory of the risk factors is used to assess whether or not professional help should be recommended (see Table 27.6).

27.4 Stress reduction methods

What can you do to prevent problems in emotional work stress? Each stress-provoking situation has a build-up period (preparation) and needs a phasing-out period (technical and human evaluation). Whether it concerns minor or significant events, you need to be prepared and given the opportunity to phase-out, so you can be actively and consciously aware of what has happened and be able to let things go that have taken up your attention. In practice, workers have developed a range of coping styles before, during and after a difficult situation. Insight into one's individual coping style forms the basis for managing distressing situations with awareness. Three types of coping styles are now further explained, notably, physical release, emotional release and realistic thinking.

27.4.1 Physical release

An old saying is 'a healthy mind in a healthy body.' Work-related stress also builds up in the body. Active physical exercise is the way to release physical tension. How great it can be to start exercising with 'a heavy head' and to return feeling energized afterwards. Relaxation exercises may also be helpful to reduce the stress in body and mind.

27.4.2 Emotional relief

Feeling emotionally upset calls for pain release. When you are experiencing emotional and physical pain, it may help to scream, burst into tears, tremble, laugh or yawn. Releasing your emotions in such ways can only be realized in a work climate where people are allowed to be vulnerable. Your environment has to be sensitive to what you are going through and to how it has affected you.

27.4.3 Realistic thinking

It's a good thing to have a realistic view of your own situation. Undervaluation and overvaluation contribute to increased stress. Therefore, you need to identify your unrealistic thoughts:

* People in my environment that are important to me have to appreciate me and love me.
* I have to be perfect in every way, successful and competent to think myself worthwhile.
* I'm not allowed to make mistakes.
* It's terrible when things in my life are not going according to plan.
* I can't influence my negative feelings and my behaviour, they are determined by external factors.
* My personality and character have been totally shaped by my past.
* I should feel guilty when I do things my way and therefore disappoint others.

Employees become frustrated if their expectations are too high. The level they expect can never be reached. Lowering these expectations – the desired goal isn't realistic yet – enables workers to work towards higher job performance. When you find yourself in a difficult situation – failed or distressing action – and tell yourself to look at things realistically – you have a better chance of putting the incident behind you. When it involves positive experiences the realistic thing to do is to reward yourself by for instance, saying to yourself 'I handled things well.' In the occurrence of negative experiences you should avoid talking to yourself in a punishing way: 'I'm not reprimanding myself for what has happened.'

27.5 Support from work and home

Employees can derive support from both colleagues and from the home situation. A well-functioning system of staff support is highly important in care and rescue work. Employees that are well taken care of by their organization are in a good condition and prepared to help others. A Dutch doctor, working in a Cambodian hospital, failed to understand why local doctors and nurses left parents to themselves when their child had died. Then she noticed that practically all workers were still dealing with so much grief themselves – resulting from the Pol Pot massacre among the Cambodian population – that they froze when facing other people's suffering. According to the Dutch doctor:

'When I comfort nurses and doctors, they can, in turn, comfort others'.

The important thing is that support is given freely, not imposed. Therefore, the motto for freely given support is 'watchful waiting'. It may be obvious that the person involved is emotionally affected. No one likes being talked into problems. Your starting point is the other person's resilience. A feature of watchful waiting is regularly checking the individual's situation. Nowadays, the usual practice for professions with high PTSD prevalence among workers is to offer staff support. We prefer the term 'business support' as delivered in hospitals by unit support teams, considering that employees are not always direct victims of work incidents. We are seeing a growing need for improved business support, not only in rescue work, but also in social work and the nursing profession. Every hospital has guidelines for aftercare following traumatic incidents and social work agencies have established support groups for colleagues.

The new corporate culture starts from the principle that colleagues need to be actively supported after a traumatic experience. However, as an employee, you are also responsible for asking for support when needed. You have to acknowledge that distressing experiences can't be erased from memory. You should accept your own vulnerability and ask for help, if necessary. Business support should be offered at every level of the organization and provide a kind of safety net (see Figure 27.3). There has been limited research into the quality of support for employees in organizations. A business support team provides care that is additional to regular business support. Members of the business support team offer their support directly following the event. They make an appointment for you if you react positively. Should you decline, they will get in touch with you again a week later. An important aspect of support is a detailed reconstruction of the distressing experience. The purpose of support is to create conditions for peace of mind, talking and emotional release (laughing, crying, and anger).

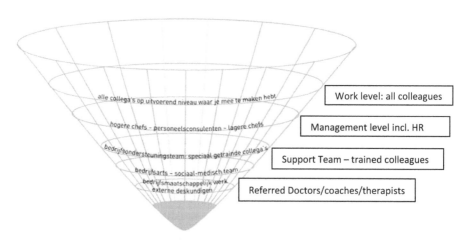

FIGURE 27.3 Safety net for social workers themselves

Source: de Mönnink (2016)

27.5.1 Support from the home environment

You can derive valuable help from a supportive home environment. Are you a couple or single? Do you have children? Do you live with together with a colleague? These factors make a difference in the availability and timing of support from the home environment. It may also occur that people at home are reluctant to get involved because of their custom to keep work and personal life separate. It is of utmost importance to ask for help when you are experiencing problems and to keep the lines of communication open at all times.

27.6 Preventive actions

A systematic approach is essential to preventing employees' development of exhausting and traumatic work stress. The important starting point is that your or your colleagues' vulnerability is perceived as a normal reaction to stressful events. An organization that supports this principle provides its workers the opportunity to share their stories with colleagues or in people's homes. In doing so, exhausting and traumatic work stress can remain manageable and there is no need for professional help.

27.6.1 Personal stress management

Suggestions are given to help prevent burnout:

*   Find ways to release your emotions to prevent numbness.
*   Do regular exercises that you enjoy.
*   Eat healthy and limit use of sugar and coffee, try to function without caffeine.
*   Enjoy life and don't sacrifice yourself at work.
*   Adopt a lifestyle that gives you satisfaction and ensure that your happiness does not depend on client satisfaction.
*   Take a break regularly.
*   Try to set your personal boundaries, learn to say no when you need time for yourself. It feels good to say yes when you genuinely wish to do what is asked.
*   Allow yourself to enjoy, laugh, even when having experienced tragic incidents.
*   Acknowledge your need for support.
*   Arrange a consultation, intervention, a place to get yourself together.
*   Develop a kind, loving attitude towards yourself, develop the ability to forgive yourself and stop punishing yourself.
*   Love yourself as a person.
*   Appreciate yourself for who you are.

A large number of basic training courses for nurses, social workers and police officers pay limited attention to grief counselling and trauma management. Fortunately, we are now seeing a growing number of trainings schools that include grief studies and stress management in their curriculum. Grief studies and stress management courses help workers to develop a realistic and constructive basic attitude towards themselves and their clients, and to face emotionally upsetting situations and deal with them.

TABLE 27.7 Five principles for support in critical incidents

Principle for support		Implementation
1	Every organization has an appointed permanent support worker.	The appointed employee contacts victim after event, gives psychological first aid
2	The support must be standardized.	A number of talking sessions are offered.
3	Adequate training of support workers is a must.	Support workers are skilled in providing grief support.
4	The support programme is ready for implementation.	A protocol is available, in which responsibilities and tasks are clearly laid down.
5	Organizational policies are to include special arrangements for victims.	Absenteeism is not perceived as sick leave but as special leave, employee can return to an equivalent post

Source: adapted from Kleber et al. (1986)

27.6.2 Support and information in the workplace

It is important for the workplace to provide support and information. Managers and confidential counsellors can fulfil a key role in supporting employees in distressing events. They can help employees deal with the practical aspects in a forthcoming way and help them blow off steam by talking with them (see Table 27.7).

27.6.3 Information

Another tool to prevent complaints from developing is providing information about the signs of burnout and PTSD and the need for early support and debriefing. An educational programme is essential to successful business support and to preventing unnecessary deterioration of problems following traumatic events. Employers are now acknowledging that organizations benefit from preventive measures that help limit exhausting and traumatic work stress and sickness absenteeism as well as work incapacity. It can therefore be concluded that attention to the emotional aspects of work is indispensable to providing quality support for employees.

27.7 Summary and questions

The current chapter has described emotional work stress as a form of stress among rescue workers and care professionals, including social workers. Practice shows that employees don't report sick as a result of a single incident at work. Reporting sick from work often involves diverse factors that contribute towards workers' reduced coping ability in (parts of) their job. It concerns long-lasting, emotionally upsetting situations – for instance, prolonged exposure to severe human suffering – which may develop into burnout syndrome. However, it may also involve acute exposure to distressing situations, possibly leading to PTSD.

Next, the signs and risk factors were discussed for developing burnout and PTSD. Then, a number of stress reduction methods were described, including coping styles, positive self-instructions, colleagues' desired and undesired responses and support by the organization. In addition, attention was given to support from both the workplace and the home situation. Finally, the focus was placed on the importance of including grief studies and work stress management in training courses for social workers. It is clear that employers would be well-advised to create not only a good working atmosphere, but also a suitable form of business support.

Questions

1   Please complete the burnout questionnaire in Appendix 4 and discuss the results with a number of colleagues/fellow students who have also filled out the question-naire. Make an overview of participants' levels of tension. Draw up a stepped plan if tension appears too high.
2   Please design your own self-care package.

APPENDICES

1

Social casework report

Explanatory notes for the social worker

Medical social work

To: Johan Heel, internist
From: Wendy van Zanten, medical social work
Date: November 25, 2008
Subject: Final report Mrs. Stack, born 24–08–1978.

Above mentioned patient was seen on an outpatient basis from May 24 until July 21

Anamnesis

Mrs. Stack has many psychosocial stress symptoms in the physical, mental and relational field. On a physical level: she experiences muscle tension complaints. Spiritually she is irritable, she has insufficient control over the situation, she feels sad and worries a lot, she feels that she is out of balance and can no longer relax. In the relational field she misses support from her network.

Tension sources and strength sources

At the start of the conversation the biggest stress seems to come from the fear of not being able to work again. She works at a company that trades in car parts, which is physically demanding work. With her back pain it seems unlikely that she will return to the same job. Mrs. Stack is worried about the future and fears dependence on social benefits. But during social work conversation, I find out there is also a lot of stress related to the divorce that took place 3 years ago. Her husband left her for an 18-year-old girl. She is disappointed in the support that her friends have provided for her. Mrs. Stack likes the fact that she is now more conscious and has a better overview of her situation using PAK.

The aforementioned stressors have contributed to Mrs. Stack's imbalance. She did not have enough personal strength or support from her environment. Because of inadequate coping she was unable to deal with this herself. The coping style is mainly aimed at changing behaviour, emotion and cognition. Stimulus is needed to activate her friends for more support.

Intervention goals

- To reduce or eliminate negative tension;
- Emotional pain needs to be discharged;
- Negative stress caused by unrealistic thinking and behavioural deficits need to be decreased;
- Support from friends needs to be activated;
- Therefore optimizing Quality of Life (QoL).

Social work took place on an individual level first and was aimed to strengthen Mrs. Stack by making her aware of her reaction style and to teach her proper coping mechanisms. The discharge method was indicated because of the bottled-up sadness and the inner anger about the divorce, but also about the way her husband had left her. With the use of the authorization technique and the mirror technique she could discharge her emotions. Given the health of Mrs. Stack there was there a real chance that she would be labelled unfit for work, with the result that she would have to rely on a disability benefit. She had a lot unrealistic thoughts, did not want to 'hold her hands up'. These thoughts only gave more stress, while the goal was to reduce the amount of stress she was feeling. Through the normalizing technique I showed her that she was entitled to disability benefits because of the premiums she paid for years. Furthermore she had so many ailments, and the work was much too hard for her, it was not for nothing that she needed to rely on this benefit. With the reframing technique she could put these harmful thoughts in a less burdensome framework so that the stress was reduced. This allowed Mrs. Stack have a more a positive view into the future and she was able to take the time she needed to recover properly. She was able to balance her strength and how much she was able to handle. The behavioural method was used because Mrs. Stack had problems with setting specific boundaries and because of her lack of social skills, especially towards her ex-husband. I have mostly focused on the conditioning technique and prompting technique by offering behavioural remedies. When Mrs. Stack was once more accustomed to the practice of setting her own limits, by applying the *feeling yes/feeling no* technique, she found a real flow in finding the right coping style, because she felt increasingly strengthened. As far as the social aspect goes, an ecogram was made with potential sources of support and a plan to activate it herself.

Conclusion

By using the cognitive method Mrs. Stack is able to think more realistically about her situation when it comes to health in conjunction with work. This gives her less harmful thoughts and she can instruct herself more positively. Because of the discharge of the emotional pain she has more energy available and her head feels less cluttered. She has a good overview and clarity of her own situation.

Because of the behavioural method Mrs. Stack is less tense, more socially adept; she is more adequate in her communication and can respond in a more assertive way.

Mrs. Stack was amazed how the tension was reduced from 9 to 3 on the scale of 0 to 10. She never expected that by having conversations with the social worker she could lose so much tension. The support of her friends has also increased.

We have completed the conversations with great satisfaction on both sides.

Sincerely,

Wendy van Zanten, extension 400

Medical social worker

2

Self-test traumatic stress

Explanation for the client

Here you will find a number of statements that may apply to you since experiencing a significant event(s). Please tick the box with the most appropriate answer for you. With each question, keep the previous 4-week period in mind: note down if the described reaction was or wasn't applicable in the past 4 weeks.

Frequent reactions or reliving the event

☐ I thought about the event often, even if I didn't want to.
☐ From time to time, images of the event popped up in my mind.
☐ I dreamed about the event repeatedly.
☐ Every now and then I woke up bathing in sweat and screaming.
☐ I've had the feeling that I was re-experiencing the event again (or certain parts of it).
☐ I felt very (sad, angry, scared, etc.) or I got upset when I was reminded of the event. For example by: listening to the radio, watching TV, reading a newspaper, seeing people or experiencing situations.

Reactions of avoidance

☐ I tried hard and forced myself not to think about the event.
☐ Which of the following apply to you after the event? (If needed: tick multiple answers)

    ☐ Alcohol use;
    ☐ Drug use;
    ☐ Gambling;
    ☐ Medication;
    ☐ Seeking refuge in work;
    ☐ No longer working;
    ☐ No interest in TV anymore;
    ☐ No strength;

☐ Wanting to read;

☐ Less interest in seeing people;

☐ Having less appetite;

☐ Roaming the streets;

☐ Since the incident I avoid people or things that remind me of the event (for example: shops, restaurants, cinemas, airports, parties);

☐ I can't remember the event;

☐ I have the feeling as if the event hasn't really happened;

☐ Since the incident I take less pleasure or interest in things that I usually find fun (e.g., hobbies, leisure activities);

☐ Since the incident I spend less time with people;

☐ Since the incident, I feel less involved with other people. My feelings are more or less gone;

☐ Since the incident, I am pessimistic about my future (e.g., 'I don't expect much from life, my work or relationships with people anymore').

Increased-vigilance reactions

☐ Since the incident, I have trouble sleeping (e.g., difficulty falling asleep, or waking up in the middle of the night and not being able to get back to sleep).

☐ Since the event, I lose my temper more often than usual or I get angry quickly.

☐ Since the event, I can hardly keep my mind on something (such as reading a book or the paper, my work).

☐ Since the incident, I've become forgetful.

☐ Since the incident, I feel less at ease or more insecure.

☐ Since the incident, I've become more nervous or quickly startled (e.g. like from an unexpected sound).

☐ When I think about the event, I feel me physically terrible (e.g. I experience chest pain, tremors, I start to sweat, I feel nauseous or get a headache).

After filling out the traumatic stress self-test

Realize that the above reactions are normal reactions to abnormal events. And also realize that if you share your feelings in an adequate way with colleagues, people close to you, a care team and professionals, those reactions will gradually decrease. If the reactions don't go away after a period of time, then professional help is recommended. Make sure to prevent it from getting worse, because it's not good for anyone if the experiences also make you sick. Take your complaints seriously. It is not a pretence!

3

Trauma-reactions checklist

Explanation for the social worker

A large number of calls for help are related to extreme situations that clients are facing. The so-called normal reactions to abnormal events – such as murder, suicide, violence, sexual abuse – are: 'Veelvuldige herbeleving, Vermijding en Verhoogde waakzaamheid' (Frequent re-experience, Avoidance and Increased vigilance). In Dutch they are called the three V's of processing shock. Being shocked is a normal reaction to an abnormal event. After a traumatic event – and therefore a shocking loss – we speak of a post-traumatic stress reaction (PTSR). According to the definition in the Diagnostic Statistical Manual-IV (DSM-IV), the standard for psychiatric classifications, there are 17 symptoms of PTSR. These reactions are considered a normal reaction to an abnormal event in the beginning, but in time – some say after 3 months, others after 6 months or 1 year or even longer – when clients keep six symptoms of the three V's, we can speak of a post-traumatic stress disorder (PTSD). People with these persistent symptoms are eligible for intensive forms of treatment. We speak of a full PTSD when three complaints of the V's are still persistently there over time, in a particular combination.

Frequent re-experience:	at least one complaint is found
Avoidance:	at least three complaints occur
Increased vigilance:	at least two complaints occur

When complaints do indeed occur, but not in above mentioned combination, we speak of partial PTSD. When there is a major incident with a lot of powerlessness and acute disruption, in which the symptoms persist over a longer period, we speak of a complicated process, which is otherwise treatable.

TABLE B5.1 Post–traumatic stress reactions (PTSR)

Three reaction types	Nr.	Stress reactions
Frequent Re-experience	1	Recurring obtrusive memories
	2	Repeatedly having bad dreams
	3	Acting and feeling as if the traumatic experience is happening again (for example: hiding)
	4	Intense sadness during a memory of the event
Avoidance	5	Avoiding relevant thoughts or feelings
	6	Avoiding relevant activities or situations
	7	Memory loss (complete or partial) because of the trauma
	8	Decreased interest
	9	Reclusive behaviour
	10	Feeling less expressive, indifferent
	11	Feeling down, sense of limited future
Increased vigilance	12	Insomnia
	13	Irritability, anger outbursts
	14	Concentration problems
	15	Being 'on his or her toes' all the time
	16	Excessive startle response
	17	Functional physical complaints (sweating with remembrance of the critical incident)

4

Quickscan UBS

Unfinished Business Syndrome

One can speak of the unfinished business syndrome (UBS) when four characteristics are present. The column 'Observations' shows an example of the fictitious case of a 45-year-old man.

Characteristics	Questions	Observations
1 *Current unexplained symptoms:* the presence of topical unexplained symptoms in biopsychosocial area.	1.1 *Complaints Inventory:* Are there unexplained symptoms (often stacked-up)? • Medical (bio) • Personal (psycho) • In relationship, own family, other family relatives, school, and work (social)	*Complaints Inventory:* • Unexplained depression • Unexplained fatigue, burnout symptoms
	1.2 *Complaint Etiology:* • Symptoms exist since when? • Is there a definite time when the symptoms have begun (time before and after the onset of symptoms)?	*Complaint Etiology:* • 15 years of complaints • More complaints at the age of 30
2 *Sensory triggers:* the presence of one or more sensory triggers that cause an increase of complaints (disruptive effect)	2.1 *Sensory stimuli:* Are there specific sensory stimuli to which the client is sensitive? • Image triggers • Sound triggers • Touch triggers • Smell triggers • Taste triggers	*Sensory stimuli:* • Arguments and dismissal from his job 15 years ago: unjustly treated, he could not deal with it, completely escalated, lead to resignation at his own request.

Characteristics	Questions	Observations
	2.2 *Trigger Recognition*: Which aspect(s) of the old pain are linked to these specific stimuli?	*Trigger Recognition:* • Injustice at work and recalls injustice of humiliations by stepfather.
3 *Unfinished life events:* the presence of several unfinished life events in the biography of the client	3.1 *Unfinished business (SUB):* Are there one or more life events that have been processed insufficiently according to the client? • Unresolved loss experience • Unresolved trauma experiences • Unfinished conflicts unfinished negative life periods	*Multi-UB:* • Unprocessed loss father (10 years) • Unfinished period of humiliation stepfather (10– 20 years) • Rift with sister (20 years)
4 Avoidance of coping and support; multiplier effect The presence of complaint perpetuating and worsening complaint coping and support.	4.1 *Avoidance*: is there an avoidance of coping or support? • Avoidance of coping (avoidance, bottling up, dramatizing, etc.) • Avoidance of support (ignoring, suppressing, disqualifying comments)	*Avoidance:* • Avoidance of coping: don't always talk but act, always work hard, self-employed (workaholic) • Avoiding social network but also avoiding outside help (social work) • Professional help with burnout stalled (not really feeling helped)
	4.2 *Complaint Aggravation*: • Does this avoidance lead to maintaining or aggravating the symptoms?	*Aggravation of complaints*: • Fantasies of jumping off a flat if it all became unbearable

UBS approach

- Focused attention on finalizing the proven unfinished business;
- Breaking from risk of 'wild fire' by the unprocessed old pain.

Also check website 'Science of Loss' (Private Practice Mönnink) (www.mmsocialwork. com)

5

Territorial inventory checklist (TICL)

Explanation for the social worker:

If the customer experiences a 'no-feeling' during a contact this may involve territorial issues. The social worker can make the following territorial inventory with the client (see also Chapter 15).

1) Territorial inventory: leading questions

Territorial aspects	Leading question
1. Irritation:	Ask yourself when you were (very) annoyed and what it was about.
2. Exploration:	When, how, about what were you annoyed?
3. Territorial area:	What theme/area is the annoyance about? (see territorial areas)
4. Property:	What do you consider yours and what someone else's?
5. Interest:	What is your interest in that area?
6. Competencies:	Are there difficulties in the area of (a) self-defence (b) acquisition (c) territorial management? (see territorial skills)
7. Solutions:	What are the possible steps towards a solution of the conflict?
8. Step 1:	What can you do from now on?

2) Explanation: territorial areas

To get an impression of your territories, questions are set for each area.

1   *Private ownership:* What is your personal property? To what extent do others have access your possessions?
2   *Your body and mind:* How do you experience it when others exceed your physical limits? To what extend do you experience it when others exceed your mental boundaries?
3   *Personal hiding place:* What is your favourite place to retire? In what kind of areas are they? Are you disturbed by others? If so, how? And by whom?

4   *Personal space:* Which physical distance from others do you prefer? When do you get the feeling that others are intruding into your private thoughts, fantasies?

5   *Psychological space:* How much and how do you draw attention to yourself, to your ideas, or to your expressions? How much time are you usually given? Are you annoyed when others interrupt you? When do you experience competition when someone else is speaking?

6   *Action area:* In what areas are you active and to what extend do you consider these areas yours? Under which control, responsibility, capacity to act, are they? Does your role and job description correspond to your true field of action? Would you like to change your field of action? Do you see any rivals?

3) Explanation: territorial skills

1   *Territorial defence:* Do you defend your territory effectively? If not, how are your:

   a   Available 'weapons of defence'?

   And what is the:
   b   Expected outcome of a conflict?
   c   The importance of the disputed area?

2   *Territorial acquisition:* If you are unable to acquire new territory, then is it due to (or because of an interplay between):

   a   The lack of skill to disarm the other person?
   b   The lack of importance the other territories have to you?
   c   The lack of hope you have in acquiring the territory?

3   *Territorial management:* Is the field of action too big or too small? Then there are multiple possibilities to solve the problem:

   a   Reduce the territory.
   b   Acquire more practice in management skills.
   c   Obtain management assistance.

6

Facing sudden death

Of all the experiences we confront in life, the toughest to face is the sudden, unexpected loss of someone we love. Loss in itself is painful enough, but sudden loss is shocking. The shock doubles our pain and intensifies our grief.

Even if on some level we understand that no one lives forever, actually losing people we love is unimaginable. When we know someone we love has a fatal disease or when we have nursed a loved one who is very ill, we have a chance to begin to prepare for their loss – at least a little. However, the unexpected death of a loved one – regardless of how that loved one dies – can leave us stunned, lost, and overwhelmed with pain. We may not know where to begin to cope.

Sudden loss gives us no chance to prepare. It is not unusual that we feel cheated by a sudden death, cheated of a chance to say the last words we would have liked to say or to do some last act that would have had meaning to us – like a hug, a kiss, a walk hand in hand. Missing out from having a way of saying some kind of good-bye can leave us feeling especially bereft for weeks or even months. Feeling cheated in this way can add to our grief, anguish and despair.

Besides our feeling cheated by it, sudden loss can make the world feel shaky or less safe. This is a natural response to any unexpected and traumatic event. When we feel as if someone we love is suddenly 'yanked' out of our lives, we are left feeling that the world isn't a safe place. We may then become fearful and uncertain, or angry and frustrated. This loss can negatively colour our view of life, but hopefully only temporarily.

When we face a sudden loss, all at once we have three overwhelming tasks to deal with: Our grief over the loss of our loved one, the absence of this special person from our daily lives, and the changes in our lives that are caused by this loss. Each is a big task to take on, and each will become a part of our mourning and healing process.

Although it may be hard to imagine at the moment, we must remember that people do recover from sudden losses, and that we too can ultimately move through this terrible pain and begin to heal.

It helps to bear in mind that emotional pain isn't constant, and that we don't have to grieve forever. We will love forever, whether our loved ones are with us in body or not, but we do not need to grieve to honour that love. We can just love.

In talking to many people who have suffered sudden loss, I have learned that there are several important, possibly universal, ways to help yourself heal:

Love yourself and take special care of yourself through your grief.

Do your mourning now. Being strong and brave is important, but I always tell those I counsel to never miss an opportunity to cry. That is not self-indulgent, but simply sensible and honest in dealing with your emotions.

Expressing your feelings will help you heal, as feelings expressed disappear. Feelings repressed don't. So give vent to your feelings.

Get support from other people – counsellors and support groups like widow's groups, bereavement groups, compassionate friends, or suicide survivors. You may find them through a hospice, your church, or a community or social service agency.

You will not only help yourself, but you may also help another and that can be a great source of strength, joy and recovery.

And, most of all, trust that the person you loved and lost would want you to recover from losing them, and would want you to remember and honour them by living a fulfilling life.

This article by Judy Tatelbaum, LCSW originally appeared in *Journeys: A Newsletter to Help in Bereavement*. Copyright, Hospice Foundation of America, Washington, DC, April 1996.

by Judy Tatelbaum, LCSW

7

Individual methods checklist: what methods match with what needs?

HUMAN NEEDS	INDIVIDUAL SOCIAL WORK METHODS *)
NEED FOR HELP	**BASIC SOCIAL WORK METHOD**
Need for contact/growing awareness	**Non-directive core method**
Lack of overview, imbalance between positive resources and negative stressors, insufficiënt social support system	*Unconditional positive regard, empathy, congruence, assessing negativity (unfulfilled needs) & positivity (fulfiled needs).* *Techniques: PFC, SBVP, sandwich, motivational interviewing*
SURVIVAL-NEEDS (biopsychosocial)	**SURVIVAL FOCUSED SOCIAL WORK METHODS**
Need for physical safety (bio)	**Body work method**
Lack of proper oxygen/water/sleep/physical rest/warmth/food/movement/sex	*Physical rest, relaxation, food, life-style improvement.* *Techniques: self touching, relaxation, activation*
Need for social security (social)	**Practical-materialistic method**
Lack of proper housing/work/money/ practical problem solving	*Strengthen resources, work on practical solutions.* *Techniques: advising, advocacy, budgeting, referral*
Need for psychological safety (psycho)	**Trauma work method**
Lack of psychic security by traumatic, sensory burned critical experiences	*Work on mental safety.* *Techniques: stabilization, reconstruction, follow-up*
AFFECTIVE NEEDS	**AFFECTIVE ORIENTED SOCIAL WORK METHODS**
Need for emotional proximity	**Cathartic method**
Lack of respect/trust/affection/inclusion/ respect/feeling seen and heard	*Emotional proximity will let go emotional pain (crying, shouting, trembling).* *Techniques: permission, exposure, flooding, empty chair*
Need for creative expression	**Expressive method**
Lack of creative/musical/art/digital and drama-expression of 'painful' experiences	*Creative, symbolic, imaginary express emotional experiences.* *Techniques: writing, plastic, biographical, play*

HUMAN NEEDS	INDIVIDUAL SOCIAL WORK METHODS *)
Need for closure, saying goodbye Lack of proper goodbye, emotional finished business	**Ritual method** *Proper goodbye, finishing unfinished business, symbolic transition from old to new life.* *Techniques: farewell, yet-still, suspension, trauma closure*
SELF-DETERMINATION NEEDS	**SELF-DETERMINATION SOCIAL WORK METHODS**
Need for realistic information processing Lack of realistic thinking/information/ overview/effective problem solving/ learning/ personal identification	**Cognitive method** *Education, realistic thinking, cognitive problem solving, sensory confrontation.* *Techniques: reality check, cognitive restructuring, problem-solving normalization, challenging unrealistic thinking, solution focused, internet support*
Need for existential re-orientation Lack of meaning making/a helping story/ identity transformation/being one with a greater perspective (spiritual)	**Narrative method** *Coming to terms, constructing a helping story, existential and spiritual re-orientation, meaning making.* *Techniques: externalization, relabeling, cost-benefit, rewriting, remembering*
Need for competence and influence Lack of assertive skills (sub-assertive of aggressive behavior)	**Behavioral method** *Social skills, stepped, exercise assertive behavior.* *Techniques: diary, SOSKI, modeling, shaping, prompting, feeling yes/feeling no*

*) A mix of individual methods can be indicated especially in multiproblem situations: when clients are in different needs struggling with poverty, migration, exclusion, worklessness, trauma, divorce, handicap, terrorism.

) Social workers additionally also use **systemic methods (helping the support network better help the client such as relationship, family, social group- or network-oriented methods) and **macro-methods** (helping empower the societal resources by monitoring, prevention and collective advocacy).*

8

The PIE-concept in the history of social work

Cornell (2006) explored the sort of 'jojo'-movement within the concept of the Person-in-Environment (PIE) in social work history either focussing on the person or the environment:

1   Mary Richmond (1922) attempted in *What Is Social Casework? An Introductory Description* to bridge the dual PIE-division by emphasizing the importance in work with individuals and families.

2   Gordon Hamilton (1940) reaffirmed in 'Theory and Practice of Social Casework' social work's traditional concern with the environment and committed not only to understand the structure and dynamics of personality but also to rediscover the use of environmental and socio-therapy.

3   Florence Hollis (1964) defined PIE in *Casework: A Psychosocial Therapy*: 'the PIE concept to a threefold configuration consisting of the person-in-his-situation: the person, the situation and the interaction between them.' Hollis limited her understanding of 'situation' to an interpersonal dynamic between the client and significant others such as friends and family rather than broader socio-political concerns.

4   Goldstein (1996) stated in 'What is clinical social work: looking back to look ahead?' that direct practice caseworkers lost status in the 1960s to turn its attention away from direct practice and towards community organization, policy design and social action. Supporters of direct practice were accused of 'blaming the victim' of oppression and pathologizing marginalized groups such as women, gays and people of color.

5   Frank J. Turner (1986) highlighted in *Social Work Treatment* the knowledge and skill direct practitioners need to make use of communities as well as skills in mobilizing available resources. He noted that the need for a multi-skilled direct service social worker was becoming evident as psychosocial therapy gained attention and highlighted a variety of needs and interventions.

6   The ecosystems perspective combined the ecological perspective as adapted for social work by Gitterman and Germain (1980) with concepts from General Systems Theory (Bertelanffy, 1968) in an attempt to more broadly integrate biopsychosocial aspects of human functioning. Within the ecosystems framework, both individuals and the

environment are understood to be physical as well as social entities. Individuals' adaptive capabilities are seen as having both psychological and biological underpinnings. Social work interventions are therefore directed at the interchanges between persons and their environments; concepts of reciprocity and mutuality between these two entities are stressed. Emphasis is on the systemic nature of relationships between individuals and on the social worker as a participant in the client system.

7 Neil Thompson (1992) stated that radical theory draws heavily from Marxist concepts and emphasizes politics, class conflict, ideological hegemony and socialism. It refocuses the attention of the social worker on the environment and would prescribe structural interventions rather than individual, family or group work. But the notion that the oppressive social order manifests itself in a variety of significant ways – social, psychological and emotional – should not lead to neglect the individual's experience by the social worker to address social issues. Neil Thompson (1992) used Sartrean existentialism to develop an existentialist framework for social work practice as a dialectic between existential freedom (person) and political liberty (environment) (see also Chapter 3).

LITERATURE

Addams, J. (1902). *Democracy and social ethics*. New York: Macmillan.

Ader, R., Felten, D. & Cohen, N. (2001). *Psychoneuroimmunology*. New York: Academic Press.

Adriani, J.H. (1932). *Voorlezingen over armenzorg en maatschappelijk werk*. Zutphen: Ruys' Uitgeversmaatschappij.

American Psychological Association. (2007). *Dictionary of psychology*. Washington, DC: Author.

Andersen, T. (1987). The reflecting team: dialogue and meta-dialogue in clinical work. *Family Process, 26*, 415–428.

Androff, D. (2016). *Practicing rights: human rights-based approaches to social work practice*. Abingdon: Routledge.

Arends, L. & Hosman, C.M.H. (1991). *Beleidsgerichte signalering in de preventieve AGGZ*. Utrecht: Trimbos-instituut.

Arntz, A. & Elgersma, H. (1999). Cognitieve therapie bij gegeneraliseerde angststoornis. In: Bögels, S.M. & Oppen, P. van (eds.), *Cognitieve therapie: theorie en praktijk*. Houten: Bohn Stafleu van Loghum.

Baarda, D.B. & Goede, M.P.M. de (2001). *Basisboek methoden en technieken. Handleiding voor het opzetten en uitvoeren van onderzoek*. Groningen: Wolters-Noordhoff.

Baars, H.M.J., Dreessen, L.J.J.M. & Uffing, J.F.T. (1995). Interventies in en met het sociale netwerk. In: *Handboek maatschappelijk werk*. Houten: Bohn Stafleu van Loghum.

Baars, M.W.M. & Hosman, C.M.H. (1990). *Preventie op waarde geschat*. Nijmegen: Bèta Boeken.

Baart, A. (2001). *Een theorie van de presentie*. Utrecht: Lemma.

Baart, A. (2005). *Aandacht. Etudes in presentie*. Utrecht: Lemma.

Baart, S. (1995). Juist de ideale werknemer raakt voortijdig opgebrand. *De Volkskrant* (11 March).

Baartman, H.E.M., Vogelvang, B.O. & Veerman, J.W. (1994). *De Vragenlijst Gezinsfunctioneren*. Amsterdam: Vrije Universiteit, vakgroep Pedagogiek/Duivendrecht: Paedologisch Instituut.

Bailey, S. (1995). *Creativity and the close of life*. Brantford, CT: Hospice Institute.

Bak, M., Os, J. van, Delespaul, P., Bie, A. de, À Campo, J.A., Poddighe, G. et al. (2007). An observational, "real life" trial of the introduction of assertive community treatment in a geographically defined area using clinical rather than service use outcome criteria. *Social Psychiatry and Psychiatric Epidemiology, 42*(2), 125–130.

Bakker, A.B. & Demerouti, E. (2007). The job demands-resources model: state of the art. *Journal of Managerial Psychology, 22*, 309–328.

Bakker, C.B. & Bakker, M.K. (1972). *Verboden toegang. Verkenning rond het menselijk territorium*. Amsterdam: De Nederlandse Boekhandel.

Bakker, M.K. & Bakker, C.B. (1978). *Workshops I, II en III*. Diepenbeek: Postuniversitair Medisch Centrum.

Barker, R.L. (1999). *The social work dictionary*. Washington, DC: NASW Press.

Barker, R.L. (2003). *The social work dictionary* (5th edition). Washington, DC: NASW Press.

Barman-Adhikari, A. & Rice, E. (2014). Social networks as the context for understanding employment services utilization among homeless youth. *Evaluation and Program Planning*, *45*, 90–101.

Barnes, J.A. (1954). Class and communication in a Norwegian island community. *Human Relations*, 7, 39–54.

BASW (2012). Social media policy. http://cdn.basw.co.uk/upload/basw_34634–1.pdf.

Baucom, D.H., Shoham, V., Mueser, K.T., Daiuto, A.D. & Stickle T.R. (1998). Empirically supported couple and family interventions for marital distress and adult mental health problems. *J Consult Clin Psychol*, *66*, 53–88.

Baumeister, R.F. (1991a). *Meanings of life*. New York: Guilford Press.

Baumeister, R.F. (1991b). *Escaping the self*. New York: Basic Books.

Beck, A. (1979). *Cognitive therapy and the emotional disorders*. New York: International University Press.

Beck, A.T. & Emery, G. (1985). *Anxiety disorders and phobias: a cognitive perspective*. New York: Basic Books.

Becvar, D.S. & Becvar, R.J. (1996). *Family therapy: a systemic integration*. Needham Heights: Allan & Bacon.

Beekers, M. (1982). *Interpersoonlijke vaardigheidstherapieën voor kansarmen*. Lisse: Swets & Zeitlinger.

Beets, N. (1905). Onmogelijke definities. In: *Jaarboek van de Maatschappij der Nederlandse Letterkunde*. The Hague: Digital Library.

Berendsen, S. (2003). *Maatschappelijk werk na rampen en calamiteiten*. Zaltbommel: Uitgeverij Thema.

Berg, I.K. (2000). *Ik wil mijn kind niet kwijt, samenwerken met ouders onder dwang van de kinderbescherming. Praktische richtlijn voor de hulpverlening*. Haarlem: De Toorts.

Berg, I.K. & Jong, P. de (2001). *De kracht van oplossingen. Handwijzer voor oplossingsgerichte gesprekstherapie*. Lisse: Swets & Zeitlinger.

Bergenhenegouwen-Van Mil, R. & Quaak, M. (1997). *Verwerking beperking. Verslag van een themagroep in het revalidatiemaatschappelijk werk*. Vlaardingen: Sophia Revalidatiecentrum.

Berne, E. (1976). *Transactionele Analyse in de psychotherapie*. New York: Grove Press.

Bern-Klug, M., Kramer, B.J. & Linder, J. (2005). All aboard: advancing the social work research agenda in end-of-life and palliative care. *Journal of Social Work in End-of-Life and Palliative Care*, *1*(2), 71–86.

Bernstein, G.A., & Garfinkel, B.D. (1988). Pedigrees, functioning, and psychopathology in families of school phobic children. *American Journal of Psychiatry*, *145*(1), 70–74.

Bernstein, G.A., Svingen, P.H. & Garfinkel, B.G. (1990). School Phobia: Patterns of Family Functioning, *29*(1), 24–30.

Bertelanffy, L. von (1968). *General system theory. foundations, developments, applications.* New York: Braziler.

Bertman, S.L. (1999). *Grief and the healing arts: creativity as therapy*. New York: Baywood.

Bettelheim, B. (1976). *The uses of enchantment: the meaning and importance of fairy tales*. New York: Vintage Books.

Blackman, M., Pitcher, S. & Rauch, F. (1986). A preliminary outcome study of a community group treatment programme for emotionally disturbed adolescents. *Canadian Journal of Psychiatry*, *31*(2), 112–118.

Blow, A.J., Sprenkle, D.H. & Davis, S.D. (2008). Is who delivers the treatment more important than the treatment itself? The role of the therapist in common factors. *Journal of Marital and Family Therapy*, *33*(3), 298–317.

Bögels, S.M. & Oppen, P. van (1999). *Cognitieve therapie: theorie en praktijk*. Houten: Bohn Stafleu van Loghum.

Bokseveld, B. (1990). *Helpen bij financiële problemen. Schuldhulpverlening vanuit het algemeen maatschappelijk werk*. Baarn: Nelissen.

Bonanno, G.A., Westphal, M. & Mancini, A.D. (2011). Resilience to loss and potential trauma. *Annual Review of Clinical Psychology*, 7, 511–535.

Bonuck, K.A. (1996). Theory and method: a social work approach to unmet needs. *Administration in Social Work*, *20*(2), 29–40.

Bosscher, R. (1996). Over de effectiviteit van runningtherapie bij depressie. *Bewegen & Hulpverlening*, *13*, 246–258.

Böszörményi-Nagy, I. & Spark, G.M. (1973). *Invisible loyalties: reciprocity in intergenerational family therapy.* New York: Harper & Row.

Bout, J. van den (1986). *Verliesgebeurtenissen in attributietheoretisch perspectief.* Delft: Eburon.

Bouwkamp, R. & Vries, S. de (1992). *Handboek psychosociale therapie.* Amersfoort: College uitgevers.

Bowlby, J. (1988). *A secure base: parent-child attachment and healthy human development.* New York: Basic Books.

Boyd, D.M. & Ellison, N.B. (2007). Social network sites: definition, history, and scholarship. *Journal of Computer-Mediated Communication, 13*(1), 210–230.

Braams, R. (1994). Verloren in het paradijs. Opvang criminele jongeren door 'Nieuwe Perspectieven'. *NRC Handelsblad* (28 May).

Brock, G. (2005). Needs and global justice. In: Reader, S. (ed.), *The philosophy of need* (pp. 51–72). Cambridge/New York: Cambridge University Press.

Broich, J. (1994). *Lichaam en beweging: meer dan 100 nieuwe gespreksspelen.* Baarn: Nelissen.

Brouwers, E., Tiemens, B., Terluin, B. & Verhaak, P. (2007). De effectiviteit van een interventie door het maatschappelijk werk bij huisartspatiënten die overspannen zijn. *Huisarts en Wetenschap, 50*, 403–411. http://www.henw.org/archief/id179-de-effectiviteit-van-een-interventie-door-het-maatschappelijk-werk-bij-huisartspatinten-die-overspannen-zijn.html.

Brown, B. (2010). *The gifts of imperfection: let go of who you think you're supposed to be and embrace who you are.* Hazelden: Center City.

Brown, B. (2012). *Daring greatly.* New York: Gotham Books. (translated as: Brown, B. (2013). *De kracht van kwetsbaarheid.* Utrecht: A.W. Bruna.)

Brown, B. (2015). *Rising strong.* New York: Gotham Books.

Brown, R. & Hill, B. (1996). Opportunity for change: exploring an alternative to residential treatment. *Child Welfare League of America, 725*, 35–57.

Bruin, E. de (2014). Een ritueel geeft gevoel van controle over verlies. *NRC Handelsblad*, 15 February. http://www.nrc.nl/next/2014/02/15/een-ritueel-geeft-gevoel-van-controle-over-verlies-1346086.

Bruns, E., Burchard, J. & Yoe, J. (1995). Evaluating the Vermont system of care: outcomes associated with community-based wraparound services. *Journal of Child and Family Studies, 4*(3), 321–339.

Buitenhuis, M.L. (1993). *Projectmatig werken. Een handreiking voor het opzetten van preventieprojecten in de (geestelijke) gezondheidszorg.* Utrecht: Trimbos-instituut.

Burnham, J.B. (1986). *Family therapy.* New York: Tavistock.

Burnham, J.B. (1994). *Inleiding in de gezinsbehandeling.* Baarn: Intro.

Busch, M. (1993). Therapeutic touch, een instrument voor zorgverbetering. *Prana* (August/September).

Buys, J. (1956). *Algemene Nederlandse systematisch ingerichte encyclopedie.* Amsterdam: Wetenschappelijke uitgeverij.

Cannon, W.B. (1932). *The wisdom of the body.* New York: Norton.

Caplan, G. (1964). *Principles of preventive psychiatry.* New York: Basic Books.

Carli, V., Hoven, C.W., Wasserman, C., Chiesa, F., Guffanti, G., Sarchiapone, M. e.a. (2014). A newly identified group of adolescents at "invisible" risk for psychopathology and suicidal behavior: findings from the SEYLE study. *World Psychiatry, 13*(1), 78–86.

Carlier, I.V.E., Lamberts, R.D. & Gersons, B.P.R. (1994). *Ingrijpende gebeurtenissen in politiewerk.* Arnhem/Gouda: Quint.

Carlier, I.V.E., Lamberts, R.D., Gersons, B.P.R. & Uchelen, A.J. van (1995). *Het lange-termijn effect van debriefen. Een vervolgonderzoek bij de Amsterdamse politie naar aanleiding van de Bijlmerramp.* Amsterdam: AMC.

Carney, M. & Buttell, F. (2003). Reducing juvenile recidivism: evaluating the Wraparound Services Model. *Research on Social Work Practice, 13*(5), 551–568.

Carter, B. & McGoldrick, M. (1989a). *The changing family life cycle: a framework for family therapy.* Boston: Allyn & Bacon.

Carter, B. & McGoldrick, M. (1989b). *The joining of families through marriage: the new couple.* Boston: Allyn & Bacon.

Carter, E.A. (1978). The transgenerational scripts and nuclear family stress: theory and clinical implications. In: Sager, R.R. (ed.), *Georgetown family symposium*. Washington, DC: Georgetown University.

Chan, C. (2015). A scoping review of social media use in social work practice. *Journal of Evidence-Informed Social Work*, (July 15),), 1–14 (e-pub ahead of print).

Chapple, A. & Ziebland, S. (2010). Viewing the body after bereavement due to a traumatic death: qualitative study in the UK. *British Medical Journal*, 340, c2032.

Cladder, H. (2000). *Oplossingsgerichte korte psychotherapie*. Lisse: Swets & Zeitlinger.

Clark, E.J. (2012). Advocacy: profession's cornerstone. http://www.socialworkers.org/pubs/news/2007/07/clark.asp.

Clark, H., Lee, B., Prange, M. & McDonald, B. (1996). Children lost within foster care system: can wraparound service strategies improve placement outcomes? *Journal of Child and Family Studies*, 5(1), 39–54.

Cobb, S. & Kasl, S. (1977). *Termination: the consequences of job loss*. New York: John Wiley & Sons.

Cohen, D., De la Vega, R. & Watson, G. (2001). *Advocacy for social justice*. Bloomfield, CT: Kumarian Press.

Cohen, S., Doyle, W.J., Skoner, D.P., Rabin, B.S., VanderPlate, C., Aral, S.O. e.a. (1988). The relationship among genital herpes simplex virus, stress, and social support. *Health Psychology*, 7, 159–168.

Cohn, R. (1979). *Thematische interactie, een methode voor hulpverlening, vorming en onderwijs*. Bloemendaal: Nelissen.

Cooper, A. (2003). Position paper. Network for Psycho-Social Practice and Policy.

Cornell, K.L. (2006). Person-in-situation: history, theory, and new directions for social work practice. *Praxis*, 6, 50–57.

Corr, C.A. (1992). A task-based approach to coping with dying. *Omega Journal of Death and Dying*, 24(2).

Corr, C.A., Nabe, C.M. & Corr, D.M. (1994). *Death and dying, life and living*. Belmont: Wadsworth.

Coulton, C.J. (1986). Implementing monitoring and evaluation systems in social work. *QRB Quality Review Bulletin*, 12(2), 72–75.

Council on Social Work Education. (2004). Educational policy and accreditation standards. [Online]. Available: http://www.cswe.org/accreditation/EPAS.

Cowen, L., Corey, M., Keenan, N., Simmons, R., Arndt, E., & Levison, H. (1985). Family adaptation and psychosocial adjustment to cystic fibrosis in the preschool child. *Social Science and Medicine*, 20(6), 553–560.

Coyle, G. (1948). *Group work with American youth*. New York: Harper & Row.

Craven, J. & Wald, F.S. (1975). Hospice care for dying patients. *American Journal of Nursing*, 75, 1816–1822.

Csikszentmihalyi, M. (1999). *Flow, psychologie van de optimale ervaring*. Amsterdam: Boom.

CSWE. (2004). http://www.cswe.org/

Cuperus, B.K., Smulders-Sloan, J.M. & Wynia, K. (1995). *Protocollen en observatieschalen medisch-technische handelingen*. Utrecht: Lemma.

Dalgleish, T.L., Johnson, S.M., Burgess Moser, M., Lafontaine, M.F., Wiebe, S.A. & Tascam, G.A. (2014). Predicting change in marital satisfaction throughout emotionally focused couple therapy. *Journal of Marital and Family Therapy*, 41(3), 276–291.

Dam, H. van (1992). Psychische belasting drukt erg zwaar op omgeving Alzheimer-patiënten. *De Volkskrant* (11 January).

Damasio, A. (1999). *The feeling of what happens*. New York: Harcourt-Brace.

Dantzig, A. van (1974). *Psychologie van de doodsangst: normaal is niet gewoon. Beschouwingen over psychiatrie en psychotherapie* (pp. 84–94). Amsterdam: De Bezige Bij.

Dantzig, A. van (1992). De hardnekkige angst voor lijden en de dood. *De Volkskrant* (4 April).

Dartel, H. van (1998). Ethiek in de organisatiestructuur. In: Timmer, S. (ed.), *Tijd voor ethiek. Handreikingen voor ethische vragen in de praktijk van maatschappelijk werkers*. Bussum: Coutinho.

Darwin, C. (1956). On the origin of species. In: Bates, M. & Humphreys, P.S. (eds.), *The Darwin Reader*. New York: Charles Scribner's Sons.

Davis, M., Robbins, E., McKay, E. & McKay, M. (2003). *Ontspan je. Oefeningen voor ontspanning en stressvermindering*. Amsterdam: Nieuwezijds.

Dean, H. (2008). Social policy and human rights: re-thinking the engagement. *Social Policy and Society*, 7(1), 1–12.

Degner, L.F. (1976). Death in disaster: implications for bereavement. *Essence*, 2, 69–77.

Dekker, T. & Biemans, H. (1994a). *Videohometraining in families*. Houten: Bohn Stafleu van Loghum.

Dekker, T. & Biemans, H. (1994b). *Videohometraining in gezinnen*. Houten: Bohn Stafleu van Loghum.

Delgado, M. (2000). *Community social work practice in an urban context: the potential of a capacity-enhanced perspective*. New York: Oxford University Press.

Delo, M. (2000). *Rouwgroepen: organisatie en voorbereiding*. Utrecht: LSR.

Detmer, C.M. & Lamberti, J.W. (1993). Models of family grief assessment and treatment. *Death Studies*, 17, 55–67.

Diener, E. & Chan, M.Y. (2011). Happy people live longer: subjective well-being contributes to health and longevity. *Applied Psychology: Health and Well-Being*, 3(1), 1–43.

Dijkstra, P. (1999). *De bindende kracht van familierelaties*. The Hague: Nederlands Interdisciplinair Demografisch Instituut.

Dohrenwend, B.S. & Dohrenwend, B.P. (ed.) (1974). *Stressful life events*. New York: Wiley.

Domes, G., Heinrichs, M., Gläscher, J., Büchel, C., Braus, D.F. & Herpertz, S.C. (2007). Oxytocin attenuates amygdala responses to emotional faces regardless of valence. *Biological Psychiatry*, 62, 1187–1190.

Donkers, G. (1999). *Zelfregulering als reflectiekader van methodiek maatschappelijk werk*. Baarn: Nelissen.

Doorn, L. van, Etten, Y. van & Gademan, M. (2008). *Outreachend werken. Handboek voor werkers in de eerste lijn*. Bussum: Coutinho.

Doorn, M.E. van & Elbers, E. (2003). Casemanagement en de casemanager. In: *Praktijkboek gezond werken*. Maarssen: Elsevier.

Dover, M. (2008). 'Human needs: overview'. *The encyclopedia of social work* (20th edition) (pp. 398–406). New York: Oxford University Press/National Association of Social Workers.

Doyal, L. & Gough, I. (1991). *A theory of human needs*. New York: Guilford Press.

DPA (1993). Stress ziekte van de eeuw. *De Volkskrant* (23 March).

Dragtsma, B.J. (2000). *Conflictmanagement in 244 vragen. Kader Cahier Praktijkantwoorden op bedrijfsvraagstukken*. Deventer: Question Library.

Dragtsma, B.J. (2002). De mediator. Mediation vóór conflictverzuim. In: *Praktijkboek gezond werken* (II 5.13–1–30). Maarssen: Elsevier.

Driedonks, G. (1993). Werken met netwerken, Een benadering voor ambulante chronische cliënten. *MGV*, 5.

Drukker, M., Maarschalkerweerd, M., Bak, M., Driessen, G., À Campo, J., Bie, A. de e.a. (2008). A real-life observational study of the effectiveness of FACT in a Dutch mental health region. *BMC Psychiatry*, 8, 93.

Duijnstee, M. (1992). *De belasting van familieleden van dementerenden*. Amsterdam: Thomas Rap.

Duncan, B.L., Miller, S.D. & Sparks, J.A. (2004). *The heroic client*. San Francisco: Wiley.

Dutch Health Council. (1999). *The effectiveness of physical modalities: Electro-therapy, laser-therapy, ultrasound*. The Hague: Dutch Health Council.

Duvall, E. (1962). *Family development*. Philadelphia: Lippincott.

Duvall, E. & Miller, C. M. (1985). *Marriage and family development*, 6th ed. New York: Harper & Row.

Dykstra, P. (1999). *De bindende kracht van familierelaties*. The Hague: Nederlands Interdisciplinair Demografisch Instituut.

Eerenbeemt, E.M. van den (1993). *De Grote Libelle Echtscheidingsenquête*. Haarlem: Libelle.

Efron, D. & Bradley, B. (2007). Emotionally Focused Therapy (EFT) and Emotionally Focused Family Therapy (EFFT): a challenge/opportunity for systemic and post-systemic therapists. *Journal of Systemic Therapies*, 26(4), 1–4.

Egan, G. (2004, 2012). *Deskundig hulpverlenen. Een model, methoden en vaardigheden*. Assen: Van Gorcum.

Eisenberger, N.I. (2012). The neural bases of social pain: Evidence for shared representations with physical pain. *Psychosomatic Medicine* 74(2), 126–135.

Einstein, A. (1946) (1879–1955). Atomic Education Urged. *New York Times* (25 May).

Eisma, M.C., Stroebe, M.S., Schut, H.A., Stroebe, W., Boelen, P.A. & Bout, J. van den (2013). Avoidance processes mediate the relationship between rumination and symptoms of complicated grief and depression following loss. *Journal of Abnormal Psychology, 122*, 961–970.

Eland, J., Roos, C. de & Kleber, R. (2000). *Kind & trauma. Een opvangprogramma.* Lisse: Swets & Zeitlinger.

Elliott, R., Greenberg, L. & Lietaer, G. (2004). Research on experiential psychotherapy. In: Lambert, M. (ed.), *Bergin and Garfield's handbook of psychotherapy and behavior change* (pp. 493–539). New York: John Wiley & Sons.

Ellis, A. (1976). *Reason and emotion in psychotherapy.* Secaucus, NJ: Citadel Press.

Ellison, J., Greenberg, L., Goldman, R.N. & Angus, L. (2009). Maintenance of gains following experiential therapies for depression. *Journal of Consulting and Clinical Psychology, 77*, 103–112.

Elsenbruch, S., Benson, S., Rucke, M., Rose, M., Dudenhausen, J., Pincus-Knackstedt, M.K. e.a. (2007). Social support during pregnancy: effects on maternal depressive symptoms, smoking, and pregnancy outcome. *Human Reproduction, 22*(3), 869–877.

Endt-Meijling, M. van (2008). *Medische kennis voor hulpverleners.* Bussum: Coutinho.

Engbersen, R. & Jansen, T. (1991). *Armoede in de maatschappelijke verbeelding (1945–1990). Een retorische studie.* Leiden: Stenfert Kroese.

Epstein, G., Weitz, L., Roback, H. & McKee, E. (1975). Research on bereavement: a selective and critical review. *Comprehensive Psychiatry, 16*, 537–546.

Epstein, M.H. & Sharma, H.M. (1998). *Behavioral and emotional rating scale: a strength-based approach to assessment.* Austin, TX: PRO-ED.

Erbes, C.R., Stillman, J.R., Wieling, E., Bera, W. & Leskela, J. (2014). A pilot examination of the use of narrative therapy with individuals diagnosed with PTSD. *Journal of Traumatic Stress, 27*(6), 730–733.

Erikson, E.H. (1968). *Identity, youth and crisis.* New York: Norton.

Erikson, G.P. (1976). *Personal networks and mental illness.* York: University of York.

Evers, A.W.M., Kraaimaat, F.W., Geenen, R., Jacobs, J.W.G. & Bijlsma, J.W.J. (2003). Pain coping and social support as predictors of long-term functional disability and pain in early rheumatoid arthritis. *Behaviour Research and Therapy, 3*, 1295–1310.

Feil, N. (1991). *Validation: Een nieuwe benadering in de omgang met gedesoriënteerde ouderen.* Dwingeloo: Kavanah.

Ferszt, G.G., Heineman, L., Ferszt, E.J. & Romano, S. (1998). Transformation through grieving: art and the bereaved. *Holist Nursing Practice, 13*(1), 68–75.

Flap, H.D. & Tazelaar, F. (1988). De rol van informele sociale netwerken op de arbeidsmarkt. *Mens en Maatschappij, 63*, 48–64.

Flikweert, M.W.M. & Melief, W.B.A.M. (2000). *Cliënten over het maatschappelijk werk. Een meta-studie naar tevredenheidsonderzoek in het maatschappelijk werk.* Utrecht: Verwey-Jonker Instituut.

Foley, V.D. (1974). *An introduction in family therapy.* New York: Grune & Stratton.

Frank, A. (1947). *The diary of a young girl.* Amsterdam: Anne Frank House.

Frankl, V. (1969). *The will to meaning.* New York: New American Library.

Fraser, N. (1989). Struggle over needs: outlines of a socialist-feminist critical theory of late-capitalist political culture. In: Fraser, N., *Fortunes of feminism: from state-managed capitalism to neoliberal crisis.* London/New York: Verso.

Fraterman, E. & Gils, T. van (2002). *Rouwgroepen. Een handleiding voor begeleiders.* Utrecht: Landelijk Steunpunt Rouwbegeleiding (LSR).

Freidson, E. (1970). *Profession of medicine.* New York: Dodds Mead.

Freire, P. (1972). *Pedagogie van de onderdrukten.* Baarn: In den Toren.

Freire, P. (1978). *Ervarend leren gebaseerd op de pedagogische ideeën van Paolo Freire.* Amersfoort: De Horstink.

Freud, S. (1917). *Trauer und Melancholie, Gesammelte Werke, Band X.* Frankfurt: Fischer Verlag GmbH.

Freud, S. (1925). *Mourning and melancholia.* Collected papers. Vol. IV. London: Hogarth Press.

Freud, S. (1952). *Het levensmysterie en de psycho-analyse.* Amsterdam: Wereldbibliotheek.

Friedländer, W.A. (1958). *Concepts and methods of social work.* Englewood Cliffs: Prentice Hall.

Frijns, J. (1997). *Werkboek herstelbemiddeling. Een project gericht op bemiddeling tussen slachtoffers en daders.* The Hague: Reclassering Nederland.

Frima, R. & Mok, L. (2001). *Partners van patiënten met niet-aangeboren hersenletsel.* Interne publicatie. Gorinchem: Revalidatiecentrum 'de Waarden'.

Fromm, E. (1955). *The sane society.* New York: Rineheart.

Gaillard, A. (2003). *Stress, productiviteit en gezondheid.* Amsterdam: Nieuwezijds.

Galtung, J. (1978). Paper presented for the Workshop on Needs, organized by the Internationales Institut für Umwelt und Gesellschaft (IIUG), Wissenschaftszentrum Berlin (27–29 mei). https://www.tran scend.org/galtung/papers/The%20Basic%20Needs%20Approach.pdf.

Garfield, C.A. (1981). Emotionele aspecten van sterven en dood. *Maandblad voor Geestelijke Volksgezondheid, 36,* 415–429.

Geerinck-Vercammen, C. (1998). *Met een goed gevoel. Het rouwproces bij doodgeboorte, reductie in meerlingenzwangerschap en zwangerschapsafbreking bij prenatale diagnostiek in relatie tot de rol van de professionele hulpverlener.* Leiden: LUMC.

Geerts, G. & Boon, C.A. den (1999). *Van Dale: Groot Woordenboek der Nederlandse Taal: 3 Dl.* (13e dr.). Utrecht: Van Dale Lexicografie.

Geldard, D. (1993). *Basic personal counseling: a training for counsellors.* London: Prentice Hall.

Gendlin, E. (1999). *Focussen, gevoel en je lijf.* Haarlem: De Toorts.

Gennep, A. van (1909). *Les rites de passage.* Parijs: Émile Nourry. (English edition: Gennep, A. van (1960), *The rites of passage.* London: Routledge & Kegan Paul.)

Germain, C.B. & Gitterman, A. (1980). *The life model of social work practice.* New York: Columbia University Press.

Gersons, B.P.R. (1995). *Acute psychiatrie.* Deventer: Van Loghum Slaterus.

Gezondheidsraad (1999). *De effectiviteit van fysische therapie; elektrotherapie, lasertherapie, ultrageluidbehandeling.* Publicatie nr. 1999/20. The Hague: Gezondheidsraad.

Gezondheidsraad (2003). *Oefentherapie.* Publicatie nr. 2003/22. The Hague: Gezondheidsraad.

Gibran, K. (1923). *The Prophet.* New York: Alfred A. Knopf. In een vertaling van Carolus Verhulst (1927) verschenen als *De Profeet.*

Gil, D. (1992). Foreword. In: Wronka, J. (ed.), *Human rights and social policy in the 21st century.* New York: University Press of America.

Gil, D.G. (2004). Perspectives on social justice. *Reflections: narratives of professional helping, 10*(Autumn), 32–39.

Glassman, U. (1991). The social work group and its distinct healing qualities in the health care setting. *Health & Social Work, 16*(3), 203–212.

Glick, I.Q., Weiss, R.S. & Parkes, M.C. (1974). *The first year of bereavement.* New York: John Wiley & Sons.

Glisson, C.A. (1994). Should social work take greater leadership in research on total systems of service? Yes. In: Hudson, W. & Nurius, P. (ed.), *Controversial issues in social work research.* Boston: Allyn & Bacon.

Goldman, R.N., Greenberg, L.S. & Angus, L. (2006). The effects of adding emotion-focused interventions to the client-centered relationship conditions in the treatment of depression. *Psychotherapy Research, 16,* 536–546.

Goldstein, E.G. (1984). *Ego psychology and social work practice.* New York: Free Press.

Goldstein, E. G. (1996). What is clinical social work? Looking back to move ahead. *Clinical Social Work Journal, 24*(1), 89–104.

Goldstein, H. (1983). Starting where the client is. *Social Casework, 64,* 267–275.

Goldstein, H. (1990). The knowledge base of social work practice: theory, wisdom, analogue or art? *Families in Society: the journal of contemporary human services, 71*(1), 32–43.

Gonçalves, M.M., Matosa, M. & Santosa, A. (2009). Narrative therapy and the nature of 'innovative moments' in the construction of change. *Journal of Constructivist Psychology, 22*(1), 1–23.

Goorhuis, F. (1999). *Rouwgroep voor homoseksuele mannen.* Amsterdam: Schorerstichting.

Gordon, S. & Davidson, N. (1981). Behavioral parent training. In: Gurman, A.S. & Kniskern, D.P. (ed.), *Handbook of family therapy* (pp. 517–555). New York: Brumer/Marel.

Gordon, Th. (1981). *Luisteren naar elkaar. Problemen uitpraten en oplossen in het gezin.* Antwerpen: De Nederlandsche Boekhandel.

Gottman, J.M. & Silver, M. (1999). *De zeven pijlers van een goede relatie. Tips uit de praktijk om er een succes van te maken.* Utrecht/Antwerpen: Kosmos-Z&K Uitgevers.

Graafsma, T., & Tieken, J. (1987). 'Leven in een condición migrante'. In P.A.Q.M. Lamers (Ed.), *Hulpverlening aan migranten: De confrontatie van culturen in de geestelijke gezondheidszorg*. Alphen a/d Rijn: Samsom Stafleu. 26–34.

Gray, N., Oré de Boehm, C., Farnsworth, A. & Wolf, D. (2010). Integration of creative expression into community based participatory research and health promotion with native Americans. *Family & Community Health, 33*(3), 186–192.

Greef, M.H.G. de (1992). *Het oplossen van problematische schuldsituaties: een analyse van de invloed van hulpverlening, interorganisationele samenwerking en huishoudkenmerken op de effectiviteit van schuldregelingen*. Groningen: s.n.

Greenberg, L.S. (2002). *Emotion-focused therapy*. Washington, DC: American Psychological Association.

Greenberg, L.S. & Pascual-Leone, A. (2006). Emotion in psychotherapy: a practice-friendly research review. *Journal of Clinical Psychology, 62*, 611–630.

Greenberg, L.S. & Watson, J. (1998). Experiential therapy of depression: differential effects of client-centered relationship conditions and process experiential interventions. *Psychotherapy Research, 8*, 210–224.

Greenberg, L.S., Warwar, S.H. & Malcolm, W.M. (2008). Differential effects of emotion-focused therapy and psychoeducation in facilitating forgiveness and letting go of emotional injuries. *Journal of Counseling Psychology, 55*, 185–196.

Greenberg, M.T., Feinberg, M.E., Johnson, L.E., Perkins, D.F., Welsh, J.A. & Spoth, R.L. (2015). Factors that predict financial sustainability of community coalitions: five years of findings from the PROSPER partnership project. *Prevention Science, 16*(1), 158–167.

Gruenberg, E.M. & Pepper, B. (1985). Definition of the terms 'chronic', 'disorder', 'disability' and 'patient'. In: Radebaugh, T.S., Gruenberg, E.M., Kramer, M. e.a. (ed.), *The chronically mentally ill: an international perspective*. Baltimore: Johns Hopkins University Press.

Grundmeijer, H.G.L.M., Reenders, K. & Rutten, G.E.H.M. (2004). *Het geneeskundig proces. Klinisch redeneren van klacht naar therapie*. Maarssen: Elsevier gezondheidszorg.

Gurman, A.S. (1983). Family therapy research and the new epistemology. *Journal of Marital Therapy, 9*(3), 227–234.

Gurman, A.S., Kniskern, D.P. & Pinsof, W.M. (1986). Research on the process and outcome of marital and family therapy. In: Garfield, S. & Bergin, A. (eds.), *Handbook of psychotherapy and behavioral change* (3rd edition). New York: John Wiley.

Gutierrez, L.M. (1994). Beyond coping: an empowerment perspective on stressful life events. *Journal of Sociology and Social Welfare, 21*, 201–219.

Guy, M. (1982). The adjustment of parents to wartime bereavement. *Clinical and Community Psychology: Stress and Anxiety, 8*, 243–247.

Hafford-Letchfield, T. (2009). *Management and organisations in social work*. London: SAGE.

Haggerty, K.P. & Shapiro, V.B. (2013). Science-based prevention through communities that care: a model of social work practice for public health. *Social Work in Public Health, 28*(3–4), 349–365.

Hamilton, G. (1940). *Theory and Practice of Social Casework*. New York: Columbia University Press.

Hargie, O.D.W. (1986). *The handbook of communication skills*. London: Croom Helm.

Harr, B.D. & Thistlethwaite, J.E. (1990). Or filter your current search: creative intervention strategies in the management of perinatal loss. *Maternal-Child Nursing Journal, 19*(2), 135–142.

Harris, M. (1997). *Een verlies voor altijd. De levenslange invloed van de vroege dood van een ouder*. Amsterdam: Bert Bakker.

Hart, O. van der (1987). *Rituelen in psychotherapie: overgang en bestendiging*. Houten: Bohn Stafleu van Loghum.

Hart, O. van der (1991). *Trauma, dissociatie en hypnose*. Amsterdam: Swets & Zeitlinger.

Hart, O. van der (1992). *Afscheidsrituelen. Achterblijven en verder gaan*. Lisse: Swets & Zeitlinger.

Hawkins, J.D., Shapiro, V.N. & Fagan, A.A. (2010). Disseminating effective community prevention practices: opportunities for social work education. *Research on Social Work Practice, 20*(5), 518–527.

Healy, K. (2012). *Social work methods and skills. The essential foundation of practice*. Hampshire: Palgrave Macmillan.

Hellinger, B. (2002). *Leven zoals het is. Werken met familieopstellingen, organisatieopstellingen en consultatieopstellingen*. Groningen: Het Noorderlicht.

Hemming, P. (1995). Working with children facing bereavement as individuals. *European Journal of Palliative Care, 1*(2), 72–77.

Hendrickx, C. (1987). De algemene systeemtheorie. In: *Handboek Gezinstherapie*. Afl. 6 B 1.1. Deventer: Van Loghum Slaterus.

Hendriks, J. (1981). *Emancipatie. Relaties tussen minoriteit en dominant*. Alphen aan den Rijn: Samsom.

Herman, J.L. (1993). *Trauma en herstel*. Amsterdam: Wereldbibliotheek.

Hermans, H. (1991). *Je piekert je suf. Over piekeren, besluiteloosheid en uitstellen*. Meppel: Boom.

Hermsen, J. (1986). Over de betekenis van co-counselen in een beroepsopleiding. In: Aerts, A., Helwig, L., Hermsen, J., Luttikholt, A. & Meulenbelt, A. (eds.), *Doelgroep: vrouwen en welzijnswerk*. The Hague: VUGA.

Heron, John (1998). *Co-counselling*. Auckland/Guildford: South Pacific Centre for Human Inquiry/ Human Potential Research Project, University of Surrey.

Hertz, D.G. (1981). Arrival and departure: theoretical considerations and clinical observations on migrants and immigrants. *Psychiatric Journal of the University of Ottawa*, 6(4), 234–238.

Heuves, W. (1991). Fors aantal pubers lijdt aan depressie. *De Volkskrant* (21 May).

Hobfall, S.E. (1985). Limitations of social support in the stress process. In: Sarason, I.G. & Sarason, B.R. (ed.), *Social support: theory, research and applications* (pp. 391–414). Dordrecht: Martinus Nijhoff.

Hochstenbach, J. (1998). *Na een beroerte: het opzetten van een nazorgprogramma voor CVA-patiënten en hun omgeving*. Maarssen: Elsevier.

Hoff, B. (1989). *Tao van Poeh: de kunst van het Zijn geopenbaard door de Beer met maar een klein beetje verstand*. The Hague: Sirius en Siderius.

Hoff, J.H.M. von den (2004). Van schuld naar schone lei. In: *Praktijkhandboek Gezond werken*. Houten: Bohn Stafleu van Loghum.

Hogan, B., Linden, W. & Najarian, B. (2002). Social support interventions: do they work? *Clinical Psychology Review*, 22(3), 381–440.

Hogan, R.A. (1964). Issues and approaches in supervision. *Psychotherapy: Theory, Research and Practice*, 1(3), 139–141.

Hollis, F. (1964, 1972). *Casework: a psychosocial therapy*. New York: Random House.

Holmes, T.H. & Rahe, R.H. (1967). The social readjustment rating scale. *Journal of Psychosomatic Research*, 11, 213–218.

Holstvoogd, R. (1995). *Maatschappelijk werk in kerntaken*. Houten: Bohn Stafleu van Loghum.

Holt-Lunstad, J., Smith, T.B. & Layton, J.B. (2010). Social relationships and mortality risk: a meta-analytic review. *PLOS Med*, 7(7), e1000316.

Hoochstraat, Pieter de (1949). *Problemen van maatschappelijk werk. Gedenkboek ter gelegenheid van het 50-jarig bestaan (1899–1949) van de school voor maatschappelijk werk. Pieter de Hoochstraat 78*. Amsterdam. Purmerend: Muusses.

Hoogendam, S. & Vreenegoor, E. (2002). *Intensief casemanagement & complexe meervoudige problemen*. Bussum: Coutinho.

Hoveling, P. (1995). *De belevingsgerichte benadering van dementerende ouderen*. Houten: Bohn Stafleu Van Loghum.

Hubble, M.A., Duncan, B.L. & Miller, S.D. (1999, 2002). *The heart & soul of change: what works in therapy*. Washington, DC: American Psychiatric Association.

Hughes, F. (1980). Reaction to loss: coping with disability and death. *Rehabilitation Counseling Bulletin*, 23(4), 251–256.

Hughes, L. & Pengelly, P. (1997). *Staff supervision in a turbulent environment: managing process and task in front-line services*. London: Jessica Kingsley.

ICODO (1987). *Het maatschappelijk werk en de hulpverlening aan oorlogsgetroffenen*. Utrecht: ICODO.

IFSW (1997). *Social exclusion and social work in Europe – facilitating inclusion. The IFSW Europe Project 1996–1997*. Bern: IFSW.

Illich, I. (1978). *Toward a history of needs*. New York: Pantheon Books.

Imber-Black, E. (1989). Idiosyncratic life cycle transitions and therapeutic rituals. In: Carter, B. & McGoldrick, M. (ed.), *The changing family life cycle. A framework for Family Therapy*. New York: Simon & Schuster.

International Association of Schools of Social Work (IASSW). (2001). https://www.iassw-aiets.org/

International Federation of Social Work (IFSW). (2001). http://ifsw.org/

Ivey, A.E. (1976). *Helpen en vormen door microcounseling. Hulpverlenings- en vormingsmodellen voor individu en groep*. Bloemendaal: Nelissen.

Jackins, H. (1965). *The human side of human beings: reevaluation counseling*. Seattle: Rational Island.

Jackins, H. (1997). *The list*. Seattle: Rational Island.

Jacobs, G. (1999). *Rationeel-emotieve therapie. Een praktische gids voor hulpverleners*. Houten: Bohn Stafleu van Loghum.

Jaff, J.C., Arnold, J. & Bousvaros, A. (2006). Effective advocacy for patients with inflammatory bowel disease: communication with insurance companies, school administrators, employers, and other health care overseers. *Inflammatory Bowel Diseases, 12*(8), 814–823.

Jagt, L. (2001). *Moet dat nou? Hulpverlening aan onvrijwillige cliënten*. Houten: Bohn Stafleu van Loghum.

Jagt, L. & Jagt, N. (1990). *Taakgerichte hulpverlening in het maatschappelijk werk*. Houten: Bohn Stafleu van Loghum.

Jagt, L. & Jagt, N. (1997). Taakgerichte hulpverlening. In: *De lerende professie*. Houten: Bohn Stafleu van Loghum.

James, H. (1920). *The letters of William James*. Vol. I. Boston: Atlantic Monthly Press.

James, W. (1907a). *Essays in pragmatism*. New York: Hafner.

James, W. (1907b). What pragmatism means. In: James, W. (ed.), *Pragmatism* (pp. 43–81). New York: Longmans, Green.

Janssen, H., Wentzel, W. & Vissers, B. (2009). *Basisboek huiselijk geweld. Signaleren, melden, aanpakken*. Bussum: Coutinho.

Janssen, R. (1977). *Welzijnswerk en maatschappelijke achterstelling*. Alphen aan den Rijn: Samsom.

Jansson, B. (2005). *The reluctant welfare state: American social welfare policies – past, present, and future* (5th edition). Belmont, CA: Brooks/Cole.

Jansson, B. (2011). *Improving healthcare through advocacy: a guide for the health and helping professions*. Belmont, CA: Brooks/Cole.

Javidi, H. & Yadollahie, M. (2012). Post-traumatic stress disorder. *International Journal of Occupational Environmental Medicine, 3*(1), 2–9.

Jehu, D. (1973). De rol van maatschappelijk werkers in de gedragstherapie. In: *Hulpverlenen en veranderen. Handboek voor psychisch gezondheids- en welzijnswerk*. Deventer: Van Loghum Slaterus.

Johnson, J.V. & Hall, E.M. (1988). Job strain, workplace, social support and cardiovascular disease: a cross-sectional study of a random sample of the Swedish working population. *American Journal of Public Health, 78*, 1336–1342.

Johnson, J.V., Hall, E.M. & Theorell, T. (1989). Combined effects of job strain and social isolation on cardiovascular disease morbidity and mortality in a random sample of the Swedish male working population. *Scandinavian Journal of Work and Environmental Health, 15*, 271–279.

Johnson, S.M. (2004). *Creating connection: the practice of emotionally focused couple therapy* (2nd edition). New York: Routledge.

Johnson, S.M. (2008). *Hold me tight: seven conversations for a lifetime of love*. New York: Little Brown.

Johnson, S.M., Hunsley, J., Greenberg, L. & Schlindler, D. (1999). Emotionally focused couples therapy: status and challenges. *Clinical Psychology: Science and Practice, 6*, 67–79.

Johnson, S.M., Moser, M.B., Beckes, L., Smith, A., Dalgleish, T., Halchuk, R. e.a. (2013). Soothing the threatened brain: leveraging contact comfort with emotionally focused therapy. *PLOS One, 8*(11), e79314.

Johnson, Y.M. (1999). Indirect werken: onderbelicht in het maatschappelijk werk. *Social Work, 44*, 323–334.

Jong, G. de & Schout, G. (2011). Family group conferences in public mental health care: an exploration of opportunities. *International Journal of Mental Health Nursing, 20*(1), 63–74.

Jong, G. de, Schout, G. & Abma, T. (2015). Examining the effects of family group conferencing with randomised controlled trials: the golden standard? *British Journal of Social Work, 45*, 1623–1629.

Jong, J.T.V.M. de (1993). *Handleiding bij psychotrauma. Een praktijkboek voor hulp in Nederland aan ontheemden en aan slachtoffers van rampen en vervolging*. Amsterdam: Tropeninstituut.

Jungmann, N. (2006). *De WSNP: bedoelde en onbedoelde effecten op het minnelijk traject*. Leiden: Leiden University Press.

Kadushin, A. (1976). *The social work interview. Het gesprek in het maatschappelijk werk.* Deventer: Van Loghum Slaterus.

Kamphuis, M. (1972). *Wat is social casework? Een eerste inleiding.* Alphen aan den Rijn: Samsom.

Kamphuis, M. & Jagt, N. (1997). Wat is social casework? In: *De lerende professie. Hoofdlijnen van het maatschappelijk werk* (pp. 46–59). Utrecht: SWP.

Kapteyn, B. (1998). *Probleemoplossing in organisaties.* Houten: Bohn Stafleu van Loghum.

Kasser, T. & Kanner, A.D. (2004). *Psychology and consumer culture: the struggle for a good life in a materialistic world.* Washington, DC: American Psychiatric Association.

Keers, C. & Wilke, H. (1978). *Oriëntatie in de sociale psychologie.* Alphen aan den Rijn: Samsom.

Keirse, M. (1981). Het slechtnieuwsgesprek. *Tijdschrift voor Ziekenverpleging,* 34(6), 262–267.

Kelley, H.H. (1971). *Attribution theory in social interaction.* Morristown, NJ: General Learning Press.

Kerson, T.S. & McCoyd, J.L. (2013). In response to need: an analysis of social work roles over time. *Social Work,* 58(4), 333–343.

Kiecolt-Glaser, J.K., McGuire, L., Robles, T.F. & Glaser, R. (2002). Emotions, morbidity, and mortality: new perspectives from psychoneuroimmunology. *Annual Review of Psychology,* 53, 83–107.

King, M.L. (1984). *Stride toward freedom.* New York: Harper & Brothers.

Kiser, L. J, Baumgardner, B. & Dorado, J. (2010) Who are we, but for the stories we tell: Family stories and healing. *Psychological Trauma,* 2(3), 243–249.

Kleber, R.J. (1982). *Stressbenaderingen in de psychologie.* Deventer: Van Loghum Slaterus.

Kleber, R.J., Brom, D. & Defares, P.B. (1986). *Traumatische ervaringen en psychotherapie.* Lisse: Swets & Zeitlinger.

Klerman, G.L. & Izen, J.E. (1977). The effects of bereavement and grief on physical health and general well-being. *Advances in Psychosomatic Medicine,* 9, 63–104.

Klompé, M.A.M. (1959). Toespraak van de minister van Maatschappelijk Werk. *Tijdschrift voor Maatschappelijk Werk,* 13, 38–39.

Kluckhohn, M.H. & Schneider, D.M. (1953). *Personality in nature, society and culture.* New York: Knopf.

Kolb, D.A. (1984). *Experiential learning, experience as the source of learning and development.* Englewood Cliffs: Prentice Hall.

Konopka, G. (1963). *Social groupwork: a helping process.* Englewood Cliffs: Prentice Hall.

Koprowska, J. (2010). *Communication and interpersonal skills in social work* (2nd edition). Exeter: Learning Matters.

Krahn, G.L. (1993). Conceptualizing social support in families of children with special health needs. *Family Process,* 32, 235–248.

Krupnick, J. & Horowitz, M.J. (1981). Stress response syndromes. *Archives of General Psychiatry,* 38, 428–435.

Kübler-Ross, E. (1969). *On death and dying.* New York: Macmillan.

Kuhn, T.S. (1996). *The structure of scientific revolutions.* London: University of Chicago Press.

Kuin, A. & Bieman, M. den (2002). *Dochters zonder moeder. Evaluatie van een eerste lotgenotengroep voor vrouwen die voor hun 20e levensjaar hun moeder verloren.* Utrecht: Humanitas.

Kuiper, K. (2008). *Je mag mij altijd bellen. 1001 dagen van rouw.* Arnhem: Terra Lannoo.

Kuiper, M. de (1994). Kinderen, pijn en cultuur. *Kind en ziekenhuis* (March), 26–27.

Kulik, J.A. & Mahler, H.I.M. (1993). Emotional support as a moderator of adjustment and compliance after coronary artery bypass surgery: a longitudinal study. *Journal of Behavioral Medicine,* 16, 45–64.

Kus, R.J. & Miller, M.A. (1999). Art therapy. In: Bulechek, G.M. & McCoskey, J.C. (eds.), *Nursing interventions.* Philadelphia: Saunders.

Laan, G. van der (1990). *Legitimatieproblemen in het maatschappelijk werk.* Utrecht: SWP.

Laere, I.R. van, Wit, M.A. de & Klazinga, N.S. (2009). Pathways into homelessness: recently homeless adults problems and service use before and after becoming homeless in Amsterdam. *BMC Public Health,* 9, 3.

Laing, R.D. (1961). *The self and others: Further studies in sanity and madness.* London: Tavistock.

Lakoff, G. & Johnson, M. (1980). *Metaphors we live by.* Chicago/London: University of Chicago Press.

Lambert, M.J. (1992). Implications of outcome research for psychotherapy integration. In: Norcross, C. & Goldfried, M.R. (ed.), *Handbook of psychotherapy integration* (pp. 94–129). New York: Basic Books.

Landelijke Commissie van de Geestelijke Volksgezondheid (2002). *Zorg van velen*. Eindrapportage van de Landelijke Commissie van de Geestelijke Volksgezondheid. The Hague.

Lang, G. & Molen, H.T. van der (1991). *Psychologische gespreksvoering*. Baarn: Nelissen.

Lange, A. (2002, 2006). *Gedragsverandering in gezinnen*. Groningen: Wolters-Noordhoff.

Lapworth, P., Sills, C. & Fish, S. (2001). *Integration in counselling & psychotherapy*. London: SAGE.

Lazarus, A. (1992). Multimodal therapy: technical eclecticism with minimal theoretical integration. In: Norcross, J. & Goldfried, M. (ed.), *Handbook of psychotherapy integration*. New York: Harper Collins.

Lazarus, R.S. & Folkman, S. (1984). *Stress, appraisal and coping*. New York: Springer.

Lazarus, R.S. & Launier, R. (1978). Stress-related transactions between person and environment. In: Pervin, L.A. & Lewis, M. (ed.), *Perspectives in interactional psychology* (pp. 287–327).

Leach, E.R. (1976). *Culture and communication: the logic by which symbols are connected*. Cambridge: Cambridge University Press.

Lederer, W.J. & Jackson, D.D. (1968). *Mirages of marriage*. New York: Norton.

LeDoux, J. (1996). *The emotional brain: the mysterious underpinning of emotional life*. New York: Simon & Schuster.

Lehman, D., Ellard, J. & Wortman, C. (1986). Social support for the bereaved: recipients' and providers' perspective on what is helpful. *Journal of Consulting and Clinical Psychology*, *54*(4), 438–446.

Leijssen, M. (2001). *Gids voor gesprekstherapie*. Utrecht: De Tijdstroom.

Lengelle, R. & Meijers, F. (2009). Mystery to mastery: an exploration of what happens in the black box of writing and healing. *Journal of Poetry Therapy*, *22*(2), 59–77.

Lenson, B. (2002). *Positieve stress en negatieve stress*. Herkennen en omgaan met spanning. Zaltbommel: Thema.

Levinson, D.J. (1978). *De tijdperken van het leven van de man*. Baarn: Ambo.

Lewin, K. (1951). *Field theory in social science*. New York: Harper Torchbooks.

Lewin, K. (1952). *Field theory in social science: selected theoretical papers by Kurt Lewin*. London: London: Tavistock.

Lewis, J. (1993). *Trauma en herstel. De gevolgen van geweld – van mishandeling thuis en politiek geweld*. Amsterdam: Wereldbibliotheek.

Lewis, K., Winsett, R.P., Cetingok, M., Martin, J. & Hathaway, K. (2000). Social network mapping with transplant recipients. *Progress in Transplantation*, *10*(4), 262–266.

Lietaer, G. (1991). Authenticiteit en onvoorwaardelijke positieve gezindheid. In: Swildens, J.C.A.G., Haas, O. de, Lietaer, G. & Balen, R. Van (ed.), *Leerboek gesprekstherapie. De cliëntgerichte benadering* (pp. 27–64). Utrecht: De Tijdstroom.

Lifton, R.J. (1969). Observations on Hiroshima survivors. In: Krystal, H. (ed.), *Massive psychic trauma* (pp. 168–189). New York: International Universities Press.

Ligthart, L. & Keyser, F. de (1993). Bieden van steun belangrijker dan begripvol klimaat scheppen. *Tijdschrift voor Jeugdhulpverlening en Jeugdwerk*, 10, 42–51.

Lindeman, E. (1944). Symptomatology and management of acute grief. *American Journal of Psychiatry*, *101*, 141–148.

Lindeman, E. (1972). *Bereavement: studies in grief adult life*. New York: International Universities Press.

Linden, M. van der (2006). *Hersenen en gedrag: evolutie, biologie & psychologie*. Amsterdam: Boom.

Lippitt, R., Waysons, S. & Westley, B. (1958). *The dynamics of planned change*. New York: Harcourt, Brace.

Logger, K. & Martens, J. (2000). *Aarden in vreemde grond. Handleiding vluchtelingen en netwerken*. Groningen: Stichting GGZ, afdeling Preventie.

Lohuis, G., Schilperoord, R. & Schout, G. (2008). *Van bemoeizorg naar groeizorg. Methodieken in de gezondheidszorg*. Groningen: Wolters-Noordhoff.

Loo, L.F. van (1981). *'Den arme geven . . .' Een beschrijving van armoede, armenzorg en sociale zekerheid in Nederland, 1784–1965*. Meppel: Boom.

Loumpa, V. (2012). Promoting recovery through peer support: possibilities for social work practice. *Social Work in Health Care*, *51*(1), 53–65.

Lowen, A. (1998). *Bio-energetica: de therapie die de taal van het lichaam gebruikt om de problemen van de geest te genezen*. Utrecht: Servire.

MacElveen-Hoehn, P. (1987). Sexual response to death. Paper presented at the meeting of the international workgroup on Death, Dying and Bereavement. London.

MacGillavry, D. (1979). *Buigen, barsten of bijstellen. Suggesties voor echtparen*. Rotterdam: Donker.

MacGillavry, D. (1981). *Zolang de kruik te water gaat*. Rotterdam: Donker.

MacGillavry, D. (1981). *Oefeningen van (echt) paren*. Rotterdam: Donker.

MacGillavry, D. (1998). *Echtscheiding en bemiddeling. Een alternatief voor escalerende ruzies*. Rotterdam: Donker.

MacLean, P.D. (1990). *The triune brain in evolution: role in paleocerebral functions*. New York: Plenum Press.

Madanes, V. (1996). *Geld in relaties. De verborgen rol van geld bij problemen in gezin en familie*. Baarn: Intro.

Malysiak, R. (1997). Exploring the theory and paradigm base for wraparound. *Journal of Child and Family Studies, 6*(4), 399–408.

Margadant-Bakker, A.P. (1966). Het social casework als methode van maatschappelijk werk. In: *Maatschappelijk werk. Krachten, terreinen, methoden. Deel III Methoden van maatschappelijk werk*. Assen: Van Gorcum.

Marris, P. (1974). *Loss and change*. New York: Pantheon Books.

Marteau, T.M., Bloc, S. & Baum, J.D. (1987). Family life and diabetic control. *Journal of Child Psychology and Psychiatry, 28*, 823–833.

Maslow, A. (1943). A theory of human motivation. *Psychological Review, 50*(4), 370–396.

Maslow, A. (1972). *Toward a psychology of being*. New York: Van Nostrand.

Max-Neef, M. (2012). *Human scale development: conception, application and further reflections*. London/New York: Apex Press.

McGoldrick, M. & Carter, B. (1980). *The changing family life cycle: a framework for family therapy*. Needham Heights: Allyn & Bacon.

McWinney, I.R. (1989). *A textbook of family medicine*. New York: Oxford University Press.

Meer, K. van, Neijenhof, J. van & Bouwens, M. (1999). *Elementaire sociale vaardigheden*. Houten: Bohn Stafleu van Loghum.

Meerum Terwogt-Kouwenhoven, K. (1998). *Psychische problemen en stress*. Amsterdam: Nieuwezijds.

Meijer, K. (2001). *Handboek psychosomatiek*. Baarn: HB Uitgevers.

Melief, W., Flikweert, M. & Vliet, K. van (2004). *Onderzoek naar het maatschappelijk werk. Inventariserende studie ten behoeve van een Onderzoeks- en Ontwikkelingsprogramma Kwaliteit Maatschappelijk Werk. Eindrapportage*. Utrecht: Verwey-Jonker Instituut. http://www.verwey-jonker.nl/doc/participatie/D7199387.pdf.

Merleau-Ponty, M. (1945). *Phénoménologie de la perception*. Parijs: La Librairie Gallimard, NRF.

Metz, T. (1994). Stillborn expectations. In: *Dutch: Stilte op het erf. De Volkskrant* (10 December).

Meulenbelt, A. (1987). *De ziekte bestrijden, niet de patiënt*. Amsterdam: Van Gennep.

Midgley, J. & Conley, A. (2010). *Social work and social development: theories and skills for developmental social work*. New York: Oxford University Press.

Migchelbrink, F. (2001). *Praktijkgericht onderzoek in zorg en welzijn*. Amsterdam: SWP.

Miley, K.K., O'Melia, M. & DuBois, B. (2001). *Generalist social work practice: an empowering approach*. Boston: Allyn & Bacon.

Miller, A. (1996). *Het drama van het begaafde kind*. Houten: Van Holkema & Warendorf.

Miller, S.D., Duncan, B.L. & Hubble, M.A. (1997). *Escape from Babel: toward a unifying language for psychotherapy practice*. New York/London: W.W. Norton.

Miller, T.K. (2009). *Forever No Lo*. San Francisco, CA: Rebel Reading Series.

Miller, W.R. & Rollnick, S. (2002). *Motivational interviewing: preparing people for change*. New York: The Guilford Press.

Milner, J. & O'Byrne, P. (2002). *Assessment in social work*. New York: Palgrave.

Ministerie van Justitie (2002). *Privé-geweld een publieke zaak*. The Hague: Hega Offset.

Minuchin, S. (1967). *Families of the slums*. New York: Basic Books.

Mönnink, H.J. de (1991). *Misvattingen over rouw bij kinderen*. Lezing studiedag Rouw. Groningen: Humanitas.

Mönnink, H.J. de (1992). *Verlieskunde in Nederlandse opleidingen voor beroepen in de gezondheidszorg, de psycho-sociale hulpverlening en het basisonderwijs. Interne publicatie*. Groningen: Rijkshogeschool.

Mönnink, H.J. de (1998a). Verlieskunde: zes taken in de verliesbegeleiding. *Maatschappelijk Werk Magazine, 2*, 12–15.

Mönnink, H.J. de (1998b). De cliënt centraal . . . en jij dan? Over zelfzorg in het maatschappelijk werk ter preventie van burnout en PTSS. *Maatschappelijk Werk Magazine, 5*, 2–6.

Mönnink, H.J. de (1999). Het Multimethodisch Praktijkmodel. Vrucht van 100 jaar MW. *Tijdschrift voor Zorg en Welzijn*, October, 18–23.

Mönnink, H.J. de (2001). *Verlieskunde*. Maarssen: Elsevier gezondheidszorg.

Mönnink, H.J. de (2002a). BMW kanaliseert stress. Smeerolie in de organisatie. *Maatwerk, 1*, 22–25.

Mönnink, H.J. de (2002b). *Verlieskunde als ondersteunend vak voor verpleegkunde. Handboek Verpleegkundig Consult*. Houten: Bohn Stafleu van Loghum.

Mönnink, H.J. de (2006). *Onverwerkt jong ouderverlies. Verkennende studie*. Groningen: Hanzehogeschool (internet publication).

Mönnink, H.J. de (2008). *Verlieskunde. Handreiking voor de beroepspraktijk* (5th edition). Maarssen: Elsevier.

Mönnink, H. de (2015). *Verlieskunde. Methodisch kompas voor de beroepspraktijk*. Amsterdam: Reed Business Education.

Mönnink, H.J. de (2016) *De gereedschapskist van de sociaal werker. Multimethodisch sociaal werk*. Maarn: BSL.

Moorter, H. van (1979). Territorialiteit en hulpverlening. *Tijdschrift voor Sociaal Welzijn en Maatschappelijk Werk, 6*(1).

Morales, A.M., Sheafor, B.W. & Scott M.E. (1989). *Social work: a profession of many faces*. Needham Heights: Allyn & Bacon.

Moreira, P., Beutler, L.E. & Gonçalves, O.F. (2008). Narrative change in psychotherapy: differences between good and bad outcome cases in cognitive, narrative, and prescriptive therapies. *Journal of Clinical Psychology, 64*(10), 1181–1194.

Morton, B. (1984). *Starting out in the Evening, as cited in Diana Schoemperlen (2001) Our Lady of the Lost and Found*. Toronto: Harper Collins Publishers Ltd, p. 141.

Morton, K. (1984). The story-telling animal. *New York Times Book Review* (23 December).

Mukhopadhyay, A. (2007). Advocacy for appropriate health policy and effective governance of the health system. *Promotion & Education, 14*(2), 88–89.

Muller-Lulofs, M.G. (1916). *Van mensch tot mensch*. Haarlem: Tijdschrift voor Armenzorg en Kinderbescherming, *17*, 43.

Munroe, E. (1998). Verbetering van het kennisniveau van maatschappelijk werkers in de Kinderbescherming. *Paspoort Maatschappelijk Werk, 1*, 45.

Myers, L.M. & Thyer, B.A. (1997). Should social work clients have the right to effective treatment? *Social Work, 42*, 288–298.

Nagy, I. & Spark, G.M. (1973). *Invisible loyalties: reciprocity in intergenerational family therapy*. New York: Harper Row.

National Association of Social Workers (1973). *Standards for social service manpower*. Washington, DC: NASW Press.

National Association of Social Workers (1996). *Code of ethics*. Washington, DC: NASW Press.

National Association of Social Workers (2008). *Code of ethics*. Washington, DC: NASW Press.

Netting, F.E., Kettner, P.M. & McMurtry, S.L. (2008). *Social work macro practice* (4th edition). Harlow: Pearson.

Neumann, I.D., Wigger, A., Torner, L., Holsboer, F. & Landgraf, R. (2000). Brain oxytocin inhibits basal and stress-induced activity of the hypothalamo-pituitary-adrenal axis in male and female rats: partial action within the paraventricular nucleus. *Journal of Neuroendocrinology, 12*, 235–243.

Nevejan, M. (1973). *Gezins- en echtparenbehandeling*. Deventer: Van Loghum Slaterus.

Nevejan, M. (1985). Multimethodische relatietherapie in fasen. *Tijdschrift voor Psychotherapie, 11*(4), 241–258.

Niemeyer, R.A. (1995). *Constructivism in psychotherapy*. Washington, DC: American Psychiatric Association.

Nijenhuis-van Weert, J. & Nijenhuis, R. (2002). *Een hulpverleningsmethodiek in de keten van zorg en welzijn*. Soest: Nelissen.

Nijnatten, C. van (2004). *Opvoeding, taal en continuïteit. Een pleidooi voor dialogisch maatschappelijk werk*. Amsterdam: Boom.

Noord, A. de (2006). *Door de bomen het bos zien. De methodische onduidelijkheid voorbij*. Intern artikel. Zwolle: Hogeschool Windesheim.

Noordanus, W.H. (1997). Indicatiestelling en professionele verantwoordelijkheid in de geestelijke gezondheidszorg. *Medisch Contact, 52*, 1456–1458.

Norton, M.I. & Gino, F. (2014). Rituals alleviate grieving for loved ones, lovers, and lotteries. *Journal of Experimental Psychology: General, 143*(1), 266–272.

NRC (2003). Veel hartinfarcten gemist met verouderde test. *NRC Handelsblad* (29 November).

Nutbeam, D., Harris, E. & Wise, M. (2010). *Theory in a nutshell: a practical guide to health promotion theories.* North Ryde: McGraw-Hill.

NVMW (2006). *Beroepsprofiel van de maatschappelijk werker.* Utrecht: NVMW.

Obar, J.A., Zube, P. & Lampe, C. (2012). Advocacy 2.0: an analysis of how advocacy groups in the United States perceive and use social media as tools for facilitating civic engagement and collective action. *Journal of Information Policy, 2*, 1–25.

Oderkerk, K. (1995). Ik moet de jas van pappa naar de hemel brengen. *Nieuwsblad van het Noorden* (10 June).

Ojeda del Pozo, N., Ezquerra-Iribarren, J.A., Urruticoechea-Sarriegui, I., Quemada-Ubis, J.I. & Muñoz-Céspedes, J.M. (2000). Training in social skills in patients with acquired brain damage. *Revista de Neurologia, 30*(8), 783–787.

Olde Hartman, T.C. & Hassink-Franke, L.J. (2014). Proactive monitoring of sickness absence for psychosocial problems. *Nederlands Tijdschrift voor Geneeskunde, 158*, A7387.

Oderkerk, K. (1997). Kinderen verwerken hun verlies op hun eigen manier. Rouwverwerking in groepen in plaats van eenzaamheid. *Nieuwsbrief Kinderwerkgroep,* nr. 3, mei.

Olson, J.J. (2007). Social work's professional and social justice projects: discourses in conflict. *Journal of Progressive Human Services, 18*(1), 45–69.

Onderwaater, A. (1986). *De onverbrekelijke band tussen ouders en kinderen.* Lisse: Swets & Zeitlinger.

O'Neill, O. (1998). Rights, obligations, and needs. In: Brock, G. (ed.), *Necessary goods: our responsibility to meet others' needs* (pp. 95–112). Lanham, MD: Rowman & Littlefield.

Orcutt, B.A. (1977). Stress in family interaction when a member is dying: a special case for family interviews. In: Prichard, E.R., Collard, J., Orcutt, B.A., Kutscher, A.H., Seeland, I. & Lefkowitz, N. (ed.), *Social work with the dying patient and the family.* New York: Columbia University Press.

Orlemans, J.W.G., Eelen, P. & Hermans, D. (1995). *Inleiding tot de gedragstherapie.* Houten: Bohn Stafleu van Loghum.

Padesky, C.A. (1993). *Socratic questioning: changing minds of guiding discovery.* Paper voor het European Congress of Behavioral and Cognitive Therapies, London (24 September).

Paivio, S.C. & Greenberg, L.S. (1995). Resolving 'unfinished business': efficacy of experiential therapy using empty-chair dialogue. *Journal of Consulting and Clinical Psychology, 63*, 419–425.

Paivio, S.C. & Nieuwenhuis, J.A. (2001). Efficacy of emotion focused therapy for adult survivors of child abuse: a preliminary study. *Journal of Traumatic Stress, 14*, 115–133.

Panksepp, J. (2010). Affective neuroscience of the emotional BrainMind: evolutionary perspectives and implications for understanding depression. *Dialogues in Clinical Neuroscience, 12*(4), 533–545.

Parad, H.J. (1965). *Crisis intervention: selected readings.* New York: Family Service Association of America.

Paradiso, S. & Rudrauf, D. (2012). Struggle for life, struggle for love and recognition: the neglected self in social cognitive neuroscience. *Dialogues in Clinical Neuroscience, 14*(1), 65–75.

Parkes, C.M. (1972). *Bereavement: studies of grief in adult life.* New York: International Press.

Parkes, C.M. (1975). Determinants of outcome following bereavement. *Omega, 6*, 303–323.

Parkes, C.M. & Brown, R.J. (1972). Health after bereavement: a controlled study of young Boston widows and widowers. *Psychosomatic Medicine, 34*, 449–461.

Pas, A. van der (1979). *Gezinsfenomenen.* Deventer: Van Loghum Slaterus.

Pas, A. van der (1992). *Visies op gezinsbehandeling.* Houten: Bohn Stafleu van Loghum.

Pas, A. van der (2008). *Handboek methodische ouderbegeleiding. De interventiefase.* Amsterdam: Uitgeverij SWP.

Pascual, L.J. & Greenberg, L. (2007). Emotional processing in experiential therapy: why 'the only way out is through'. *Journal of Consulting and Clinical Psychology, 75*, 875–887.

Pennebaker, J. (1994). Openhartigheid als medicijn. *NRC Handelsblad* (9 June).

Pennebaker, J.W. & Evans, J.F. (2014). *Expressive writing: Words that heal.* Enumclaw, WA: Idyll Arbor.

Pennebaker, J.W., Kiecolt-Glaser, J. & Glaser, R. (1988). Disclosure of traumas and immune function: Health implications for psychotherapy. *Journal of Consulting and Clinical Psychology, 56,* 239–245.

Perach, W.D. (1989). *Advances in art therapy.* New York: Wiley-Interscience.

Perez, R. (1982). Provisions of mental health services during a disaster: the Cuban immigration of 1980. *Journal of Community Psychology, 10*(1), 40–47.

Perlman, H.H. (1959). *Social casework.* Deventer: Van Loghum Slaterus.

Perloff, L.S. (1983). Perceptions of invulnerability to victimization. *Journal of Social Issues, 39*(2), 41–46.

Perls, F. (1969). *Gestalt Therapy Verbatim.* Lafayette (Cal.): Real People Press.

Perls, F. (1996). *Gestaltbenadering. Gestalt in actie: illustratieve teksten van sessies.* Haarlem: De Toorts.

Perls, F., Hefferline, R.F. & Goodman, P. (1951). *Gestalt therapy: excitement and growth in the human personality.* New York: Dell.

Phillips, L.J., Reid-Arndt, S.A. & Pak, Y. (2010). Effects of a creative expression intervention on emotions, communication, and quality of life in persons with dementia. *Nurse Research, 59*(6), 417–425.

Pierce, D. (1989). *Social work and society: an introduction.* New York: Longman.

Pillai, V.K. & Gupta, R. (2015). *The greening of social work. A paper developed for the Council on Social Work Education Global Commission.* Arlington/San Francisco: University of Texas/San Francisco State University.

Polster, E. & Polster, M. (1973). *Gestalt therapy integrated. Contours of theory and practice.* New York: Brunner-Mazel.

Poutré, B. la & Boelrijk, M. (2001). *Bemiddeling als alternatief. Handreiking voor hulp- en dienstverleners.* Houten: Bohn Stafleu van Loghum.

Pouwer, F., Snoek, F.J., Ploeg, H.M. van der, Adèr, H.J. & Heine, R.J. (2001). Monitoring of psychological well-being in outpatients with diabetes: effects on mood, HbA(1c), and the patient's evaluation of the quality of diabetes care: a randomized controlled trial. *Diabetes Care, 24*(11), 1929–1935.

Powell, E. (2013). *Catharsis in psychology and beyond. A historic overview.* Baltimore, MD: IPA. http://primal-page.com/cathar.htm.

Prins, P.J.M. & Bosch, J.D. (1998). *Methoden en technieken van gedragstherapie bij kinderen en jeugdigen.* Houten: Bohn Stafleu van Loghum.

Quality of Life Research Unit of the University of Toronto (2014). http://sites.utoronto.ca/qol/

Querido, B. & Querido, N. (2008). *Hulpgids: de gids voor de geestelijke gezondheidszorg (2008).* Hilversum: Praktijk Querido. http://www.hulpgids.nl.

Rakoff, V. (1985). A psychiatric odyssey. *Saturday Night* (February).

Radical Therapist Collectief (1974). *Radicale therapie.* Amsterdam: Bert Bakker.

Ramsay, R.W. (1979). Rouwtherapie. In: *Handboek gedragstherapie* (p. 5). Deventer: Van Loghum Slaterus.

Rando, T.A. (1984). *Grief, dying and death: clinical interventions for caregivers.* Champaign, IL: Research Press.

Rando, T.A. (1993). *Treatment of complicated mourning.* Champaign, IL: Research Press.

Rapaport, L. (1962). The state of crisis: some theoretical considerations. *Social Service Review, 36*(June), 211–217.

Raphael, B. (1983). *The anatomy of bereavement.* New York: Basic Books.

Rasheed, J.M., Rasheed, M.N. & Marley, J.A. (2011). *Family therapy models and techniques.* Thousand Oaks: SAGE.

Reckman, P. (1971). *Naar een strategie en methodiek voor socialisatie.* Baarn: Anthos.

Redmond, L.M. (1989). *Surviving when someone you loved was murdered.* Clearwater: Education Services, Inc.

Reichert, E. (2003, 2011). *Social work and human rights: a:a foundation for policy and practice.* New York: Columbia University Press.

Reid, W.J. (1978). *The task-centered system.* New York: Columbia University Press.

Reid, W.J. (1982). *Het taakgericht systeem. Theorie en praktijk van de taakgerichte benadering in de sociale dienstverlening.* Deventer: Van Loghum Slaterus.

Reid, W.J. (1995). *Taakgerichte strategieën, een hulpverleningsmodel gericht op het activeren van cliënten*. Houten: Bohn Stafleu van Loghum.

Reid, W.J. (1997). Evaluating the dodo's verdict: do all interventions have equivalent outcomes? *Social Work Research, 21*(1), 5–16.

Renwick, R., Brown, I. & Nagler, M. (1996). *Quality of lifel in health promotion and rehabilitation; conceptual approaches, issues and applications*. Toronto: SAGE.

Reynolds, B.C. (1932). *The discovery of need, 1880–1914: a casestudy of the development of an idea in social welfare thought*. New York: Oriole.

Richmond, M.E. (1917). *Social diagnosis*. New York: Russell Sage Foundation.

Richmond, M.E. (1922). *What is social casework? An introductory description*. New York: Russell Sage Foundation.

Ricotti, S. (2015). *Bounce back*. eBOOK.

Riet, N. van (1987). *Groepswerk in het maatschappelijk werk als bijdrage tot emancipatie. Handboek maatschappelijk werk*. Alphen aan den Rijn: Samsom.

Riet, N. van (2006). *Social work. Mensen helpen tot hun recht te komen*. Assen: Van Gorcum.

Riet, N. van & Wouters, H. (1985). *Helpen = leren. Politiserend maatschappelijk werk als bijdrage tot emancipatie*. Nijmegen: Dekker & Van der Vegt.

Riet, N. van & Wouters, H. (2000). *Casemanagement. Een leer-werkboek over de organisatie van de zorg en hulp- en dienstverlening*. Assen: Van Gorcum.

Robertson, A. (1998). Critical reflections on the politics of need: implications for public health. *Social Science and Medicine, 47*(10), 1419–1430.

Roeck, B.P. de (1977). *De loernoot. Therapie en maatschappij*. Haarlem: De Toorts.

Roelens, A. (1983). *Job stress and burnout among staff nurses in acute-care hospitals*. Niet-gepubliceerde doctoraatsthesis. New York: New York University, Department of Psychology.

Roelens, A. (1991). Leren functioneren in complexe en veeleisende situaties – het geval van burnout in de verpleging. *Acta Hospitalia, 2*, 17–26.

Rogers, C.R. (1942). *Counseling and psychotherapy. Newer concepts in practice*. Boston, MA: Houghton Mifflin.

Rogers, C.R. (1951). *Client-centered therapy: its current practice, implications and theory*. Boston, MA: Houghton Mifflin.

Roggema, R. (1979). Co-counseling: een zelfhelp-therapie. In: *Leren en leven met groepen. Handleiding voor het werken met groepen*. Alphen aan den Rijn: Samsom.

Römkens, R. (2015). Wat de politie wél had kunnen doen voor verpleegkundige Linda. *NRC*. http://www.nrc.nl/next/2015/08/25/wat-de-politie-wel-had-kunnen-doen-voor-verpleegku-1526237 (25 August).

Roos, S. de (2001). *Diagnostiek en planning in de hulpverlening. Een dynamische cyclus*. Bussum: Coutinho.

Roscam Abbing, E.W. (1994). *Het hoort er gewoon bij*. Bunnik: Landelijke Vereniging van Thuiszorg.

Rosmalen, J. van (1999). *Het woord aan de verbeelding. Spel en kunstzinnige middelen in het sociaal-agogisch werk*. Houten: Bohn Stafleu van Loghum.

Rothman, J. (2002). Approaches to community intervention. In: Rothman, J., Ehrlich, J. & Tropman, J. (eds.), *Strategies of community intervention*. Itasca, IL: Peacock.

Rubak, S., Sandbaek, A., Lauritzen, T. & Christensen, B. (2005). Motivational interviewing: a systematic review and meta-analysis. *British Journal of General Practice, 55*(513): 305–312.

Rubenstein, R.E. (1999). Conflict resolution and the structural sources of conflict. In: Jeong, H.-W. (ed.), *Conflict resolution: dynamics, process, and structure* (pp. 173–195). Aldershot: Ashgate.

Rubin, L.B. (1997). *Het onverwoestbare kind*. Amsterdam: Ambo.

Rubin, R. (1990). Social networks and mourning: a comparative approach. *Omega, 21*(2), 113–127.

Rudestam, K.E. (1977). The impact of suicide among the young. *Essence, 1*, 221–224.

Rumbaut, R.D. & Rumbaut, R.G. (1976). The family in exile: Cuban expatriates in the US. *American Journal of Psychiatry, 133*(4), 395–399.

Saleebey, D. (2006). *The strengths perspective in social work practice* (4th edition). Boston: Pearson/Allyn & Bacon.

Sarafino, E.P. (1998). *Health psychology: biopsychosocial interactions*. New York: Wiley.

Sartre, J.-P. (1960). *Critique de la raison dialectique* [Kritiek van de dialectische rede]. Parijs: Gallimard.

SATER (2002). *Self Administered Treatment Evaluation Rating*. Utrecht: Verwey-Jonker Instituut.

Satir, V. (1975). *Mensen maken mensen*. Deventer: Van Loghum Slaterus.

Satir, V. (1978). *Mensen maken mensen. De kunst om een gezin beter te laten functioneren*. Houten: Bohn Stafleu van Loghum.

Satir, V. (1982). The therapist and family therapy: process model. In: Horne, A.M. & Ohlsen, M.M. (ed.), *Family counseling and therapy* (pp. 12–42). Itasca, IL: F.E. Peacock.

Satir, V. (1983). *Conjoint family therapy*. Palo Alto, CA: Science and Behavior Books.

Satir, V. (1988). *New peoplemaking*. Palo Alto: Science and Behavior Books.

Satir, V. (1990). *Peoplemaking*. London: Souvenir Press.

Satir, V. & Baldwin, M. (1984). *Satir step by step: a guide to creating change in families*. Palo Alto, CA: Science and Behavior Books.

Schaaf, J. (2007). *Dialectiek en praktijk*. Budel: Uitgeverij Damon.

Schaap, C.P.D.R., Widenfelt, B.M. van & Gerlsma, C. (2000). *Behandelprotocol bij partnerrelatieproblematiek*. Nijmegen: Cure & Care.

Scheff, T.J. (2001). *Catharsis in healing, ritual, and drama*. Lincoln, NE: Universe.com.

Scheller-Dikkers, S.M. (1998). Waar woorden tekortschieten. *Systeemtherapie, 10*(3), 157–174.

Scholte, M. (1995). *Wegen en overwegen*. Utrecht: NIZW.

Scholte, M. (1998). *Psycho-sociale screening in de arbeidssituatie*. Utrecht: NIZW.

Scholte, M. (2002). Mediation in maatschappelijk werk. *Maatwerk, 3*.

Scholte, M. & Menger, R. (1999). Mediation: onafhankelijke geschilbeslechting. *Maatwerk: vakblad voor maatschappelijk werk, 5*, 16–19.

Scholte, M. & Splunteren, P. van (1997). *Opgelet! Systematisch signaleren in het maatschappelijk werk*. Utrecht: NIZW.

Schön, D.A. (1983). *The reflective practitioner: how professionals think in action*. New York: Basic Books/Harper Collins.

Schön, D.A. (1983). *The reflective practitioner: How professionals think in action*. New York: Basic Books. (Reprinted in 1995).

Schrameijer, F. (1990). *Sociale steun. Analyse van een paradigma*. Utrecht: NcGv.

Schreurs, M. & Wiersma, D. (1992). Chronische psychiatrische patiënten in Midden-Twente: een epidemiologisch onderzoek naar hun functioneren en hun zorgbehoefte. *Tijdschrift voor Psychiatrie, 34*, 255–267.

Schröer, K. (1991). *Ziekteverzuim wegens overspanning. Een onderzoek naar de aard van overspanning, de hulpverlening en het verzuimbeloop*. Maastricht: Universitaire Pers.

Schultz, D.P. & Schultz, S.E. (2004). *A history of modern psychology* (8th edition). Belmont, CA: Wadsworth/Thompson.

Schut, H.A., Keijser, J. de, Bout, J. van den & Stroebe, M.S. (1996). Cross-modality grief therapy: description and assessment of a new program. *Journal of Clinical Psychology, 52*(3), 357–365.

Schutz, W. (1975). *Allemaal! Lichaamsgeest en encounter-cultuur*. The Hague: Bakker.

Schwartz, W. (1971). Social group work: the interactionist approach. In: *Encyclopedia of social work*. Vol. II (pp. 1252–1263). New York: Columbia University Press.

Scott, T. & Eber, L. (2003). Functional assessment and wraparound as systemic school responses. Primary, secondary, and tertiary systems examples. *Journal of Positive Behaviour Interventions, 5*(3), 131–149.

Seeman, T.E., Lusignolo, T.M., Albert, M. & Berkman, L. (2001). Social relationships, social support, and patterns of cognitive aging in healthy, high-functioning older adults: MacArthur studies of successful aging. *Health Psychology, 20*, 243–255.

Seligman, M.E.P. (1975a). *Human helplessness: theory applications*. New York: Academic Press.

Seligman, M.E.P. (1975b). *Helplessness*. San Francisco: Freeman.

Selye, H. (1956). *The stress of life*. New York: McGraw-Hill.

Selye, H. (1974). *Stress without distress*. Toronto: McClelland & Stewart.

Shaffer, J.B.D. & Galinsky, M.D. (1977). *Groepstherapie en sensitivitytraining*. Deventer: Van Loghum Slaterus.

Shapiro, A.K. (1976). The behavior therapies: therapeutic breakthrough or latest fad? *American Journal of Psychiatry, 133,* 154–159.

Sheafor, B.W. & Horejsi, C.R. (2003). *Techniques and guidelines for social work practice* (6th edition). Boston, MA: Allyn & Bacon.

Sheldon, B. & Macdonald, G. (2009). *A textbook of social work*. Abingdon: Routledge.

Shontz, F.C. (1965). Reaction to crisis. *Volta Review, 67*(5), 364–370.

Shontz, F.C. & Fink, S. (1961). A method for evaluating psychosocial adjustment of chronically ill. *American Journal of Physical Medicine, 40,* 63–69.

Shoup, R. & Lenson, B. (2000). *Take control of your life: how to control fate, luck, chaos, karma, and life's other unruly forces*. New York: McGraw-Hill.

Silver, R.L., Boon, C. & Stones, M.H. (1983). Searching for meaning in misfortune: Making sense of incest. *Journal of Social Issues* 39, 81–102.

Silver, R.L. & Wortman, C.B. (1980). Coping with undesirable life events. In: Garaber, J. & Seligman, M.E.P. (ed.), *Human helplessness: theory and applications* (pp. 279–340). New York: Academic Press.

Simon, B.L. (1970). Theorieën van social casework: een overzicht. In: Roberts, R.W. & Nee, R.H. (ed.), *Theorieën van social casework*. Deventer: Van Loghum Slaterus.

Simon, B.L. (1994). *The empowerment tradition in American social work: a history*. New York: Columbia University Press.

Siporin, M. (1972). Situationele beoordeling en interventie. *Social Casework* (February), febr. 93–109.

Sipsma, D.H. (1973). Het wankele evenwicht. *Nederlands Tijdschrift voor Gerontologie, 4*(1), 13–22.

S'Jacob, R., Melief, W. & Broenink, N. (1997). *Maatschappelijk belang Algemeen Maatschappelijk Werk*. Utrecht: Verwey-Jonker Instituut.

Skinner, H., Steinhauer, P. & Sitarenios, G. (2000). Family assessment measure (FAM) and process model of family functioning. *Journal of Family Therapy, 22,* 190–210.

Sluiter, S., Zijderveld, M. van & Traas, M. (1996). *Signalering in het maatschappelijk werk*. Houten: Bohn Stafleu van Loghum.

Smits, W.C.M., Cassee, A.F. e.a. (1977). Gestalttherapie. In: *Psychotherapie in Nederland*. Deventer: Van Loghum Slaterus.

Snellen, A. (2000). *Basismodel voor methodisch hulpverlenen in het maatschappelijk werk*. Bussum: Coutinho.

Snellen, A. (2002). Vijftig jaar methodiek. Naar een eclectisch-integratieve benadering. *Maatwerk, 2,* april.

Social Work Policy Institute (2010). *Hospice social work: linking policy, practice, and research*. Washington, DC: National Association of Social Workers.

Spicer, C.C., Stewart, D.N. & Winser, D.M. (1942). Incidence of perforated peptic ulcer: effects of heavy air raids. *Lancet, 239,* 259–261.

Steiner, C.M. (1975). *Radicale psychiatrie*. Amsterdam: Bert Bakker.

Steinfort, A. (1999). *Herwaarderingscounselen. Heeft het HC een toegevoegde waarde voor het maatschappelijk werk in de ogen van maatschappelijk werkers? Eindwerkstuk*. Groningen: Hanzehogeschool Groningen.

Steinhauer, P.D., Santa-Barbara, J. & Skinner, H. (1984). The process model of family functioning. *Canadian Journal of Psychiatry, 29*(2), 77–88.

Stroebe, M.S. & Stroebe, W. (1985). Social support and the alleviation of loss. In: Sarason, I.G. & Sarason, B.R. (ed.), *Social support: theory, research and applications* (pp. 439–462). Dordrecht: Martinus Nijhoff.

Sulman, J., Savage, D., Vrooman, P. & McGillivray, M. (2004). Social group work: building a professional collective of hospital social workers. *Social Work in Health Care, 39*(3–4), 287–307.

Sundel, M. & Sundel, S. (1999). *Behavorial change in the human services*. Thousand Oaks: SAGE.

Sundell, K. & Vinnerljung, B. (2004). Outcomes of family group conferencing in Sweden. A 3-year follow-up. *Child Abuse & Neglect, 28*(3), 267–287.

Suzuki, S. (1980). *Zen mind, beginner's mind*. Los Altos, CA: Weatherhill.

Sweet, E., Nandi, A., Adam, E.K. & McDade, T.W. (2013). The high price of debt: household financial debt and its impact on mental and physical health. *Social Science & Medicine, 91,* 94–100.

Swildens, H. (1999). *Leerboek gesprekstherapie. De cliëntgerichte benadering*. Maarssen: Elsevier gezondheidszorg.

Taylor, S.E. (1989). *Positive illusions: creative selfdeception and the healthy mind.* New York: Basic Books.

Taylor, S.E. (2011). Social support: a review. In: Friedman, M.S. (ed.), *The handbook of health psychology* (pp. 189–214). New York: Oxford University Press.

TCC Group (Raynor, J., York, P. & Sim, S.) (2009). *Effective advocacy organization.* San Francisco: TCC Group.

Teleac (1992). *Omgaan met stress.* Baarn: Tirion.

Thompson, N. (1992). *Existentialism and social work.* Aldershot: Averbury.

Thompson, N. (2004). *Theory and practice in human services.* Buckingham: Open University Press.

Thompson, N. (2009). *People skills.* Basingstoke: Palgrave Macmillan.

Thompson, N. (2011). *Promoting equality: Working with diversity and difference*, 3rd edition. Basingstoke: Palgrave Macmillan.

Thompson, N. (2015). *People skills*, 2nd edition. Basingstoke: Palgrave.

Thompson, N. (2016). *Anti-discriminatory practice*, 6th edition. London: Palgrave Macmillan.

Thyer, B.A. & Wodarski, J.S. (1998). *Handbook of empirical social work practice.* New York: Wiley.

Thyer, B.A. & Wodarski, J.S. (ed.) (2006). *Social work in mental health: an evidence-based approach.* Hoboken, NJ: Wiley.

Thyer, B.A. (2001). *The handbook of social work research practice.* New York: Sage.

Tienen, A.J.M. van & Zwanikken, W.A.C. (1972). *Opbouwwerk als sociaal-agogische methode.* Deventer: Van Loghum Slaterus.

Tinnemans, W. (1993). Burnout onder hulpverleners. *De Gazet*, 7.

Tomm, K. (1980). Towards a cybernetic approach to family therapy at the University of California. In: Freeman, D.S. (ed.), *Perspectives on Family Therapy.* Vancouver: Butterworth Co.

Towl, C. (1945). *Human behavior in the social environment: common human needs.* Silver Spring, MD: National Association of Social Workers.

Trevithick, P. (2012). *Social work skills and knowledge: a practice handbook.* Berkshire: Open University Press.

Tuckman, B.W. (1965). Development sequence in small groups. *Psychological Bulletin, 63*(6), 384–399.

Turner, F.J. (1986). *Social work treatment.* New York: Free Press.

Turner, K.M.T., Sanders, M.R. & Dadds, C.M. (2007). *Handboek voor begeleiders van Triple P Basiszorg.* Utrecht: Nederlands Jeugdinstituut.

Uchino, B. (2009). Understanding the links between social support and physical health: a lifespan perspective with emphasis on the separability of perceived and received support. *Perspectives on Psychological Science, 4*, 236–255.

Ussel, J. van (1975). *Intimiteit.* Deventer: Van Loghum Slaterus.

Vaihinger, H. (1913). *Die Philosophie des Als Ob.* Berlijn: Reuther & Reichard. (English translation: Vaihinger, H. (1924), *The philosophy of as if: a system of the theoretical, practical and religious fictions of mankind.* London: Routledge & Kegan.)

Vahtera, J., Kivimäki, M., Pentti, J., Linna, A., Virtanen, M., Virtanen, P. & Ferrie, J.E. (2004). Organizational downsizing, sickness absence, and mortality: 10-town prospective cohort study. *British Medical Journal* (6 March): 328–338.

Vandereycken, W. (1990). *Handboek psychopathologie.* Houten: Bohn Stafleu van Loghum.

Vandereycken, W. & Deth, R. van (2003). *Psychotherapie. Van theorie tot praktijk.* Houten: Bohn Stafleu van Loghum.

Vandereycken, W., Hoogduin, C.A.L. & Emmelkamp, P.M.G. (2008). *Handboek psychopathologie* (4th edition). Houten: Bohn Stafleu van Loghum.

Vansteenwegen, A. (1999). *Liefde is een werkwoord. Spelregels voor een relatie.* Rielt: Lannoo.

Vansteenwegen, A. (2001). *Helpen bij partnerrelatieproblemen.* Houten: Bohn Stafleu van Loghum.

Vasalis, M. (1954). Vergezichten en gezichten van Oorschot. See also: James Brockway, 'Seven Poems by M. Vasalis'. In: *The Low Countries.* Jaargang 5. Stichting Ons Erfdeel, Rekkem 1997–1998.

Velden, K. van der (1980). Een indeling van directieve interventies. In: *Directieve therapie 2.* Houten: Van Loghum Slaterus.

Velden, P.G. van der (1997). *Handboek voor opvang na rampen.* Utrecht: Instituut voor Psychotrauma.

Velden, P.G. van der, Eland, J. & Kleber, R.J. (1997). *Handboek voor opvang na rampen en calamiteiten.* Zaltbommel: Thema.

Velink-Roosjen, H. (1998). *Het nut van de vraag naar medicijngebruik in de anamnese*. Interne publicatie auteur.

Verhofstad-Denève, L. (1994). *Zelfreflectie en persoonlijkheidsontwikkeling*. Leuven: Acco.

Vermeulen, E. (2001). Eerste hulp bij familievetes. *Libelle, 34*, 38.

Vervoort, M. & Weiland, M. (2003). *Therapiewijzer. Theorie en praktijk van 21 psychotherapieën*. Amsterdam: De Arbeiderspers.

Vinter, E.D. (1967). Program activities: an analysis of their effects on participant behavior. In: Vinter, R.D. (ed.), *Readings in group work practice* (pp. 95–109). Ann Arbor: Campus Publishers.

Vinter, E.D. & Galinski, M.J. (1967). Extra-group relations and approaches. In: Vinter, R.D. (ed.), *Readings in group work practice* (pp. 110–122). Ann Arbor: Campus Publishers.

Viorst, J. (1989). *Noodzakelijk verlies. De liefdes, illusies, afhankelijkheid en irreële verwachtingen die wij allen moeten opgeven om te kunnen groeien*. Baarn: Anthos.

Viscott, D. (1977). *The language of feelings: a wise doctor's unique prescription for putting more joy and freedom into your life!* New York: Pocket Books.

Viscott, D. (1996). *Emotional resilience: simple truths for dealing with the unfinished business of your past*. New York: Three Rivers Press.

Visser, A.H. (1997). Trauma en ouderschap. Over hoe het verleden kan 'rondzingen' in het heden. *Maandblad voor de Geestelijke Volksgezondheid, 6* (June).

Vitalo, A., Fricchione, J., Casali, M., Berdichevsky, Y., Hoge, E.A., Rauch, S.L. e.a. (2009). Nest making and oxytocin comparably promote wound healing in isolation reared rats. *PLOS One, 4*(5), e5523.

Vonk, W. (1995). De kracht van schouderklopjes. *Intermediair, 31*, 37, 51.

Vosler, N. (1990). Assessing family access to basic resources. An essential component of social work practice. *Social Work, 35*(5), 434–441.

Vries, S. de (1997). Ervaringsgerichte psychosociale hulpverlening. In: *De lerende professie. Hoofdlijnen van het maatschappelijk werk* (pp. 84–97). Utrecht: SWP.

Vries, S. de (2002). Kortdurende oplossingsgerichte therapie. *Maatwerk* (juni).

Waaldijk, B. (1996). *Het Amerika der vrouw; sekse en geschiedenis van het maatschappelijk werk in Nederland en de Verenigde Staten*. Groningen: Studio Woltersgroep.

Wagner, B., Knaevelsrud, C. & Maercker, A. (2006). Internet-based cognitive-behavioral therapy for complicated grief: a randomized controlled trial. *Death Studies, 30*(5), 429–453.

Wakefield, J.C. (1988). Psychotherapy, distributive justice, and social work – part 1: distributive justice as a conceptual framework for social work. *Social Service Review, 62*(2), 187–211.

Wallerstein, J.S. (1991). The long-term effects of divorce on children: a review. *Journal of the American Academy of Child & Adolescent Psychiatry*, 30(3), 349–360.

Wallerstein, J.S. & Blakeslee, S. (1989). *Second chances: men, women, and children a decade after divorce*. New York: Ticknor & Fields.

Walsh, F. (Ed.). (2012). *Normal family processes*. New York: Guilford Press.

Warren G. Bennis, Kenneth D. Benne and Robert Chin (Editors). *The Planning of Change*. New York: Holt, Rine-hart & Winston.

Wasserman, C., Hoven, C.W., Wasserman, D., Carli, V., Sarchiapone, M., Al-Halabi, S. e.a. (2012). Suicide prevention for youth – a mental health awareness program: lessons learned from the Saving and Empowering Young Lives in Europe (SEYLE) intervention study. *BMC Public Health, 12*, 776.

Wasserman, D., Hoven, C.W., Wasserman, C., Wall, M., Eisenberg, R., Hadlaczky, G. e.a. (2015). School-based suicide prevention programmes: the SEYLE cluster-randomised, controlled trial. *Lancet, 385*(9977), 1536–1544.

Watson, J.C., Gordon, L.B., Stermac, L., Kalogerakos, F. & Steckley, P. (2003). Comparing the effectiveness of process-experiential with cognitive-behavioral psychotherapy in the treatment of depression. *Journal of Consulting and Clinical Psychology, 71*, 773–781.

Watzlawick, P., Beavin, J.H. & Jackson, D.D. (1970). *De pragmatische aspecten van de menselijke communicatie*. Deventer: Van Loghum Slaterus.

Webber, M., Reidy, H., Ansari, D., Stevens, M. & Morris, D. (2015). Enhancing social networks: a qualitative study of health and social care practice in UK mental health services. *Health & Social Care in the Community, 23*(2), 180–189.

Weiner, G. (2012). A call for evidence based standards for mediator quality. *Professional Standards and Ethics.* Paper 2. http://www.civiljustice.info/profstan/2.

Wellman, B. (1985). From social support to social network. In: Sarason, I.G. & Sarason, B.R. (ed.), *Social support: theory, research and applications* (pp. 205–222). Dordrecht: Martinus Nijhoff.

Wertheim-Cahen, T. (1994a). De klei heeft mij mondig gemaakt. *Maandblad voor Geestelijke Volksgezondheid, 4.*

Wertheim-Cahen, T. (1994b). *Getekend bestaan. Beeldend-creatieve therapie met oorlogsgetroffenen.* Utrecht: ICODO.

Westerink, D. (2014). Online rouwen. De kracht van social media in tijden van verlies. In: Maes, J. & Modderman, H. (ed.), *Handboek rouw, rouwbegeleiding en rouwtherapie: tussen presentie en interventie.* Antwerpen: Witsand Uitgevers.

Whan, M.W. (1979). Accounts, narratives, and case histories. *British Journal of Social Work, 27,* 389–499.

White, M. & Epston, D. (1990). *Narrative means to therapeutic ends.* New York: Norton.

WHO (1948). *The WHO definition of health.* Preamble to the Constitution of the World Health Organization as adopted by the International Health Conference, New York, 19–22 June, 1946; signed on 22 July 1946 by the representatives of 61 states (Official Records of the World Health Organization, no. 2, p. 100) and entered into force on 7 April 1948.

Williams, J.E. (1984). Secondary victimization – confronting public attitudes about rape. *Victimology, 9*(1), 66–81.

Winn, R.L. (1981). *Retrospective evaluations of marital interaction and post bereavement adjustment in widowed individuals.* Dissertatie. Evanston, IL: Northwest University.

Winnubst, J.A.M. (2002). *Praktijkboek gezond werken. Succesvolle oplossingen voor de professional bij somatische, psychische en psychosociale klachten in organisaties.* Maarssen: Elsevier.

Winter, F. (2003). *De pijn de baas.* Z.p.: Ruitenberg Boek.

Witkin, S.L. (1998). Human rights and social work. *Social Work, 43*(3), 197–201.

Witte, L. (1997). *Materiële hulpverlening.* Houten: Bohn Stafleu van Loghum.

Wittgenstein, L. (1990). *Tractatus logico-philosophicus.* Oxford: Routledge.

Wodarski, J.S. & Feit, M.D. (2011). Adolescent preventive health and team-games-tournaments: five decades of evidence for an empirically based paradigm. *Social Work in Public Health, 26*(5), 482–512.

Wolf, S. (1971). Psychosocial forces in myocardial infarction and sudden death. In: Levi, E. (ed.), *Society, stress and disease.* Vol. I (pp. 324–330). London: Oxford University Press.

Worden, J.W. (1992). *Verdriet en rouw: gids voor hulpverleners en therapeuten.* Amsterdam: Swets & Zeitlinger.

Wortman, C.B. & Lehman, D.R. (1985). Reactions to victims of life crises: support attempts that fail. In: Sarason, I.G. & Sarason, B.R. (ed.), *Social support: theory, research and applications* (pp. 463–489). Dordrecht: Martinus Nijhoff.

Wronka, J. (1992). The relation between needs and rights. In: Wronka, J. (ed.), *Human rights and social policy in the 21st century. A history of the idea of human rights and comparison of the United Nations Universal Declaration of Human Rights with United States federal and state constitutions* (revised edition) (pp. 23–25). Lanham, MD: University Press of America.

Wronka, J. (2008). *Human rights and social justice: action and service for the helping and health professions.* Lanham, MD: SAGE.

Wyatt, T.H. & Hauenstein, E. (2008). Enhancing children's health through digital story. *Computers Informatics Nursing, 26*(3), 142–148.

Wyckoff, H. (1979). *Vrouwenpraatgroepen. Feministische Oefengroepen Radikale Therapie.* Amsterdam: Bert Bakker.

Young, J.E. (1999). *Cognitieve therapie voor persoonlijkheidsstoornissen. Een schemagerichte benadering.* Vertaling: Pijnaker, H. Houten: Bohn Stafleu van Loghum.

Young, J.E., Klosko, J.S. & Weishaar, M. (2003). *Schema Therapy: a practitioner's guide.* New York: Guilford.

Zang, Y., Hunt, N. & Cox, T. (2013). A randomised controlled pilot study: the effectiveness of narrative exposure therapy with adult survivors of the Sichuan earthquake. *BMC Psychiatry, 13,* 41.

Zimmerman, M.A. (1990). Toward a theory of learned hopefulness: a structural model analysis of participation and empowerment. *Journal of Research in Personality, 24,* 71–86.

INDEX

Note: Italicized page numbers indicate a figure on the corresponding page. Page numbers in bold indicate a table on the corresponding page.

4G technique (cognitive method) 216

absolution technique (family method) 341–2
ACT (Acceptance Commitment Therapy) 6
action technique (collective advocacy) 413–14
activation technique (body work method) 121–2
active listening 86
active process 98
addictive behavior 251–2
addressing technique (family method) 338
advising technique (practical material method) 136
advocacy by social workers 45
Advocacy Core Capacity Assessment Tool (Advocacy CCAT) 416
advocacy reports (collective advocacy method) 414–15
advocacy technique (practical material method) 136–7
affection brain 160–2, 444–5
affection-focused methods 79, 157
affection needs 41–2, 285
affirmation, defined 277–8
aggressive behavior 253
American Academy of Hospice and Palliative Medicine (AAHPM) 433
American Psychological Association 164
amusement technique (group work method) 355
amygdala function 110–11, *111*
appraisal technique (mediation method) 373
aquarium technique (group work method) 355
assessment technique (family method; case management method) 364–5

attention, defined 276–7
attention balance technique (cathartic method) 170
attention technique (relationship focused method) 305, **306**
autonomous nervous system 110–11
avoidance: behavior 251–2; coping/support 497–9, *498*, 506–10
awareness needs 39–40

bad news interviews **457**, 457–8
basic resources checklist (monitoring method) 383, **383–4**
Beck, Aaron 209
behavior, defined 250–3
Behavioral Change in the Human Services (Sundel, Sundel) 254
behavioral method: behavior, defined 250–3; case example 247; conditioning technique 260; constructive criticism (CC) technique 261; contraindications 256; diary technique 257; evidence 262–3; feeling yes-feeling no technique 260; general goal 256; history of 253–5, *254*; indications 256; informal carer 248–9; introduction 24–5, 247; modelling technique 259; nurturing technique 260–1, **261**; personal territories 249; pitfalls 263; prompting technique 259; self-control technique 260; shaping technique 259; skill deficiency questions 248–53; social work results 262; SOSKI technique 250, 257–9; specific goals 256; standardization technique 261; summary 263; task-oriented

technique 260; territorial defence skills 249–50

Bell, Norman 330

bibliotherapy 176

Binding Force of Family Relationships, The (Dykstra) 330

bio-energetics therapy 118

biofeedback technique (body work method) 123

biographical technique (expression method) 179–80

biopsychological (BPS) thinking 59

blamer, in destructive communication 323

blind spot in social work 119

blood ties 314–15

blow-off-steam technique (mediation method; relationship-focused method) 307, 374

body image technique (body work method) 122–3

body language in SBVP technique (non-directive core method) 94, **94**

body of knowledge 421

body response to loss 112–13

body territory 300–1

bodywork method: activation technique 121–2; biofeedback technique 123; body image technique 122–3; breathing technique with visualization 121; case example 109–10, 121, 127; contraindications 119–20; decontamination technique 125; diary technique 123–4; evidence for 127; fight-flight-freeze response 110–11, *111*; focusing technique 123; general goals 119; history of 118–19; indications 119–20; introduction 109; physical awareness technique 122; pitfalls with 127; relaxation technique 120–1; scaling techniques 126; segment reflex and psychosomatics 115; self-touching technique 120; SNARE technique 125–6; social work results 127; specific goals 119; stress with loss and trauma 111–14, *114*; survival brain and survival reflex 110–18; touching technique 124

brain functioning: affection brain 160–2, 444–5; oxytocin hormone 161; rational brain 444–5; rational brain function 197–9, *198*; survival brain and survival reflex 110–18

brain matrix **443**, 443–4

breathing technique with visualization (body work method) 121

British Association of Social Workers 414

Brown, Brené 50

budgeting technique (practical material method) **137**, 137–8

burnout syndrome: failure to recognize 517–18; lack of autonomy 518; lack of growth opportunities 518; lack of knowledge/skills 520; not recognizing signs of 520; over/under-burdening **515**, 515–16; overview 514–15; personal factors 519; risk factors **516**, 516–17; signs of 515; stressful work climate 518; transitions in life 520; unrealistic expectations 520; workload factors 517

Capability Approach 6

case management (CM) method: assessment technique 364–5; case example 361; contraindications 364; defined 361; evidence 366–9; general goal 363; history of 361–3; indications 363–4; introduction 15, 360; linking technique 365; pitfalls 369; planning technique 365; process evaluation technique 366; social work results 366; specific goal 363; summary 369

cathartic method: affection brain and attachment 160–2; attachment, defined 161; attention balance technique 170; case example 160; contradiction technique 170–1; contraindications 168–9; contrast technique 170; definition and elucidation 162–3; emotional stress 162; empty chair technique 171; evidence 171–2; exposure technique 169; general goal 168; history of 163–8, *166*; indications 168; introduction 159; normalizing technique 169; oxytocin hormone 161; permission technique 169; pitfalls 172; reflective technique 169; repetition technique 171; replacement technique 171; role model technique 171; scanning technique 170; seven affective systems 161–2; social work results 171; specific goal 168; summary 172–3

challenge technique (cognitive method) 214–15

checklists: basic resources checklist 54–5, **55**, **383**–4; building a social work research report 430; checklist: levels of unfinished business indicated for specific social work methods **502**–3; checklist for therapeutic viewing of photos **485**–6; checklist of social support competencies 288, **288**; group work checklist 350–1; individual methods checklist 544–5; Needs awareness checklist 14; needs of children checklist 334, **334**–5; problem solving checklist: step-by-step approach to practical stress 131, **131**–2; relational support checklist 304, **304**–5; rituals checklist: the 9w's of a proper goodbye 189, **189**; Social support checklist **295**; trauma-reactions checklist 536–7; Territorial inventory checklist (TICL) 540–1

checklist of social support competencies 288, **288**

child abuse prevention **392**, 393–4

Child Protective Services (CPS) 293

chronically tense muscle tissue 114

chronicity as stress factor 115–16

chronic stress 117, 499–500

circle of loss 455–7, *456*
circular causal thinking 59–60
Civil Rights Movement 403
Client-Centered (CC) therapy 172
client-centred approach **88**, 88–9
client progress measures 20
closure 41, 501–2, **502–3**
co-counseling 165
codification technique (group work method) 356
Cognitive-Behavioural Therapy (CBT) 172
cognitive method: 4G technique 216; case
  example 214; challenge technique 214–15;
  contraindications 212; control checking
  technique 215–16; diary technique
  213–14; education about mental health
  technique 212–13; evidence 218–19; feeling
  yes-feeling no technique 217; general goal
  211; history of 209–11; indications 211;
  internet-related techniques 218; introduction
  197; normalization technique 213; pitfalls
  219; positive self-imaging technique 215;
  problem-solving cycle 199, **200**, 200–9,
  208; rational brain function 197–9, *198*;
  reality-check technique 213; re-labelling
  technique 216–17; setting norms technique
  217; social work results 218; solution-focused
  technique 217–18; specific goal 211;
  summary 219
cognitive stress and unhelpful thoughts:
  brainstorming solutions 206–7;
  decision-making and 207; goal-setting and
  helpful perspectives 205–6; helpful action
  needs 207; learning cycle 207–9, *208*;
  learning from experience 207; overview
  200; problem-solving cycle 199, **200**, 200–7;
  realistic information needs 201; realistic
  interpretation needs 202–5
cognitive work method 24, 25, 34
Cohn, Ruth 349
collective advocacy (CA) method: action
  technique 413–14; advocacy reports 414–15;
  contraindications 409; defined 401–3;
  disadvantaged groups 404–7, *405*; evidence
  416, 416–19; force field analysis technique
  409, 409–10; general goal 408; health care
  418; health policy 418–19; history of 403–8;
  indications 409; introduction 400; lobbying
  technique 411–13; macro practice, defined
  402; pitfall 419; self-organization technique
  410; social empowerment 407; social media
  technique 413–14, 418; social policy technique
  410–11, **411**; social work results 415; specific
  goals 408; summary 419
collective agreements (CAOs) 54
common factor research 69
communication patterns and grief
  support 464–5

communication technique (family method,
  mediation method, relationship-focused
  method) 5, 305, 337–8, 374
Communities That Care (CTC) practice 396
community care team 366–7
community improvement 380
community organization (CO) method 403
computer/super-reasonable, in destructive
  communication 324
concentration problems stress 205
conditioning technique (behavioral method) 260
connection principle 65
conscious process 98
constructive communication 323
constructive coping 237
constructive criticism (CC) technique
  (behavioral method; relationship-focused
  method) 261, 308
constructivism 87, 223–4
content analysis technique (practice research
  method) 427
contextual approach 314
contract technique (mediation method) 373
contraindications in methodological profiles 76
contrast technique (cathartic method) 170
control, in DUNC needs **232**, 232–4, **234**
control checking technique (cognitive method)
  215–16
convening technique (family method) 333
conversational skills 254
conversion complaints 115
COPE model 262–3
coping aspects with grief 458–9, 461, 463, 464
coping factor in QoL 36, 49–50, 72
core method in social work 68
cost-benefit technique (narrative method) 241
counter-transference 88
covenant technique (mediation method) 374
CPR Institute for Dispute Resolution 372
creative expression 41, 175–6
Creutzfeldt-Jakob's Disease 476
critical attitude principle 66
Critical Incident Stress Debriefing (CISD)
  technique 154
Critique of Dialectical Reason (Sartre) 64
cue recognition 273, 275–6, 280–3
cultural resources 6

decontamination technique (body work
  method) 125
defence mechanism 147–8
Delphi Technique (practice research method) 429
dementia and grief support 475–80, **477**, **478**
dementia carers 367–8
depression 51, 112, 479
destructive communication 323–5
determinism 64

developmental family framework model 322
dialectical existentialism 64–6, **65**
dialectical reasoning principle 66
dialecticism of changes 64
diary technique (behavioral method, body work
    method, cognitive method) 123–4, **124**, 178,
    213–14, 257, **544–5**
differential diagnosis 14
dignity, in DUNC needs **226**, 226–8
direct effect theory 283–5, **284**, **285**
directive individual methods 2, 421
director technique (trauma work method) 152
disadvantaged groups 404–7, *405*
disaster trauma 144
distancing in catharsis 164–5
distractor/irrelevant, in destructive
    communication 324–5
divorce, grief support 464–6
domestic violence prevention 391, *392*
dream stress 204–5
DUNC needs (Dignity, Understanding of Justice,
    Now-in-relation-to-later and Control) 221,
    222–3
Dutch Health Council 425
Dutch Medical Educational Agencies 330
Dutch Mourning Support Association 413
Dutch National Mental Health Day 213
Dutch victim support organization (SHN) 150
dynamic diagnosis hypothesis 14
Dynamics of Planned Change, The (Lippitt) 403
dynamism principle 63
dysfunctional thoughts 210

eating disorders 51
ecomap technique (social network method)
    287–8
education about mental health technique
    (cognitive method) 212–13
effective support 279
Egan, Gerard 17, 87
Ellis, Albert 209, 255
emancipatory approach to social work 5, 98, 405,
    407–8
embarrassment feelings stress 204
emotional bodywork (EB) 118
emotional closeness need 41
Emotional Debt 167
emotionally focused family therapy (EFFT)
    326–7
emotionally focused therapy (EFT) 172, 299,
    309–10, 326–7
*Emotional Resilience: Simple Truths for Dealing With
    the Unfinished Business of Your Past* (Viscott) 167
emotional stress 162
empathy in client-centred approach 89
empowerment technique (non-directive
    core-method) 45, 101–2

empty chair technique (cathartic method) 171
energy meter technique 126
environment enrichment (EE) therapy **53**, 53–4
Epston, David 238–9
ethical foundations of social work 2
European Council Convention 394
evidence-based medicine 424–5
evidence-based physiotherapy 425–6
evidence-based social work 421, 424
evidence in methodological profiles 77
evidence in NDC method 103–4
exclusivity myth 422
exhausting job stress **513**, 513–14
exposure technique 169
expression method: biographical technique
    179–80; case example 175; contraindications
    178; creative expression 175–6; diverse
    techniques 180; evidence 180–2; general
    goal 177; history of 177; indications 177–8;
    introduction 25, 174; phases 176–7; pitfalls
    182; plastic technique 178–9; play technique
    180; social work results 180; specific goal 177;
    summary 182; writing technique 178
expressive writing 180–1
extended-family method 314
externalizing technique (narrative method)
    240–1

Family Access to Basic Resources (FABR) 383,
    383–4
Family Assessment Measure (FAM III) 344
family constellations (family method) 331, 342
family education technique (family method) 341
Family Group Conferences (FGC) 293
family-life cycle perspective 317–18, *318*
family method: absolution technique 341–2;
    addressing technique 338; blood ties 314–15;
    case example 312; communication technique
    337–8; contraindications 332; convening
    technique 333; deficits to strengths 315–17,
    316; defined *313*, 313–18, *316*, *318*; evidence
    343–4; family constellation technique 342;
    family education technique 341; family-life
    cycle perspective 317–18, *318*; general goal
    331; genogram technique *338*, 338–9, *339*,
    340; Growth in Family Functioning Model
    312, *319*, 319–31, **320**; history of 328–31;
    indications 332; introduction 311–12;
    joining technique 333; multifaceted partiality
    technique 341; need assessment technique
    333–4, **334–5**; pitfalls 344; restructuring
    technique 340; rules setting technique 340;
    social work results 343; specific goals 331–2;
    summary 344; systemic/individual techniques
    342; turn taking technique 340–1; wellbeing
    indicators technique *336*, 336–7
Family Network Conference 289–91

family work method 25
farewell stress 184–6
farewell technique (ritual method) 188–90
fatal accident trauma 191
feelings testing 14
feeling yes-feeling no technique (behavioral
  method; cognitive method) 217, 260
fight-flight-freeze response 110–11, *111*, 116,
  147–50, 224
Fighting the Illness, Not the Patient
  (Meulenbelt) 407
final scaling 21
five stages of dying 481
Flexible-ACT (Assertive Community Treatment)
  368–9
focusing technique (body work technique) 123
follow-up technique 153
force field analysis technique (collective advocacy
  method) *409*, 409–10
Foundation Dutch Mediation Institute
  (NMI) 372
Freud, Sigmund 40, 88, 118
Fromm, Erich 40
Fronto-Temporal Dementia (FTD) 476

Gendlin, Gene 87
genogram technique (family method) *338*,
  338–9, *339, 340*
Gestalt therapy 17, 330
'Getting It Right for Every Child'
  programme 313
Global Definition of the Social Work
  Profession 445
goal-setting and helpful perspectives 205–6
goals in methodological profiles 75
grief counselling 254–5
grief groups 182
grief labour 225
grief support: aspects of coping 458–9, 461,
  463, 464, 467, 470–3, **473**, 477; bad news
  interviews **457**, 457–8; for children and young
  people 458–61; circle of loss 455–7, *456*;
  dementia 475–80, **477, 478**; disabled children
  461–3; divorce 464–6; HIV/AIDS 463–4;
  hospice programmes 482–4, **483**; impactful
  work changes 466–9, *468*; introduction 454–7,
  456; loss types/degrees 455; migration issues
  469–75, **471, 472, 473**; palliative social work
  480–4, **481, 483**; photo viewing after trauma
  484–7, **485–6**; pitfalls 461, 462–3, 464, 466,
  469, 475, 480, 484; social work tasks 459–61,
  478, 482; summary 487–8; therapy 163
group crisis intervention 351–3
group education programmes (prevention
  method) 390
group interview technique 427–8, *428*
group phase technique (group work
  method) 353

group work method: amusement technique 355;
  approach to social work 406–7; aquarium
  technique 355; case example 346; central
  area of 352; codification technique 356;
  completion of 352–3; contraindication 349;
  defined 346–7; evidence 357–8; general
  goal 349; group crisis intervention 351–3;
  group phase technique 353; history of
  347–9; indication 349; individual/systemic
  techniques 356–7; introduction 345; pitfalls
  358; problematizing technique 356; recovery
  groups 358; reflecting team technique
  354–5; role-playing technique 355; sandwich
  technique 351; scripting technique 350–1;
  social work results 357; specific goals 349;
  start of 352; summary 358–9; task-oriented
  technique 355; thematic interactional
  technique 353–4, *354*
Growth in Family Functioning Model (GFFM):
  communication between family members
  320, 322–5; emotional involvement of family
  members 320; family structure 325–6; five
  factors 320–8; history of 328–31; introduction
  312, *319*, 319–20, **320**; needs fulfilment of
  family members 320, 321–2, **322**; self-esteem
  of family members 320, 321; structure of
  family members 320
guilty feelings stress 204

hallucination stress 204–5
Handbook of Empirical Social Work Practice (Thyer,
  Wodarski) 254
Health Behaviour Model (HBM) 430
health care advocacy 418
health information 182
health policy advocacy 418–19
Heraclitus (Greek philosopher) 47
highly tense muscle tissue 114
HIV/AIDS, grief support 463–4
HIV patients, unmet needs 430–1
Hollis, Florence 40
homeless and practical material method
  139–40
homicide trauma 144
hospice programmes 482–4, **483**
human freedom concept 64
human needs and rights (HNR) perspective:
  affection brain/rational brain 444–5; case
  example 439, 446–7; classification of 440–1,
  441; defined 447–8; history of 445–6, 451–2;
  introduction 437–8, *438*; neuroscience
  and 441–4, *442, 443*; social justice pursuits
  449–50; social work and 439–44, **441, 442,
  443**, 446–52; summary 452–3; sustainable
  social work 452
Human Rights Commission 448
hurt and loss 166–7
hydraulic model of emotions 163

identification technique (non-directive core
    method) 100
immune system weakness *116*, 116–18, 499–500
impact factor 36, 46–9, *47*, *49*
improvement programs 55–6
inadequate knowledge/skills stress 203–4
inclusion function 280
indications in methodological profiles 76
individual coping 78–9
individually tailored competency 273, 278–9
individual methods of coping 20
individual social work methods 15, 544–5
ineffective support 279–80
informal carer 248–9
information/consultation centres 395
information technique (practical material
    method) 136
Innovative Moments Coding System 245
input-throughput-output cycle 198, *198*
instrumental professionalism 437
interactive social work methods 34
intergenerational method 314
International Association of Schools of Social
    Work (IASSW) 45
International Classification of Human
    Functioning 59
International Declaration of Human Rights 448
International Federation of Social Work (IFSW)
    45, 408
International Labour Organization (ILO) 513
internet-related techniques (cognitive
    method) 218
inventory technique (non-directive core method;
    practical material method) 97, 99, 135–6
Ivey, Allen 87

Jackins, Harvey 165
James, William 62
job stress among social workers: burnout
    syndrome 514–20, **515**, **516**, *519*; introduction
    511–13, *512*; post-traumatic job stress
    520–1; post-traumatic stress disorder 521–2,
    522; preventative actions 525–6, **526**;
    stress-reduction methods 522–3; summary
    526–7; support from work/home 523–5, *524*;
    types of **513**, 513–14
job search support technique (practical material
    method) 138
joining technique (family method) 333
joint social work theory 4

Kadushin, Alfred 87
Kant, Immanuel 224
Kennedy Poverty Program 403

lacking behavior 253
ladder of reflection in social work 3–4, *4*
landscape of action 242

landscape of identity 243
Language, Ordering, Perspectives, Organization
    and Influence/Effort (LOPOI) 474
Language of Feelings, The (Viscott) 166
Leadership Development Program 432
learning cycle 207–9, *208*
learning in SBVP technique (non-directive core
    method) 96–7, **97**
leveler, in constructive communication 323
Lewin, Kurt 48, 420
life-threatening diseases 181
life transitions 46, 185–6, *186*
lightly tense muscle tissue 113–14
limbic brain 160
linking technique (case management
    method) 365
Listening, Summarizing and Empathizing (LSE)
    technique 305–6
Listening, Summarizing and Further Questioning
    (LSFQ) 92
listening and mirroring techniques (SBVP) 90
living on process 49
lobbying technique (collective advocacy method)
    411–13
Lowen, Alexander 118
loyalty problems in families 315
LSE technique (relationship-focused technique)
    299, 305–6

MacGillavry, Donald 298, 299
macro level of intervention 2
macro methods of coping 20, 377
macro practice, defined 402
macro social work methods 15
main theme technique (non-directive core
    method) 100–1
Matryoshka doll technique 92
meaning making in narrative method 234–5
meaning making mechanism 221
media screening (monitoring method) 383
mediation method: appraisal technique 373;
    blow-off steam technique 374; case example
    371; communication technique 374; contract
    technique 373; contraindications 373; covenant
    technique 374; defined 371–2; evidence 375;
    general goal 372; history of 372; indications
    373; introduction 370–1; pitfalls 375; social
    work results 374; specific goals 372; summary
    375; territorial negotiation technique 373, **374**
mental health and social support 51
Mental Health Awareness Programme
    (MHAP) 397
metaphor technique 241–2
metatheoretical level of reflection 4
meters **22**, 23; condition meter **22**; coping meter;
    energy meter 21–2, **22**, 126; impact meter
    22; progress meter 21–3; provisions meter **22**;
    quality-of-life meter condition meter **22**; stress

level meter 21–2, **101**; support meter **22**, 55–6;
tension meter 126
methodological profiles 73–8
migration issues and grief support 469–75, **471,
472, 473**
mind territory 301
Minuchin, Salvador 330
Mirages of Marriage (Lederer, Jackson) 298
modelling technique (behavioral method) 259
monitoring method: basic resources checklist
383, **383**–4; contraindications 382; defined
379–81; development of monitoring systems
386; evidence 385–7; general goal 382;
history of 381; indications 382; introduction
379; media screening 383; peer screening
382–3; pitfalls 387; problem identification
cards 382; for psychological wellbeing 386;
for psychosocial problems 386–7; registration
screening 383; social work results 385; specific
goals 382; summary 387
mood disorders 51
motivational interviewing 104
motivational interview technique (non-directive
core method) 102
multi-causal thinking 59
multicomponent intervention 69–70
multifaceted partiality technique (family
method) 341
multi-infarct dementia 476
multimethodical loss guidance 181
multimethod paradigm 5–6
multimethod social work (MMSW) 47, 70
muscle tension and loss 113–14
musical expression 176
'My World Triangle' resource 333–4

Nagy, Ivan 314, 330
Narrative Exposure Therapy (NET) 245
Narrative Means to Therapeutic Ends (White,
Epston) 238–9
narrative method: case example 222, 225–6,
242, 243; conceptual definition and
elucidation 238–9; constructive coping
237; contraindications 239–40; cost-benefit
technique 241; DUNC needs, control **232**,
232–4, **234**; DUNC needs, dignity **226**, 226–8;
DUNC needs, now-in-relation-to-later **230**,
230–2; DUNC needs, overview 221, 222–3;
DUNC needs, understanding **228**, 228–30;
evidence 244–5; externalizing technique
240–1; general goal 239; history of 237–8;
impact *vs.* helping narrative 223–6; indications
239; introduction 221; meaning making
234–5; metaphor technique 241–2; overview
87; pitfalls 245; reassessment technique 244;
re-labelling technique 241; re-membering
technique 243–4; rewriting technique 242–3;

self-appreciation technique 241; social work
result 244; specific goals 239; summary 246;
zero-dimension 221, *235*, 235–7
National Association of Social Workers 431
National Center for Social Work Research
Act 432
National Health Service (NHS) 414
National Hospice and Palliative Care
Organization (NHPCO) 433
National Institutes of Health (NIH) 432
National Longitudinal Study of Adolescent
Health 140
need assessment technique (family method)
333–4, **334–5**
need for affection 13, 37–8, 39, 41–2
need for an existential (re)orientation 42
need for awareness 39–40; self-awareness 40
need for competency and influence 42
need for physical safety (bio) 39, 40–1
need for psychological safety (psycho) 39, 40–1
need for realistic information processing 42
need for safety
need for self-determination 13, 37–8, 39, 42–3
need for social safety (social) 39, 40–1
need for survival 13, 37–8, 40
needs testing 14
neocortex function 197–9, *198*
network conference (NC) technique (social
network method) 289–91
neuroscience and human needs and rights 441–4,
442, **443**
nominal group technique (non-directive core
method) 429
non-directive core method (NDC method): case
study 24–8; client-centred approach **88**, 88–9;
conceptual definition 84; contraindications 91;
elucidation 84–7, *85*; empowerment technique
101–2; evidence 103–4; general goals 90, 102;
history of 87–90; identification technique
100; identifying client needs 89–90; impact
factor 70–1, *71*; indicators 91; interviewing
techniques 17; introduction 2, 83; inventory
technique 99; main theme technique 100–1;
motivational interview technique 102;
personal filing cabinet (PFC) as structural
tool 97–102, *101*; pitfalls 104; psychosocial
assessment 15; safeguarding confidentiality
technique 99; sandwich technique 99;
SBVP technique **92–3**, 92–7, **94**, **95–6**, **97**,
104; scanning technique 100; social casework
87–8; social worker's toolkit 70; social work
results 102–3; specific goals 90–1, 102–3;
summary 104–5; techniques of 91
non-specific factors 67
non-verbal skills 254
normalization technique 213
normalizing technique (cathartic method) 169

normal muscle tissue 113
normative aspect of professionalism 3
Not Filling in for the Other Person (NFOP) 92
now-in-relation-to-later, DUNC needs **230**, 230–2
nursing home care 181
nurturing technique (behavioral method) 260–1, **261**
Nussbaum, Martha 40

occupational social work (OSW) 408
ontology principle 65
open interview technique (practice research method) 427
Open Society Institute 432
organizational improvement 380–1
outcome-focused methods 20–3, *21*, **22**, 66–70
outreach work 17–19
oxytocin hormone 161

palliative care 432–3
Palliative Social Work (Green, Green) 482–3
palliative social work and grief support 480–4, **481**, **483**
panic disorder 51
parental loss trauma 244, 503–10
participating observations (practice research method) 429–30
Partnerships to Enhance Resilience (PROSPER) partnership 396–7
peer screening (monitoring method) 382–3
Perlman, Helen 40
permission technique (cathartic method) 169
persistent stress 500
personal aspect of professionalism 3
personal failure stress 202–3
personal filing cabinet (PFC): client as expert *12*, 12–13; impact factor 13; introduction 10, 11–13, *12*; narrative method 240; overview 10, 11–13, *12*; as structural tool 97–102, *101*; unfinished business syndrome 509
personal freedom of choice and responsibility principle 65
personal property territory 300
personal space territory 301
personal stress management 525–6
Person-in-Environment Empowerment Theory (PIE-ET) 57–8; affection needs 41–2; awareness needs 39–40; biopsychological thinking 59; case study 31, 32, 34, 37, 39, 40, 41, 43–4; circular causal thinking 59–60; direct effect theory 284; history of social work 546–7; intertwining of QoL factors 56–60, *58*; introduction 3, 31; overview *35*, 35–45, *38*; person-in-environment concept 44–5, 163; pseudo-satisfier needs 43–4; psychosocial assessment 15; psychosocial empowerment

45; Quality of Life *35*, 35–7, 45–56; safety needs 40–1; self-determination need 38, 42–3; social network theory 31–4, *33*; summary 60; support factor importance 267; universal human needs 5–6, 37–44
Phénoménologie de la perception (Merleau-Ponty) 65
photo viewing after trauma 484–7, **485–6**
physical abuse 163
physical awareness technique (body work method) 122
physical complaints 500–1
physical contact by social worker 94
physical health and social support 51–4, **53**
physical safety need 40
pitfalls in methodological profiles 77–8
placator, in destructive communication 323
planning technique (case management method) 365
plastic expression 175–6
plastic technique (expression method) 178–9
play technique (expression method) 180
pluralism principle 63
policy practice, defined 411
positive associations 88
Positive Pedagogical Programme 260–1, **261**
positive self-imaging technique (cognitive method) 215
post-traumatic job stress 520–1
post-traumatic stress disorder (PTSD) 51, 143, 147, 245, 512, 521–2, **522**
post-traumatic stress reaction (PTSR) 143, **143**, **146**, 146–7, 521, **537**
practical assistance in SBVP technique (non-directive core method) 96–7, **97**
practical material method: advising technique 136; advocacy technique 136–7; budgeting technique **137**, 137–8; contraindications 135; debt management 132–3; evidence for 138–40; general goal 135; history of 133–5; homeless and 139–40; indications 135; information technique 136; introduction 24, 129–33, **131–2**; inventory technique 135–6; job search support technique 138; pitfalls 140; referral technique 138; social work results 138; specific goal 135; stress and 130; summary and questions 140
practical research method: content analysis technique 427; contraindications 427; defined 420–2; Delphi Technique 429; evidence 430–3, **432**; evidence-based medicine 424–5; evidence-based physiotherapy 425–6; general goal 426; group interview technique 427–8, *428*; history of 422–6; indications 426; introduction 420; nominal group technique 429; open interview technique 427; participating observations 429–30; pitfalls 433; questionnaire technique 428–9;

scientific research 423–4; social work results 430; specific goals 426; summary 433–4; types of 424

pragmatism **62**, 62–3

preliminary scaling 21

preservation technique (relationship-focused method) 307

prevention method: Communities That Care (CTC) practice 396; contraindications 390; defined 389; efficacy of 398; evidence 395–8, **398**; general goal 390; group education programmes 390; history of 389; indications 390; information/consultation centres 395; introduction 388; Partnerships to Enhance Resilience (PROSPER) partnership 396–7; pitfall 399; project technique 391–4, **392**, *392*; safety net technique 395; schooling programmes 391; social worker engagement in 395–6; social work results 395; specific goal 390; standardization 395; suicide prevention 397–8; summary 399; support groups 391; Teams-Games-Tournaments (TGT) project 397; volunteer support 394–5

private hideout territory 301

problematizing technique (group work method) 356

problem identification cards 382

problem-solving cycle 199, **200**, 200–7, 200–9, *208*

process evaluation technique (case management method) 366

professional expertise in social work 2–3

progress meter in scaling 22–3

Project on Death in America (PDIA) 432

project technique (prevention method) 391–4, **392**, *392*

prompting technique (behavioral method) 259

pseudo-satisfier needs 43–4

psychiatric patients, multidisciplinary collaboration 368–9

psychological complaints 500

psychological safety need 40

psychological space territory 301

psychoneuroimmunology 115–18, *116*, 127

psychopharmaceuticals *166*

psychosocial assessment (PSA): dynamic diagnosis hypothesis 14; outreach work 17–19; overview 10, 14–19, **16**, 72; summary 28

psychosocial empowerment 45

psychosocial intervention (PSI) 10, 19–20, 28

psycho social stress interventions (PSI) 509

psychosomatic reactions 112, 115

psychotherapeutic interventions 67

psychotherapy, outcome research 66–7, **67**

Quality of Life (QoL): case management method 360; coping factor 49–50; human needs and 440; impact factor 46–9, *47*, *49*; interrelated factors in 31; intertwining of factors 56–60, *58*; introduction 1–2, 9; overview of factors 45–56; PIE concept 44–5; PIE-Empowerment Theory *35*, 35–7; social network method 268; stumbling blocks for 11; support factor 36, 51–6, **53**, **55**, 72

Question, Persuade, Refer (QPR) 398

questionnaire technique (practice research method) 428–9

Radical Therapist Collective 406

radical therapy approach to social work 405–6

rational brain 197–9, *198*, 444–5

rational emotive therapy (RET) 209, 210, 255

realistic information needs 201

realistic interpretation needs 202–5

reality-check technique (cognitive method) 213

Reality Orientation Training (ROT) 478–9

reality testing 14

reassessment technique (narrative method) 244

recommendation, defined 422

reconstruction technique (trauma work method) 153

recovery groups 358

referral technique (practical material method) 138

reflecting team technique (group work method) 354–5

reflective technique (cathartic method) 169

reframing technique (cognitive method; narrative method) 216–17, 241

registration screening (monitoring method) 383

Reid, William 254

rejection, defined 278

relational support checklist 304–5, **304–5**

relationship-focused method: attention technique 305, **306**; blow-off-steam technique 307; communication technique 305; constructive criticism (CC) technique 308; contraindications 303–4; definition elucidation 297; evidence 308–9; example case 297; general goal 303; history of 298–9; indications 303; introduction 296–7; LSE technique 305–6; pitfalls 310; preservation technique 307; relational support checklist 304–5, **304–5**; social work results 308; specific goal 303; SRC technique 307; summary 310; territorial aggression 300–2; territorial negotiation technique 307–8; transgressional behaviour 302–3

relaxation technique 120–1

re-membering technique (narrative method) 243–4

repetition technique (cathartic method) 171

replacement technique (cathartic method) 171

restructuring technique (family method) 340

rewriting technique (narrative method) 242–3

Richmond, Mary Ellen 362

RISE (Re-integrative Shaming
   Experiments) 372
Rising Strong (Rubin) 50
ritual method: case example 183, 189–90;
   contraindications 188; custom-made rituals
   184–5; evidence 191; farewell stress 184–6;
   farewell technique 188–90; general goal 187;
   grief instinct 185; history of 186–7; indications
   188; introduction 27, 183; life transitions
   185–6, *186*; pitfalls 193; ritual, defined 184;
   sense of control from rituals 192–3; social
   work results 191; specific goal 187; summary
   193; suspension technique 190; trauma closure
   technique 190; yet-still technique 190
Rogerian counselling 86
Rogers, Carl 17, 40, 88
role model technique 171
role-playing technique (group work method) 355
Rubin, Lilian 50
rules setting technique 340

safeguarding confidentiality technique
   (non-directive core method) 99
safety net technique (prevention method) 395
sandwich technique (non-directive core method,
   group work method) 99, 351
Sartre, Jean-Paul 64
Satir, Virginia 330
Satisfaction Research of Social Work 431
Saving and Empowering Young Lives in Europe
   (SEYLE) 397–8
scaling: functions of 23; outcome-focused
   working with 20–3, *21*, **22**; preliminary
   and final scaling 21; progress meter 22–3;
   techniques 126; techniques and measurements
   21, 21–2, **22**
scanning technique (cathartic method,
   non-directive core method) 100, 170
schema therapy 211
schooling programmes in prevention method 391
Schopenhauer, Arthur 224
Schwartz, William 348
scientific philosophy of reflection 4
scientific research 423–4
Scottish Development Centre for Mental Health
   (SDC) 414
Screening by Professionals (Profscreen)
   programme 398
scripting technique (group work method) 350–1
secondary victimization 34, 490–1
segment reflex and psychosomatics 115
self-appreciation technique (narrative
   method) 241
self-control technique (behavioral method) 260
self-deception 163
self-determination methods 38, 42–3, 79, 195
self-organization technique (collective advocacy
   method) 410

self-statements 206
self-talk 209
self-test traumatic stress 534–5
self-touching technique 120
Sen, Amartya 40
sensory triggers 495–6
setting norms technique (cognitive method) 217
sexual abuse 163
sexual violence prevention 391–2
shaping technique (behavioral method) 259
showing proximity competency 273, 276–8
silence, body language, verbalization and practical
   assistance (SBVP) **92–3**, 92–7, **94**, **95–6**,
   97, 104
skeptical open-mindedness principle 63
skill deficiency questions in behavioral method
   248–53
Skilled Helper, The (Egan) 87
SNARE technique (body work method) 125–6
social casework 87–8, 531–3
social cohesiveness theory 53
social empowerment 407
social isolation 52
social justice pursuits 449–50
social media technique (collective advocacy
   method; social network method) 291–2,
   413–14
social network method: case example 268–9;
   contraindications 287; cue recognition and
   proximity 280–3; cue recognition competency
   273, 275–6; defined 270–1; direct effect
   theory 283–5, **284**, **285**; ecomap technique
   287–8; evidence 292–4; failure of social
   networks 271–3; focus on 269–73, *270*;
   general goal 287; history of 285–7, *286*;
   indications 287; individual approach 270;
   individually tailored competency 273, 278–9;
   introduction 267–8; network conference
   (NC) technique 289–91; pitfalls 294; showing
   proximity competency 273, 276–8; social
   media technique 291–2; social work results
   292; specific goal 287; summary 294; support
   checks competency 273, 279–80; supportive
   environment characteristics 273–5, *274*; tree
   technique 287, 289, *290*
social networks: availability of 283; density of
   283; diversity of 282; size of 281–2; support 6,
   54–5, **55**
social network theory 31–4, *33*
social phobias 51
social policy technique (collective advocacy
   method) 410–11, **411**
Social Presence Theory 6
social safety need 40
social security function 280
social skills groups (SSG) 346–7
social support: meeting affective needs 285;
   meeting self-determination needs 285, **285**;

meeting survival needs 284, **284**; mental health 51–4, **53**; overview 283–4
Social support checklist 295
social work: blind spot in 119; grief support tasks 459–61; human needs and rights (HNR) perspective 439–44, **441**, *442*, **443**, 446–52; methods 2; outcome research 67–8; overview of methods 70–2, 74; research 423; results with NDC method 102–3; survival reflex and 107–8; theory 4
social worker's toolbox: conclusion 78; coping factor in QoL 36, 49–50, 72; dialectical existentialism 64–6, **65**; empowering service users 45; improving coping factor 72; individual coping 78–9; introduction 1, 61–2; ladder of reflection in social work 3–4, *4*; multimethod paradigm 5–6; outcome focused methods 66–70; overview of methods 70–2, *71*; paradigm shift 4–5; pragmatism **62**, 62–3; professional expertise in social work 2–3; structure of 1–2; support factor in QoL 36, 51–6, **53**, **55**, 72; taxonomic principles per method 73–8
Social Work Hospice and Palliative Care Network (SWHPN) 432, 433
social work interventions 23, **23**
Social Work Interview From 1976, The (Kadushin) 87
Social Work Policy Institute 431
Socratic dialogue 214
solution-focused brief therapy (SFBT) 6, 210–11
solution-focused technique (cognitive method) 201
Soros Foundation 432
SOSKI technique (behavioral method) 250, 257–9
SOS narrative 224
specificity myth 422
SRC technique (relationship-focused method) 307
stabilization technique (trauma work method) 152
standard, defined 421
standardization in prevention method 395
standardization technique (behavioral method) 261
strength-based assessment and intervention 316
stress buffering theory 53, 280–3
stress with loss and trauma 111–14, *114*
structure in methodological profiles 75–6
sudden death 542–3
Suicide Aftercare (SUNA) project 275
suicide prevention 397–8
suicide trauma 144
support checks competency 273, 279–80
support factor in QoL 36, 51–6, **53**, **55**, 72
support groups 391

suppression theory 5
survival brain and survival reflex 110–18
survival-focused methods 78
survival needs 284, **284**
survival reflex 107–8
suspension technique (ritual method) 190
sustainable multimethod social work 10–20
Swedish Association of Local Authorities 293
systemic perspective: introduction 2, 5, 44; level of intervention 2; methods of client support 265; methods of coping 20; overview 57–8; social work methods 15, 34; understanding of human functioning 44

task-oriented approach to dying **481**, 481–2
task-oriented technique (behavioral method; group work method) 260, 355
taxonomic principles per method 73–8
Teams-Games-Tournaments (TGT) project 397
technical-instrumental aspect of professionalism 3
techniques of methodological profiles 76–7
tension meter technique 126
territorial aggression 300–2
territorial inventory checklist (TICL) 540–1
territorial negotiation technique (mediation method, relationship-focused method) 307–8
Thematic Interactional Method (TIM) 349
thematic interactional technique (group work method) 353–4, *354*
therapist–client relationship 67
this hurts technique 170–1
three-step social work approach: case study 10, 11, 12, 24–8, **27**; introduction 9; outcome-focused working with scaling 20–3, *21*, **22**; personal filing cabinet 10, 11–13, *12*; psychosocial assessment 10, 14–19, **16**; psychosocial intervention 10, 19–20; social work interventions 23, **23**; summary 28; sustainable multimethod social work 10–20
Thyer, Bruce 32
tie-score effect 68
TOPOI approach 474
touching technique (body work method) 124
toxic nostalgia 167
traffic accidents 144
training schools 87
Transcendent Child, The (Rubin) 50
transference 88
transgressional behaviour 302–3
transition theory 46–8, *47*
trauma: bodywork method for 111–14, *114*; closure technique (ritual method) 190; intake technique (trauma work method) 152; job stress 514; parental loss trauma 244, 503–10; photo viewing after 484–7, **485**–6; self-test traumatic stress 534–5
trauma reactions checklist 536–7, **537**

trauma work method: case example 142; contraindications 151; director technique 152; disasters 144; evidence for 154; follow-up technique 153; general goals 151; history of 150–1; homicide 144; indications 151; introduction 141; pitfalls 154; posttraumatic stress reaction 143, **143**, **146**, 146–7; reconstruction technique 153; social work results 153–4; specific goals 151; stabilization technique 152; suicide 144; summary and questions 154–5; survival reactions 147–50; traffic accidents 144; trauma intake technique 152; traumatic experience characteristics 145–6; traumatic loss situations 143, **143**; traumatic stress 142–50; war 144
trauma-work method 26, 27
tree technique (social network method) 287, 289, *290*
triggers and loss 496, 504
tunnel vision in social work 34
turn taking technique (family method) 340–1

unaddressed loss of parent (UPY) 503–10
uncertainty principle 66
unconditional positive regard 89
understanding, in DUNC needs **228**, 228–30
unexplained complaints/behavior 491, 494–5
unfinished business syndrome (UBS): avoidance coping/support 497–9, *498*, 506–10; case example 493–4; case examples 26, 504–5, 507–8; combination approach to 490; defined 491–2, *492*; introduction 2, 489–90; physical disorders through old pain 499–501; quickscan **538–40**; secondary victimization 490–1; sensory triggers 495–6; signs of 491; summary 510; treatment 501–2, **502–3**; types of 499, **499**; unaddressed loss of parent 503–10; unexplained complaints/behavior 491, 494–5; unfinished life experiences 496–7, **497**

unfinished life experiences 496–7, **497**
unfreezing-moving-freezing process 48–9, *49*
uniformity myth 422
uniquely personal aspects 6
United Nations General Assembly (UNGA) 448
United Nations treaties 448–9
Universal Declaration of Human Rights 448
universal human needs/rights 5–6, 37–44, 450
universal responsibilities 450–1
unmet needs 43–4
unpleasant behavior 253
usefulness principle 63

Vaihinger, Hans 224
valuation function 280
verbalization in SBVP technique (non-directive core method) 95, **95–6**
victimism 50
Victim-Offender Reconciliation Programs 372
Vinter, Robert 347–8
VORP *see* Victim-Offender Reconciliation Programs

war trauma 144
wellbeing indicators technique (family method) *336*, 336–7
White, Michael 238–9
Whittaker, Carl 330
wishes testing 14
withdrawn behavior 252–3
work changes and grief support 466–9, *468*
World Health Organization 394
writing technique (expression method) 178

yet-still technique (ritual method) 190
Youth Aware of Mental Health (YAM) 397–8

zero-dimension 221, *235*, 235–7
Zhuangzi (Chinese philosopher) 252